Oxford Handbook of
Psychiatry

THIRD EDITION

David Semple

Consultant Psychiatrist,
Hairmyres Hospital, East Kilbride
and Honorary Fellow,
Division of Psychiatry,
University of Edinburgh

Roger Smyth

Consultant Psychiatrist,
Department of Psychological Medicine,
Royal Infirmary of Edinburgh
and Honorary Clinical Senior Lecturer,
University of Edinburgh

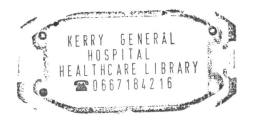

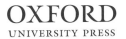

OXFORD
UNIVERSITY PRESS

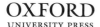

OXFORD
UNIVERSITY PRESS

Great Clarendon Street, Oxford, OX2 6DP
United Kingdom

Oxford University Press is a department of the University of Oxford.
It furthers the University's objective of excellence in research, scholarship,
and education by publishing worldwide. Oxford is a registered trade mark of
Oxford University Press in the UK and in certain other countries

© Oxford University Press, 2013

The moral rights of the authors have been asserted

First edition published 2005
Second edition published 2009
Third edition published 2013, Reprinted 2014, 2016, 2017
Impression: 6

British Library Cataloguing in Publication Data

Data available

Library of Congress Cataloging in Publication Data
Library of Congress Control Number: 2012944040

ISBN 978-0-19-969388-7

Printed in China by
C&C Offset Printing Co. Ltd

Dedication

To Fiona
(D.M.S.)

Preface to the first edition

Every medical student and doctor is familiar with that strange mixture of panic and perplexity which occurs when, despite having spent what seems like endless hours studying, one is completely at a loss as to what to do when confronted with a real patient with real problems. For doctors of our generation that sense of panic was eased somewhat by the reassuring presence in the white coat pocket of the original *Oxford Handbook of Clinical Medicine*. A quick glance at one of its pages before approaching the patient served to refresh factual knowledge, guide initial assessment, and highlight 'not to be missed' areas, allowing one to enter the room with a sense of at least initial confidence which would otherwise have been lacking.

The initial months of psychiatric practice are a time of particular anxiety, when familiar medical knowledge seems of no use and the patients and their symptoms appear baffling and strange. Every new psychiatrist is familiar with the strange sense of relief when a 'medical' problem arises in one of their patients—'finally something I know about'. At this time, for us, the absence of a similar volume to the *Oxford Handbook of Clinical Medicine for Psychiatrists* was keenly felt. This volume attempts to fulfil the same function for medical students and doctors beginning psychiatric training or practice. The white coat pocket will have gone, but we hope that it can provide that same portable reassurance.

2004

D.M.S.
R.S.S.
J.K.B.
R.D.
A.M.M.

Preface to the second edition

It is entirely unoriginal for authors to think of their books as their 'children'. Nonetheless, during the process of creating the first edition of this handbook we found ourselves understanding why the comparison is often made: experiencing the trials of a prolonged gestation and a difficult delivery, balanced by the pride of seeing one's offspring 'out in the world'. And of course, the rapid forgetting of the pain leading to agreement to produce a second a few years later.

We have updated the handbook to reflect the substantial changes in mental health and incapacity legislation across the UK, updated clinical guidance, the continuing service changes across psychiatric practice and the more modest improvements in treatments and the evidence base for psychiatric practice.

The main audience for this handbook has been doctors in training. Unfortunately the most recent change experienced by this group has been profoundly negative, namely the ill-starred reform of medical training in the UK. This attempt to establish a 'year zero' in medical education is widely agreed to have been a disaster. A 'lost generation' of juniors has been left demoralized and bewildered—some have left our shores for good.

Despite this, we have been impressed and heartened by the cheerful optimism and stubborn determination shown by the current generation of trainees and we have been tremendously pleased when told by some of them that they have found our handbook useful. To them and their successors we offer this updated version.

2008

D.M.S.
R.S.S.

Preface to the third edition

One of the ironies of writing books is that the preface, that part to which the reader comes first, is the very part to which the writers come last of all. Once the rest of the book is finished, composing the preface can allow the authors an opportunity for reflection and an attempt at summing-up their initial aims and current hopes for the book as it leaves their hands for the final time.

While writing this third preface we found it interesting to examine its two predecessors, to see what they revealed about our thoughts at those times. Reading the first preface it's clear we were writing to ourselves, or at least to our slightly younger selves, reflecting on the book we wished we'd had during our psychiatric training. The emotions conveyed are those of anxiety and hope. Moving on to the second, it is addressed to our junior colleagues, and seems to us to convey a mixture of indignation and pride.

In this third edition we have continued to revise and update the book's contents in line with new developments in clinical practice. While these changes reflect ongoing and incremental improvement, one cannot fail to be struck by how unsatisfactory the state of our knowledge is in many areas and how inadequate many of our current treatments are. On this occasion we finished the book with the hopes that it would continue to serve as a useful guide to current best practice and an aid in the management of individual patients, and that these current inadequacies would inspire, rather than discourage, the next generation of clinicians and researchers. Our feelings at the end of a decade of involvement with this handbook are therefore of realism mixed with optimism.

2012

D.M.S.
R.S.S.

Acknowledgements

First edition

In preparing this Handbook, we have benefited from the help and advice of a number of our more senior colleagues, and we would specifically like to thank Prof. E.C. Johnstone, Prof. K.P. Ebmeier, Prof. D.C.O. Cunningham-Owens, Prof. M. Sharpe, Dr S. Gaur, Dr S. Lawrie, Dr J. Crichton, Dr L. Thomson, Dr H. Kennedy, Dr F. Browne, Dr C. Faulkner, and Dr A. Pelosi for giving us the benefit of their experience and knowledge. Also our SpR colleagues: Dr G. Ijomah, Dr D. Steele, Dr J. Steele, Dr J. Smith, and Dr C. McIntosh, who helped keep us on the right track.

We 'piloted' early versions of various sections with the SHOs attending the Royal Edinburgh Hospital for teaching of the MPhil course in Psychiatry (now reborn as the MRCPsych course). In a sense they are all contributors, through the discussions generated, but particular thanks go to Dr J. Patrick, Dr A. Stanfield, Dr A. Morris, Dr R. Scally, Dr J. Hall, Dr L. Brown, and Dr J. Stoddart.

Other key reviewers have been the Edinburgh medical students who were enthusiastic in reading various drafts for us: Peh Sun Loo, Claire Tordoff, Nadia Amin, Stephen Boag, Candice Chan, Nancy Colchester, Victoria Sutherland, Ben Waterson, Simon Barton, Anna Hayes, Sam Murray, Yaw Nyadu, Joanna Willis, Ahsan-Ul-Haq Akram, Elizabeth Elliot, and Kave Shams.

Finally, we would also like to thank the staff of OUP for their patience, help, and support.

Second edition

In the preparation of the first edition of this handbook we were joined by three colleagues who contributed individual specialist chapters: Dr R. Darjee (Forensic psychiatry, Legal issues, and Personality disorders), Dr J. Burns (Old age psychiatry, Child and adolescent psychiatry, and Organic illness) and Dr A. McIntosh (Evidence-based psychiatry and Schizophrenia). They continue to contribute to this revised version.

For this second edition we have been joined by four additional colleagues who revised and updated specialist sections: Dr L. Brown (Child and adolescent psychiatry), Dr A. McKechanie (Learning disability) and Dr J. Patrick and Dr N. Forbes (Psychotherapy). We are grateful to them for their advice and help.

We are also pleased to acknowledge the assistance of Dr S. MacHale, Dr G. Masterton, Dr J. Hall, Dr N. Sharma, and Dr L. Calvert with individual topics and thank them for their advice and suggestions.

Other helpful suggestions came from our reviewers and those individuals who gave us feedback (both in person or via the feedback cards).

Once again we thank the OUP staff for their encouragement and help.

Third edition

The contributors named above were joined for this third edition by Dr S. Jauhar (Substance misuse), Dr S. Kennedy (Sexual disorders),

Dr F. Queirazza (Therapeutic issues), Dr A. Quinn and Dr A. Morris (Forensic psychiatry), and Dr T. Ryan (Organic illness and Old age psychiatry). We are also pleased to acknowledge the assistance of Prof. J. Hall and Prof. D. Steele who provided helpful suggestions and engaged in useful discussions. We remain indebted to the staff at OUP for their support of this book and its authors over the last decade.

Contributors

Sameer Jauhar
Clinical Research Worker,
Psychosis Studies,
Institute of Psychiatry,
London, UK

Sarah Kennedy
Locum Consultant Psychiatrist,
St John's Hospital,
Livingston,
West Lothian, UK

Filippo Queirazza
ST4 in General Adult Psychiatry,
Hairmyres Hospital,
Glasgow, UK

Alex Quinn
Consultant forensic psychiatrist,
The Orchard Clinic,
The Royal Edinburgh Hospital,
Edinburgh, UK

Tracy Ryan
Consultant Liaison Psychiatrist,
Department of Psychological
Medicine,
Royal Infirmary of Edinburgh,
Edinburgh, UK

David Semple
Consultant Psychiatrist,
Hairmyres Hospital,
East Kilbride, UK

Honorary Fellow
Division of Psychiatry,
University of Edinburgh,
Edinburgh, UK

Roger Smyth
Consultant Psychiatrist,
Department of Psychological
Medicine,
Royal Infirmary of Edinburgh.
Honorary Clinical Senior Lecturer,
University of Edinburgh,
Edinburgh, UK

Contents

Symbols and abbreviations

Abbreviations can be a useful form of shorthand in both verbal and written communication. They should be used with care however, as there is the potential for misinterpretation when people have different understandings of what is meant by the abbreviation (e.g. PD may mean personality disorder or Parkinson's disease; SAD may mean seasonal affective disorder or schizoaffective disorder).

⚠	Warning
▶	Important
▶▶	Don't dawdle
♂	Male
♀	Female
∴	Therefore
~	Approximately
≈	Approximately equal to
±	Plus/minus
↑	Increased
↓	Decreased
→	Leads to
1°	Primary
2°	Secondary
α	Alpha
β	Beta
γ	Gamma
δ	Delta
σ	Sigma
®	Registered trademark
💣	Bomb (controversial topic)
5-HT	5-hydroxytryptamine (serotonin)
5-HTP	5-hydroxytryptophan
6CIT	Six-item Cognitive Impairment Test
A & E	Accident and Emergency
AA	Alcoholics Anonymous
AAIDD	American Association of Intellectual and Developmental Disability
AASM	American Academy of Sleep Disorders
ABC	Airway/breathing/circulation (initial resuscitation checks); antecedents, behaviour, consequences; Autism Behaviour Checklist

ABG	Arterial blood gas
ACC	Anterior cingulate cortex
ACE—R	Addenbrooke's Cognitive Examination—Revised
ACh	Acetylcholine
AChE(Is)	Acetylcholinesterase (inhibitors)
ACTH	Adrenocorticotrophic hormone
AD	Alzheimer's disease
ADDISS	Attention Deficit Disorder Information and Support Service
ADH	Alcohol dehydrogenase; antidiuretic hormone
ADHD	Attention deficit hyperactivity disorder
ADI—R	Autism Diagnostic Interview—Revised
ADLs	Activities of daily living
ADOS	Autism Diagnostic Observation Schedule
ADPG	ALS–dementia–Parkinson complex of Guam
AED	Anti-epileptic drug
AF	Atrial fibrillation
AFP	Alpha-fetoprotein
AIDS	Acquired immunodeficiency syndrome
AIMS	Abnormal Involuntary Movement Scale
AJP	*American Journal of Psychiatry*
aka	Also known as
ALD	Alcoholic liver disease
ALDH	Acetaldehyde dehydrogenase
AMHP	Approved mental health professional
AMP	Approved medical practitioner
AMT	Abbreviated Mental Test
AN	Anorexia nervosa
ANF	Antinuclear factor
AP	Anterioposterior
APA	American Psychiatric Association
APD	Antisocial personality disorder
ApoE	Apolipoprotein E
APP	Addicted Physicians' Programme; amyloid precursor protein
ARDS	Acute respiratory distress syndrome
ARR	Absolute risk reduction
ASD	Autism spectrum disorders
ASPS	Advanced sleep phase syndrome
ASW	Approved social worker
AUDIT	Alcohol Use Disorders Identification Test
BAC	Blood alcohol concentration

BAI	Beck Anxiety Index
bd	Bis die (twice daily)
BDI	Beck Depression Inventory
BDP-SCALE	Borderline personality disorder scale
BDNF	Brain derived neurotrophic factor
BDZ	Benzodiazepine
BIMC	Blessed Information Memory Concentration Scale
BiPAP	Bi-level positive airways pressure
BJP	*British Journal of Psychiatry*
BMI	Body mass index
BMJ	*British Medical Journal*
BNF	*British National Formulary*
BP	Blood pressure
BPD	Borderline personality disorder
BPRS	Brief Psychiatric Rating Scale
BPSD	Behavioural and psychological symptoms in dementia
BSE	Bovine spongiform encephalopathy
C&A	Child and adolescent
C(P)K	Creatine (phospho)kinase
Ca^{2+}	Calcium
CADASIL	Cerebral autosomal dominant arteriopathy with subcortical infarcts and leukoencephalopathy
CAGE	Cut down? Annoyed Guilty? Eye opener
CAMHS	Child and Adolescent Mental Health Services
cAMP	Cyclic adenosine monophosphate
CARS	Childhood Autism Rating Scale
CAT	Cognitive analytical therapy
CBD	Cortico-basal degeneration
CBF	Cerebral blood flow
CBT	Cognitive behavioural therapy
CC	Creatinine clearance
CCF	Congestive cardiac failure
CCK	Cholecystokinin
CD	Conduct disorder
CDD	Childhood disintegrative disorder
CDI	Children's Depression Inventory
CDT	Carbohydrate-deficient transferrin
CER	Control event rate
CFS	Chronic fatigue syndrome
CJD	Creutzfeldt–Jakob disease
CK	Creatinine kinase

Cl⁻	Chloride
CMV	Cytomegalovirus
CNS	Central nervous system
CO	Carbon monoxide
CO_2	Carbon dioxide
COAD	Chronic obstructive airways disease
COPD	Chronic obstructive pulmonary disorder
COPE	Calendar of premenstrual experiences
CPA	Care programme approach; Criminal Procedures Act; Care Programme Approach
CPAP	Continuous positive airway pressure
CPMS	Clozapine Patient Monitoring Service
CPN	Community psychiatric nurse
CPS	Complex partial seizure
CR	Conditioned response
CRF	Corticotropin-releasing factor; chronic renal failure
CRH	Corticotropin-releasing hormone
CRP	C-reactive protein
CS	Conditioned stimulus
CSA	Childhood sexual abuse
CSF	Cerebrospinal fluid
CT	Computed tomography
CTO	Community Treatment Order; Compulsory Treatment Order (Scotland)
CVA	Cerebrovascular accident
CVS	Cardiovascular system
CXR	Chest X-ray
d	Day(s)
DA	Dopamine
DAH	Disordered action of the heart
DAMP	Deficits in attention, motor control, and perception
DAOA	d-amino acid oxidase activator
DAT	Dementia of the Alzheimer type
DBS	Deep brain stimulation
DBT	Dialectical behavioural therapy
DCD	Developmental coordination disorder
DESNOS	Disorders of extreme stress not otherwise specified
DIB	Diagnostic interview for borderline personality
DIPD-IV	Diagnostic Interview for dsm Personality Disorders
DIS	Diagnostic Interview Schedule
DISC 1	Disrupted in Schizophrenia 1

DKA	Diabetic Ketoacidosis
DLB	Dementia with Lewy bodies
DLPFC	Dorsolateral Prefrontal Cortex
DMP	Designated medical practitioner
DMS	Denzapine Monitoring System
DMST	Dexamethasone suppression test
DMT	dimethyltryptamine
DNA	Deoxyribonucleic acid
DNRI	Dopamine-norepinephrine reuptake inhibitor
DOM	2,5-di-methoxy4-methylamfetamine
DP	Depressive
DRSP	Daily record of severity of problems
DSH	Deliberate self-harm
DSM-IV	*Diagnostic and Statistical Manual*, 4th edition
DSPS	Delayed sleep phase syndrome
DTs	Delirium tremens
DTTOS	Drug testing and treatment orders
DZ	Dizygotic
E/P	Extrapyramidal
EBM	Evidence-based medicine
EBMH	Evidence-based mental health
EBV	Epstein–Barr virus
ECA	Epidemiological Catchment Area Programme (NIMH)
ECG	Electrocardiogram
echo	Echocardiogram
ECT	Electro-convulsive therapy
EDC	Emergency detention certificate
EDS	Excessive daytime sleepiness
EEG	Electroencephalogram
EER	Experimental event rate
ELISA	Enzyme-linked immunosorbent assay
EMDR	Eye movement desensitization and reprocessing
EMG	Electromyograph
EMW	Early morning wakening
EOG	Electro-oculogram
EPA	Enduring power of attorney
EPC	Epilepsy partialis continuans
EPSEs	Extra-pyramidal side-effects
ERIC	Enuresis Resource and Information Centre
ERP	Exposure response prevention
ESR	Erythrocyte sedimentation rate

FAB	Frontal assessment battery
FAS	Foetal alcohol syndrome
FBC	Full blood count
FFT	Family-focused therapy
FGA	First generation antipsychotic
FGF	Frenzied guilt and fear
FIIS	Factitious or induced illness syndrome
FISH	Fluorescence *in situ* hybridization
fMRI	Functional magnetic resonance imaging
FPG	Fasting plasma glucose
FSH	Follicle-stimulating hormone
FT	Family therapy
FTD	Fronto-temporal dementia
FTM	Female to male
g	Gram
GABA	Gamma-aminobutyric acid
GAD	Generalized anxiety disorder
GAF	Global Assessment of Functioning Scale
GAG	Glycosaminoglycans
GARS	Gilliam Autism Rating Scale
GBL	Gammabutyrolactone
GCS	Glasgow Coma Scale
GDS	Geriatric Depression Scale
GENDEP	Genome-based Therapeutic Drugs for Depression
GET	Graded exercise therapy
GFR	Glomerular filtration rate
GGT	Gamma glutamyl transferase
GH	Growth hormone
GHB	Gamma-hydroxybutyrate
GHQ	General Health Questionnaire
GI(T)	Gastrointestinal tract
GMC	General Medical Council
GnRH	Gonadotrophin-releasing hormone
GP	General practitioner
GSH	Guided self-help
GU	Genitourinary
GWA	Genome-wide association
GWAS	Genome-wide association Studies
h	Hour
HAD	HIV-associated dementia; Hamilton anxiety and depression rating scale

HADS	Hospital Anxiety and Depression Scale
HAM-A	Hamilton Anxiety Rating Scale
HAM-D	Hamilton Rating Scale for Depression
HALO	Hampshire Assessment for Living with Others
HAV	Hepatitis A virus
Hb	Haemoglobin
HBV	Hepatitis B virus
Hct	Haematocrit
HCV	Hepatitis C virus
HD	Huntington's disease (chorea)
HDL-C	High-density lipoprotein cholesterol
HDV	Hepatitis D virus
HIV	Human immunodeficiency virus
HLA	Human leucocyte antigen
HPA	Hypothalamic–pituitary–adrenal (axis)
HR	Heart rate
HRT	Hormone replacement therapy
HSV	Herpes simplex virus
HVA	Homovanillic acid
HVS	Hyperventilation syndrome
Hz	Hertz (cycles per second)
IADL	Instrumental Activities of Daily Living
IBS	Irritable bowel syndrome
ICD	Impulse-control disorder
ICD-10	International Classification of Diseases, 10th revision
ICER	Incremental cost-effectiveness ratio
ICP	Intracranial pressure
ICU	Intensive care unit
IDDM	Insulin-dependent diabetes mellitus
IED	Intermittent explosive disorder
IHD	Ischaemic heart disease
IM	Intramuscular
IMHA	Independent mental health advocacy
INR	International normalized ratio (prothrombin ratio)
Intcp	Integrated Care Pathways
IPCU	Intensive psychiatric care unit
IPDE	International Personality Disorder Examination
IPT	Interpersonal therapy
IQ	Intelligence quotient
IQCODE	Informant Questionnaire on Cognitive Decline
ITU	Intensive care unit

iu	International unit
IV(I)	Intravenous (infusion)
IVDU	Intravenous drug user
JAMA	*Journal of the American Medical Association*
K⁺	Potassium
kg	Kilogram
L	Litre; left
LAC	Looked-after child
LD	Learning disability
LFTs	Liver function tests
LH (RH)	Luteinizing hormone (releasing hormone)
LOC	Loss of consciousness
LP	Lumbar puncture
LPA	Lasting powers of attorney
LR	Likelihood ratio
LRTI	Lower respiratory tract infection
LSD	Lysergic acid diethylamide
LTM	Long-term memory
LTP	Long-term potentiation
MADRas	Montgomery-Asberg Depression Rating Scale
mane	In the morning
MAOI	Monoamine oxidase inhibitor
MARS	Munich Antidepressant Response Signature
MCMI	Millon Clinical Multiaxial Inventory
MCMs	Major congenital malformations
MCT	Magneto-convulsive therapy
MCV	Mean cell volume; mean corpuscular volume
MD	Mental disorder
MDD	Major depressive disorder
MDMA	Methylenedioxymethamfetamine (ecstasy)
MDQ	Mood Disorders Questionnaire
ME	Myalgic encephalomyelitis
MEG	Magnetoencephalogram
MERRF	Myoclonic epilepsy with ragged red fibres
mg	Milligram
Mg^{2+}	Magnesium
mGluR	Regional metabolism of glucose
MHA	Mental Health Act
MHAC	Mental Health Act Commission
MHC	Mental Health Commission (RoI)
MHCNI	Mental Health Commission for Northern Ireland

MHO	Mental health officer
MHRT	Mental Health Review Tribunal
MHRTNI	Mental Health Review Tribunal for Northern Ireland
MHTS	Mental Health Tribunal for Scotland
MI	Myocardial infarction
MID	Multi-infarct dementia
min(s)	Minute(s)
mL	Millilitre
mmHg	Millimetres of mercury
MMPI	Minnesota Multiphasic Personality Inventory
MMSE	Mini Mental State Examination
MND	Motor neurone disease
mPFC	Medial prefrontal cortex
MR	Modified release
MRI	Magnetic resonance imaging
MRS	Magnetic resonance spectroscopy
MS	Multiple sclerosis
MSA	Multiple system atrophy
MSE	Mental state examination
MSLT	Multiple sleep latency test
MTF	Male to female
Mth(s)	Month(s)
MUS	Medically unexplained symptoms
MWC	Mental Welfare Commission (Scotland)
MZ	Monozygotic
n	Sample size, number of subjects
N&V	Nausea and vomiting
NA	Narcotics Anonymous
Na^{2+}	Sodium
NAD	No abnormality detected
NARI	Noradrenaline reuptake inhibitor
NaSSA	Noradrenaline and specific serotonin antagonist
NCS	National Comorbidity Survey (1990–92)
NCS-R	National Comorbidity Survey – Replication (2001–02)
NDRI	Noradrenergic and dopaminergic reuptake inhibitor
NE	Norepinephrine (noraderenaline)
NEJM	*New England Journal of Medicine*
NFT	Neurofibrillary tangles
ng	Nanogram
NG(T)	Nasogastric (tube)
NICE	National Institute for Health and Clinical Excellence

NIDDM	Non-insulin dependent diabetes mellitus
NIH	National Institutes of Health
NIMH	National Institute of Mental Health (US)
NMD	Neurosurgery for mental disorder
NMDA	*N*-methyl-*D*-aspartate
NMR	Nuclear magnetic resonance
NMRS	Nuclear magnetic resonance spectroscopy
NMS	Neuroleptic malignant syndrome
NNT	Number needed to treat
NO	Nitric oxide
NP	Nocturnal panic attacks
NPH	Normal pressure hydrocephalus
NPV	Negative predictive values
NR	Nearest relative
NSAIDs	Non-steroidal anti-inflammatory drugs
nvCJD	New variant Creutzfeldt–Jakob disease
OASys	Offender assessment system
OCD	Obsessive–compulsive disorder
OCP	Oral contraceptive pills
od	Omni dei (once daily)
OD	Overdose
ODD	Oppositional defiant disorder
OFC	Orbitofrontal cortex
OGRS	Offender Group Reconviction Scale
OGTT	Oral glucose tolerance test
OPD	Outpatient department
OPG	Office of the Public Guardian
OR	Odds ratio
OSA	Obstructive sleep apnoea
OT	Occupational therapy
P_aCO_2	Partial pressure of carbon dioxide in arterial blood
PAG	Periaqueductal grey matter
PAN	Polyarteritis nodosa
PANDAS	Paediatric autoimmune neurological disorder associated with streptococcus
PANSS	Positive and Negative Symptom Scale
P_aO_2	Partial pressure of oxygen in arterial blood
PAS	Personal assessment schedule
PCL-R	Psychopathy checklist—revised
PCL-SV	Psychopathy checklist—screening version
PCP	*Pneumocystis carinii* pneumonia; phencyclidine

PD	Personality disorder; panic disorder; Parkinson's disease
PDD	Pervasive developmental disorder; premenstrual dysphoric disorder
PDQ-IV	Personality Disorder Questionnaire IV
PE	Pulmonary embolism
PECS	Picture exchange communication system
PET	Positron emission tomography
pHVA	Plasma homovanillic acid
PKU	Phenylketonuria
PL	Prolactin
PLMS	Periodic limb movement (in sleep)
PMDD	Premenstrual dysphoric disorder
PMH	Past medical history
PMS	Premenstrual syndrome
PMT	Parent management training; premenstrual tension
PND	Paroxysmal nocturnal dyspnoea; postnatal depression
PO	*Per os* (by mouth, orally)
PO_4	Phosphate
PPV	Positive predictive values
PR	*Per rectum* (by the rectum); pulse rate
PRIME-MD	Primary Care Evaluation of Mental Disorder
PRISM	Prospective record of the impact and severity of menstruation
PRL	Prolactin (or PrL)
PRN	*Pro re nata* (as required)
PrP	Prion protein
PSA	Prostate-specific antigen
PSE	Present state examination
PSNP	Progressive supranuclear palsy
PTA	Post-traumatic amnesia
PTD	Post-traumatic delirium
PTE	Post-traumatic epilepsy
PTH	Parathyroid hormone
PTSD	Post-traumatic stress disorder
PTT	Prothrombin time
PV	*Per vagina* (by the vagina)
PWS	Prader–Willi syndrome
qds	*Quarter die sumendus* (four times daily)
qid	*Quarter in die* (four times daily)
QOLI	Quality of Life Interview

R	Right
RA	Rheumatoid arthritis; retrograde amnesia
RAGF	Risk assessment guidance framework
RAMAS	Risk assessment, management, and audit systems
RAS	Reticular activating system
RBC	Red blood cell
rCBF	Regional cerebral blood flow
RCP	Royal College of Psychiatrists
RCT	Randomized controlled trial
RDC	Research diagnostic criteria
REM	Rapid eye movement (sleep)
RET	Rational emotive therapy
RIMA	Reversible inhibitor of monoamine oxidase
RMO	Responsible medical officer
ROR	Risk of reconviction (score)
RPG	Random plasma glucose
RPS	Reconviction prediction score
RR	Relative risk
RRASOR	Rapid risk assessment of sex offender recidivism
RRR	Relative risk reduction
RSBD	REM sleep behaviour disorder
RSVP	Risk of sexual violence protocol
RTA	Road traffic accident
RTI	Respiratory tract infection
rTMS	Repetitive transcranial magnetic stimulation
R_x	Recipe (treat with)
s	Second (or sec)
S	Section (of MHA)
SAD	Seasonal affective disorder
SANS	Scale for the Assessment of Negative Symptoms
SAP	Standardized assessment of personality
SAPS	Scale for the Assessment of Positive Symptoms
SARA	Spousal assault risk assessment
SARI	Serotonin antagonist and reuptake inhibitor
SBE	Subacute bacterial endocarditis
SC	Subcutaneous
SCARED	Anxiety Screen for Child Anxiety-Related Emotional Disorders
SCID-II	Structured Clinical Interview for DSM-IV personality disorder
SCT	Supervised community treatment

SD	Standard deviation
SDH	Subdural hematoma
SDQ	Strengths and differences questionaire
SE	Sleep efficiency
SGA	Second generation antipsychotic
SIADH	Syndrome of inappropriate antidiuretic hormone secretion
SIB	Structured interview for borderlines
SIDP-IV	Structured interview for DSM-IV personality disorder
SL	Sublingual
SLE	Systemic lupus erythematosus
SLL	Stereotactic limbic leucotomy
SM	Selective mutism
SNOAR	Sleep and nocturnal obstructive apnoea redactor
SNRI	Serotonin and noradrenaline reuptake inhibitor
SOAD	Second opinion appointed doctor
SORAG	Sexual offending risk appraisal guide
SOREMP	Sleep onset REM period
SP	Social phobia
SPECT	Single photon emission computed tomography
SPET	Single photon emission tomography
SR	Systematic review
SRS	Sex reassignment surgery
SS	Serotonin syndrome
SSP	Schedule for schizoid personalities
SSPE	Subacute sclerosing panencephalitis
SSRI	Selective serotonin reuptake inhibitor
SST	Stereotactic subcaudate tractotomy
STAR*D	Sequenced Treatment Alternatives to Relieve Depression
stat	*Statim* (immediately)
STD	Sexually transmitted disease
STDO	Short-term detention order
STI	Sexually transmitted infection
STM	Short-term memory
SWS	Slow wave sleep
SXR	Skull X-ray
T	Temperature
$t_{1/2}$	Biological half-life
T_3	Tri-iodothyronine
T_4	Thyroxine
TA	Total abstinence

TB	Tuberculosis
TCA	Tricyclic antidepressant
TD	Tardive dyskinesia
tds	*Ter die sumendus* (three times daily)
TeCA	Tetracyclic antidepressant
TENS	Transcutaneous electrical nerve stimulation
TFTs	Thyroid function tests
TG	Triglycerides
TGA	Transient global amnesia
THC	Tetrahydrocannabinol
TIA	Transient ischaemic attack
tid	*Ter in die* (three times daily)
TLE	Temporal lobe epilepsy
ToRCH	Toxoplasmosis, rubella, cytomegalovirus, herpes simplex virus
TPR	Temperature, pulse, respirations (general observations)
TRH	Thyroid-releasing hormone
TRS	Treatment-resistant schizophrenia
TS	(Gilles de la) Tourette's syndrome
TSC	Tuberous sclerosis
TSH	Thyroid-stimulating hormone
TST	Total sleep time
U	Units
U&Es	Urea and electrolytes
UG	Urine glucose
UPPP	Uvulopalatopharyngoplasty
UR	Unconditioned response
URT	Upper respiratory tract
URTI	Upper respiratory tract infection
US	Unconditioned stimulus
US(S)	Ultrasound (scan)
UTI	Urinary tract infection
vCJD	Variant Creutzfeldt–Jakob disease
VDRL	Venereal Disease Research Laboratory (test for syphilis)
VEP	Visual evoked potential
VHL	Von Hippel–Lindau
VMA	Vanillyl mandelic acid
vmPFC	Ventromedial prefrontal cortex
VNS	Vagus nerve stimulation
WBC	White blood cell

WCC	White cell count
WD	Wilson's disease
WFMH	World Federation for Mental Health
WHO	World Health Organization
WISPI	Wisconsin Personality Inventory
wk(s)	Week(s)
WM	Working memory
WPA	World Psychiatric Association
XR	X-ray
Y–BOCS	Yale–Brown Obsessive–Compulsive Scale
YMRS	Young Mania Rating Scale
yr(s)	Year(s)
ZTAS	Zaponex Treatment Access System

Thinking about psychiatry

First thoughts

In the stanzas (Box 1.1) satirist Alexander Pope captured the essence of the then ongoing European Enlightenment, inspiring his readers to use their sense of reason to replace irrationality in their exploration of the world. This period also saw the re-emergence of attempts to use the same methods of thinking to study mental illness, whose sufferers had then spent more than a thousand years as objects of fear and superstition. Pope's words resonate even today, nearly three centuries later, when—confronted with patients thinking 'too little or too much' or in 'chaos of thought and passion all confused'—we are still struggling to use science to guide the exploration of this 'riddle of the world'.

Psychiatry has often been derided as the Cinderella specialty: poorly funded, exiled to outside hospitals, a victim of rushed political experiments, castigated by anti-psychiatrists, its intellectual basis ridiculed, and the self-confidence of its practitioners lowered. As a trainee psychiatrist you will have to cope with questions like 'are you a real doctor?' In addition, the general public (and sometimes other medical professionals) frequently misunderstand the types and severity of illnesses that you deal with. Either they picture you spending all of your time tending to Woody Allen-like self-obsessed, befuddled neurotics, or guarding Hannibal Lecter-like murdering psychopaths. The reality is that psychiatrists deal with the most common human disorders which cause the greatest morbidity worldwide.

Psychiatry considers all aspects of human experience over the whole of the lifespan: elation, grief, anxieties, flights of fancy, confusion, despair, perception and misperception, and memory and its loss. We see the mother with a healthy baby, perplexed and frightened by her tearfulness and inability to cope, and terrified by her thoughts of harming her child. We see the family of a young man who have watched him become a stranger, muttering wild accusations about conspiracies, and we aim to be the doctors who know what best to do in these circumstances. The specialty of psychiatry is (or should be) the most 'human' specialty—devoted to the understanding of the whole person in health and illness. Indeed, it is the only medical specialty without a veterinary counterpart.

It is certainly true that the level of knowledge about causation and treatment of mental disorders is less advanced than for other branches of medicine. In some ways, however, this is an attraction. In other specialties much of what was formerly mysterious is now understood, and interventions and diagnostic methods once fantastic are now quotidian. Psychiatry offers a final frontier of diagnostic uncertainty and an undiscovered country of aetiology to explore. Perhaps the lack of progress made in psychiatry, compared with the other specialties, is not because of lack of will or intelligence of the practitioners but due to the inherent toughness of the problems. To put this another way, all scientists 'stand on the shoulders of giants': in psychiatry we have no fewer and no shorter giants, just a higher wall to peer over.

Box 1.1 The proper study of mankind

Know then thyself, presume not God to scan
The proper study of mankind is man
Placed on this isthmus of a middle state
A being darkly wise, and rudely great
With too much knowledge for the sceptic side
With too much weakness for the stoic's pride
He hangs between, in doubt to act, or rest
In doubt to deem himself a God, or Beast
In doubt his mind or body to prefer
Born but to die, and reasoning but to err
Alike in ignorance, his reason such
Whether he thinks too little, or too much
Chaos of thought and passion, all confused
Still by himself abuse, or disabuse
Created half to rise, and half to fall
Great lord of all things, yet a prey to all
Sole judge of truth, in endless error hurled
The glory, jest, and riddle of the world
Go, wondrous creature!
Mount where Science guides
Go, measure earth, weigh air and state the tides
Instruct the planets in what orbs to run
Correct old time, and regulate the sun
Go, soar with Plato to the empyreal sphere
To the first good, first perfect, and first fair
Or tread the mazy round his followers trod
And quitting sense call imitating God
As Eastern priests in giddy circles run
And turn their heads to imitate the Sun
Go, teach Eternal Wisdom how to rule
Then drop into thyself, and be a fool
Superior being, when of late they saw
A mortal man unfold all Nature's law
Admired such wisdom in an earthly shape
And showed a Newton as we show an Ape
Could he, whose rules the rapid comet bind
Describe or fix one movement of his mind
Who saw its fires here rise, and there descend,
Explain his own beginning, or his end?
Alas what wonder! Man's superior part
Unchecked may rise, and climb from art to art
But when his own great work is but begun
What reason weaves, by passion is undone
Trace science then, with modesty thy guide
First strip off all her equipage of pride
Deduct what is but vanity, or dress
Or learning's luxury, or idleness
Or tricks to show the stretch of human brain
Mere curious pleasure, ingenious pain
Expunge the whole, or lop the excrescent parts
Of all, our vices have created arts
Then see how little the remaining sum
Which served the past, and must the times to come!

From Alexander Pope (1688–1744). *An Essay on Man.*
As reproduced in *Poetical Works*, ed. Cary HF (London: Routledge, 1870), 225–6.

What is disease?

Most mental diagnoses have had their validity questioned at several points in their history. Diagnosed by doctors on the basis of symptoms alone, some people find their presence difficult to accept in a field which has been almost universally successful in finding demonstrable physical pathology or infection.

Disease in medicine as a whole was not always based on pathology. The microscope was developed long after doctors began to make disease attributions. Thomas Sydenham developed the medico-pathological model based on symptoms, but it has grown to incorporate information obtained from post-mortem and tissue examination. This model of disease has become synonymous in many people's minds with a model based solely on demonstrably abnormal structure. Thomas Szasz (📖 p. 25) has criticized psychiatry in general by suggesting that its diseases fail when this model is applied.

This argument that psychiatric diagnoses are invalid still strikes a chord with many doctors and non-medical academics. When the *BMJ* conducted a survey of non-disease[1,2] (see Fig. 1.1), many people thought depression to be a non-disease, although schizophrenia and alcoholism fared somewhat better. It is clear from the graph that many conditions rated as real diseases have a characteristic pathology, although some do not (alcoholism, epilepsy). Similarly, many people regard head injury and duodenal ulcer as non-disease, although their pathology is well described.

There are several models of disease in existence (see Table 1.1). No single model is adequate by itself and diseases may move from one group to another. Models based on aetiology or pathology have been found to be the most useful, but the reality may be that 'disease' is a concept which will tend to change over time and has no real existence in itself.

Table 1.1 Models of disease

Model	Summary of assumptions
Medical-pathological definition (Sydenham 1696; Szasz 1960)	Assumes diseases are associated with a necessary cause (e.g. bacterial infection) or have a replicable morbid anatomy.
Biological disadvantage (Scadding 1972)	Assumes that sufferers from a disease have a common characteristic to place them at a biological disadvantage.
Plan of action (Linder 1965)	Assumes disease labels are justifications for treatments and further investigations.
Syndrome with characteristic symptoms/ outcome (Kendell 1975)	Assumes diseases represent circumscribed concepts distinguished from others by a bimodal distribution of scores on a discriminant function.
Disease as imperfection (Cohen 1943, 1953)	Assumes diseases are quantitative or qualitative deviations from a desirable norm.
Disease as 'concept' (Aristotle)	Assumes diseases are man-made abstractions with no independent existence.

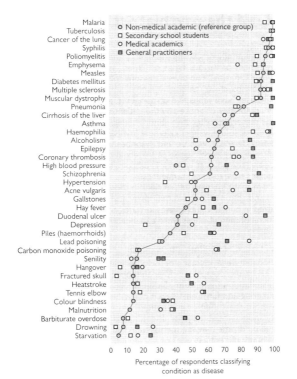

Fig. 1.1 Percentage of respondents classifying a condition as a disease. Reproduced from Smith (2002)[1] with permission of BMJ Publishing Group.

1 Smith R (2002) In search of 'non-disease'. *Br Med J* **324**: 883–5.
2 Campbell EJ, Scadding JG, Roberts RS (1979) The concept of disease. *Br Med J* **2**(6193): 757–62.

The role of the psychiatrist

What is illness?

Doctors, being generally practical people, busy themselves with the diagnosis and treatment of various types of illness. They rarely ask 'what is illness?' or 'what is health?' For several reasons this type of questioning is more germane for psychiatrists:

- While all illnesses have subjective components, psychiatric disorders are usually completely diagnosed by the patient's subjective experiences rather than objective abnormalities.
- There is a non-absolute, value judgement involved in the diagnosis of mental disorder—e.g. wheeze and dyspnoea are abnormal and a sign of disease, but some degree of anxiety at times is a common experience and the point at which it is pathological is debatable.
- Mental illnesses have legal consequences.
- It is important that psychiatrists are clear in themselves about which behaviours and abnormalities are their province. Psychiatrists have been involved in human rights abuses in states around the world when the definitions of mental illness were expanded to take in political insubordination.

Disease, sickness, and illness behaviour

The distinction between disease (or disorder) and sickness should be understood. Disease encompasses either the specific tissue lesion or characteristic constellation of symptoms. Sickness, on the other hand, encompasses the suffering and functional deficit consequent on symptoms. One may exist without the other—e.g. a patient with undiagnosed, asymptomatic breast cancer undoubtedly has disease but is not sick; a patient with chronic fatigue syndrome may see themselves (and be considered) as sick, but does not have an identifiable lesion.

Patients generally present complaining of symptoms, and this process is called illness or illness behaviour. Patients need not be suffering from a disease or disorder in order to do this, and sometimes illness behaviour may be abnormal (even when the patient does have a disease). Subject to certain social conventions (e.g. attending a doctor), they are then afforded the 'sick role' which allows them to relinquish some of their normal obligations. This is a man-made concept, encompassing the special rights and expected behaviour of both someone who is sick and the doctor who is treating them (see Table 1.2). Difficulties arise when a person adopts the sick role to gain the rights afforded to them, whilst neglecting their duties. Another concern relates to the process of diagnosis—causing someone who is not currently ill to adopt the 'sick role'. Doctors should understand their special responsibility to act in the patient's best interests and not to stray outside their area of expertise.

Clarity of roles

It is all too easy for psychiatrists to slip into other roles than that which is properly theirs—an expert in mental disorder. These may include: substitute parent, 'friend', guardian of public morals, predictor of future criminality, arbiter of normal behaviour. Psychiatrists have special training and

Table 1.2 The rights and duties of patients and doctors

Patient	Doctor
Rights	
Exemption from blame	To be considered an expert
Exemption from normal duties whilst in the sick role	To have privileged access to patient information and person
To expect the doctor to act in their best interests	To direct (and sometimes insist on) a course of action
	To validate the sick role
Duties	
To seek help	To act in the patient's best interests
To be open and honest	To maintain confidentiality
To comply with treatment	To keep up to date
To give up the sick role once well	To act, where possible, in society's interests

experience in mental disorder, and should avoid being drawn outside this remit in their professional role.

Mental health and mental illness

Psychiatrists are properly occupied in the business of diagnosing and treating significant psychiatric disorders. As gatekeepers to mental health resources there are often pressures to validate distress or medicalize normal experience. Saying that someone does not satisfy criteria for a specific mental disorder does not mean that they do not have significant problems; rather, the problems do not fall within the scope of psychiatry and would probably be best dealt with by help or advice elsewhere. In general, psychiatrists should not spend their time advising people on 'good mental health' or how to live their lives—this is the self-appointed remit of popular psychology.

Good mental health is more than simply the absence of mental disorder, it requires:

- A sense of self-sufficiency, self-esteem, and self-worth.
- The ability to put one's trust in others.
- The ability to give and receive friendship, affection, and love.
- The ability to form enduring emotional attachments.
- The ability to experience deep emotions.
- The ability to forgive others and oneself.
- The ability to examine oneself and consider change.
- The ability to learn from experience.
- The ability to tolerate uncertainty and take risks.
- The ability to engage in reverie and fantasy.

Diagnosis in psychiatry

Labels People have a natural enthusiasm to be seen as individuals rather than members of a class: 'I'm a person, not a label'. This desire for the recognition of individuality and uniqueness is a part of the public reaction against race-, class-, and gender-related value judgements. Doctors, on the other hand, appear to love labels and classification, and in their enthusiasm can sometimes appear like the stereotypical Victorian butterfly collector who cannot deal with life unless it is named, categorized, and safely inert behind glass. Labels in medicine are based on characteristic combinations of symptoms and signs, but these are viewed differently by patient and doctor. Symptoms are important to patients because of their *individual* nature; that this strange and atypical thing is happening to them. Symptoms are important to doctors because they indicate diagnosis and are features which make this patient similar to others we have seen or read about.

Diagnosis The naming of a thing is the first step towards understanding it. We seek to identify disorders (diagnosis) in order that we should be able to suggest treatments (management) and predict their course (prognosis). Ultimately, the aim is to identify the physical abnormality (pathology) and the cause of the disease (aetiology) and so develop means of prevention and cure. The ideal diagnostic system labels diseases according to aetiology. The aetiology of most mental disorders is unknown and so we tend towards a diagnostic system based upon common clinical features, shared natural history, common treatment response, or a combination of all three. Diagnosis leads to the consideration of individual diseases as members of groups contained within a hierarchy: a form of classification system.

Why make a diagnosis? Why allocate the patient, with his individual and unique history, experience, and range of signs to a single label, with the inevitable compromises and loss of information this entails? Diagnosis must be justified on a general and an individual basis. Generally, the process of establishing a diagnosis is essential to allow succinct communication with colleagues, to help predict prognosis, and to carry out valid research on pathological mechanisms and on treatments. Remember, however, that allocation of a patient to a diagnostic category can only be justified if it will bring him benefit, not harm.

Classification in psychiatry Over the past century within psychiatry there has been a debate about the value of, and method of, psychiatric classification. On one hand the academic and biological psychiatrists worried that psychiatric diagnosis was insufficiently reliable and valid, with a wide variety of terms being used in imprecise or idiosyncratic ways; on the other hand psychodynamic practitioners emphasized the importance of unique patient factors and the degree of detail lost by the reductionism of the diagnostic method. The first concern was tackled by the development of *operational criteria*—clearly defined clinical descriptions of the disorders, together with explicit inclusion and exclusion criteria and details of the number and duration of symptoms required for diagnosis. The second concern was met by the development of *multi-axial diagnosis*, where, in addition to the primary mental disorder coded on axis-I, additional axes code information about the patient's psychosocial problems, personality factors, medical health, and degree of disability (Box 1.2).

Box 1.2 International classification

In psychiatric classification, there are two systems in use worldwide: the International Classification of Diseases (ICD-10), produced by the World Health Organization; and the *Diagnostic and Statistic Manual of Mental Disorders (DSM-IV)*, produced by the American Psychiatric Association.

The International Classification of Diseases (ICD-10)

The ICD-10 is a general medical classification system intended for world-wide, multi-specialty use. It includes 21 chapters, each identified by a roman numeral and a letter. Psychiatric disorders are described in chapter V, and are identified by the letter F. An index of the disorders described in this book, together with their ICD-10 coding, is given on 📖 pp. 1023–42.

Coding The disorders are identified using an open alpha-numeric system in the form Fxx.xx. The letter 'F 'identifies the disorder as a mental or behavioural disorder; the first digit refers to the broad diagnostic grouping (e.g. psychotic, organic, substance-induced); and the second digit refers to the individual diagnosis. The digits which follow the decimal point code for additional information specific to the disorder such as subtype, course, or type of symptoms. When used as second or third digits, 8 codes for 'other' disorders while 9 codes for 'unspecified'.

Versions Four versions of the ICD-10 classification of mental disorders exist, suitable for different purposes. ICD-10: *Clinical descriptions and diagnostic guidelines* ('the blue book') is used by psychiatric practitioners and gives clinical descriptions of each disorder together with the diagnostic criteria. ICD-10: *Diagnostic criteria for research* ('the green book') contains more restrictive and clearly defined clinical features with explicit inclusion, exclusion, and time-course criteria, and is suitable for identification of homogeneous patient groups for research purposes. The *primary care version* focuses on those disorders prevalent in primary care settings and contains broad clinical descriptions, diagnostic flow-charts, and treatment recommendations. A *short glossary* containing the coding together with brief descriptions can be used as a quick reference by practitioners, as well as by administrative and secretarial staff.

Axial-diagnosis The multi-axial version of ICD-10 uses three axes to broaden the assessment of the patient's condition. Axis 1 describes the mental disorder (including personality disorder and mental handicap); axis 2 describes the degree of disability; and axis 3 describes current psychosocial problems.

The Diagnostic and Statistical Manual of Mental Disorders (DSM-IV)

While ICD-10 is a wider general medical classification, DSM-IV describes only mental disorders. The two classifications are broadly similar, having undergone a degree of convergence and cross-fertilization with subsequent revisions. Relevant DSM-IV codes corresponding to ICD-10 disorders are given on 📖 pp. 1023–42. DSM-IV uses a closed, numeric coding system of the form xxx.xx (mostly in the range 290–333.xx). A single version of DSM-IV is used for both clinical and research purposes. DSM-IV is a multi-axial diagnostic system using five axes. Axis 1 describes the clinical disorder or the current clinical problem; axis 2 describes any personality disorder and any mental handicap; axis 3, general medical conditions; axis 4, current psychosocial problems; and axis 5, a global assessment of functioning.

Why don't psychiatrists look at the brain?

Psychiatrists, with the exception of those doing academic research projects, are the only medical specialists who rarely directly examine the organ they treat. The chances that a patient with a serious psychiatric disorder (e.g. schizophrenia, bipolar disorder, severe depression) has ever had a brain scan are fairly slim. Psychiatrists prescribe antipsychotics, antidepressants, mood stabilizers, electroconvulsive therapy (ECT)—all of which have a major impact on brain function—but do not know beforehand which areas of the brain are working well, and which are not functioning properly. Why is this?

As a medical student, a medical practitioner, or even as a trainee psychiatrist, this situation does seem somewhat at odds with the medical training we receive. Imagine the outcry if an orthopaedic surgeon were to set fractures without first taking an X-ray, or a cardiologist diagnosed coronary artery disease without an electrocardiogram (ECG), angiography, or computed tomography (CT). Imagine if, based on your description of the problem, a car mechanic replaced the radiator in your car (at great expense to you) without even bothering to look under the bonnet first. How can it be that the state of the art in psychiatry is not to look at the brain?

Looking at this issue another way it is perhaps not surprising. If I were a patient, who presented to a psychiatrist with a catalogue of recent losses (including both my parents, and a recent redundancy), low mood, sleep problems, loss of appetite, and a feeling of general hopelessness about the future, I would probably be somewhat perturbed if my psychiatrist declared that they could not help me until they had taken half an armful of blood, performed a painful lumbar puncture (LP), and arranged a magnetic resonance image (MRI)/single photon emission computed tomography (SPECT) of my brain (which might take a few months). I might be impressed at their thoroughness, but over the following weeks as I fretted even more about the results of my brain scan, I might contemplate the wisdom of approaching someone who just seems to have added to my worries. When the final results came in and the psychiatrist declared that I was suffering from depression, I might seriously question their abilities, when I could have told them that 3mths ago!

In the main, psychiatrists base diagnosis and treatment on symptom clusters, not brain imaging or other investigations. This is not to say that it is not good clinical practice to perform a physical examination and some routine blood tests (or even an electroencephalograph [EEG] or CT/MRI when indicated by the history or clinical signs). Rather, these are generally investigations of *exclusion* (sometimes a *negative* result can be useful—a point that is often lost on other clinicians when psychiatrists do request investigations which are reported as 'normal'). Psychiatric disorders (with the exception of the organic brain disorders, e.g. dementia) are predominantly disorders of brain *function*; there are rarely observable changes in brain *structure* which would aid diagnosis. At present there are no gold standard diagnostic tests for psychiatric disorders. This is not to say that in the future functional imaging of the brain might not play a role in psychiatric diagnosis, but at present (and despite the fact that high-resolution SPECT and positron emission tomography [PET] scans of the brain have been available for more than 20yrs) it's not yet time to use these imaging tools in *routine* psychiatric practice. More research is needed to determine the specificity and sensitivity of these imaging tools, even though there are hundreds of articles on functional brain imaging in a variety of psychiatric disorders (as a Medline search will quickly reveal).

Does this relegate psychiatry to the lower divisions of medical specialties? No. Rather, the doctor practising in psychiatry needs a firm grounding in general medicine (to recognize *when* a condition may have an organic basis), sharply honed interviewing skills (to elicit important psychiatric symptoms), a firm grasp of psychopharmacology (to differentiate between symptoms of disease and drug-related problems), and an appreciation of the psychosocial problems that may affect an individual in the society in which they live.

Psychiatry is not about *medicalizing* normal experience; it is the ability to recognize *symptoms of disease*, as they are manifest in abnormalities of emotion, cognition, and behaviour. Psychopathology reveals as much to a trained psychiatrist as *pathology* does to his medical or surgical colleagues. Psychiatrists may not (yet) examine the brain directly, but they are certainly concerned with the functioning of the brain in health and disease.

Can psychotherapy change the brain?

Descartes' error is never more apparent than when confronted with explanations of *how* exactly the psychotherapies bring about often profound changes in a patient's beliefs, ways of thinking, affective states or behaviour. If we are ever to bridge the mind–brain divide, then a neurobiological understanding of the mechanisms by which the psychotherapies exert their actions is vital. This would not only provide a sound theoretical foundation for these treatment approaches, but also aid the improvement of psychotherapeutic interventions by opening up the possibility of *objectively* measuring potential benefits and comparing one approach with another.

Psychotherapy has been beset with accusations of being non-scientific. Even Freud had the good sense to abandon his Project for a Scientific Psychology which he started in 1895. He just did not have the tools he needed to detect functional changes in the living brain. However, Freud's early experiments with cocaine—mainly on himself—convinced him that his putative libido must have a specific neurochemical foundation. Now that we do have the ability to reliably detect training- and learning-related changes in brain activation patterns using non-invasive functional imaging,[1] Freud's unfinished Project may be finally realizable. Research in this area is never likely to attract the funding that major drug companies can invest in neurobiological research. Nevertheless, evidence is emerging for alterations in brain metabolism or blood flow that relate to therapeutic effects. A recent review article[2] identified a number of studies assessing the effects of cognitive behavioural therapy (CBT) in obsessive–compulsive disorder (OCD) and phobic disorders and of CBT and interpersonal therapy in depression.

In OCD, psychological intervention led to reduced metabolism in the caudate and a decreased correlation of right orbitofrontal cortex with ipsilateral caudate and thalamus. Interestingly, similar changes are observed in OCD treatment with fluoxetine, suggesting common or at least converging mechanisms in the therapeutic benefits of psycho- and pharmacotherapies. In phobia, the most consistent effect of CBT was reduced activation in limbic and paralimbic areas. Reducing amygdala activation appears to be a common final pathway for both psycho- and pharmacotherapy of phobic disorders. Whether different functional networks are responsible for this common end point remains to be determined, although animal research does suggest this may well be the case.

Studies of depression are more difficult to interpret, showing both increases and decreases in prefrontal metabolism associated with successful treatment. It does appear that depression is a much more heterogeneous disorder and the functional networks implicated in the treatment effects of the different therapies are not as straightforward as for the anxiety disorders.

Future studies need to address issues including larger patient numbers, use of standardized imaging protocols, and utilization of molecular markers. However, it is clear that modulation of brain activity through psychotherapeutic interventions not only occurs, but also may explain the benefits that patients experience. It may be time to put old prejudices aside and properly study alternative non-pharmacological interventions. As the neurobiologist Jaak Panksepp has said, modern research into the aetiology of disorders of emotion and behaviour 'is not a matter of proving Freud right or wrong, but of finishing the job'.

1 Linden DEJ (2003) Cerebral mechanisms of learning revealed by functional neuroimaging in humans. In R Kühn et al. (eds) *Adaptivity and learning—an interdisciplinary debate*, pp. 49–57. Heidelberg, Springer.
2 Linden DEJ (2006) How psychotherapy changes the brain—the contribution of functional imaging. *Mol Psychiat* **11**: 528–38.

The power of placebo

'the passions of the mind [have a wonderful and powerful influence] upon the state and disorder of the body.'
Haygarth (1801)

'Placebo' from the Latin 'placare', 'to please', entered the medical lexicon in *Hooper's Medical Dictionary* in 1811, as 'an epithet given to any medicine adopted to please rather than benefit the patient'. However, the modern study of the 'placebo effect' began when anaesthetist Henry K. Beecher described patient responses to oral analgesics in 1953 and later discussed 'the powerful placebo' in the often quoted JAMA article of 1955.[1] In these largely uncontrolled studies he found that around 30% of the clinical effect could be attributed to the effect of placebo. Over 50yrs later, research has generated many theories of *how* placebos may exert their effects (see Box 1.3) but it still remains a controversial area.

For psychiatry, understanding the reality of the placebo effect is critical when it comes to examining the evidence for (and against) interventions. A good example is the recent controversy that 'Antidepressants are no better than a sugar pill'. This statement conceals an assumption that giving placebo ('sugar pills') is the same as no treatment at all. This could not be further from the truth, and in mild to moderate depression placebo exerts a powerful effect. Nobody is likely to run the headline 'Psychiatrists agree antidepressants should not be first-line treatment for mild to moderate depression'. In fact, clear separation of antidepressant medication benefit from placebo is only seen for moderately severe depression as defined by the Hamilton Depression Rating Scale (i.e. scores of 25+).[2]

Another telling illustration of the power of placebo in psychiatry is Johnstone *et al.*'s[3] ECT trial comparing sham-ECT (anaesthesia plus paralysis) to active treatment. It is no surprise that placebo treatment with sham-ECT was very effective, reducing Hamilton Depression scores by around 50%. The real result was that ECT *was* superior to sham-ECT but only for *psychotic* depression (i.e. clinically much more severe).

Should we be surprised that placebos can exert such powerful effects? Research on pain[4] (see Box 1.3) suggests that humans and other animals have neurobiological systems that evolved to utilize activation through cognitive mechanisms, including expectation, preconditioning, and contextual-related assessment, that are capable of inducing physiological change. (Just imagine the physical effects of exam nerves.) This certainly presents a challenge when designing RCTs and interpreting efficacy of active treatments but it also offers the potential of invoking these resiliency mechanisms to effectively aid in the recovery of an organism from injury, infection, distress, and functional impairment.

The potency of such techniques has been well known to practitioners of traditional medicine for millennia. This is not to suggest we should pipe in soothing music, don Mesmeresque purple robes, and mutter incantations in Latin. Rather, we ought to be circumspect in how we interpret and present the evidence for the treatments we recommend to our patients. We also ought to be aware that our attitude towards the patient and the setting in which they are seen will affect the real benefits of any intervention.

Box 1.3 Proposed mechanisms for the placebo effect

- **Natural remission** Improvement would have occurred anyway due to the nature of the condition.
- **Regression to the mean** If a measurement is outwith normal parameters, later testing is more likely to be closer to the mean than to be more extreme.
- **Anxiety reduction** Alleviation of anxiety following a therapeutic encounter leads to diminution of symptoms, particularly when they are painful or emotionally distressing.
- **Expectations** Cognitive factors—*past influences*: direct experience (of the intervention, practitioner, setting), experience of others' accounts, media influences, and cultural factors; and *current influences*: logic, verbal information, non-verbal cues, attitude (towards the intervention, practitioner, setting), perception of the practitioner (attitude, personality, temperament, experience), and knowledge.
- **Transference** Psychoanalytical theory would suggest placebo works due to the unconscious projection of feelings, attitudes and wishes, initially formed towards a significant figure early in development, onto another person, such as the doctor. e.g. the patient's response may be a simulacrum of the child's need to please the parent.
- **Meaning effects** Whereas 'expectations' are generally explicit and accessible, sometimes the meaning or context of an interaction may be more complex and not directly expressible. Researchers separate *microcontext* (setting or physical environment) from *macrocontext* (wider culture pertaining to the practitioner, patient, and setting).
- **Conditioning** Previous exposure to active treatment engages learned response mechanisms when followed by placebo. Conditioning processes help explain 'expectations' and 'meaning effects' but there are also circumstances when conditioning operates on physiological responses (e.g. heart rate, blood pressure, hormone excretion, immune response) without explicit expectation or even conscious awareness of the response occurring.
- **Neurobiology** Functional brain imaging studies of pain implicate a distributed network (anterior cingulate, periaqueductal grey, DLPFC, orbitofrontal cortex, insula, nucleus accumbens, amygdala, and medial thalamus) modulated by both opioid and dopamine neurotransmission in various elements of the placebo effect: e.g. its subjective value, expectations over time, affective state, and subjective qualities of pain.

1 Beecher HK (1955) The powerful placebo. *JAMA* **159**: 1602–6 ℘ http://www.ncbi.nlm.nih.gov/pubmed/13271123
2 Fournier JC, DeRubeis RJ, Hollon SD, *et al.* (2010) Antidepressant drug effects and depression severity: a patient meta-level analysis. *JAMA* **303**: 47–53 ℘ http://jama.ama-assn.org/cgi/content/full/303/1/47
3 Johnstone EC, Deakin JF, Lawler P, *et al.* (1980) The Northwick park electroconvulsive therapy trial. *Lancet* **2**: 1317–20.
4 Zubieta JK & Stohler CS (2009) Neurobiological mechanisms of placebo responses. *Ann N Y Acad Sci* **1156**: 198–210.

Treating patients against their will

Psychiatric patients may have treatment, hospitalization, and other measures imposed on them against their wishes. The power to impose such measures does not sit comfortably with the usual doctor–patient relationship, and psychiatrists may find 'sectioning' patients unpleasant. The existence of these powers means that under some circumstances psychiatrists will be damned if they do (criticized for being agents of social control, disregarding a person's autonomy, and being heavy handed) and damned if they don't (neglecting their duties, not giving patients the necessary care, and putting the public at risk). Although it may not seem so, sectioning a patient may, in fact, be a very caring thing to do: akin to lifting and holding a two-year-old having a tantrum and at risk of hurting themselves and then soothing them. Such a (literally) paternalistic view may appal some people, but historically, paternalism has had a major influence in this area.

When we consider why it is that we have such powers, we might argue that because psychiatric illness may affect insight and judgement (i.e. a person's *capacity*) sometimes patients might not be capable of making appropriate decisions about their care and treatment. Although to modern ears this may sound ethically sensible, we have had mental health legislation for over 200yrs, and it is only recently that explicit consideration of such matters has influenced mental health legislation.

Mental health legislation has its origins in eighteenth-century laws allowing for the confinement of 'lunatics' and the regulation of private madhouses. The main concerns at that time were the proper care of lunatics, fear of lunatics wandering free, and paternalistic sentiments that lunatics as a group did not know what was best for them and so others should determine this. Large county asylums were built in the nineteenth century and became the old mental hospitals of the twentieth. Until 1930, all patients were detained; there was no such thing as a voluntary or informal patient. If you were insane your relatives (if you were rich) or the poor law receiving officer (if you were poor) would apply to a justice of the peace with the necessary medical certification and you would be confined to an asylum—because this was deemed to be the best place for you. Our current legislation has its ancestral roots in such procedures—reform has rarely led to redrafting from scratch; vestiges of old laws are passed on through the centuries.

Another question often raised is why should we deal with psychiatric illnesses any differently from physical illnesses? After all, physicians cannot detain their patients in order to manage their medical problems, can they? Interestingly, in certain circumstances, they can. Although it is unusual, under Sections 37 and 38 of the Public Health Act, the compulsory detention of patients with infectious tuberculosis of the respiratory tract is allowed—however, the patient cannot be treated against their wishes. Patients with physical illness can only be treated against their wishes if they lack capacity (which may be due to psychiatric disorder).

Is it right that psychiatric patients can be treated against their wishes even when they have capacity to make such decisions? In the twenty-first century paternalism is dead and autonomy rules. A patient with motor neuron disease is allowed to have their life support machine turned off, despite the wishes of their doctors—why not the same right for psychiatric patients?

This does seem to raise interesting ethical questions about whether interventions can ever be justified by principles of paternalism or public protection, when a mentally disordered person has capacity. A pertinent example is that of a currently well patient with a diagnosis of bipolar disorder, who wishes to stop their mood stabilizer, despite past episodes of dangerous driving when unwell.

Let's return to the public health argument of public protection. Infectious patients with tuberculosis may pose a risk to others, and some psychiatric patients may also pose a risk to others. However, most people with mental disorder (even severe cases) are never violent; violence is difficult to predict, and many other people who pose a public risk (those who drink heavily or drive fast) are not subject to such special measures. Potentially dangerous behaviour is not *in itself* a justification for the existence of mental health legislation, but instead provides one criterion for the use of such measures when a person meets other criteria (namely having a mental disorder) and needs care and treatment.

We need to be very wary of how our special powers to detain and treat patients against their wishes might be extended and misused. It is not the role of psychiatric services (including forensic psychiatric services) to detain dangerous violent offenders and sex offenders just to prevent them from re-offending. That is not to argue that psychiatrists should not have a role in the assessment and management of such individuals; just that we should not have primary responsibility for their care.

In the twenty-first century we should be clear of our role: to care for individuals with psychiatric illnesses, without necessarily being paternalistic. We should treat our patients in such a way as to prevent harm to them and to others, but this should not be our raison d'être. The primary justification for the existence of mental health legislation should be to ensure the provision of care and treatment for people who, because of mental disorder, have impaired ability to make appropriate decisions for themselves. We should not be able to forcibly intervene unless this is the case and, when we do, our interventions should be for *their* benefit.

Perceptions of psychiatry

Since the beginning of recorded history, the public imagination has been fascinated and provoked by the mentally afflicted. Of equal interest have been the social and political responses to mental illness and the mechanisms that have emerged to manage and control the 'mad' among us. In general, public perceptions have tended towards polar extremes: on the one hand fear, ignorance, ridicule, and revulsion; on the other, idealization, romanticism, and a voyeuristic curiosity. The social constructions of madness throughout history have coloured both lay and professional notions of mental illness and its treatment in the present age. These varying perceptions are represented in the arts, the media, and the political discourse of our societies.

In the ancient world, mental illness came from the Gods. Nebuchadnezzar's delusions, the senseless violence of Homer's Ajax, and the suicidal depression of Saul were the result of angry or meddling deities and 'furies'. In Deuteronomy (vi: 5) it is written 'The Lord will smite thee with madness.' The first to situate mental suffering within the brain were the sages of the classic world: Hippocrates, Aristotle, and Galen. However, the dark age of medieval Europe saw a return to magical and spiritual interpretations of mental disturbance—madness was the work of demonic forces and witchcraft. Thus, Joan of Arc and countless others were burnt at the stake or drowned for their sins. With the dawn of the Enlightenment, Cartesian notions of rationality and a mind that resided separate from the body displaced the supernatural and laid a foundation for modern concepts of mental illness. Insanity represented the 'flight of reason' and religious moralism gave way to scientific moralism—instead of being one possessed the unfortunate sufferer was now a 'degenerate'. The Romantic era provided a foil to the empiricist veneration of reason. Byron, Blake, Rousseau, Shelley—these were the figures that epitomized in the public mind the archetypal union of madness and genius. 'Great wits are sure to madness near allied;/And thin partitions do their bounds divide' wrote Dryden, while in a 17th-century etching, Melancolicus proclaims 'the price of wisdom is melancholy'. The age of asylums and shackles (portrayed by Hogarth in his series depicting 'The Rake's Progress' through Bedlam and condemned by Foucault as 'the great confinement') came to an end when, in the spirit of the French Revolution, Pinel struck off the chains from his charges.

The beginning of the twentieth century witnessed Freud's description of the unconscious and the birth of medical psychiatry. It was to be a century of controversy and intense soul-searching as psychiatry became equated in the public imagination with 'shock therapy', lobotomies, and the political abuses of Nazi and Soviet regimes. This provided fodder for Laing and Cooper and the anti-psychiatry movement (pp. 24–5), while skirmishes continue to this day between psychoanalytic and biological paradigms. Finally, in the age of mass media, the actions of a handful of mentally ill stalkers and assassins such as Hinckley (who shot President Reagan), Mark David Chapman (who killed John Lennon), and Tsafendas (who killed Verwoerd, the architect of apartheid) have kindled the public's image of the crazed killer into a blaze of prejudice and stigma.

In the second decade of the third millennium we are the inheritors of these historical constructs of mental illness. Our individual notions of madness and perceptions of psychiatry are derived in part from this varied bequest. Supernatural, romantic, biological, and psychological notions of madness abound, while the historic tensions between the belief that psychiatry is fundamentally benevolent and the conviction that it is inherently repressive continue into the present. The public mind is exposed to portrayals of madness and psychiatry in art, literature, film, and the media, and these are powerful influences in shaping individual and collective perceptions. There are many examples of our contrasting notions within popular art. For example, *The Crucible* illustrates the mentally afflicted as cursed and invokes witchcraft as the agent of causation. By comparison, *Quills* and *The Madness of George III* portray the sick as mentally impaired, disordered, degenerate (with differing degrees of historical accuracy). Similarly, in literature, *Don Quixote* and *King Lear* depict the anti-hero as simple or incomplete. The neurologist Oliver Sacks has done much to counter this stereotype with his sympathetic portrayal of neuropsychiatric conundrums, for example in *Awakenings*. The mad genius archetype appears in *A Beautiful Mind*, *The Hours*, and *Shine*, while Joyce's 'Nighttown' chapter of *Ulysses* and Nietzsche's *Thus Spake Zarathustra* celebrate the gift of unfettered thought. Nietzsche defines madness as the 'eruption of arbitrariness in feeling, seeing and hearing, the enjoyment of the mind's lack of discipline, the joy in human unreason'.[1] In Hannibal Lecter *(Silence of the Lambs)*, Raskolnikov *(Crime and Punishment)*, and the villainous Hyde of *Dr Jekyll and Mr Hyde*, we see the stereotype of the crazed and dangerous killer. Finally, artistic critiques of psychiatry abound, but the champions surely include *One Flew Over the Cuckoo's Nest*, *The Snake Pit*, and Sylvia Plath's *The Bell Jar*.

The challenge for us in this postmodern era is to consider our own constructs of what mental suffering means and to reflect upon how we should portray our psychiatric profession in society. In doing so, it is worth remembering the ideas we have inherited from our ancestors and how these ideas pervade current discourse. In sifting the grain from the chaff we would do well to proceed cautiously: most ideas contain at least some grains of wisdom.

---

1 Nietzsche F (1974) *The gay science*. Trans W, Kaufman. New York, Vintage.

Psychomythology

'Science must begin with myths and with the criticism of myths.'
Sir Karl Popper (1963)

Myths matter. Throughout history myths have served the central function of explaining the inexplicable: creating the illusion of understanding. Human nature seems to defy explanation and yet we constantly make value judgements of people and ourselves – inferring motivation and causation on relatively little evidence – in an attempt to make sense of the world. Most of the time erroneous beliefs matter little and may even be comforting, but some of the time they can make us prejudicial or lead us to act unwisely. Whilst it may be acceptable in our private lives to be more liberal with the truth, in our professional lives we are afforded the benefits of authority based upon our expertise. This is why there are professional examinations and qualifications. We must guard against misinformation and protect ourselves and our patients from treatments and explanatory models for which evidence is decidedly lacking.

Pseudoscience

Fortunately we have the scientific method to help us sift the evidence (see EBM 📖 pp. 107–27) and the testable biopsychosocial model of the aetiology of psychiatric illness (📖 p. 245). Nevertheless we can be fooled when a set of ideas is presented in a scientific way, even though it does not bear scrutiny. These *pseudoscientific* theories may be based upon *authority* rather than empirical observation (e.g. old-school psychoanalysis, New Age psychotherapies, Thought Field Therapy), concern the *unobservable* (e.g. orgone energy, chi), confuse metaphysical with empirical claims (e.g. acupuncture, cellular memory, reiki, therapeutic touch, Ayurvedic medicine), or even maintain views that contradict known scientific laws (e.g. homeopathy). Some theories are even maintained by adherents despite empirical testing clearly showing them to be false (e.g. astrology, biorhythms, ESP). Others cannot even be tested. As Carl Sagan pointed out in his excellent book 'The Demon Haunted World: Science as a Candle in the Dark' (1995): any hypotheses should, at least in principle, be falsifiable. In fact the scientific method has this at its heart: the rejection of the null hypothesis. More worrying perhaps is the unthinking promotion of some of these methods by physicians who really should know better. Chi imbalance is not the same as serotonin dysregulation (no, really it isn't).

'Men are from Mars, Women are from Venus'[1]

Our culture is infused with popular myths about psychology and psychiatry. From personality profiling to violence and mental illness, there is no end to confusion. The media lap up the newest theory, treatment or drug even when the scientific evidence is shaky. Emotive anecdotes and stirring personal accounts lodge themselves into the public imagination. Modern Barnums promote their wares in bookshops, on the Internet, and TV. Autism is on the rise, they say; hospital admissions go up during a full moon; people are more depressed at Christmas; antidepressants cause suicide; I can make you do X,Y and Z; this is what your dreams *really* mean. There are many reasons why myths persist (see Box 1.4) and they are very difficult to challenge once they are established. This is one reason why psychoeducation is a vital component of most psychological therapies. Most people find that the antidote to the influence of pseudoscience on them is knowledge of real science. The twist in all of this is that understanding the truth of how the brain functions in health and disease is more remarkable, more amazing, and more life-changing than any fiction could ever be.

Box 1.4 Mythbusting

The 10 sources of error:

- **Word of mouth** If we hear something repeated enough times, we begin to believe it is true.
- **Desire for easy answers and the quick fix** If something sounds too good to be true, it probably is.
- **Selective perception and memory** We all suffer from *naïve realism* and believe that how we see the world is exactly how it is. We also have a tendency to remember hits and forget misses which leads to *illusionary correlation*: the mistaken perception that two statistically unrelated event are actually related.
- **Inferring causation from correlation** For example, although it may be true that a history of CSA is highly correlated with schizophrenia it does not necessarily follow that schizophrenia is caused by CSA.
- **Post hoc, ergo propter hoc reasoning ('after this, therefore because of this')** Just because someone appears to get better after receiving a homeopathic remedy does not necessarily mean the remedy was effective.
- **Exposure to a biased sample** Psychiatrists usually see treatment-resistant patients and may assume treatment is less effective than it actually is for the majority of patients.
- **Reasoning by representativeness** Just because two things appear similar does not make them the same.
- **Misleading film and media portrayals** ECT perceptions have never recovered from *One Flew Over the Cuckoo's Nest*.
- **Exaggeration of a kernel of truth**
- **Terminology confusion** The etymology of words like 'schizophrenia' can lead to confusion with most people believing it means patients have multiple personalities.

---

1 '...and most popular psychology is from Uranus.' When John Gray, author of 'Men are from Mars, Women are from Venus' appeared on Season 2, Episode 3 of Penn & Teller's *Bullshit!* Penn quipped 'I guess the title "We're all people and should be treated with love and respect" just wouldn't fit on the book spine'.

2 Adapted from the Introduction of So, Lynn SJ, Ruscio J, Beverstein BL (2010) Lilienfeld *50 Great myths of popular psychology*. Oxford: Wiley-Blackwell.

Stigma

Stigma is a Greek word meaning 'mark' and originally referred to a sign branded onto criminals or traitors in order to identify them publicly. The plural, stigmata, when used in medical settings, means the collection of symptoms and signs by which a particular disorder may be identified. In its wider, modern sense, stigma refers to the sense of collective disapproval and group of negative perceptions attached to a particular people, trait, condition, or lifestyle. Stigmatization describes the process by which the characteristics of the group in question are identified and discriminated against.

Stigmatization can be thought of as a three-stage process: first, the individual is marked out as different by his actions or appearance; secondly, society develops a series of beliefs about the affected individual; finally, society changes its behaviour towards these individuals in a way consistent with those beliefs, often to the detriment of the stigmatized individuals. Stigma can become self-reinforcing as it can be associated with avoidance of the stigmatized individuals, leaving no opportunity for society to confront and change its beliefs.

Fear of the unknown, fear of contamination, and fear of death or the sight of death have led to diseases of all kinds being stigmatized throughout history. This is particularly true of infectious diseases, diseases causing disfigurement, and mental disorders. As the infectious and disfiguring diseases have become both more treatable and better understood, sufferers from mental disorders have remained uniquely vulnerable to stigmatization.

One marker of this has been the ease with which originally neutral, descriptive terms for mental disorders have taken on a pejorative and disparaging meaning: cretin, maniac, spastic, imbecile. All have been abandoned in an attempt to free affected individuals from the approbation the name had acquired. Unfortunately, stigmatization involves fundamental and widely held beliefs and is not usually amenable to simple cures such as changes of name of conditions or organizations.

For the person affected by mental illness, the name of the condition and their abnormalities of experience and behaviour will mark them out as different, and are the root cause of their distress. However, the wider societal beliefs, expressed as stigmatization, will add to the burden of morbidity, and may in themselves prolong the condition. For example, the belief that depression is 'all in the mind' and could be resolved if the affected individual would only 'pull themselves together' may cause people to behave less sympathetically towards the sufferer, but it may also hinder the sufferer from seeking appropriate help.

There is no simple answer to the problem of stigma. We can certainly learn from the increasingly successful approach to the problem of the stigmatization which initially attached to those individuals suffering from HIV infection. Increased public awareness of the cause of the disease, its method of transmission, the plight of its sufferers, and its means of treatment appear to be associated with less, not more stigmatization. The Royal College of Psychiatrists, with its 'Defeat Depression' campaign, has been active in this regard.

On an individual basis we can:
- **Challenge our own prejudices** These may exist, particularly in connection with patients with personality disorder and patients with substance misuse problems.
- **Avoid stigmatizing language** There is no place for forced political correctness in medicine, but we should consider whether calling an individual 'a schizophrenic' describes them as a single, unfavourable characteristic, rather than as a person with an illness.
- **Challenge lack of knowledge within the profession** A surprising lack of knowledge of mental disorders is often seen in our colleagues in other specialties. This may be expressed in, for example, a lower aspiration for treatment in individuals with mental handicap or chronic psychotic illness.
- **Be advocates for political change** Professional conservatism should not halt us from being at the forefront of moves to improve the autonomy of patients, their involvement in society, and their legal protection.

Anti-psychiatry

One view of medicine is that it is an applied science whose object of scientific curiosity is the understanding of the causes and processes of human illness and the study of methods of preventing or ameliorating them. In the scientific method there are no absolute truths, only theories which fit the observed facts as they are currently known. All scientists must be open to the challenging of firmly established theories as new observations are made and new experiments reported.

All psychiatrists should retain this healthy scientific scepticism and be prepared to question their beliefs about the causes and cures of mental illness. Developments (and hence improvements in patient care) come from improvement in observation methods and trials of new treatment modalities. A result of this may be the enforced abandonment of cherished beliefs and favoured treatments. Always remember that insulin coma therapy[1] was at one time believed to be an effective treatment for psychotic illnesses.

While rigorous examination of the basic and clinical sciences of psychiatry is essential if the specialty is to progress, psychiatry as a medical specialty has, over the last 50yrs, been subject to a more fundamental criticism—that the empirical approach and the medical model are unsuited to the understanding of mental disorder and that they cause harm to the individuals they purport to treat. This basic belief, known as 'anti-psychiatry', has been expressed by a variety of individuals over the years, reaching a peak in the late 1960s. Although the central arguments of the anti-psychiatry movement have largely been discredited in the mainstream scientific literature, they have retained currency in some areas of the popular press, within some patient organizations, and in certain religious cults. They are presented here for historic interest and so that the sources for modern-day advocates of these ideas can be identified (see Box 1.5).

Central anti-psychiatry beliefs

- The mind is not a bodily organ and so cannot be diseased.
- The scientific method cannot explain the subjective abnormalities of mental disorder as no direct observation can take place.
- Mental disorder can best be explained by social, ethical, or political factors.
- The labelling of individuals as 'ill' is an artificial device used by society to maintain its stability in the face of challenges.
- Medication and hospitalization are harmful to the individual so treated.

The anti-psychiatry movement did raise some valid criticisms of then contemporary psychiatric practice; in particular, pointing out the negative effects of institutional living, criticizing stigma and labelling, and alerting psychiatrists to the potential use of political change in improving patient care.

It was, however, fatally flawed by a rejection of empiricism, an over-reliance on single case reports, domination by a small number of personalities with incompatible and deeply held beliefs, and an association with half-baked political theory of the Marxist–Leninist strain.

Box 1.5 Prominent anti-psychiatrists

- **Szasz** Rejected compulsory treatment. Author of *Pain and pleasure* and *The myth of mental illness*. Viewed disease as a bodily abnormality with an observable pathology to which, by its nature, the brain was immune. Saw mental illness as conflict between individuals and society. Rejected the insanity defence and committal to hospital. Accepted patients for voluntary treatment for drug-free analysis on payment of fee and acceptance of treatment contract.
- **Scheff** Worked in labelling theory. Wrote *Being mentally ill*. Hypothesized that mental illness was a form of social rule-breaking. Labelling such individuals as mentally ill would stabilize society by sanctioning such temporary deviance.
- **Goffman** Wrote *Asylums*. Described the 'total institution' observed as a result of an undercover study. Commented on the negative effects of institutions segregated from the rest of society and subject to different rules.
- **Laing** Author of *The divided self*, *Sanity, madness and the family*, and *The politics of experience*. Developed probably the most complete anti-psychiatry theory. He saw the major mental illnesses as arising from early family experiences, in particular from hostile communication and the desire for 'ontological security'. He saw newborns as housing potential which was diminished by the forced conformity of the family and the wider society. Viewed normality as forced conformity and illness as 'the reality which we have lost touch with'.
- **Cooper** Revived anti-psychiatry ideas. A committed Marxist, he saw schizophrenia as a form of social repression.
- **Buscaglia** Wrote *The deviant majority*. Held that diagnosis didn't aid understanding of the patient's experience. Believed that social and economic factors were crucial. Successful in pressing for significant reform of the Italian mental health system.
- **Scull** Wrote *Museums of madness*. Saw mental health systems as part of 'the machinery of the capitalist system'.
- **Breggin** Modern advocate of anti-psychiatry views. Author of *Toxic psychiatry* which views psychopharmacology as 'disabling normal brain function'. Rejects results of systematic reviews.

---

1 In 1933 Manfred Sakel introduced insulin coma therapy for the treatment of schizophrenia. This involved the induction of a hypoglycaemic coma using insulin, the rationale being that a period of decreased neuronal activity would allow for nerve cell regeneration. In the absence of alternative treatments, this was enthusiastically adopted by practitioners worldwide. However, with the advent of antipsychotics in the 1950s and the emergence of randomized controlled trials (RCTs), it became clear that the treatment had no effect above placebo and it was subsequently abandoned.

A brief history of psychiatry

Ancient times **~4000 BC** Sumerian records describe the euphoriant effect of the poppy plant. **~1700 BC** First written record concerning the nervous system. **460–379 BC** Hippocrates discusses epilepsy as a brain disturbance. **387 BC** Plato teaches that the brain is the seat of mental processes. **280 BC** Erasistratus notes divisions of the brain. **177** Galen lectures *On the brain.*

Pre-modern **1649** Descartes describes the pineal gland as a control centre of body and mind. **1656** Bicêtre and Salpêtrière asylums established by Louis XIV in France. **1755** Perry publishes *A mechanical account and explication of the hysteric passion.* **1758** Battie publishes his *Treatise on madness.* **1773** Cheyne publishes his book *English malady,* launching the idea of 'nervous illness'. **1774** Mesmer introduces 'animal magnetism' (later called hypnosis). **1793** Pinel is appointed to the Bicêtre and directs the removal of chains from the 'madmen'. **1794** Chiarugi publishes *On insanity,* specifying how a therapeutic asylum should be run.

1800–1850 **1808** Reil coins the term 'psychiatry'. **1812** Rush publishes *Medical inquiries and observations upon the diseases of the mind.* **1813** Heinroth links life circumstances to mental disorders in the *Textbook of mental hygiene.* **1817** Parkinson publishes *An essay on the shaking palsy.* ● Esquirol lectures on psychiatry to medical students. **1825** Bouillaud presents cases of aphonia after frontal lesions. ● Todd discusses localization of brain functions. **1827** Heinroth appointed as the first professor of psychological therapy in Leipzig. **1832** Chloral hydrate discovered. **1843** Braid coins the term 'hypnosis'. **1848** Phineas Gage has his brain pierced by an iron rod with subsequent personality change.

1850–1900 **1856** Morel describes 'démence précoce'—deteriorating adolescent psychosis. **1863** Kahlbaum introduces the term 'catatonia'. ● Friedreich describes progressive hereditary ataxia. **1864** Hughlings Jackson writes on aphonia after brain injury. **1866** Down describes 'congenital idiots'. **1868** Griesinger describes 'primary insanity' and 'unitary psychosis'. **1869** Galton claims that intelligence is inherited in *Hereditary genius.* **1871** Hecker describes 'hebephrenia'. **1872** Huntington describes symptoms of a hereditary chorea. **1874** Wernicke publishes *Der aphasische symptomenkomplex* on aphasias. **1876** Ferrier publishes *The functions of the brain.* ● Galton uses the term 'nature and nurture' to describe heredity and environment. **1877** Charcot publishes *Lectures on the diseases of the nervous system.* **1883** Kraepelin coins the terms 'neuroses' and 'psychoses'. **1884** Gilles de la Tourette describes several movement disorders. **1885** Lange proposes use of lithium for excited states. **1887** Korsakoff describes characteristic symptoms in alcoholics. **1892** American Psychological Association formed. **1895** Freud and Breuer publish *Studies on hysteria.* **1896** Kraepelin describes 'dementia praecox'. **1899** Freud publishes *The interpretation of dreams.*

1900s **1900** Wernicke publishes *Basic psychiatry* in Leipzig. **1903** Barbiturates introduced. ● First volume of *Archives of neurology and psychiatry* published in USA. ● Pavlov coins the term 'conditioned reflex'. **1905** Binet and Simon develop their first IQ test. **1906** Alzheimer describes 'presenile degeneration'. **1907** Adler's *Study of organ inferiority and its physical compensation* published. ● Origins of group therapy in Pratt's work supporting TB patients in Boston. **1909** Brodmann describes 52 cortical areas. ● Cushing electrically stimulates human sensory cortex. ● Freud publishes the case of Little Hans in Vienna.

1910s 1911 Bleuler publishes his textbook *Dementia praecox or the group of schizophrenias*. **1913** Jaspers describes 'non-understandability' in schizophrenia thinking. ● Syphilitic spirochaete established as cause of 'generalized paresis of the insane'. ● Jung splits with Freud forming the school of 'analytic psychology'. ● Mental Deficiency Act passed in UK. ● Goldmann finds blood–brain barrier impermeable to large molecules. **1914** Dale isolates acetylcholine. ● The term 'shell shock' is coined by British soldiers. **1916** Henneberg coins the term 'cataplexy'. **1917** Epifanio uses barbiturates to put patients with major illnesses into prolonged sleep. ● Wager-Jauregg discovers malarial treatment for neurosyphilis.

1920s 1920 Moreno develops 'psychodrama' to explore individual problems through re-enactment. ● Watson and Raynor demonstrate the experimental induction of phobia in 'Little Albert'. ● Crichton-Miller founds the Tavistock Clinic in London. ● Klein conceptualizes development theory and the use of play therapy. ● Freud's *Beyond the pleasure principle* published. **1921** Rorschach develops the inkblot test. **1922** Klaesi publishes results of deep-sleep treatment, which is widely adopted. **1923** Freud describes his 'structural model of the mind'. **1924** Jones uses the first example of systematic desensitization to extinguish a phobia. **1927** Jacobi and Winkler first apply pneumoencephalography to the study of schizophrenia. ● Wagner-Jauregg awarded the Nobel Prize for malarial treatment of neurosyphilis. ● Cannon-Bard describes his 'theory of emotions'. **1929** Berger demonstrates first human electroencephalogram.

1930s 1930 First child psychiatry clinic established in Baltimore, headed by Kanner. **1931** Hughlings-Jackson describes positive and negative symptoms of schizophrenia. ● Reserpine introduced. **1932** Klein publishes *The psychoanalysis of children*. **1933** Sakel introduces 'insulin coma treatment' for schizophrenia. **1934** Meduna uses chemical convulsive therapy. **1935** Moniz and Lima first carry out 'prefrontal leucotomy'. ● Amfetamines synthesized. **1936** Mapother appointed as England's first Professor of Psychiatry. ● Dale and Loewi share Nobel Prize for work on chemical nerve transmission. **1937** Kluver and Bucy publish work on bilateral temporal lobectomies. ● Papez publishes work on limbic circuits and develops 'visceral theory' of emotion. **1938** Cerletti and Bini first use 'electroconvulsive therapy'. ● Skinner publishes *The behaviour of organisms* describing operant conditioning. ● Hoffmann synthesizes LSD.

1940s 1942 Freeman and Watts publish *Psychosurgery*. **1943** Antihistamines used in schizophrenia and manic depression. **1946** Freeman introduces 'transorbital leucotomy'. ● Main publishes *Therapeutic communities*. **1948** Foulkes' *Introduction to group analytical psychotherapy* published. ● *International classification of diseases* (ICD) first published by WHO. ● Jacobsen and Hald discover the use of disulfiram. **1949** Cade introduces lithium for treatment of mania. ● Penrose publishes *The biology of mental defect*. ● Moniz awarded Nobel Prize for treatment of psychosis with leucotomy. ● Hess receives Nobel Prize for work on the 'interbrain'. ● Magoun defines the reticular activating system. ● National Institute of Mental Health is established. ● Hebb publishes *The organization of behaviour: a neuropsychological theory.*

1950s 1950 First World Congress of Psychiatry held in Paris. ● Chlorpromazine (compound 4560 RP) synthesized by Charpentier. ● Roberts and Awapara independently identify GABA in the brain. **1951** Papaire and Sigwald report efficacy of chlorpromazine in psychosis. **1952** *Diagnostic and statistical manual* (DSM-I) introduced by the APA. ● Eysenck publishes *The effects of psychotherapy.* ● Delay and Deniker treat patients with psychological disturbance using chlorpromazine. ● Delay, Laine, and Buisson report isoniazid use in the treatment of depression. **1953** Lurie and Salzer report use of isoniazid as an 'antidepressant'. **1954** Kline reports that reserpine exerts a therapeutic benefit on both anxiety and obsessive–compulsive symptoms. ● Delay and Deniker, Noce and Steck report favourable effects of reserpine on mania. ● First community psychiatric nurse post established in UK. **1955** Chlordiazepoxide, the first benzodiazepine, synthesized by Sternbach for Roche. ● Kelly introduces his 'personal construct therapy'. ● Shepherd and Davies conduct the first prospective placebo-controlled, parallel-group randomized controlled trial in psychiatry, using reserpine in anxious-depressive outpatients (with definite benefit). **1957** Imipramine launched as an antidepressant. ● Iproniazid launched as an antidepressant. ● Delay and Deniker describe the characteristics of neuroleptics. **1958** Carlsson *et al.* discover dopamine in brain tissues and identify it as a neurotransmitter. ● Janssen develops haloperidol, the first butyrophenone neuroleptic. ● Lehman reports first (successful) trial of imipramine in USA. **1959** Russell Barton's *Institutional neurosis in England* draws attention to the adverse effects of institutional regimes. ● Diazepam first synthesized by Roche. ● Schneider defines his 'first-rank symptoms' of schizophrenia. ● English Mental Health Act of 1959 allows voluntary admission to psychiatric hospitals.

1960s 1960 Merck, Roche, and Lundbeck all launch versions of amitriptyline. **1961** Knight, a London neurosurgeon, pioneers stereotactic subcaudate tractotomy. ● Founding of the World Psychiatric Association. ● Thomas Szasz publishes *The myth of mental illness.* **1962** Ellis introduces 'rational emotive therapy'. ● US Supreme Court declares addiction to be a disease and not a crime. **1963** Beck introduces his 'cognitive behavioural therapy.' ● Carlsson shows that neuroleptics have effects on catecholamine systems. **1966** Gross and Langner demonstrate effectiveness of clozapine in schizophrenia. **1968** Strömgren describes 'brief reactive psychosis'. ● Ayllon and Azrin describe the use of 'token economy' to improve social functioning. ● Publication of DSM-II and ICD-8.

1970s 1970 Laing and Esterson publish *Sanity, madness and the family.* ● Rutter publishes the landmark Isle of Wight study on the mental health of children. ● Janov publishes *Primal scream.* ● Maslow describes his 'hierarchy of needs'. ● Axelrod, Katz, and Svante von Euler share Nobel Prize for work on neurotransmitters. **1971** British Misuse of Drugs Act passed. ● Carlsson, Corrodi *et al.* develop zimeldine, the first of the SSRIs. **1972** Feighner *et al.* describe the St Louis criteria for diagnosis of schizophrenia. **1973**

International pilot study of schizophrenia uses narrow criteria and finds similar incidence of schizophrenia across all countries studied. **1974** Hughes and Kosterlitz discover enkephalin. **1975** Research diagnostic criteria (RDC) formulated by Spitzer *et al.* in the USA. • Clozapine withdrawn following episodes of fatal agranulocytosis. **1976** Johnstone uses CT to study schizophrenic brains. **1977** Guillemin and Schally share Nobel Prize for work on peptides in the brain. **1979** Russell describes bulimia nervosa.

1980s 1980 DSM-III published by the APA. • Crow publishes his two-syndrome (type I and type II) hypothesis of schizophrenia. **1984** Klerman and Weissman introduce 'interpersonal psychotherapy'. • Smith *et al.* first use MRI to study cerebral structure in schizophrenia. • Andreasen develops scales for the assessment of positive and negative symptoms in schizophrenia (SAPS/SANS ⊞ p. 81). **1987** Liddle describes a three-syndrome model for schizophrenia. • Fluvoxamine introduced. • Mednick publishes first prospective cohort study of schizophrenia using CT. **1988** The 'harm minimization' approach to drug misuse introduced in Britain. • Kane *et al.* demonstrate efficacy of clozapine in treatment-resistant schizophrenia.

1990s 1990 Sertraline introduced. • Ryle introduces 'cognitive analytical therapy'. **1991** Paroxetine introduced. **1992** Moclobemide introduced as first reversible inhibitor of monoamine oxidase (RIMA). • The False Memory Syndrome Society Foundation formed in the USA. • Publication of ICD-10. **1993** Huntington's disease gene identified. • Launch of risperidone as an 'atypical' antipsychotic. • Linehan first describes her 'dialectical behaviour therapy'. **1994** Publication of DSM-IV. • Launch of olanzapine. • Gilman and Rodbell share the Nobel Prize for their discovery of G-protein coupled receptors and their role in signal transduction. **1995** Citalopram, a selective serotonin reuptake inhibitor (SSRI), nefazodone (dual-action SSRI), venlafaxine, a serotonin and noradrenaline reuptake inhibitor (first SNRI) all introduced. **1999** Hodges publishes first results from prospective Edinburgh High Risk (Schizophrenia) Study using MRI.

2000s 2000 Carlsson, Greengard, and Kandel share Nobel Prize for their work on neurotransmitters. **2002** Neuregulin-1 and dysbindin identified as susceptibility genes for schizophrenia. **2003** Aripiprazole, the first dopamine partial agonist antipsychotic, launched. • Caspi and colleagues show that genetic and environmental factors interact to modulate risk for depression and antisocial behaviour. **2005** The DISC1 gene, implicated in psychotic and affective illness, is shown to regulate cyclic adenosine monophosphate (cAMP) signalling. • The first non-commercial large-scale trial compares new and old antipsychotics—Clinical Antipsychotic Trials of Intervention Effectiveness (CATIE). **2006** Hall and co-workers show that the Neuregulin-1 gene is associated with changes in brain function and psychosis in the Edinburgh High Risk (Schizophrenia) Study. **2007** A glutamate agonist (LY2140023) is found by Patel and colleagues to have antipsychotic effects in patients with schizophrenia—potentially the first genuinely new (i.e. non-dopamine-based) treatment for psychosis. **2009** Genome-wide genetic analysis reveals both common and rare genetic variants involved in schizophrenia. **2011** Neural stem cells derived from peripheral samples reveal cellular changes in patients with schizophrenia and related disorders.

The future

Attempting to predict the future is a dangerous business. Predictions tend to be based upon contemporary ideas and have a tendency to overestimate some types of change and underestimate others. Wild inaccuracy is the usual rule. This is particularly so in medical science where change is often a result of chance discoveries (e.g. penicillin) and sweeping reforms which make most then-current knowledge redundant (e.g. the germ theory of disease).

Currently practising psychiatrists are (or should be) keenly aware of the deficiencies of current psychiatric practice. We lack knowledge of the aetiology and pathogenesis of most psychiatric disorders; we have no objective diagnostic or prognostic investigations; and our drug and psychological treatments are often minimally or only partially effective. While we welcome the ongoing gradual progress in knowledge and treatments, we are naturally impatient for rapid and fundamental improvements—we hope to join the other medical specialties in moving 'from the descriptive to the analytical'. Now at last it seems the tools are becoming available to develop a true understanding of psychiatric disease.

We are, however, cautious—there have been false dawns before. The insights into mental mechanisms provided by the psychoanalytical pioneers in the first half of the twentieth century gave rise to hope that these methods would prove therapeutic in many mental illnesses. The discovery of effective antipsychotic and antidepressant drugs in the 1950s raised hopes that examination of drug effects would reveal the pathological mechanisms of the underlying diseases. The move to community care which followed Enoch Powell's 'Water Tower Speech' in 1961 was driven by the hope that many of the deficits experienced by sufferers from mental disorder were not intrinsic to the disorders themselves, but were related to institutional living. None of these hopes were fulfilled. However, in the first decades of the twenty-first century, we have a number of genuine reasons for optimism and excitement.

Genetics

The information provided by the Human Genome Project, and large linkage and association studies, combined with techniques of high-throughput genetic screening, allow identification of susceptibility genes for complex polygenic disorders. Advances in molecular biology will allow the functions of these gene products to be understood, potentially generating new therapies. We are increasingly coming to understand how susceptibility genes interact with the environment to cause illness, including the potential role of epigenetic factors in mediating the impact of environmental stresses on gene expression.

Novel treatment approaches

In the last century discovery of effective treatments led to aetiological hypotheses. In this century the hope is that understanding of the molecular and chemical pathways involved in risk for illness will lead to the development of novel treatment approaches, therapeutics becoming hypothesis driven rather than hypothesis creating. Rational drug design will be aided by computer modelling and screening of large numbers of potential drug molecules. There will be further investigation of stem cell therapy in neurodegenerative disorders.

Functional and diagnostic imaging

Current structural scanning methods (e.g. CT and MRI) reveal changes across cohorts of patients with major mental disorders but do not allow objective diagnosis in individuals. Many psychiatric disorders show no measurable abnormalities at all using current structural methods. In the future, functional imaging (e.g. PET, functional MRI), either alone or in combination with structural scanning, may allow an understanding of how changes in neural systems contribute to illness and possibly true diagnostic imaging.

Large-scale treatment trials

In current practice, even relatively common treatment decisions are not clearly evidence-based. The current evidence base is overly reliant on small randomized trials, uncontrolled trials and 'expert opinion'. Now, however, psychiatry researchers are following their peers in cardiology and oncology and recruiting to large-scale treatment trials.

Every generation enjoys the use of a vast hoard bequeathed to it by antiquity, and transmits that hoard, augmented by fresh acquisitions, to future ages.

Thomas Babington Macaulay

I like the dreams of the future better than the history of the past.

Thomas Jefferson

There are fish in the sea better than have ever been caught.

Irish proverb

Psychiatric assessment

The clinical interview

In most branches of clinical medicine, diagnoses are made largely on the basis of the patient's history, with physical examination and investigation playing important but subordinate roles. In psychiatry, physical examination and investigations are of lesser diagnostic value and diagnosis is based on the clinical interview and, to a lesser extent, the later course of the patient's illness. Clinical interviewing is thus the central skill of the psychiatrist and development of clinical interviewing skills is the main aim of basic psychiatric training.

The clinical interview includes both history taking and mental state examination. The mental state examination is a systematic record of the patient's current psychopathology. In addition to its role in diagnosis, the clinical interview begins the development of a therapeutic relationship and is, in many cases, the beginning of treatment.

Clinical interview skills cannot be learned from a textbook. This chapter is intended as a guide to the doctor developing skills in interviewing psychiatric patients. As a trainee psychiatrist you should also take the opportunity to observe experienced clinicians as they interview patients; to review your own videotaped consultations with a tutor; and most importantly, carry out many clinical interviews and present the results to your seniors. Skills in this area, as with all others, come with experience and practice.

This chapter describes a model for the assessment of general adult and old-age psychiatry patients on the wards or in the outpatient clinic. For special patient populations, modifications or extensions to the standard interview are described in the appropriate chapter: alcohol and drug problems (📖 p. 552, p. 592); forensic (📖 p. 692, p. 710); child and adolescent (📖 pp. 612–17); learning disability (📖 p. 738); and psychotherapy (📖 p. 822).

The student or doctor coming to psychiatric interviewing for the first time is likely to be apprehensive. The symptoms which the patient describes may seem bizarre or incomprehensible, and the examiner may struggle for understanding and knowledge of which further questions to ask. Remember that the interviewer is not like a lawyer or policeman trying to 'get at the truth' but rather an aid to the patient telling the story in their own words. Start by listening, prompting only when necessary, and aim to feel at the end of the interview that you really understand the patient's problems and their perception of them.

The following pages describe the standard structure for a routine history, mental state examination, and case summary; there are then pages devoted to the different symptom areas in adult psychiatry with suggested probe questions. These are intended as guides to the sort of questions to ask the patient (or to ask yourself about the patient) and may be rephrased in your own words. See Box 2.1 for advice on personal safety.

Box 2.1 Always consider your personal safety when interviewing

There is a risk of aggression or violence in only a small minority of psychiatric patients. In the vast majority of patients the only risk of violence is towards themselves. However, the fact that violence is rare can lead to doctors putting themselves at risk due to thoughtlessness. To combat this it is important to think about the risk of violence before every consultation with a new patient or with a familiar patient with new symptoms.

Before interviewing a patient, particularly for the first time, consider: who you are interviewing, where you are interviewing, and with whom. Ensure that the nursing staff have this information.

- If possible, review the patient's records noting previous symptomatology and episodes of previous violence (the best predictor of future violence).
- A number of factors will increase the risk of violence, including: previous history of violence, psychotic illness, intoxication with alcohol or drugs, frustration, feeling of threat (which may be delusional or relate to real-world concerns).
- The ideal interview room has two doors, one for you and one for the patient. If this is not available sit so that the patient is not between you and the door. Remove all potential weapons from the interview room.
- Familiarize yourself with the ward's panic alarm system before you first need to use it.
- If your hospital organizes break-away or aggression management training courses, attend these regularly to keep your skills up to date.

Setting the scene

Introductions Observe the normal social forms when meeting someone for the first time. Introduce yourself and any accompanying staff members by name and status. Ensure that you know the names and relationships of any people accompanying the patient (and ask the patient if they wish these persons to be present during the interview). It is best to introduce yourself by title and surname and refer to the patient by title and surname. Do not use the patient's Christian name except at their request.

Seating The traditional consultation room, with the patient facing the doctor across a desk, is inappropriate in psychiatry. Use two or more comfortable chairs, of the same height, orientated to each other at an angle. This is less confrontational but allows direct eye contact as necessary. A clipboard will allow you to write notes as you go along.

Explanation Inform the patient of your status and specialty and explain the purpose of the interview. Explain the reasons for referral as you understand them and inform the patient of the information you have been told by the referrer. Patients often imagine you know more about them than you do. It is helpful to indicate to the patient how long the interview will last; this will allow both of you to plan your time so as not to omit vital topics. Advise them that you may wish to obtain further information after the interview from other sources, and obtain their consent to talk to any informants accompanying them if this would add to your assessment.

Documentation For all clinical interviewing a written account is crucial, both as a way of recording and communicating information and as a medico-legal record. It is best to write up the account as you go along. This saves time afterwards and allows for a more accurate account of the patient's own words. The record should be legible, signed, and dated, and ordered in a standard fashion. Initially you may find it helpful to write out the standard headings on sheets of paper beforehand.

Interviewing non-English speaking patients Where the doctor and the patient do not speak a common language, an interpreter is essential. Even in situations where the patient appears to speak some English, sufficient for day-to-day conversation, an interpreter is still highly desirable because idiomatic language and culturally specific interpretations of psychological phenomena may confuse understanding. Where possible the interpreter should share not only a language but also a cultural background with the patient, as many descriptions of psychiatric symptoms are culture-specific. Do not use members of a patient's family as interpreters except where unavoidable (e.g. in emergency situations). It is unethical to use children as interpreters.

Interviewing psychiatric patients

Interview structure

The exact internal structure of the interview will be decided by the nature of the presenting complaint. However, the interview will generally go through a number of more or less discrete phases:

Initiation Introduce yourself and explain the nature and purpose of the interview. Describe how long the interview will last and what you know about the patient already.

Patient-led history Invite the patient to tell you about their presenting complaint. Use general opening questions and prompt for further elaboration. Let the patient do most of the talking: your role is to help them to tell the story in their own words. During this phase you should note down the major observations in the mental state examination (MSE). Having completed the history of the present complaint and the MSE you will be able to be more focused when taking the other aspects of the history.

Doctor-led history Clarify the details in the history thus far with appropriate questions. Clarify the nature of diagnostic symptoms (e.g. are these true hallucinations? Is there diurnal mood variation?). Explore significant areas not mentioned spontaneously by the patient.

Background history Complete the history by direct enquiry. This is similar to standard medical history-taking, with the addition of a closer enquiry into the patient's personal history.

Summing-up Recount the history as you have understood it back to the patient. Ensure there are no omissions or important areas uncovered. Indicate if you would like to obtain other third-party information, emphasizing that this would add to your understanding of the patient's problems and help you in your diagnosis.

Questioning techniques

Open vs. closed questions An open question does not suggest the possible answers; a closed question expects a limited range of replies (cf. 'can you tell me how you are feeling?' and 'is your mood up or down at the moment?'). In general, begin the interview with open questions, turning to more closed questions to clarify details or factual points.

Non-directive vs. leading questions A leading question directs a patient towards a suggested answer (e.g. 'is your mood usually worse in the mornings?' rather than 'is your mood better or worse at any time of day?') Just as lawyers are reprimanded for 'leading a witness' we should in general avoid leading our patients to certain replies, as the desire to please the doctor can be a very powerful one.

Giving advice

Aim to leave at least the last quarter of the available interview time for discussion of the diagnosis, your explanation to the patient of your understanding of the nature and cause of their symptoms, and your detailing of your plans for treatment or further investigation or referral as indicated. The patient's confidence in your diagnosis will be improved by their belief that you really understand 'what is going on' and spending time detailing exactly what you want them to do will pay dividends in increased compliance. As a junior trainee you may have to break at the end of the history-taking segment in order to present the case to your senior and get advice on management.

After the interview

The process of assessment does not of course end with the initial clinical interview. In psychiatry, all diagnoses are to some extent provisional. You should follow your initial interview by gathering information from relatives, GP, previous case records, and clarifying symptoms observed by nursing staff. In the emergency situation a modification of this technique, focusing mainly on the acute problem, is more appropriate, with re-interviewing later to fill in the blanks if required.

Discussing management

In psychiatry, more than any other specialty, it is essential for successful management that the patient has a good understanding of their disorder and its treatment. There is no equivalent in psychiatry of the simple fracture where all that is required of the patient is to lie back and take the medicine. The treatment of any psychiatric disorder begins at the initial interview, where in addition to the assessment, the doctor should aim to establish the therapeutic alliance, effectively communicate the management plan, instil a sense of hope in the patient, and encourage self-help strategies.

Establish a therapeutic relationship

- Aim to listen more than you speak (especially initially).
- Show respect for the patient as an individual (e.g. establish their preferred mode of address; ask permission for anyone else to be present at the interview).
- Explicitly make your actions for the benefit of the patient.
- Do not argue; agree to disagree if consensus cannot be reached.
- Accept that in some patients trust may take time to develop.

Communicate effectively

- **Be specific** Explain what you think the diagnosis is and what the management should be.
- **Avoid jargon** Use layman's language or explain specialist terms which you use.
- **Avoid ambiguity** Clarify precisely what you mean and what your plans are. Be explicit in your statements to patients (e.g. say 'I will ask one of our nurses to visit you at home on Monday morning', rather than 'I'll arrange some community support for you').
- **Connect the advice to the patient** Explain why you think what you do and what it is about the patient's symptoms that suggests the diagnosis to you.
- **Use repetition and recapitulation** Use the 'primacy/recency' effect to your advantage. Restate the important information first and repeat it at the end.
- **Break up/write down** Most of what is said to patients in medical interviews is rapidly forgotten or distorted. Make the information easier to remember by breaking it up into a numbered list. Consider providing personalized written information, in addition to any advice leaflets etc. that you give the patient. This is imperative if the advice is complex and specific (e.g. dosage regimes for medication).

Instil hope

- Patients with mental health problems often feel extremely isolated and cut off from others, and may feel that they are the only people ever to experience their symptoms. Reassure them that you recognize their symptoms as part of a pattern representing a treatable illness.
- Convey to the patient your belief that this illness is understandable and that there are prospects for recovery.
- Counteract unrealistic beliefs (e.g. fear of 'losing my mind' or 'being locked away forever').
- Where cure is not possible, emphasize that there is still much that can be done to manage the illness and ameliorate symptoms.

Encourage self-help

- Be clear to the patient what they can do to help themselves, for example, maintain treatment adherence (📖 p. 924), avoid exacerbating factors (e.g. drug or alcohol misuse), consider lifestyle changes (e.g. house move, relationship counselling).
- Provide written self-help materials appropriate to the current disorder (📖 pp. 1010–17).
- Where appropriate, encourage contact/attendance at voluntary treatment organizations, self-help groups, or patient organizations (📖 pp. 1010–17). Develop knowledge of, and links with, local resources and aim to have their contact numbers and location information available at the consultation.

History

The history should, as far as possible, be gathered in the standard order presented here. This provides structure and logical coherence to the questioning, both for the doctor and the patient, and it is less likely that items will be omitted.

Basic information Name, age, and marital status. Current occupation. Route of referral. Current legal status (detained under Mental Health Act?).

Presenting complaints Number and brief description of presenting complaints. Which is the most troublesome symptom?

History of presenting complaints For each individual complaint record its nature (in the patient's own words as far as possible); chronology; severity; associated symptoms and associated life events occurring at or about the same time. Note precipitating, aggravating, and relieving factors. Have these or similar symptoms occurred before? To what does the patient attribute their symptoms?

Past psychiatric and medical history Previous psychiatric diagnoses. Chronological list of episodes of psychiatric inpatient, day hospital, and outpatient care. Current medical conditions. Chronological list of episodes of medical or surgical illness. Episodes of symptoms for which no treatment was sought. Any illnesses treated by GP.

Drug history List names and doses of current medication (have they been taking it?) Previous psychiatric drug treatments. History of adverse reactions or drug allergy. Any non-prescribed or alternative medications taken.

Family history Family tree (see Fig. 2.1) detailing names, ages, relationships, and illnesses of first- and second-degree relatives. Are there any familial illnesses?

Personal history

Childhood Were there problems during their pregnancy or delivery? Did they reach development milestones normally? Was their childhood happy? In what sort of family were they raised?

Education Which primary and secondary schools did they attend? If more than one of each, why was this? Did they attend mainstream or specialist schools? Did they enjoy school—if not, why? At what age did they leave school and with what qualifications? Type of further education and qualifications attained. If they left higher education before completing the course—why was this?

Employment Chronological list of jobs. Which job did they hold for the longest period? Which job did they enjoy most? If the patient has had a series of jobs—why did they leave each? Account for periods of unemployment in the patient's history. Is the type of job undertaken consistent with the patient's level of educational attainment?

Relationships Sexual orientation. Chronological account of major relationships. Reasons for relationship breakdown. Are they currently in a relationship? Do they have any children from the current or previous relationships? Who do the children live with? What relationship does the patient have with them?

Forensic (📖 p. 692, p. 710) Have they been charged or convicted of any offences? What sentence did they receive? Do they have outstanding charges or convictions at the moment?

Social background information Current occupation. Are they working at the moment? If not, how long have they been off work and why? Current family/relationship situation. Alcohol and illicit drug use (📖 p. 552, p. 592). Main recreational activities.

Premorbid personality How would they describe themselves before they became ill? How would others have described them?

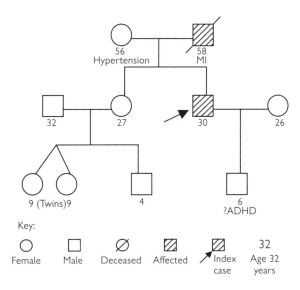

Fig. 2.1 A family tree diagram.

Mental state examination

The mental state examination (MSE) is an ordered summary of the examining doctor's observations as to the patient's mental experiences and behaviour at the time of interview. Its purpose is to suggest evidence for and against a diagnosis of mental disorder, and if mental disorder is present, to record the current type and severity of symptoms. The information obtained should, together with the psychiatric history, enable a judgement to be made regarding the presence of and severity of any mental disorder and the risk of harm to self or others.

The required information can be obtained during the course of history taking or in a systematic fashion afterwards. The MSE should be recorded and presented in a standardized format, although the information contained may derive from material gained in different ways. It is helpful to record the patient's description of significant symptoms word for word.

Appearance
- Apparent age
- Racial origin
- Style of dress
- Level of cleanliness
- General physical condition
- Abnormal involuntary movements including tics, grimaces, stereotypies, dyskinetic movements, tremors etc.

Behaviour
- Appropriateness of behaviour
- Level of motor activity
- Apparent level of anxiety
- Eye contact
- Rapport
- Abnormal movement or posture
- Episodes of aggression
- Distractibility

Speech
- Volume, rate, and tone
- Quantity and fluency
- Abnormal associations, clang and punning
- Flight of ideas

Mood
- Subjective and objective assessment of mood
- Mood evaluation should include the quality, range, depth, congruence, appropriateness and communicability of the mood state
- Anxiety and panic symptoms
- Obsessions and compulsions

Perception
- Hallucinations and pseudo-hallucinations
- Depersonalization and derealization. Illusions and imagery

Thought form
- Linearity
- Goal-directedness
- Associational quality
- Formal thought disorder

Thought content
- Delusions
- Over-valued ideas
- Preoccupations
- Obsessive thoughts, ideas, and impulses
- Thoughts of suicide or deliberate self-harm
- Thoughts of harm to others. Assess intent, lethality of intent, plan, and inimicality. Does the patient show any urge to act upon the plan?

Cognition
- Attention and concentration
- Orientation to time, place and person
- Level of comprehension
- Short-term memory

Insight
- Does the patient feel his experiences are as the result of illness?
- Will he accept medical advice and treatment?

Case summary

The written and oral presentation of the results of clinical interview should follow a standard format—history, MSE, results of physical examination, and case summary. The case summary can take a variety of forms but the structure suggested here is suitable for most situations. You should include a brief synopsis of the case, a differential diagnosis with your favoured working diagnosis, and a comment on aetiological factors in this patient.

Synopsis This should be a short paragraph summarizing the salient points of the preceding information and covering:
- basic personal information
- previous psychiatric diagnosis
- description of presentation
- description of current symptoms
- positive features on MSE
- suicide risk
- attitude to illness

Differential diagnosis This will usually be a short list of two or three possibilities. In an exam situation, mention other less likely possibilities you would consider in order to exclude. Your presentation should have directed you towards choosing one as your working diagnosis.

Formulation For general psychiatric patients the formulation should include comment on why the person has become ill and why now. You should identify the 'three P's'—predisposing, precipitating, and perpetuating factors for the current illness. This information will be important in guiding a suitable management plan. So, for example, in a patient with depressed mood following the birth of a baby: predisposing factors could be family history of depressive illness, female sex; precipitating factors could be the postnatal period, job loss, change of role, and feelings of inadequacy; and prolonging factors could be disturbed sleep, unsupportive partner.

Management plan Following the presentation of history, MSE, physical examination, and formulation you would normally go on to present or to document your initial management plan, including necessary investigations, initial drug treatment, instructions to nursing staff, and comment on potential risks and whether or not, in your opinion, the patient is currently detainable under the Mental Health Act.

Observations of appearance and behaviour

The greater part of the MSE consists of empathic questioning about the patient's internal experiences. Nonetheless, important information regarding mental state can be obtained from careful observation of the patient's appearance, behaviour, and manner, both during the interview and in some cases, later on the ward. This is particularly important in some situations, for example with a patient who may be concealing the presence of psychotic symptoms, or where there is reason to doubt the patient's account.

Take time to observe the patient during the interview and ask yourself the following questions. If possible, ask nursing staff about behaviour on the ward (e.g. does he have any abnormal movements or mannerisms; how does he interact with other patients; does he appear to be responding to unseen voices or commands?).

What is the patient's appearance? Describe the patient's physical appearance and racial origin. Compare what age they appear with their actual age (i.e. biological vs. chronological age). What is their manner of dress? Patients with manic illnesses may dress in an excessively formal, flamboyant, or sexually inappropriate manner. Patients with cognitive impairment may have mismatched or wrongly buttoned clothing.

What is the patient's behaviour during the interview? Are there episodes of tearfulness? Do they attend to the interview or do they appear distracted? Do they maintain an appropriate level of eye contact? Do you feel that you have established rapport?

What is the patient's level of activity during the interview? Does the patient appear restless or fidgety? Do they settle to a chair or pace during interview? Is there a normal level of gesticulation during conversation?

Is there any evidence of self-neglect? Does the patient have lower than normal standards of self-care and personal hygiene? Are they malodorous, unshaven, or dishevelled? Are their clothes clean? Are there cigarette burns or food stains on their clothes?

Is the patient's behaviour socially inappropriate? Is there embarrassing, overly familiar, or sexually forward behaviour? All are seen in manic illness or where there is cognitive impairment.

Is the patient's behaviour threatening, aggressive, or violent? In manner or in speech does the patient appear hostile or threatening? Do you feel at risk? Is there aggressive or violent behaviour on display during the interview? What prompts it?

Are there any abnormal movements? Does the patient have repetitive or rocking movements or bizarre posturing (stereotypies)? Do they perform voluntary, goal-directed activities in a bizarre way (mannerisms)? What is their explanation for this? For patients on neuroleptic medication, is there evidence of side-effects (e.g. stiffness, rigidity, tremor, akathisia)?

Is the patient distractible or appearing to be responding to hallucinations? Does the patient appear to be attending to a voice other than yours? Are they looking around the room as if for the source of a voice? Are they murmuring or mouthing soundlessly to themselves? Are there episodes of giggling, verbal outbursts, or other unexplained actions?

Speech

The content of the patient's speech (i.e. what they say) will be our major source of information for their history and mental state. The form of their speech (i.e. how they say it) is abnormal in a number of mental disorders and should be observed and commented upon.

Is there any speech at all? A small number of patients are mute during interview. Here the doctor should aim to comment on apparent level of comprehension (does the patient appear to understand what is said, e.g. shakes or nods head appropriately), level of alternate communication (can they write answers down, do they point or use gestures?), and level of structural impairment of the organs of speech (a patient who can cough on demand is demonstrably able to oppose both vocal cords normally).

What is the quantity of speech? Are answers unduly brief or monosyllabic? Conversely, are they inappropriately prolonged? Does the speech appear pressured? (i.e. there is copious, rapid speech, which is hard to interrupt)?

What is the rate of speech? There is a wide variation in normal rates of speech across even the regions of the UK. Is the patient's speech unusually slow or unusually rapid, given the expected rate? This may reflect acceleration or deceleration in the speed of thought in affective illnesses.

What is the volume and quality of speech? Does the patient whisper? Or speak inappropriately loudly? Is there stuttering or slurring or speech?

What is the tone and rhythm of speech? Even in a non-tonal language like English, normal speech has a musical quality with the intonation of the voice and rhythm of the sentences conveying meaning (i.e. the rise in tone at the end of a question). Loss of this range of intonation and rhythmic pattern is seen in chronic psychotic illnesses.

How appropriate is the speech? Is the content of the speech appropriate to the situation? Does the patient answer questions appropriately? Are there inappropriate or pointless digressions? Can the meaning of the speech always be followed?

Is there abnormal use of language? Are there word-finding difficulties, which may suggest an expressive dysphasia? Are there neologisms (i.e. made-up words, or normal words used in an idiosyncratic manner)?

Abnormal mood

In describing disorders of mood we draw a distinction between affect (the emotional state prevailing at a given moment) and mood (the emotional state over a longer period). To use a meteorological analogy, affect represents the weather, where mood is the climate. Variations in affect, from happiness to sadness, irritability to enthusiasm are within everyone's normal experience. Assessment of pathological abnormality of affect involves assessing the severity, longevity, and ubiquity of the mood disturbance and its association with other pathological features suggestive of mood disorder.

Depressed mood is the most common symptom of the mood disorders and in its milder forms has been experienced by most people at some point. Its experience is personal and is described in a variety of ways by different people: sometimes as a profound lowering of spirits, subjectively different from normal unhappiness; sometimes as an unpleasant absence of emotions or emotional range; and sometimes as a more physical symptom of 'weight' or 'blackness' weighing down on the head or chest. Increasingly, severe forms of depressed mood are indicated by the patient's rating of greater severity as compared with previous experience, increased pervasiveness of the low mood to all situations, and decreased reactivity of mood (i.e. decreased ability of the mood to be lightened by pleasurable or encouraging events).

The two central clinical features of depressive illness are (1) pervasively depressed and unreactive mood and (2) anhedonia—the loss of pleasure in previously pleasurable activities. The clinical picture also includes the 'biological features of depression', thoughts of self-harm, and, in more severe cases, mood-congruent psychotic features. The biological features include disturbance of sleep (particularly early morning waking and difficulty getting off to sleep), reduced appetite, loss of libido, reduced energy levels, and subjective impression of poorer concentration and memory. Many depressed patients will have thoughts of deliberate self-harm or ending their lives as a way of ending their suffering. With increasingly severe depressed mood there are increasingly frequent and formed plans of suicide. The development of a sense of hopelessness towards the future is a worrying sign.

Mania and depression are often thought of as two extremes of illness with normality or euthymia in the middle. Morbid change in mood (either elevation or depression) can more accurately be considered as being on one side of a coin with normality on the other. Some patients display both manic and depressive features in the one episode—a mixed affective state. Manic and depressive illnesses have, in common, increased lability (i.e. susceptibility to change) of mood, increased irritability, decreased sleep, and an increase in subjective anxiety.

The core clinical features of manic illnesses are sustained and inappropriate elevation in mood (often described as feeling on top of the world) and a distorted or inflated estimate of one's importance and abilities. The clinical picture also includes increased lability of mood, increased irritability, increased activity levels, disturbed sleep pattern with a sense of diminished need for sleep, and subjectively improved memory and concentration despite objective deterioration in these skills. With increasingly severe episodes of manic illness there is loss of judgement, an increase in inappropriate and risky behaviour, and the development of mood-congruent delusions.

Asking about depressed mood

'**How has your mood been lately?**' Patients vary in their ability to introspect and assess their mood. Beginning with general questioning allows a more unbiased account of mood problems. Report any description of depression in the patient's own words. Ask the patient to assess the depth of depression (e.g. 'on a scale of one to ten, where ten is normal and one is as depressed as you have ever felt, how would you rate your mood now?'). How long has the mood been as low as this? Enquire about any notable discrepancy between the patient's report of mood and objective signs of mood disturbance.

'**Does your mood vary over the course of a day?**' Clarify if the mood varies as the day goes on. If mood improves in the evening, does it return completely to normal? Does anything else change as the day goes on to account for the mood change (e.g. more company available in the evenings)?

'**Can you still enjoy the things you used to enjoy?**' By this point of the interview you should have some idea about the activities the patient formerly enjoyed. Depressed patients describe lack of interest in their previous pursuits, decreased participation in activities, and a sense of any participation being more of an effort.

'**How are you sleeping?**' Many patients will simply describe their sleep as 'terrible'. They should be asked further about time to bed, time falling asleep, wakefulness throughout the night, time of waking in the morning, quality of sleep (is it refreshing or not?), and any daytime napping.

'**What is your appetite like at the moment?**' Patients reporting a change in their appetite should be asked about reasons for this (loss of interest in food, loss of motivation to prepare food, or swallowing difficulties?). Has there been recent weight loss? Do their clothes still fit?

'**How is your concentration?**' Clarify any reported decline by asking about ability to perform standard tasks. Can they read a newspaper? Watch a TV show? Ask about work performance.

'**What is your memory like at the moment?**' Again, clarify any reported decline.

'**How is the sexual side of your relationship?**' Potentially embarrassing topics are best approached in a professional and matter-of-fact way. It is important to enquire about this directly as the symptom of loss of libido can cause considerable suffering for patient and partner and is less likely than other symptoms to be mentioned spontaneously. During treatment this symptom should again be asked about as many psychotropic drugs negatively affect sexual performance.

'**Do you have any worries on your mind at the moment?**' Characteristic of depressive illness is a tendency to preferentially dwell on negative issues.

'**Do you feel guilty about anything at the moment?**' Patients with depressive illnesses often report feelings of guilt or remorse about current or historical events. In severe illnesses these feelings can become delusional. Aim to assess the presence and nature of guilty thoughts.

Asking about thoughts of self-harm

Completed suicide is an unfortunately common outcome in many psychiatric conditions. Thoughts of deliberate self-harm occur commonly and should always be enquired about. The majority of patients with illness of any severity will have had thoughts of deliberate self-harm at some stage. It should be emphasized that asking about deliberate self-harm does not 'put the idea in their head', and indeed many patients will welcome the opportunity to discuss such worrying thoughts.

The assessment is not only of the presence of suicidal thoughts, but also their severity and frequency and the likelihood of them being followed by suicidal action. One suggested method involves asking about behaviours and thoughts associated with increasing suicide risk. This tactful enquiry can be made in addition to an estimate of risk. The aim is not to trap the patient into an unwanted disclosure but to assess the severity of suicidal intent and hence the attendant risk of completed suicide.

'How do you feel about the future?' Many patients will remain optimistic of improvement despite current severe symptoms. A description of hopelessness towards the future and a feeling that things will never get better is worrying.

'Have you ever thought that life was not worth living?' A consequence of hopelessness is the feeling that anything, even nothingness, would be better.

'Have you ever wished you could go to bed and not wake up in the morning?' Passive thoughts of death are common in mental illness and can also be found in normal elderly people towards the end of life, particularly after the deaths of spouses and peers.

'Have you had thoughts of ending your life?' If yes, enquire about the frequency of these thoughts—are they fleeting and rapidly dismissed; or more prolonged? Are they becoming more common?

'Have you thought about how you would do it?' Enquire about methods of suicide the patient has considered. Particularly worrying are violent methods that are likely to be successful (e.g. shooting, hanging, or jumping from a height).

'Have you made any preparations?' Aim to establish how far the patient's plans have progressed from ideas to action—have they considered a place, bought pills, carried out a final act (e.g. suicide note, or begun putting their affairs in order).

'Have you tried to take your own life?' Has there been a recent concealed attempt (e.g. overdose)? If so, consider whether current medical assessment is required.

Self-injurious behaviours Some patients report causing harm to themselves, sometimes repeatedly, without reporting a desire to die (e.g. lacerate their arms, legs, or abdomen; burn themselves with cigarettes). In these cases, enquire about the reasons for this behaviour, which may be obscure even to the person concerned. In what circumstances do they harm themselves? What do they feel and think before harming themselves? How do they feel afterwards?

Asking about elevated mood

'How has your mood been lately?' As for enquiries about depressed mood, begin with a very general question. Report the patient's description of their mood in their own words. Clarify what the patient means by general statements such as 'on top of the world'.

'Do you find your mood is changeable at the moment?' Besides general elevation in mood, patients with mania often report lability of mood, with tearfulness and irritability as well as elation. The pattern and type of mood variation should be noted if present.

'What is your thinking like at the moment?' Patients with mania often report a subjective increase in the speed and ease of thinking, with many ideas occurring to them, each with a wider variety of associated thoughts than normal. This experience, together with the nature of their ideas, should be explored and described.

'Do you have any special gifts or talents?' A characteristic feature of frank mania is the belief that they have exceptional abilities of some kind (e.g. as great writers or painters), or that they have some particular insight to offer the world (e.g. the route to achieving world peace). These beliefs may become frankly delusional, with the patient believing they have special or magical powers. The nature of these beliefs and their implications and meaning for the patient should be described.

'How are you sleeping?' Manic patients describe finding sleep unnecessary or a distraction from their current plans. Enquire about the length and quality of sleep.

'What is your appetite like at the moment?' Appetite is variable in manic illnesses. Some patients describe having no time or patience for the preparation of food; others eat excessively and spend excessively on food and drink. Ask about recent weight gain or loss and about a recent typical day's food intake.

'How is your concentration?' Typically, manic patients have impaired concentration and may report this; in this case the complaint should be clarified by examples of impairment. Some manic patients overestimate their concentration, along with other subjective estimates of ability. Report on objective measures of concentration (e.g. attention to interview questioning or ability to retain interest in newspapers or TV while on the ward).

'How is the sexual side of your relationship?' Again, this topic should be broached directly and straightforwardly. Manic patients sometimes report increased interest in sexual activity. Clarify the patient's estimate of his or her own sexual attractiveness and recent increase in sexual activity or promiscuity.

Anxiety symptoms

Anxiety symptoms are the most common type of symptoms seen in patients with psychiatric disorders. They are the core clinical features of the ICD-10 neurotic disorders (which are indeed called anxiety disorders in DSM-IV), and are also prominent clinical features in psychotic illnesses, affective illness, organic disorders, and in drug and alcohol use and withdrawal.

Anxiety has two components: **psychic anxiety**—an unpleasant effect in which there is subjective tension, increased arousal, and fearful apprehension; and **somatic anxiety**—bodily sensations of palpitations, sweating, dyspnoea, pallor, and abdominal discomfort. The sensations of anxiety are related to autonomic arousal and cognitive appraisal of threat which were adaptive primitive survival reactions.

Anxiety symptoms are part of normal healthy experience, particularly before novel, stressful, or potentially dangerous situations. Moderate amounts of anxiety can optimize performance (the so-called 'Yerkes–Dobson' curve—plotting performance level against anxiety shows an inverse-U shape). They become pathological when they are abnormally severe, abnormally prolonged, or if they are present at a level out of keeping with the real threat of the situation.

Anxiety symptoms may be present at a more or less constant level—**generalized anxiety**; or may occur only episodically—**panic attacks**. Anxiety symptoms may or may not have an identifiable stimulus. Where a stimulus can be identified it may be very specific, as in a simple phobia (e.g. fear of cats or spiders); or may be more generalized, as in social phobia and agoraphobia. In phobias of all kinds there is avoidance of the feared situation. Because this avoidance is followed by a reduction in unpleasant symptoms it is reinforced and is liable to be repeated. Breaking of this cycle is the basis of desensitization methods of treating phobias (p. 848).

The repetition of behaviours in order to achieve reduction in the experience of anxiety is also seen in the symptoms of **obsessions** and **compulsions**. Here, the patient regards the thoughts (obsessions) and/or actions (compulsions) as purposeless, but is unable to resist thinking about them or carrying them out. Resistance to their performance produces rising anxiety levels, which are diminished by repeating the resisted behaviour.

Asking about anxiety symptoms

In enquiring about anxiety symptoms, aside from the nature, severity, and precipitants of the symptoms, it is important to establish in all cases the impact they are having on the person's life. Record what particular activities or situations are avoided because of their symptoms and, in the case of obsessional symptoms, note how much time the patient spends on them.

'**Would you say you were an anxious person?**' There is a wide variation in the normal level of arousal and anxiety. Some people are inveterate 'worriers', while others appear relaxed at all times.

'**Recently, have you been feeling particularly anxious or on edge?**' Ask the patient to describe when the symptoms began. Was there any particular precipitating event or trauma?

'**Do any particular situations make you more anxious than others?**' Establish whether the symptoms are constant or fluctuating. If the latter, enquire about those situations that cause worsening or improvement.

'**Have you ever had a panic attack?**' Ask the patient to describe to you what they mean by this. A classical panic attack is described as sudden in onset with gradual resolution over 30–60 min. There are physical symptoms of dyspnoea, tachycardia, sweating, chest tightness/chest pain, and paraesthesia (related to over-breathing); coupled with psychological symptoms of subjective tension and apprehension that 'something terrible is going to happen'.

'**Do any thoughts or worries keep coming back to your mind even though you try to push them away?**'

'**Do you ever find yourself spending a lot of time doing the same thing over and over—like checking things, or cleaning—even though you've already done it well enough?**' Besides identifying the type of repetitive thought or action involved it is important to establish that the thoughts or impulses are recognized as the person's own (in contrast with thought insertion in psychotic illness) and that they are associated with resistance (although active resistance may diminish in chronic OCD). Patients with obsessional thoughts often worry that they are 'losing their mind' or that they will act on a particular thought (e.g. a mother with an obsessional image of smothering her baby). Where the symptom is definitively that of an obsession the patient can be reassured that they will not carry it out.

Abnormal perceptions

Abnormal perceptual experiences form part of the clinical picture of many mental disorders. Equally, the range of normal perceptual experience is very wide. Patients vary in their ability to explain their subjective perceptual experiences.

The brain constantly receives large amounts of perceptual information via the five special senses of vision, hearing, touch, taste, and smell; the muscle, joint, and internal organ proprioceptors; and the vestibular apparatus. The majority of this information is processed unconsciously and only a minority reaches conscious awareness at any one time. An *external object* is represented internally by a *sensory percept* that combines with memory and experience to produce a *meaningful internal percept* in the conscious mind. In health, we can clearly distinguish between percepts which represent real objects and those which are the result of internal imagery or fantasy, which may be vividly experienced in the mind but are recognized as not real.

Abnormal perceptual experiences may be divided into two types:
- Altered perceptions—including sensory distortions and illusions—in which there is a distorted internal perception of a real external object.
- False perceptions—including hallucinations and pseudo-hallucinations—in which there is an internal perception without an external object.

Sensory distortions are changes in the perceived intensity or quality of a real external stimulus. They are associated with organic conditions and with drug ingestion or withdrawal. **Hyperacusis** (experiencing sounds as abnormally loud) and **micropsia** (perceiving objects as smaller and further away, as if looking through the wrong end of a telescope) are examples of sensory distortions.

Illusions are altered perceptions in which a real external object is combined with imagery to produce a false internal percept. Both lowered attention and heightened affect will predispose to experiencing illusions.

Affect illusions occur at times of heightened emotion (e.g. while walking through a dangerous area late at night a person may see a tree blowing in the wind as an attacker lunging at them).

Completion illusions rely on our brain's tendency to 'fill in' presumed missing parts of an object to produce a meaningful percept and are the basis for many types of optical illusion. Both these types of illusions resolve on closer attention.

Pareidolic illusions are meaningful percepts produced when experiencing a poorly defined stimulus (e.g. seeing faces in a fire or in clouds).

Hallucinations A hallucination is defined as 'a percept without an object' (Esquirol 1838). As symptoms of major mental disorder, hallucinations are the most significant type of abnormal perception. It is important to appreciate that the subjective experience of hallucination is that of experiencing a normal percept in that modality of sensation. A *true hallucination* will be perceived as being in external space, distinct from imagined images, outside conscious control, and as possessing relative permanence.

A *pseudo-hallucination* will lack one or all of these characteristics and be subjectively experienced as internal or 'in my head'. The only characteristic of true perceptions which true hallucinations lack is publicness; hallucinating patients may accept that their experiences are not shared by others around them in the same way as a normal sensory experience.

Auditory hallucinations are most frequently seen in functional psychoses. Three experiences of auditory hallucinations are first-rank symptoms in schizophrenia. These are:
- Hearing a voice speak one's thoughts aloud.
- Hearing a voice narrating one's actions.
- Hearing two or more voices arguing.

Visual hallucinations are associated with organic disorders of the brain and with drug and alcohol intoxication and withdrawal. They are very rarely seen in psychotic illness alone but are reported in association with dementias, cortical tumours, stimulant and hallucinogen ingestion, and, most commonly, in delirium tremens. The visual hallucinations seen in delirium tremens are characteristically 'Lilliputian hallucinations' of miniature animals or people.

Olfactory and gustatory hallucinations may be difficult to distinguish and occur in a wide range of mental disorders. Olfactory hallucinations occur in epileptic auras, in depressive illnesses (where the smell is described as unpleasant or repulsive to others), and in schizophrenia. They may also occur in association with a persistent delusion of malodourousness.

Hypnagogic/hypnopompic hallucinations are transient false perceptions which occur on falling asleep (hypnagogic) or on waking (hypnopompic). They may have the characteristics of true or pseudo-hallucinations and are most commonly visual or auditory. While they are sometimes seen in narcolepsy and affective illnesses they are not indicative of ill health and are frequently reported by healthy people.

Elemental hallucinations are the hallucinatory experience of simple sensory elements, such as flashes of light or unstructured noises. They are associated with organic states.

Extracampine hallucinations are those false perceptions where the hallucination is of an external object beyond the normal range of perception of the sensory organs.

Functional hallucinations are hallucinations of any modality that are experienced simultaneously with a normal stimulus in that modality (e.g. a patient who only experiences auditory hallucinations when he hears the sound of the ward's air conditioning).

Reflex hallucinations are hallucinations in one modality of sensation experienced after experiencing a normal stimulus in another modality of sensation.

Asking about abnormal perceptions

Asking patients about their experience of abnormal perceptions and abnormal beliefs (e.g. hallucinations and delusions) presents a number of problems for the examiner. Unlike symptoms such as anxiety, these symptoms are not part of normal experience, and so the examiner will not have the same degree of empathic understanding. Patients will often fear the reaction of others to the revelation of psychotic symptoms (fear of being thought 'mad') and so conceal them. When such symptoms are not present, patients may resent such questioning or regard it as strange or insulting.

As with most potentially embarrassing topics, the best approach is frankness, lack of embarrassment, and straightforwardness. If the interview thus far has not led to report of psychotic symptoms, the examiner should begin by saying something like:

'Now I want to ask you about some experiences which some-times people have, but find difficult to talk about. These are questions I ask everyone.' This makes clear that these questions are not as a result of suspicion in the examiner's mind or an indicator of how seriously he regards the patient's problems.

'Have you ever had the sensation that you were unreal—or that the world had become unreal?' The symptoms of depersonalization and derealization are non-specific symptoms in a variety of affective and psychotic conditions. Many patients find them difficult or impossible to explain clearly, commonly describing the experience as 'like being in a play'. Patients often worry about these experiences fearing they presage 'going mad'. They may therefore be reluctant to mention them spontaneously.

'Have you ever had the experience of hearing noises or voices when there was no-one about to explain it?' If the patient agrees, then this experience should be further clarified: When did this occur? Was the patient fully awake? How often? Where did the sound appear to come from? If a voice was heard, what did it say? Did the patient recognize the voice? Was there more than one? How did the voice refer to the patient (e.g. as 'you' or 'him')? Can the patient give examples of the sort of things the voice said?

'Have you seen any visions?' Again, clarify when and how often the experience occurred. What were the circumstances? Was the vision seen with the 'mind's eye' or perceived as being in external space? Was it distinct from the surroundings or seen as part of the wallpaper or curtain pattern?

'Do you ever notice smells or tastes that other people aren't bothered by?' Again, clarify the details surrounding any positive response. Aim to distinguish olfactory hallucinations (where there is the experience of an abnormal odour) from a patient who has a delusion that he is malodorous.

Abnormal beliefs

Examination of the patient's ideas and beliefs will form an important part of the MSE. Abnormal or false beliefs include primary and secondary delusions and over-valued ideas. More so than other symptoms of mental ill health, a patient with delusions fits the common preconceptions of 'madness'. Delusions are important symptoms in the diagnosis of the major psychoses.

Delusions

A delusion is a pathological belief which has the following characteristics:
- It is held with absolute subjective certainty and cannot be rationalized away.
- It requires no external proof and may be held in the face of contradictory evidence.
- It has personal significance and importance to the individual concerned.
- It is not a belief which can be understood as part of the subject's cultural or religious background.

Note: Although the content of the delusion is usually demonstrably false and bizarre in nature, this is not invariably so.

A **secondary delusion** is one whose development can be understood in the light of another abnormality in mental state (e.g. the development of delusions of poverty in a severely depressed patient).

A **primary delusion** cannot be understood in this way and must be presumed as arising directly from the pathological process. Delusions can be categorized by their content or by the manner in which they are perceived as having arisen.

Over-valued ideas

An over-valued idea is a non-delusional, non-obsessional abnormal belief. Here, the patient has a belief which is in itself acceptable and comprehensible but which is preoccupying and comes to dominate their thinking and behaviour. The idea is not perceived as external or senseless but will generally have great significance to the patient. Over-valued ideas may have a variety of contents in different disorders (e.g. concern over physical appearance in dysmorphophobia; concern over weight and body shape in anorexia nervosa; concern over personal rights in paranoid personality disorder).

Asking about abnormal beliefs

Both at the initial interview and during subsequent treatment, professional staff dealing with a deluded patient should avoid colluding in the delusional belief system. The doctor should not be drawn into arguments about the truth of the delusion—by their nature delusions cannot be argued or rationalized away and arguments of this type will damage rapport. Nonetheless, the doctor should always make clear to the patient that he regards the delusional symptom as a symptom of mental ill health, albeit one which is very real and important to the patient concerned.

Delusional ideas vary in their degree of detail and in their intensity over the course of an illness episode. In evolving psychotic illness there will often be a perplexing sense of 'something not being right' and ill-formed symptoms such as a vague sense that they are being spied upon or persecuted in some way. As the delusion becomes more fully formed it comes to dominate the person's thinking and becomes more **elaborated**—more detailed and with more 'evidence' produced to support the belief. With treatment the delusion will hopefully fade in importance and the person may come to appreciate the belief as false or, despite holding to its initial truth, will regard it as no longer important.

'Do you have any particular worries preying on your mind at the moment?' Beginning with a very general question like this offers the patient an opportunity to broach a topic which may have been concerning them but which they have been putting off mentioning.

'Do you ever feel that people are watching you or paying attention to what you are doing?' Ask the patient to describe this sensation and an episode of its occurrence. Distinguish normal self-consciousness or a patient's awareness of genuinely notable abnormality from referential delusions. A delusion will generally have further elaboration of the belief—there will be some 'reason' why the reported events are happening. Elaboration may take the form of other beliefs about cameras, bugs, etc.

'When you watch the television or read the newspapers, do you ever feel that the stories refer to you directly, or to things that you have been doing?' Invite the patient to elaborate further on a positive response. Again, probe for further elaboration of the belief and seek examples of when it has occurred.

'Do you ever feel that people are trying to harm you in any way?' Persecutory delusions are among the most common features of psychotic illness. There is potential for diagnostic confusion with paranoid personality traits, with suspicion and resentfulness towards medical and nursing staff and with genuine fears, understandable in the context of the patient's lifestyle (e.g. of retribution from drug dealers or money lenders). Explore the nature and basis of the beliefs and the supporting evidence that the patient advances for them.

'Do you feel that you are to blame for anything, that you are responsible for anything going wrong?' Delusions of guilt are seen in psychotic depression, in addition to the psychotic disorders. The affected individual may believe that they are responsible for a crime, occasionally one which has been prominently reported. On occasions these individuals may 'turn themselves in' to the police rather than seeking medical help.

'Do you worry that there is anything wrong with your body or that you have a serious illness?' Hypochondriacal delusions show diagnostic overlap with normal health concerns, hypochondriacal over-valued ideas, and somatization disorder. Clarify this symptom by examining the patient's evidence for this belief and the firmness with which it is held.

Asking about the first-rank symptoms of schizophrenia

The first-rank symptoms are a group of symptoms which have special significance in the diagnosis of schizophrenia. There is no symptom that is pathognomic of schizophrenia. The first-rank symptoms are useful because they occur reasonably often in schizophrenia and more rarely in other disorders and it is not too difficult to tell whether they are present or not. They can all be reported in other conditions (e.g. organic psychoses, manic illnesses). They do not give a guide to severity or prognosis of illness (i.e. a patient with many first-rank symptoms is not 'worse' than one with few) and they may not occur at all in a patient who undoubtedly has schizophrenia. There are eleven first-rank symptoms, organized into four categories according to type.

Auditory hallucinations
- 'Voices heard arguing'
- Thought echo
- 'Running commentary'

Delusions of thought interference
- Thought insertion
- Thought withdrawal
- Thought broadcasting

Delusions of control
- Passivity of affect
- Passivity of impulse
- Passivity of volitions
- Somatic passivity

Delusional perception
- A primary delusion of any content that is reported by the patient as having arisen following the experience of a normal perception

'Do you ever hear voices commenting on what you are doing? Or discussing you between themselves? Or repeating your own thoughts back to you?' For this symptom to be considered first-rank, the experience must be that of a true auditory hallucination where the hallucinatory voice refers to the patient in the third person (i.e. as 'him' or 'her' rather than 'you'). Distinguish these experiences from internal monologues.

'Do you ever get the feeling that someone is interfering with your thoughts—that they are putting thoughts into your head or taking them away? Or that your thoughts can be transmitted to others in some way?' It is the experience itself that renders this symptom first-rank. The patient may describe additional delusional elaboration (e.g. involving implanted transmitters or radio waves). The important point to clarify with the patient is that the experience is really that of thoughts being affected by an external agency and that it is not simple distraction or absent-mindedness. For thought broadcasting, ensure that the patient is not simply referring to the fact that they are 'easily read' or that they give away their emotions or thoughts by their actions.

'Do you ever get the feeling that you are being controlled? That your thoughts or moods or actions are being forced on you by someone else?' Again, there may be delusional elaboration of this symptom but it is the experience itself, of an external controller affecting things which are normally experienced as totally under one's own control, which makes this symptom first-rank. Clarify that the actions are truly perceived as controlled by an outside agency, rather than, for example, being directed by auditory hallucinations.

Disorders of the form of thought

In describing psychopathology we draw a distinction between the content and the form of thought.

Content and form

Content describes the meaning and experience of belief, perception, and memory as described by patients, while form describes the structure and process of thought. In addition to abnormalities of perception and belief, mental disorders can produce abnormality in the normal form of thought processes. This may be suggested by abnormalities in the form of speech, the only objective representation of the thoughts, or may be revealed by empathic questioning designed to elicit the patient's subjective experiences. When patients mutter to themselves, listen closely to see if it is comprehensible or not. The latter is usually indicative of disorder of form of thinking. See Box 2.2 for methods of assessing symptoms of thought disorder.

Thought disorder

Among the psychiatric symptoms that are outside normal experience, thought disorder is challenging to understand and perhaps the most difficult for the clinician to have empathy with. Consider a model of normal thought processes and use this to simplify discussions of abnormalities. In this model we visualize each thought, giving rise to a constellation of associations (i.e. a series of related thoughts). One of these is pursued, which gives rise to a further constellation and so on. This sequence may proceed towards a specific goal driven by a determining tendency (colloquially the 'train of thought') or may be undirected as in daydreaming. Disturbances in the form of thought may affect the rate or internal associations of thought.

Accelerated tempo of thought

Accelerated tempo of thought is called flight of ideas. It may be reflected in the speech as pressure of speech or may be described by the patient. The sensation is of the thoughts proceeding more rapidly than can be articulated and of each thought giving rise to more associations than can be followed up. Flight of ideas can be a feature of a manic episode. In the majority of cases of flight of ideas, some form of association of each thought can be discerned. For example, it could be a superficial clang association, alliteration and punning that proceeds like the game of dominoes where the last move determines the next move. In milder forms, called prolixity, the rate is slow and eventually reaches the goal if allowed adequate time.

Decelerated tempo of thought

Decelerated tempo of thought, or psychic retardation, occurs in depressive illnesses. Here the subjective speed of thought and the range of associations are decreased. There may be decreased rate of speech and absence of spontaneous speech. In addition, the remaining thoughts tend towards gloomy themes. In both accelerated and decelerated thought there may be an increased tendency for the determining tendency of thought to be lost (referred to as increased distractibility).

Schizophrenic thought disorder

Disturbances of the associations between the thoughts are closely associated with schizophrenia and may be referred to as *schizophrenic thought disorder*. Four disturbances are classically described: snapping-off (*entgleiten*), fusion (*verschmelzung*), muddling (*faseln*), and derailment (*entgleisen*).

- Snapping-off or thought blocking describes the subjective experience of the sudden and unintentional stop in a chain of thought. This may be unexplained by the patient or there may be delusional elaboration (e.g. explained as *thought withdrawal*).
- Derailment or *knight's move thinking* describes a total break in the chain of association between the meanings of thoughts.
- Fusion is when two or more related ideas from a group of associations come together to form one idea.
- Muddling is a mixture of elements of fusion and derailment. *Drivelling* refers to the resulting speech.
- In mild forms the determining tendency in the thoughts can be followed (increased follow-up of side associations is referred to as circumstantiality).

Box 2.2 Assessing symptoms of thought disorder

Patients will rarely directly complain of the symptoms of thought disorder. In assessing the first-rank symptoms of schizophrenia the doctor will have enquired about delusions of the control of thought and about the passivity delusions. Both these symptom areas require the patient to introspect their thought processes; however, they will more rarely be aware of disorders which affect the form as opposed to the content of their thoughts. They can be asked directly about the symptoms of acceleration and deceleration of thought and these symptoms may be directly observable in acceleration or deceleration of speech. Observation and recording of examples of abnormal speech is the method by which formal thought disorder is assessed. Record examples of the patient's speech as verbatim quotes, particularly sentences where the meaning or the connection between ideas is not clear to you during the interview. Following recovery, patients can sometimes explain the underlying meaning behind examples of schizophrenic speech.

Abnormal cognitive function

All mental disorders affect cognition as expressed in affect, beliefs, and perceptions. The organic mental illnesses directly affect the higher cognitive functions of conscious level, clarity of thought, memory, and intelligence.

Level of consciousness This can range from full alertness through to clouding of consciousness, sopor, and coma (**pathological unconsciousness**); or from full alertness through to drowsiness, shallow sleep, and deep sleep (**physiological unconsciousness**).

Confusion Milder forms of brain insult are characterized by a combination of disorientation, misinterpretation of sensory input, impairment in memory, and loss of the normal clarity of thought—together referred to as confusion. It is the main clinical feature of delirium (📖 p. 790) and is also present during intoxication with psychotropic substances and occasionally as part of the clinical picture of acute psychotic illnesses.

- **Disorientation** An unimpaired individual is aware of who he is and has a constantly updated record of where he is and when it is. With increasing impairment there is disorientation for time, then place, and lastly, with more severe confusion, disorientation for person.
- **Misinterpretation** With confusion there is impairment of the normal ability to perceive and attach meaning to sensory stimuli. In frank delirium there may be hallucinations, particularly visual, and secondary delusions, particularly of a persecutory nature.
- **Memory impairment** With confusion there is impairment in both the registration of new memories (anterograde amnesia) and recall of established memories (retrograde amnesia). Events occurring during the period of confusion may be unable to be recalled, or may be recalled in a distorted fashion, indicating a failure of registration.
- **Impaired clarity of thought** The layman's 'confusion'. A variable degree of impairment in the normal process of thought with disturbed linkages between meaning, subjective and objective slowing of thought, impaired comprehension, and bizarre content.

Memory Beyond the ephemeral contents of our minds, containing our current thoughts and current sensorium, our memory contains all records of our experience and personality.

- **Working memory** Synonymous with short-term memory, which is responsible for the immediate recall of small amounts of verbal (as in digit span) or visuospatial information. Used for such purposes as holding a telephone number while dialling it. Most people have between 5 and 9 'spaces' available, with an average of 7 (the 'magic number'). New information will enter at the expense of the old. It has been traditionally held that storage of information in long-term memory is dependent on short-term memory. This is now no longer thought to be true; rather these two memory components are thought to function independently of each other. For example, patients with even severe impairment of episodic memory (e.g. persons with Korsakoff's syndrome) can present with normal short-term memory.

Long-term memory System for storage of permanent memories with apparently unlimited capacity. There appear to be separate storage systems for different types of information: memory for events (**episodic memory**), learned skills (**procedural memory**), memory of concepts and ideas unrelated to personal experience (**semantic memory**), which can be differentially affected by disease process.

Intelligence A person's intelligence refers to their ability to reason, solve problems, apply previous knowledge to new situations, learn new skills, think in an abstract way, and formulate solutions to problems by internal planning. It is stable through adult life unless affected by a disease process. Intelligence is measured by the intelligence quotient (IQ), a unitary measure with a population mean of 100 and a normal distribution. There is a 'hump' on the left-hand side of the population curve for IQ representing those individuals with congenital or acquired lowered IQ. No pathological process produces heightened IQ.

Acute vs. chronic brain failure Despite its great complexity the brain tends to respond to insults, whatever their source, in a variety of stereotyped ways (e.g. delirium, seizure, coma, dementia). These present as clinically similar or identical whatever their underlying cause. Acute brain failure (delirium) and chronic brain failure (dementia) are two characteristic and stereotyped responses of the brain to injury. In common with other organ failure syndromes there is an 'acute on chronic' effect, where patients with established chronic impairment are susceptible to developing acute impairment following an insult which would not cause impairment in a normal brain (e.g. the development of florid delirium in a woman with mild dementia who develops a urinary tract infection [UTI]).

Assessing cognitive function 1

Assessing level of consciousness The Glasgow Coma Scale (GCS) is a rapid, clinical measure of the conscious level (see Box 2.3). In delirium both the conscious level and the level of confusion may vary rapidly on an hour-by-hour basis and may present as apparently 'normal' on occasions. Patients with symptoms suggestive of delirium should therefore be re-examined regularly.

Assessing confusion Assess orientation by direct questioning. Some degree of uncertainty as to date and time can be expected in the hospitalized individual who is away from their normal routine. Directly enquire about episodes of perceptual disturbance and their nature. Document examples of confused speech and comment on the accompanying affect.

Assessing memory Working memory can be assessed by giving the patient a fictitious address containing six components, asking them to repeat it back or by testing digit span, spelling of WORLD backwards, etc. Clinicians traditionally used the term 'short-term memory' to reflect material held over a short period (e.g. 5–30 min) or some time to refer to retention over the ensuing days or week. There is no evidence, however, from a neuropsychological perspective of a memory system with these characteristics, and one is better occupied in thinking of memory as defined here, and thereafter considering anterograde and reterograde aspects of same.

Level of intelligence In most cases formal IQ testing will not be used and the IQ is assessed clinically. Clinical assessment of IQ is by consideration of the highest level of educational achievement reached and by assessment of the patient's comprehension, vocabulary, and level of understanding in the course of the clinical interview. To some extent this technique relies upon experience giving the doctor a suitable cohort of previous patients for comparison, and allowance should be made for apparent impairment that may be secondary to other abnormalities of the mental state. In any case, if there is significant doubt about the presence of mental impairment more formal neuropsychological testing should be undertaken.

Box 2.3 Glasgow Coma Scale (GCS)

The GCS is scored between 3 and 15, 3 being the worst (you cannot score 0), and 15 the best. It is composed of three parameters:

[E] Best eye response (maximum score = 4)
1. No eye opening
2. Eye opening to pain
3. Eye opening to verbal command
4. Eyes open spontaneously

[V] Best verbal response (maximum score = 5)
1. No verbal response
2. Incomprehensible sounds
3. Inappropriate words
4. Confused but converses
5. Orientated and converses

[M] Best motor response (maximum score = 6)
1. No motor response
2. Extension to pain
3. Flexion to pain
4. Withdrawal from pain
5. Localizing pain
6. Obeys commands

Notes:
- The phrase 'GCS of 11' is essentially meaningless; the figure should be broken down into its components (e.g. E3 V3 M5 = GCS 11).
- A GCS of 13 or more correlates with a mild brain injury; 9–12 is a moderate injury; and 8 or less, a severe brain injury.

Reproduced from Teasdale G, Jennett B (1974) Assessment of coma and impaired consciousness. A practical scale. *Lancet* **304**(7872): 81–4, with kind permission from Elsevier.

Assessing cognitive function 2

A wide range of standardized instruments is available for use in screening for cognitive impairment and for measuring severity and progression in established cases of dementia. There is currently no clear consensus on the best screening instrument, but in general, shorter screening tests are favoured in primary care or general medical settings.

Bedside screening instruments

Six-item Cognitive Impairment Test (6CIT) (Katzman 1983) A 6-question, abbreviated form of the older Blessed Information Memory Concentration Scale (BIMC) (1968) which examines orientation, memory and concentration. Its usage is increasing following its use as one component in a standardized assessment (Easycare©) recognized by The Royal College of General Practitioners. A computerized version is also available (Kingshill Version 2000). It is inversely scored and weighted so that a score of 8 or more out of 28 is suggestive of significant cognitive impairment (sensitivity 78–90%, specificity 100%).

Abbreviated Mental Test (AMT) (Hodkinson 1972) A 10-item questionnaire testing orientation, memory and concentration originally developed by geriatricians as an abbreviated form of the mental test score from the BIMC. Useful for rapid screening for cognitive impairment—indicated by a score of 7 or less out of 10 (sensitivity 70–80%, specificity 71–90%).

Mini Mental State Examination (MMSE)

In psychiatric settings there is almost universal use of the Mini Mental State Examination (Folstein 1975). It is included in many guidelines for dementia diagnosis and there is a large body of research providing reference ranges for a variety of clinical situations and premorbid levels of functioning. Copies of the questions and scoring system are usually readily available in wards and clinics (*Note*: as with many psychological tests the MMSE is subject to copyright). A low sensitivity makes it less suitable as a screening test in primary care, but it is often used as a relatively short test to monitor changes in cognitive function over time, particularly in response to treatment. It should be remembered that the MMSE is based almost entirely on verbal assessment of memory and attention. It is insensitive to frontal-executive dysfunction and visuospatial deficits. A score of 23–25 or less out of 30 is considered impaired; however, note low sensitivity, and clinical experience which finds not uncommonly cognitive impairment in individuals with scores of 30/30 (sensitivity 30–60%, specificity 92–100%).

Addenbrooke's Cognitive Examination—Revised (ACE—R) (2005)

When time permits, or clinical presentation is more complex, the ACE-R provides a more detailed, 100-item, clinician-administered bedside test of cognitive function. It is a superset of the MMSE and will therefore also generate an MMSE score. Questions cover five areas of function: attention and orientation, memory, verbal fluency, language and visuospatial awareness. Detailed data is available to allow interpretation of scoring, and specific training on administration of the test is recommended.

The ACE-R version A (2005) gives a sensitivity of 94% and a specificity of 89% for dementia with a cut-off score of 88/100.

Collateral information

It is always useful to have third-party information when assessing cognitive function—usually from a spouse, partner, family member, or carer. Third-party information can be more formally assessed using standardized instruments, e.g. the Informant Questionnaire on Cognitive Decline (IQCODE).

Recommended further reading

Hodges JR (2007) *Cognitive assessment for clinicians*, 2nd edn. Oxford: Oxford University Press.

Supplementary tests of cerebral functioning

Where there is clinical suspicion of specific functional impairment, it is often useful to directly test the functioning of the different cerebral lobes. This provides more detailed supplementary information to the MMSE (which is essentially a screening test). More formal neuropsychological assessment may be required with additional, well-established psychological tests, although these will usually be administered by psychologists.

Frontal lobe functioning

Frontal assessment battery (FAB) A brief (10-min) test of executive function, which essentially regroups tests often used when testing executive function at the bedside. These tests are associated with specific areas of the frontal lobes (i.e. conceptualization with dorsolateral areas; word generation with medial areas), and inhibitory control with orbital or medial areas. The maximum score is 18 and a cut-off score of 12 in patients with dementia has been shown to have a sensitivity of 79% for frontotemporal dementia vs. Alzheimer's disease. However, any performance below 17 may indicate frontal lobe impairment.

The Wisconsin card sorting task The patient has to determine the rule for card allocation and allocate cards accordingly. When the rule changes, a patient with frontal lobe dysfunction is likely to make more errors (tests response inhibition and set shifting).

Digit span Short-term verbal memory is tested with progressively longer number sequences, first forwards (normal maximum digit span 6 ± 1) and, subsequently, in reverse order (normal maximum 5 ± 1).

Trail-making test A 'join the dots' test of visuomotor tracing testing conceptualization and set shifting. Test A is a simple number sequence; Test B is of alternating numbers and letters (more sensitive for frontal lobe dysfunction).

Cognitive estimate testing The patient is asked a question that requires abstract reasoning and cannot be answered by general knowledge alone (e.g. 'how many camels are there in the UK?').

Testing of interpretation of proverbs can be helpful in uncovering concreteness of thought—e.g. 'People in glass house shouldn't throw stones'—asking the patient 'are you aware of this proverb?', 'can you tell me what this means/give me a life scenario in which this would apply?' It is important to note that persons with more orbito-medial frontal lobe damage may present with completely normal neurocognitive assessment, but clinically with histories that are consistent with frontotemporal dementia-behavioural variant.

Parietal lobe functioning

Tests for dominant lesions

Finger agnosia Patient cannot state which finger is being touched with their eyes closed.

Astereoagnosia Patient unable to recognize the feel of common objects (e.g. coin, pen) with their eyes closed.

Dysgraphaesthesia Inability to recognize letters or numbers written on the hand.
Note: Although of disputed clinical value, Gerstmann syndrome is classically described as: right-left disorientation, finger agnosia, dysgraphia, and dyscalculia; due to a lesion of the dominant (usually left) parietal lobe.

Tests for non-dominant lesions
Asomatognosia Patient does not recognize parts of their body (e.g. hand, fingers).
Constructional dyspraxia Inability to draw shapes or construct geometrical patterns.

Other problem areas
- Visual fields (as optic tracts run through the parietal lobe to reach the occipital lobe).
- Speech—alexia, receptive dysphasia (Wernicke's area); conduction aphasia (cannot repeat a phrase, but does understand the meaning).
- Reading/writing (angular gyrus lesions).

Insight

The question of whether the patient has insight into the nature of their symptoms tends only to arise in psychiatric illnesses. In general, a patient with physical illness knows that their symptoms represent abnormality and seeks their diagnosis and appropriate treatment. In contrast, a variety of psychiatric illnesses are associated with impairment of insight and the development of alternative explanations by the patient as to the cause of their symptoms, for example:

- An elderly man with early dementia who is unable to recall where he leaves objects and attributes this to someone stealing them. He angrily accuses his son of the 'crime'.
- An adolescent, with developing schizophrenia, who believes his auditory hallucinations and sense of being watched are caused by a neighbour who has planted cameras and loudspeakers in his flat. He repeatedly calls the police and asks them to intervene.
- A middle-aged woman with worsening depression who develops the delusion that she is bankrupt and is shortly to be evicted from her home in disgrace.

Impairment of insight is not specific to any one psychiatric condition and is not a generally a diagnostically important symptom. It tends to occur in psychotic and organic illnesses and the more severe forms of depressive illness. Neurotic illnesses and personality disorders are generally not associated with impairment of insight. Impairment of insight can give a crude measure of severity of psychotic symptoms. Regaining of insight into the pathological nature of psychotic beliefs can give a similarly crude measure of improvement with treatment.

Insight can be defined succinctly as 'the correct attitude to morbid change in oneself'. It is a deceptively simple concept that includes a number of beliefs about the nature of the symptoms, their causation, and the most appropriate way of dealing with them. Insight is sometimes reported as an all or nothing measure—as something an individual patient either does or does not have. In fact, insight is most usefully inquired about and reported as a series of health beliefs:

- Does the patient believe that their abnormal experiences are symptoms?
- Does the patient believe their symptoms are attributable to illness?
- Do they believe that the illness is psychiatric?
- Do they believe that psychiatric treatment might benefit them?
- Would they be willing to accept advice from a doctor regarding their treatment?

Beyond the simple question of whether the patient has impairment of insight or not it is vital to understand how the patient views their symptoms as this will tend to influence their compliance and future help-seeking behaviour. It is important to emphasize that disagreement with the doctor as to the correct course of action does *not* necessarily indicate lack of insight. A patient may very well not agree to be admitted to hospital or to take a particular medication despite having full insight into the nature of their symptoms. In these cases the doctor should be sure to clarify that the patient has all the necessary information to make a suitable decision before considering the possible need for compulsory treatment.

Physical examination

Examination of the patient's physical condition is an integral part of a comprehensive psychiatric assessment. There are five main reasons why this is so:

- Physical symptoms may be a direct result of psychiatric illness (e.g. alcohol dependency—see 📖 p. 574; eating disorders—see 📖 p. 402; physical neglect in severe depression, schizophrenia, etc.).
- Psychiatric drugs may have physical side-effects (e.g. extra-pyramidal side-effects [EPSEs] and antipsychotics, hypothyroidism and lithium, withdrawal syndromes).
- Physical illnesses can cause or exacerbate mental symptoms.
- Occult physical illness may be present.
- In the case of later development of illness (or more rarely, medico-legal issues) it is helpful to have baseline physical findings documented.

Physical examination is all too often deferred and then not done, or not done as thoroughly as is indicated. It may well be acceptable to defer full examination on occasions (e.g. a distressed and paranoid man seen in A&E), but a minimal investigation can be done and completed as the situation allows.

A routine physical examination has the aim of documenting the patient's baseline physical state, noting the presence or absence of abnormal signs which could be associated with mental or physical illness, and highlighting areas requiring further examination or investigation.

General condition Note height and weight. Does the patient look well or unwell? Are they underweight or are there signs of recent weight loss? Note bruising or other injuries and estimate their age.

Cardiovascular Radial pulse—rate, rhythm, and character. Blood pressure. Carotid bruits? Heart sounds. Pedal oedema.

Respiratory Respiratory rate. Expansion. Percussion note. Breath sounds to auscultation.

Abdominal Swelling or ascites. Masses. Bowel sounds. Hernias.

Neurological Pupillary response and other cranial nerves. Wasting. Tone. Power. Sensation. Reflexes. Gait. Involuntary movements.

Some physical signs in psychiatric illness, and possible causes (Table 2.1)

General examination

Table 2.1 Some physical signs in psychiatric illness, and possible causes.

Parkinsonian facies	Antipsychotic drug treatment
	Psychomotor retardation (depression)
Abnormal pupil size	Opiate use
Argyll–Robertson pupil	Neurosyphilis
Enlarged parotids ('hamster face')	Bulimia nervosa (secondary to vomiting)
Hypersalivation	Clozapine treatment
Goitre	Thyroid disease
Multiple forearm scars	Borderline personality disorder
Multiple tattoos	Dissocial personality disorder
Needle tracks/phlebitis	IV drug use
Gynaecomastia	Antipsychotic drug treatment
	Alcoholic liver disease
Russell's sign (knuckle callus)	Bulimia nervosa (secondary to inducing vomiting)
Lanugo hair	Anorexia nervosa
Piloerection ('goose flesh')	Opiate withdrawal
Excessive thinness	Anorexia nervosa

Cardiovascular

Rapid/irregular pulse	Anxiety disorder
	Drug/alcohol withdrawal
	Hyperthyroidism
Slow pulse	Hypothyroidism

Abdominal

Enlarged liver	Alcoholic liver disease
	Hepatitis
Multiple surgical scars ('chequerboard' abdomen)	Somatization disorder
Multiple self-inflicted scars	Borderline personality disorder

Neurological

Resting tremor	Increased sympathetic drive (anxiety, drug/alcohol misuse)
	Antipsychotic drug treatment
Involuntary movements	Lithium treatment
	Antipsychotic drug treatment
	Tic disorder
Abnormal posturing	Huntingtons's/Sydenham's chorea
	Antipsychotic-induced dystonia
Festinant (shuffling) gait	Catatonia
Broad-based gait	Antipsychotic drug treatment
	Cerebellar disease (alcohol, lithium toxicity)

Clinical investigation

Clinical investigations, including blood testing, imaging techniques, and karyotyping, play a smaller role in psychiatry than in other medical specialties. They are mainly carried out to exclude medical conditions which may be part of the differential diagnosis (such as hypothyroidism as a cause of lethargy and low mood) or which may be comorbid. They should generally be carried out as a result of positive findings in the history or physical examination or in order to exclude serious and reversible occult disorders (such as syphilis as a cause of dementia).

Routine investigations may be carried out to assess general physical health, and to provide a baseline measure prior to commencing medication known to have possible adverse effects, for example full blood count (FBC), liver function tests (LFTs) and antipsychotic medication; urea and electrolytes (U&Es), creatinine clearance, thyroid function tests (TFTs) prior to lithium therapy. Specific screening and monitoring tests are detailed in specific sections. It is good practice to screen new patients with some standard tests, and the usual test battery will include: FBC (and differential), U&Es, LFTs, TFTs, glucose. Where there is suspicion of drug or alcohol misuse/dependency, mean cell volume (MCV), B12/folate, and toxicology screening may be added.

Other physical investigations are rarely requested (with perhaps the exception of ECG for patients on specific or high-dose antipsychotics) unless clinical examination indicates the possibility of an underlying (undiagnosed) physical disorder. Performance of a lumbar puncture, for example, is reserved for situations where there is clear evidence to suggest a neurological disorder presenting with psychiatric symptoms (e.g. suspected meningitis or encephalitis; multiple sclerosis) and, more often than not, in these circumstances a referral will be made for a medical review.

Use of other tools, such as EEG, CT, or MRI (and SPECT or PET where available) requires justification on the grounds of diagnostic need. EEG is frequently overused by psychiatrists, and may be difficult to interpret as psychotropic medications may 'muddy the waters'. EEG may be useful where epilepsy is suspected (on clinical grounds), to monitor some acute (toxic) confusional states, to assess atypical patterns of cognitive impairment, to aid diagnosis in certain dementias (e.g. HIV, variant Creutzfeldt–Jakob disease [vCJD]), to evaluate particular sleep disorders, or as the gold standard for seizure monitoring during ECT. EEG should not be used as a general screening tool.

Similarly, brain imaging adds little to the diagnosis of primary psychiatric disorders, and should only be used where there is good evidence for possible neurological problems (e.g. history of significant head injury, epilepsy, multiple sclerosis, previous neurosurgery) or where history and clinical examination indicate the possibility of a space-occupying lesion (e.g. localizing neurological signs, unexplained fluctuating level of consciousness, severe headache, marked and unexplained acute behavioural change). With the exception of organic disorders (e.g. the dementias—where diagnostic imaging techniques may add useful information to inform diagnosis, management, and prognosis), the sensitivity and specificity of imaging findings for most psychiatric conditions have yet to be established.

As a general rule comorbid or causative disorders will be suspected due to other symptoms and signs or by the atypical nature of the psychiatric picture, and the likelihood of revealing a totally unexpected diagnosis is small.

Common assessment instruments 1

The diagnosis of psychiatric disorders is largely clinical, although assessment tools are increasingly used for both clinical and research purposes. A huge variety of assessment tools is available for the diagnosis and assessment of severity of individual disorders, and for the monitoring of progress and treatment response in established cases.

Their primary use is as an aid in diagnosis and to provide an objective measurement of treatment response. They should not be considered as a primary means of diagnosis. A secondary use is in research, in order to ensure heterogeneous patient groupings and reliably standardized diagnosis.

Scales are often available in several versions, are either clinician- or patient-administered and vary in required skill and experience of the administrator. Some are available for free by searching on the Internet, while others are copyrighted and are available from purchase from the manufacturer. Examples of the more commonly found general and specific tests are given here.

General

General Health Questionnaire (GHQ) Self-rated questionnaire used as screening instrument for presence of psychiatric illness. Patient is asked to report the presence of a list of symptoms in the preceding weeks. Four versions are available using 12, 28, 30, and 60 items.

Diagnostic Interview Schedule (DIS) Can be used by non-clinicians to administer a fully structured interview to diagnose the major psychiatric illnesses for research purposes.

Global Assessment of Functioning Scale (GAF) 100-item, self-report rating scale measuring overall psychosocial functioning.

Minnesota Multiphasic Personality Inventory (MMPI) Self-report questionnaire consisting of 567 questions covering 8 areas of psychopathology, 2 additional areas of personality type, and 3 scales assessing truthfulness. Results are compared with normative data from non-clinical populations. Results generate information useful for a broad range of clinical applications.

Primary Care Evaluation of Mental Disorders (PRIME-MD) One-page patient-completed questionnaire focusing on psychiatric illness commonly encountered in primary care. Has a corresponding Clinician Evaluation Guide.

Quality of Life Interview (QOLI) Non-clinician-administered fully structured interview available in full and brief versions with 158 and 78 items respectively. Suitable for assessment of quality of life in those with enduring and severe mental illnesses.

Structured Clinical Interview for DSM-IV (SCID-I/SCID-II) Clinician-administered semi-structured clinical interview for use with patients in whom a psychiatric diagnosis is suspected. Primarily used in research with trained interviewers to inform the operationalized diagnosis of Axis I and II disorders.

Mood disorders

Beck Depression Inventory (BDI) Self-rated questionnaire containing 21 statements with four possible responses for each. Total score is quoted with >17 indicating moderate and >30 indicating severe depression.

Hospital Anxiety and Depression Scale (HADS) 14-item, self-rated questionnaire, producing an anxiety and a depression subscore.

Hamilton Rating Scale for Depression (HAM-D) Interviewer-rated, 17-item rating scale for depressive illness. Not a diagnostic instrument; used to measure changes (e.g. as a result of drug treatment), 17 items scored according to severity, producing total score.

Montgomery-Asberg Depression Rating Scale (MADRaS) 10-item observer-rated scale. Each item rated 0–6 with total score obtained.

Mood Disorders Questionnaire (MDQ) Self-rated screen for bipolar disorder. 13 yes/no questions, and two others. Positive screen is 'yes' 7/13, and 'yes' to question 2, moderate/serious to question 3.

Young Mania Rating Scale (YMRS) Assesses mania symptoms and weighted severity over the past 48 hr.

Anxiety spectrum

Hamilton Anxiety Rating scale (HAM-A) Clinician-administered rating scale for generalized anxiety disorder. 14 items rated on a 5-point scale.

Yale–Brown Obsessive–Compulsive Scale (Y–BOCS) Clinician-administered semi-structured interview allowing rating of severity in patients with a pre-existing diagnosis of OCD.

Schizophrenia

Brief Psychiatric Rating Scale (BPRS) Measures major psychotic and non-psychotic symptoms, primarily used for schizophrenia patients. Clinician rated based on observation.

Positive and Negative Symptom Scale (PANSS) Clinician-administered rating scale for assessment of severity and monitoring of change of symptoms in patients with a diagnosis of schizophrenia. Items covering positive symptoms, negative symptoms, and general psychopathology.

Scale for the Assessment of Positive/Negative Symptoms (SAPS/SANS) Administered together, and completed from history and clinician observation. It breaks down into three divisions: psychoticism, negative symptoms and disorganization.

Abnormal Involuntary Movement Scale (AIMS) Clinician-administered scale for assessing the severity of anti-psychotic side-effects. 12 items rated 0–4.

Common assessment instruments 2

Substance use

Cut down? Annoyed? Guilty? Eye opener? (CAGE) Brief screening test for alcohol problems consisting of 4 yes/no questions, a score of 2 or more indicating the need for further assessment.

Alcohol Use Disorders Identification Test (AUDIT) Completed by skilled clinician to reveal if there is a need for further evaluation. Questions cover quantity and frequency of alcohol use, drinking behaviours, adverse psychological symptoms, and alcohol-related problems.

Assessment instruments specific to children

ADHD (SNAP, Vanderbilt, Conners' Rating Scale) Used to assess presence and severity of ADHD symptoms in multiple settings. Completed by adults who know the child well (parents, teachers). Also have subscales to measure other symptoms, such as disruptive behaviour.

Anxiety Screen for Child Anxiety-Related Emotional Disorders (SCARED) A self-report instrument designed to measure anxiety symptoms in children.

Autism Spectrum Childhood Autism Rating Scale (CARS) Ages 2 and up, scored by clinicians based on observation. Gilliam Autism Rating Scale (GARS) Ages 3 to 22, scored by teachers and parents as well as clinicians. Autism Diagnostic Observation Schedule (ADOS) A semi-structured and lengthy diagnostic interview given by specially trained clinicians. It uses standardized data to aid in diagnosis of pervasive developmental disorders.

Children's Depression Inventory (CDI) Self-report of depression symptoms for ages 7 to 17 (first-grade reading level).

Structured interviews such as KSADS-PL are semi-structured diagnostic interviews covering the spectrum of psychiatric illness in children, administered by trained clinicians only.

Older adults

Geriatric Depression Scale (GDS) Self-reported screen for depression using a series of yes/no questions.

Instrumental Activities of Daily Living (IADL) Used to evaluate the day-to-day living skills in an older population. It can be used to evaluate treatment effectiveness or help identify placement needs of the individual.

Recommended further reading

Sajatovic M, Ramirez L, Ramirez LF (2003) *Rating scales in mental health*, 2nd edn. Hudson: Lexi Comp.

Symptoms of psychiatric illness

Symptoms of psychiatric illness

In general medicine, *symptom* refers to an abnormality reported by the patient, while *sign* refers to an abnormality detected by the doctor by observation or clinical examination. In psychiatry, the terms symptom and sign tend to be used synonymously because abnormalities of mental state can only be elicited by exploring, with the patient, their internal experiences.

Psychopathology is the study of abnormalities in mental state and is one of the core sciences in clinical psychiatry. *Descriptive psychopathology* is one method for describing the subjective experience and behaviour of patients and is the basis for our current clinical descriptions of mental disorder. It is atheoretical, and does not rest on any particular explanation for the cause of the abnormal mental state. In this it contrasts with *dynamic (Freudian) psychopathology* which attempts to describe and then to explain these states.

Descriptive psychopathology includes close observation of the patient's behaviour and empathic exploration of their subjective experience. The latter is called *phenomenology*. The following general terms are used as qualifiers for symptoms described in the following pages:

- **Subjective vs. objective** Objective signs are those noted by an external observer; subjective signs are those reported by the patient.
- **Form vs. content** A distinction is drawn between the *form* and *content* of *abnormal* internal experiences. For example, a patient may believe that he is continually under surveillance by agents of MI5 who are plotting to frame him for another's crimes. Here, the *content* of the symptom is the belief about the name and methods of the persecutor; the *form* is that of a persecutory delusion. *Content* is culture- and experience-related, whereas *form* is attributable to the type of underlying mental illness.
- **Primary vs. secondary** Primary symptoms are considered as arising directly from the pathology of the mental illness; secondary symptoms arise as an understandable response to some aspect of the disordered mental state (e.g. a patient with severe depression developing a *secondary delusion* of being wicked and deserving punishment). Secondary symptoms can be understood in the light of knowledge of the patient's symptoms; primary symptoms can be empathized with but not fully understood.
- **Endogenous vs. reactive** These terms have been largely made redundant by developments in understanding of mental disorders, but are still seen occasionally. It was formerly thought that some conditions arose in response to external events (e.g. depression arising after job loss) (*reactive*), while others arose spontaneously from within (*endogenous*).
- **Psychotic vs. neurotic** In present classifications these terms are used purely descriptively to describe two common types of symptoms that may occur in a variety of mental disorders. Previously, they were used to distinguish those disorders characterized by impairment of insight, abnormal beliefs, and abnormal perceptual experiences from those where there was preserved insight but abnormal affect.

- **Congruent vs. incongruent** This is an observation made regarding the apparent appropriateness of a patient's affect towards their symptoms or their symptoms to their mood. A patient with apparent cheerfulness despite persecutory beliefs is described as having *incongruent* affect; a patient with profoundly depressed mood developing a delusion that they were mortally ill is described as possessing a *mood-congruent* delusion.
- **Structural vs. functional** A distinction formerly made between those brain disorders with observable structural abnormalities on post-mortem (e.g. Alzheimer's disease) and those without (e.g. schizophrenia). This usage has diminished since the discovery of definite observable brain changes in those disorders formerly called *functional psychoses*. Nowadays, the term is more often used in neurology/neuropsychiatry to distinguish syndromes which generally have abnormal investigation findings (e.g. multiple sclerosis) from those without (e.g. conversion paralysis).

Dictionary of psychiatric symptoms

Abnormal beliefs A category of disturbance which includes **delusions** and **overvalued ideas**.

Abnormal perceptions A category of disturbance which includes **sensory distortions** and **false perceptions**.

Acute confusional state See **Delirium**.

Affect The emotional state prevailing in a patient at a particular moment and in response to a particular event or situation. Contrasted with **mood** which is the prevailing emotional state over a longer period of time.

Affect illusion See **Illusion**.

Agitated depression A combination of depressed **mood** and **psychomotor agitation**, contrasting with the more usual association of depressed mood with **psychomotor retardation**. A common presentation of depressive illness in the elderly.

Agitation See **Psychomotor agitation**

Agoraphobia A generalized **phobia** in which there is fear of open spaces, social situations, crowds, etc. Associated with **avoidance** of these stimuli.

Akathisia A subjective sense of uncomfortable desire to move, relieved by repeated movement of the affected part (usually the legs). A side-effect of treatment with neuroleptic drugs.

Alexithymia The inability to describe one's subjective emotional experiences verbally. May be a personality characteristic but is also associated with **somatization**.

Alogia Poverty of thoughts as observed by absence of spontaneous speech. A **negative symptom** of schizophrenia and a symptom of depressive illness.

Ambitendency A **motor symptom** of schizophrenia in which there is an alternating mixture of **automatic obedience** and **negativism**.

Amnesia Loss of the ability to recall memories for a period of time. May be **global** (complete memory loss for the time period), or **partial** (patchy memory loss with 'islands' of preserved memory).

Anergia The subjective feeling of lack of energy and sense of increased effort required to carry out tasks. Associated with depressive illness.

Anhedonia The feeling of absent or significantly diminished enjoyment of previously pleasurable activities. A core symptom of depressive illness, also a **negative symptom** of schizophrenia.

Anorexia Loss of appetite for food. Seen in depressive illness and many general medical conditions. Interestingly, patients with anorexia nervosa often do not have anorexia as so defined. They commonly describe themselves as very hungry—controlling their desire for food by supreme effort in order to control their weight.

Anterograde amnesia The period of **amnesia** between an event (e.g. head injury) and the resumption of continuous memory. The length of anterograde amnesia is correlated with the extent of brain injury.

Anxiety A normal and adaptive response to stress and danger which is pathological if prolonged, severe, or out of keeping with the real threat of the external situation. Anxiety has two components: psychic anxiety, which is an affect characterized by increased arousal, apprehension, sense of vulnerability, and **dysphoria**; and somatic anxiety, in which there are bodily sensations of palpitations, sweating, dyspnoea, pallor, and abdominal discomfort.

Aphonia Loss of the ability to vocalize. May occur with structural disease affecting the vocal cords directly, the 9th cranial nerve, or higher centres. May also occur in functional illness where the underlying vocal cord function is normal. This can be demonstrated by asking the patient to cough—a normal cough demonstrates the ability of the vocal cords to oppose normally.

Asyndesis Synonym for **loosening of associations**.

Ataxia Loss of coordination of voluntary movement. Seen in drug and alcohol intoxication and organic disorders, particularly cerebellar.

Athetosis Sinuous, writhing involuntary movements.

Aura Episode of disturbed sensation occurring before an epileptic event. Wide range of manifestations although usually stereotyped for each individual.

Autistic thinking An abnormal absorption with the self, distinguished by interpersonal communication difficulties, a short attention span, and inability to relate to others as people.

Autochthonous delusion A primary **delusion** which appears to arise fully formed in the patient's mind without explanation (e.g. a patient suddenly becomes aware that he has inherited a large estate in the Scottish Highlands and will thus have the funds to settle scores with all those who have ever wronged him).

Automatic obedience A **motor symptom** of schizophrenia in which the patient obeys the examiner's instructions unquestioningly. This cooperation may be 'excessive', with the patient going beyond what is asked (e.g. raising both arms and both legs when asked to raise an arm).

Automatism Behaviour which is apparently conscious in nature which occurs in the absence of full consciousness (e.g. during a temporal lobe seizure).

Autoscopy The experience of seeing a visual **hallucination** or **pseudo-hallucination** of oneself. Also known as 'phantom mirror image'. Uncommon symptom reported in schizophrenia and in temporal lobe epilepsy.

Autotopagnosia Condition where one cannot identify or describe their own body parts. Individuals can dress and move appropriately, but cannot talk about their bodies.

Avoidance The action of not exposing oneself to situations which generate anxiety, for example a patient with **agoraphobia** remaining at home or a patient with post-traumatic stress disorder (PTSD) following a road traffic accident (RTA) refusing to drive. Can be understood in terms of an operant conditioning model where actions with reward—in this case reduction of anxiety—are repeated.

Belle indifference A surprising lack of concern for, or denial of, apparently severe functional disability. It is part of classical descriptions of hysteria and continues to be associated with operational descriptions of conversion disorder. It is also seen in medical illnesses (e.g. cerebrovascular accident [CVA]) and is a rare and non-specific symptom of no diagnostic value.

Biological features of depression Symptoms of moderate to severe depressive illness which reflect disturbance of core vegetative function. They are **depressive sleep disturbance**, **anorexia**, **loss of libido**, anergia, and subjective impression of deterioration in memory and concentration.

Blunting of affect Loss of the normal degree of emotional sensitivity and sense of the appropriate emotional response to events. A **negative symptom** of schizophrenia.

Broca's dysphasia A type of **expressive dysphasia** due to damage to the posterior part of the inferior frontal gyrus of the dominant hemisphere (Broca's language area).

Bulimia Increased appetite and desire for food and/or excessive, impulsive eating of large quantities of usually high-calorie food. Core symptom of bulimia nervosa and may also be seen in mania and in some types of learning disability.

Capgras syndrome A type of **delusional misidentification** in which the patient believes that a person known to them has been replaced by a 'double' who is to all external appearances identical, but is not the 'real person'.

Catalepsy A rare **motor symptom** of schizophrenia. Describes a situation in which the patient's limbs can be passively moved to any posture which will then be held for a prolonged period of time. Also known as **waxy flexibility** or **flexibilitas cerea**. See also **Psychological pillow.**

Cataplexy Symptom of narcolepsy in which there is sudden loss of muscle tone leading to collapse. Usually occurs following emotional stress.

Catastrophic reaction Response occasionally seen in patients with **dementia** who are asked to perform tasks beyond their, now impaired, performance level. There is sudden agitation, anger, and occasionally violence.

Catatonia Increased resting muscle tone which is not present on active or passive movement (in contrast to the rigidity associated with Parkinson's disease and **extra-pyramidal side-effects**). A **motor symptom** of schizophrenia.

Chorea Sudden and involuntary movement of several muscle groups with the resultant action appearing like part of a voluntary movement.

Circumstantial thinking A disorder of the form of thought where irrelevant details and digressions overwhelm the direction of the thought process. This abnormality may be reflected in the resultant speech. It is seen in mania and in anankastic personality disorder.

Clang association An abnormality of speech where the connection between words is their sound rather than their meaning. May occur during manic **flight of ideas**.

Clouding of consciousness Conscious level between full consciousness and coma. Covers a range of increasingly severe loss of function with drowsiness and impairment of concentration and perception.

Command hallucination An auditory hallucination of a commanding voice, instructing the patient towards a particular action. Also known as **teleological hallucination**.

Completion illusion See **Illusion**.

Compulsion A behaviour or action which is recognized by the patient as unnecessary and purposeless but which he cannot resist performing repeatedly (e.g. hand washing). The drive to perform the action is recognized by the patient as his own (i.e. there is no sense of 'possession' or passivity) but it is associated with a subjective sense of need to perform the act, often in order to avoid the occurrence of an adverse event. The patient may resist carrying out the action for a time at the expense of mounting **anxiety**.

Concrete thinking The loss of the ability to understand abstract concepts and metaphorical ideas leading to a strictly literal form of speech and inability to comprehend allusive language. Seen in schizophrenia and in dementing illnesses.

Confabulation The process of describing plausibly false memories for a period for which the patient has **amnesia**. Occurs in Korsakoff psychosis, dementia, and following alcoholic **palimpsest**.

Confusion The core symptom of delirium or acute confusional state. There is **disorientation**, **clouding of consciousness** and deterioration in the ability to think rationally, lay down new memories, and to understand sensory input.

Conversion The development of features suggestive of physical illness but which are attributed to psychiatric illness or emotional disturbance rather than organic pathology. Originally described in terms of psychoanalytic theory where the presumed mechanism was the 'conversion' of unconscious distress to physical symptoms rather than allowing its expression in conscious thought.

Coprolalia A 'forced' vocalization of obscene words or phrases. The symptom is largely involuntary but can be resisted for a time, at the expense of mounting **anxiety**. Seen in Gilles de la Tourette's syndrome.

Cotard syndrome A presentation of psychotic depressive illness seen particularly in elderly people. There is a combination of severely depressed mood with **nihilistic delusions** and/or **hypochondriacal delusions**. The patient may state that he is already dead and should be buried, that his insides have stopped working and are rotting away, or that he has stopped existing altogether.

Couvade syndrome A **conversion** symptom seen in partners of expectant mothers during their pregnancy. The symptoms vary but mimic pregnancy symptoms and so include nausea, vomiting, abdominal pain, and food cravings. It is not delusional in nature; the affected individual does not believe they are pregnant (cf. **pseudocyesis**). This behaviour is a cultural norm in some societies.

Craving A subjective sense of need to consume a particular substance (e.g. drugs or alcohol) for which there may be **dependence.**

Cyclothymia A personality characteristic in which there is cyclical mood variation to a lesser degree than in bipolar disorder.

De Clérambault syndrome A form of **delusion of love**. The patient, usually female, believes that another, higher-status individual is in love with them. There may be an additional **persecutory delusional** component where the affected individual comes to believe that individuals are conspiring to keep them apart. The object may be an employer or doctor, or in some cases a prominent public figure or celebrity.

Déjà vu A sense that events being experienced for the first time have been experienced before. An everyday experience but also a non-specific symptom of a number of disorders including temporal lobe epilepsy, schizophrenia, and anxiety disorders.

Delirium A clinical syndrome of **confusion**, variable degree of **clouding of consciousness**, visual **illusions**, and/or visual **hallucinations, lability of affect**, and disorientation. The clinical features can vary markedly in severity hour by hour. Delirium is a stereotyped response by the brain to a variety of insults and is similar in presentation whatever the primary cause.

Delirium tremens The clinical picture of acute confusional state secondary to alcohol withdrawal. Comprises **confusion, withdrawals,** visual **hallucinations,** and, occasionally, **persecutory delusions** and **Lilliputian hallucinations.**

Delusion An abnormal belief which is held with absolute subjective certainty, which requires no external proof, which may be held in the face of contradictory evidence, and which has personal significance and importance to the individual concerned. Excluded are those beliefs which can be understood as part of the subject's cultural or religious background. While the content is usually demonstrably false and bizarre in nature, this is not invariably so.

Primary delusions are the direct result of psychopathology, while *secondary* delusions can be understood as having arisen in response to other primary psychiatric conditions (e.g. a patient with severely depressed mood developing delusions of poverty, or a patient with progressive memory impairment developing a delusion that people are entering his house and stealing or moving items). Primary delusions can be subdivided by the method by which they are perceived as having arisen or into broad classes based on their content.

If the patient is asked to recall the point when they became aware of the delusion and its significance to them, they may report that the belief arose: 'out of the blue' (**autochthonous delusion**); on seeing a normal percept (**delusional perception**); on recalling a memory (**delusional memory**); or on a background of anticipation, odd experiences, and increased awareness (**delusional mood**).

Based on their content, 12 types of primary delusion are commonly recognized: persecutory, grandiose, delusions of control, of thought interference, of reference, of guilt, of love, delusional misidentification, jealousy, hypochondriacal delusions, nihilistic delusions, and delusions of infestation.

Delusional atmosphere Synonym for delusional mood.

Delusional elaboration Secondary delusions which arise in a manner which is understandable as the patient attempting to find explanations for primary psychopathological processes (e.g. a patient with persistent auditory hallucinations developing a belief that a transmitter has been placed in his ear).

Delusional jealousy A delusional belief that one's partner is being unfaithful. This can occur as part of a wider psychotic illness, secondary to organic brain damage (e.g. following the 'punch drunk syndrome' in boxers), associated with alcohol dependence, or as a monosymptomatic delusional disorder ('**Othello syndrome**'). Whatever the primary cause, there is a strong association with violence, usually towards the supposedly unfaithful partner. For this type of delusion the content is not bizarre or inconceivable and the central belief may even be true.

Delusional memory A primary **delusion** which is recalled as arising as a result of a memory (e.g. a patient who remembers his parents taking him to hospital for an operation as a child becoming convinced that he had been implanted with control and monitoring devices which have become active in his adult life).

Delusional misidentification A delusional belief that certain individuals are not who they externally appear to be. The delusion may be that familiar people have been replaced with outwardly identical strangers (**Capgras syndrome**) or that strangers are 'really' familiar people (**Frégoli syndrome**). A rare symptom of schizophrenia or of other psychotic illnesses.

Delusional mood A primary **delusion** which is recalled as arising following a period when there is an abnormal mood state characterized by anticipatory anxiety, a sense of 'something about to happen', and an increased sense of the significance of minor events. The development of the formed delusion may come as a relief to the patient in this situation.

Delusional perception A primary **delusion** which is recalled as having arisen as a result of a perception (e.g. a patient who, on seeing two white cars pull up in front of his house became convinced that he was therefore about to be wrongly accused of being a paedophile). The percept is a real external object, not a hallucinatory experience.

Delusions of control A group of delusions which are also known as **passivity phenomena** or delusions of bodily passivity. They are considered **first-rank symptoms** of schizophrenia. The core feature is the delusional belief that one is no longer in sole control of one's own body. The individual delusions are that one is being forced by some external agent to feel emotions, to desire to do things, to perform actions, or to experience bodily sensations. Respectively these delusions are called: **passivity of affect, passivity of impulse, passivity of volition**, and **somatic passivity**.

Delusions of guilt A delusional belief that one has committed a crime or other reprehensible act. A feature of psychotic depressive illness (e.g. an elderly woman with severe depressive illness who becomes convinced that her child, who died by cot death many years before, was in fact murdered by her).

Delusions of infestation A delusional belief that one's skin is infested with multiple, tiny mite-like animals. As a monosymptomatic delusional disorder this is called **Ekbom syndrome**. It is also seen in acute confusional states (particularly secondary to drug or alcohol withdrawal), in schizophrenia, in dementing illnesses, and as **delusional elaboration** of tactile hallucinatory experiences.

Delusions of love A delusion where the patient believes another individual is in love with them and that they are destined to be together. A rare symptom of schizophrenia and other psychotic illnesses, one particular subtype of this delusion is **de Clérambault syndrome**.

Delusions of reference A delusional belief that external events or situations have been arranged in such a way as to have particular significance for, or to convey a message to, the affected individual. The patient may believe that television news items are referring to him or that parts of the Bible are about him directly.

Delusions of thought interference A group of delusions which are considered **first-rank symptoms** of schizophrenia. They are **thought insertion, thought withdrawal**, and **thought broadcasting**.

Dementia Chronic brain failure—in contrast with delirium (which is acute brain failure). In dementia, there is progressive and global loss of brain function. It is usually irreversible. Different dementing illnesses will show different patterns and rate of functional loss but, in general, there is impairment of memory, loss of higher cognitive function, perceptual abnormalities, **dyspraxia**, and disintegration of the personality.

Dependence The inability to control intake of a substance to which one is addicted. The dependence syndrome (□ p. 542) is characterized by primacy of drug-seeking behaviour, inability to control intake of the substance once consumption has started, use of the substance to avoid **withdrawals**, increased tolerance to the intoxicating effects of the substance, and re-instigation of the pattern of use after a period of abstinence. Dependence has two components: **psychological dependence**, which is the subjective feeling of loss of control, cravings, and preoccupation with obtaining the substance; and **physiological dependence**, which is the physical consequences of withdrawal and is specific to each drug. For some drugs (e.g.

alcohol) both psychological and physiological dependence occur; for others (e.g. LSD) there are no marked features of physiological dependence.

Depersonalization An unpleasant subjective experience where the patient feels as if they have become 'unreal'. A non-specific symptom occurring in many psychiatric disorders as well as in normal people.

Depressed mood The core feature of depressive illness. Milder forms of depressed mood are part of the human experience, but in its pathological form it is a subjective experience. Patients describe variously: an unremitting and pervasive unhappiness; a loss of the ability to experience the normal range of positive emotions ('feeling of a lack of feeling'); a sense of hopelessness and negative thoughts about themselves, their situation, and the future; somatic sensations of 'a weight' pressing down on head and body; and a sort of 'psychic pain' or wound.

Depressive sleep disturbance Characteristic pattern of sleep disturbance seen in depressive illness. It includes **initial insomnia** and **early morning waking**. In addition, sleep is described as more shallow, broken, and less refreshing. There is increased rapid eye movement (REM) latency, where the patient enters REM sleep more rapidly than normal and REM sleep is concentrated in the beginning rather than the end of the sleep period.

Derailment A symptom of **schizophrenic thought disorder** in which there is a total break in the chain of association between the meaning of thoughts. The connection between the two sequential ideas is apparent neither to the patient nor to the examiner.

Derealization An unpleasant subjective experience where the patient feels as if the world has become unreal. Like **depersonalization** it is a non-specific symptom of a number of disorders.

Diogenes syndrome Hoarding of objects, usually of no practical use, and the neglect of one's home or environment. May be a behavioural manifestation of an organic disorder, schizophrenia, depressive disorder, or obsessive–compulsive disorder; or reflect a reaction late in life to stress in a certain type of personality.

Disinhibition Loss of the normal sense of which behaviours are appropriate in the current social setting. Symptom of manic illnesses and occurs in the later stages of dementing illnesses and during intoxication with drugs or alcohol.

Disorientation Loss of the ability to recall and accurately update information as to current time, place, and personal identity. Occurs in delirium and dementia. With increasing severity of illness, orientation for time is lost first, then orientation for place, with orientation for person usually preserved until dysfunction becomes very severe.

Dissociation The separation of unpleasant emotions and memories from consciousness awareness with subsequent disruption to the normal integrated function of consciousness and memory. **Conversion** and **dissociation** are related concepts. In conversion the emotional abnormality produces physical symptoms; while in dissociation there is impairment of mental functioning (e.g. in **dissociative fugue** and **dissociative amnesia**).

Distractibility Inability to maintain attention or the loss of vigilance on minimal distracting stimulation.

Diurnal variation A variation in the severity of a symptom depending on the time of day (e.g. depressed mood experienced as most severe in the morning and improving later in the day).

Double depression A combination of **dysthymia** and depressive illness.

Dysarthria Impairment in the ability to properly articulate speech. Caused by lesions in brainstem, cranial nerves, or pharynx. Distinguished from **dysphasia** in that there is no impairment of comprehension, writing, or higher language function.

Dyskinesia The impairment of voluntary motor activity by superimposed involuntary motor activity.

Dyslexia Inability to read at the level normal for one's age or intelligence level.

Dysmorphophobia A type of **over-valued idea** where the patient believes one aspect of his body is abnormal or conspicuously deformed.

Dysphasia Impairment in producing or understanding speech (**expressive dysphasia** and **receptive dysphasia** respectively) related to cortical abnormality, in contrast with **dysarthria** where the abnormality is in the organs of speech production.

Dysphoria An emotional state experienced as unpleasant. Secondary to a number of symptoms (e.g. **depressed mood, withdrawals**).

Dyspraxia Inability to carry out complex motor tasks (e.g. dressing, eating) although the component motor movements are preserved.

Dysthymia Chronic, mildly depressed mood and diminished enjoyment, not severe enough to be considered depressive illness.

Early morning waking (EMW) Feature of **depressive sleep disturbance**. The patient wakes in the very early morning and is unable to return to sleep.

Echo de la pensée Synonym for **thought echo**.

Echolalia The repetition of phrases or sentences spoken by the examiner. Occurs in schizophrenia and mental retardation.

Echopraxia Motor symptom of schizophrenia in which the patient mirrors the doctor's body movements. This continues after being told to stop.

Eidetic imagery Particular type of exceptionally vivid visual memory. Not a hallucination. More common in children than adults, cf. **flashbacks**.

Ekbom syndrome A monosymptomatic delusional disorder where the core delusion is a **delusion of infestation**.

Elation Severe and prolonged **elevation of mood**. A feature of manic illnesses.

Elemental hallucination A type of hallucination where the false perceptions are of very simple form (e.g. flashes of light or clicks and bangs). Associated with organic illness.

Elevation of mood The core feature of manic illnesses. The mood is preternaturally cheerful, the patient may describe feeling 'high', and there is subjectively increased speed and ease of thinking.

Entgleisen Synonym for **derailment**.

Entgleiten Synonym for **thought blocking** or **snapping off**.

Erotomania Synonym for **delusions of love**.

Euphoria Sustained and unwarranted cheerfulness. Associated with manic states and organic impairment.

Euthymia A 'normal' mood state, neither depressed nor manic.

Expressive dysphasia Dysphasia affecting the production of speech. There is impairment of word-finding, sentence construction, and articulation.
   Speech is slow and 'telegraphic', with substitutions, null words, and **perseveration**. The patient characteristically exhibits considerable frustration at his deficits. Writing is similarly affected. Basic comprehension is largely intact and emotional utterances and rote learned material may also be surprisingly preserved.

Extracampine hallucination A hallucination where the percept appears to come from beyond the area usually covered by the senses (e.g. a patient in Edinburgh 'hearing' voices seeming to come from a house in Glasgow).

Extra-pyramidal side-effects (EPSEs) Side-effects of rigidity, tremor, and dyskinesia caused by the anti-dopaminergic effects of psychotropic drugs, particularly neuroleptics. Unlike in idiopathic Parkinson's disease, bradykinesia is not prominent.

Ey syndrome Synonym for **Othello syndrome**.

False perceptions *Internal* perceptions which do not have a corresponding object in the external or 'real' world. Includes **hallucinations** and **pseudo-hallucinations**.

Faseln Synonym for **muddling**.

First-rank symptoms (of schizophrenia) A group of symptoms originally described by Schneider which are useful in the diagnosis of schizophrenia. They are neither pathognomic for, nor specific to, schizophrenia and are also seen in organic and affective psychoses. There are 11 symptoms in 4 categories:

Auditory hallucinations
- 'Voices heard arguing'.
- Thought echo.
- 'Running commentary'.

Delusions of thought interference
- Thought insertion.
- Thought withdrawal.
- Thought broadcasting.

Delusions of control
- Passivity of affect.
- Passivity of impulse.
- Passivity of volitions.
- Somatic passivity.

Delusional perception
- A primary delusion of any content that is reported by the patient as having arisen following the experience of a normal perception.

Flashbacks Exceptionally vivid and affect-laden re-experiencing of remembered experiences. Flashbacks of the initial traumatic event occur in PTSD and flashbacks to abnormal perceptual experiences initially experienced during lysergic acid diethylamide (LSD) intoxication can occur many years after the event.

Flattening of affect Diminution of the normal range of emotional experience. A **negative symptom** of schizophrenia.

Flexibilitas cerea Synonym for **catalepsy**.

Flight of ideas Subjective experience of one's thoughts being more rapid than normal, with each thought having a greater range of consequent thoughts than normal. Meaningful connections between thoughts are maintained.

Folie à deux Describes a situation where two people with a close relationship share a delusional belief. This arises as a result of a psychotic illness in one individual with development of a delusional belief, which comes to be shared by the second. The delusion resolves in the second person on separation, the first should be assessed and treated in the usual way.

Formal thought disorder A term which is confusingly used for three different groups of psychiatric symptoms:
- To refer to all pathological disturbances in the form of thought.
- As a synonym for **schizophrenic thought disorder**.
- To mean the group of first-rank symptoms which are delusions regarding thought interference (i.e. **thought insertion, thought withdrawal**, and **thought broadcasting**).

The first of these uses is to be preferred.

Formication A form of tactile **hallucination** in which there is the sensation of numerous insects crawling over the surface of the body. Occurs in alcohol or drug withdrawal, particularly from cocaine.

Free-floating anxiety **Anxiety** occurring without any identifiable external stimulus or threat (cf. **Phobia**).

Frégoli syndrome A type of **delusional misidentification** in which the patient believes that strangers have been replaced with familiar people.

Fugue A **dissociative** reaction to unbearable stress. Following a severe external stressor (e.g. marital break-up) the affected individual develops global **amnesia** and may wander to a distant location. Consciousness is unimpaired. Following resolution there is amnesia for the events which occurred during the fugue.

Functional hallucination A hallucination experienced only when experiencing a normal percept in that modality (e.g. hearing voices when the noise of an air conditioner is heard).

Fusion A symptom of **schizophrenic thought disorder** in which two or more unrelated concepts are brought together to form one compound idea.

Ganser symptom The production of 'approximate answers'. Here the patient gives repeated wrong answers to questions which are nonetheless 'in the right ballpark' (e.g. 'what is the capital of Scotland?'—'Paris'). Occasionally associated with organic brain illness it is much more commonly seen as a form of **malingering** in those attempting to feign mental illness (e.g. in prisoners awaiting trial).

Gedankenlautwerden Synonym for **thought echo**.

Globus hystericus The sensation of a 'lump in the throat' occurring without oesophageal structural abnormality or motility problems. A symptom of anxiety and somatization disorders.

Glossolalia 'Speaking in tongues'. Production of non-speech sounds as a substitute for speech. Seen in dissociative and neurotic disorders and accepted as a subcultural phenomenon in some religious groups.

Grandiose delusion A delusional belief that one has special powers, is unusually rich or powerful, or that one has an exceptional destiny (e.g. a man who requested admission to hospital because he had become convinced that God had granted him 'the greatest possible sort of mind' and that coming into contact with him would cure others of mental illnesses). Occurs in all psychotic illnesses but particularly in manic illnesses.

Grandiosity An exaggerated sense of one's own importance or abilities. Seen in manic illnesses.

Hallucination An internal percept without a corresponding external object. The subjective experience of hallucination is that of experiencing a normal percept in that modality of sensation. A true hallucination will be perceived as in external space, distinct from imagined images, outside conscious control, and as possessing relative permanence. A **pseudo-hallucination** will lack one or all of these characteristics.

Hallucinations are subdivided according to their modality of sensation and may be auditory, visual, gustatory, tactile, olfactory, or kinaesthetic. Auditory hallucinations, particularly of voices, are characteristic of schizophrenic illness, while visual hallucinations are characteristic of organic states.

Hemiballismus Involuntary, large-scale, 'throwing' movements of one limb or one body side.

Hypersomnia Excessive sleepiness with increased length of nocturnal sleep and daytime napping. Occurs as core feature of narcolepsy and in atypical depressive states.

Hypnagogic hallucination A transient false perception experienced while on the verge of falling asleep (e.g. hearing a voice calling one's name which then startles you back to wakefulness to find no-one there). The same phenomenon experienced while waking up is called **hypnopompic hallucination**. Frequently experienced by healthy people and so not a symptom of mental illness.

Hypnopompic hallucination See **Hypnagogic hallucination**.

Hypochondriacal delusion A delusional belief that one has a serious physical illness (e.g. cancer, AIDS). Most common in psychotic depressive illnesses.

Hypochondriasis The belief that one has a particular illness despite evidence to the contrary. Its form may be that of a primary **delusion**, an **over-valued idea, a rumination**, or a **mood-congruent** feature of depressive illness.

Hypomania Describes a mild degree of mania where there is elevated mood but no significant impairment of the patient's day-to-day functioning.

Illusion A type of false perception in which the perception of a real world object is combined with internal imagery to produce a false internal percept. Three types are recognized: **affect**, **completion**, and **pareidolic illusions**. In **affect illusion** there is a combination of heightened emotion and mis-perception (e.g. whilst walking across a lonely park at night, briefly seeing a tree moving in the wind as an attacker). **Completion illusions** rely on our brain's tendency to 'fill in' presumed missing parts of an object to produce a meaningful percept and are the basis for many types of optical illusion. Both these types of ilusions resolve on closer attention. **Pareidolic illusions** are meaningful percepts produced when experiencing a poorly defined stimulus (e.g. seeing faces in a fire or clouds).

Imperative hallucination A form of **command hallucination** in which the hallucinatory instruction is experienced as irresistible, a combination of **command hallucination** and **passivity of action**.

Impotence Loss of the ability to consummate sexual relationships. Refers to inability to achieve penile erection in men and lack of genital prepared-ness in women. It may have a primary medical cause, be related to psycho-logical factors, or can be a side-effect of many psychotropic medications.

Incongruity of affect Refers to the objective impression that the displayed affect is not consistent with the current thoughts or actions (e.g. laughing while discussing traumatic experiences). Occurs in schizophrenia.

Initial insomnia Difficulty getting off to sleep. Seen as a symptom of primary insomnia as well as in **depressive sleep disturbance**.

Insightlessness See **Lack of insight**.

Irritability Diminution in the stressor required to provoke anger or ver-bal or physical violence. Seen in manic illnesses, organic cognitive impair-ment, psychotic illnesses, and drug and alcohol intoxication. Can also be a feature of normal personality types and of personality disorder.

Jamais vu The sensation that events or situations are unfamiliar, although they have been experienced before. An everyday experience but also a non-specific symptom of a number of disorders including temporal lobe epilepsy, schizophrenia, and anxiety disorders.

Knight's move thinking Synonym for **derailment**.

Lability of mood Marked variability in the prevailing affect.

Lack of insight Loss of the ability to recognize that one's abnormal experiences are symptoms of psychiatric illness and that they require treatment.

Lilliputian hallucination A type of visual **hallucination** in which the subject sees miniature people or animals. Associated with organic states, particularly delirium tremens.

Logoclonia Symptom of Parkinson's disease where the patient gets 'stuck' on a particular word of a sentence and repeats it.

Logorrhoea Excess speech or 'verbal diarrhoea'. Symptom of **mania**.

Loosening of associations A symptom of **formal thought disorder** in which there is a lack of meaningful connection between sequential ideas.

Loss of libido Loss of the desire for sexual activity. Common in depressive illness and should be inquired about directly as it is usually not mentioned spontaneously. Should be distinguished from **impotence**.

Magical thinking A belief that certain actions and outcomes are connected although there is no rational basis for establishing a connection (e.g. 'if you step on a crack, your mother will break her back'). Magical thinking is common in normal children and is the basis for most superstitions. A similar type of thinking is seen in psychotic patients.

Malingering Deliberately falsifying the symptoms of illness for a secondary gain (e.g. for compensation, to avoid military service, or to obtain an opiate prescription).

Mania A form of mood disorder initially characterized by **elevated mood**, **insomnia**, loss of appetite, increased libido, and **grandiosity**. More severe forms develop **elation** and **grandiose delusions**.

Mannerism Abnormal and occasionally bizarre performance of a voluntary, goal-directed activity (e.g. a conspicuously dramatic manner of walking. Imagine John Cleese's 'the minister of funny walks').

Mental retardation Diminished intelligence below the second standard deviation (IQ <70). Increasing severity of retardation is associated with decreased ability to learn, to solve problems, and to understand abstract concepts. Subdivided as: mild: 50–69; moderate 35–49; severe 20–34; profound 0–19.

Micrographia Small 'spidery' handwriting seen in patients with Parkinson's disease; a consequence of being unable to control fine movements. This is most easily recognized by comparing their current signature with one from a number of years previously.

Middle insomnia Wakefulness and inability to return to sleep occurring in the middle part of the night.

Mirror sign Lack of recognition of one's own mirror reflection with the perception that the reflection is another individual who is mimicking your actions. Seen in **dementia.**

Mitgehen An extreme form of **mitmachen** where the patient's limbs can be moved to any position by very slight or fingertip pressure ('angle-poise lamp sign').

Mitmachen A **motor symptom** of schizophrenia where the patient's limbs can be moved without resistance to any position (cf. **mitgehen**). The limbs return to their resting state once the examiner lets go, in contrast with **catalepsy**, where the limbs remain in their set positions for prolonged periods.

Mood The subjective emotional state over a period of time, in contrast to **affect** which describes the emotional response to a particular situation or event.

Mood congruent A secondary symptom which is understandable in the light of an abnormal mood state (e.g. a severely depressed patient developing a **delusion** that they are in severe debt, or a manic patient developing a delusion that they are exceptionally wealthy).

Morbid jealousy Synonym for **delusional jealousy**.

Motor symptoms of schizophrenia. Schizophrenic illness is associated with a variety of soft neurological signs and motor abnormalities. In the modern era many motor abnormalities will be attributed to the side-effects of neuroleptic drugs, but all were described in schizophrenic patients prior to the introduction of these drugs in 1952.

Recognized motor symptoms in schizophrenia include: **catatonia, catalepsy, automatic obedience, negativism, ambitendency, mitgehen, mitmachen, mannerism, stereotypy, echopraxia,** and **psychological pillow.**

Muddling A feature of **schizophrenic thought disorder** caused by simultaneous **derailment** and **fusion**. The speech so produced may be very bizarre.

Multiple personality The finding of two or more distinct 'personalities' in one individual. These personalities may answer to different names, exhibit markedly different behaviours, and describe amnesia for periods when other personalities were active. This symptom is most probably an iatrogenic condition produced during exploratory psychotherapy in suggestible individuals.

Mutism Absence of speech without impairment of consciousness.

Negative symptoms (of schizophrenia) The symptoms of schizophrenia which reflect impairment of normal function. They are: lack of volition, lack of drive, apathy, **anhedonia, flattening of affect, blunting of affect**, and **alogia**. Believed to be related to cortical cell loss.

Negativism A **motor symptom** of schizophrenia where the patient resists carrying out the examiner's instructions and his attempts to move or direct the limbs.

Neologism A made-up word or normal word used in an idiosyncratic way. Neologisms are found in schizophrenic speech.

Nihilistic delusions A delusional belief that the patient has died or no longer exists or that the world has ended or is no longer real. Nothing matters any longer and continued effort is pointless. A feature of psychotic depressive illness.

Nystagmus Involuntary oscillating eye movements.

Obsession An idea, image, or impulse which is recognized by the patient as their own, but which is experienced as repetitive, intrusive, and distressing. The return of the obsession can be resisted for a time at the expense of mounting anxiety. In some situations the **anxiety** accompanying the obsessional thoughts can be relieved by associated **compulsions** (e.g. a patient with an obsession that his wife may have come to harm feeling compelled to phone her constantly during the day to check she is still alive).

Othello syndrome A monosymptomatic delusional disorder where the core delusion has the content of **delusional jealousy**.

Over-valued ideas A form of **abnormal belief**. These are ideas which are reasonable and understandable in themselves but which come to unreasonably dominate the patient's life.

Palimpsest Episode of discrete amnesia related to alcohol or drug intoxication. The individual has no recall for a period when, although intoxicated, he appeared to be functioning normally. This is also commonly known as 'blackout', but the term palimpsest is preferable as it avoids confusion with episodes of loss of consciousness.

Panic attack Paroxysmal, severe **anxiety**. May occur in response to a particular stimulus or occur without apparent stimulus.

Paranoid delusion Strictly speaking this describes self-referential delusions (i.e. **grandiose delusions** and **persecutory delusions**). It is however more commonly used as a synonym for **persecutory delusion**.

Paraphasia The substitution of a non-verbal sound in place of a word. Occurs in organic lesions affecting speech.

Passivity phenomena Synonym for **delusions of control**.

Persecutory delusion A delusional belief that one's life is being interfered with in a harmful way.

Perseveration Continuing with a verbal response or action which was initially appropriate after it ceases to be apposite (e.g. 'Do you know where you are?'—'in the hospital'; 'do you know what day it is?'—'in the hospital'. Associated with organic brain disease and is occasionally seen in schizophrenia).

Phantom mirror image Synonym for **autoscopy**.

Phobia A particular stimulus, event, or situation which arouses **anxiety** in an individual and is therefore associated with **avoidance**. The concept of 'biological preparedness' is that some fears (e.g. of snakes, fire, heights) had evolutionary advantage and so it is easier to develop phobias for these stimuli than other, more evolutionarily recent threats (e.g. of guns or electric shock).

Physiological dependence See **Dependence.**

Pica The eating of things which are not food or of food items in abnormal quantities.

Positive symptoms (of schizophrenia) The symptoms of schizophrenia which are qualitatively different from normal experience (i.e. **delusions**, **hallucinations**, **schizophrenic thought disorder**). Believed to be related to neuro-chemical abnormalities.

Posturing The maintenance of bizarre and uncomfortable limb and body positions. Associated with psychotic illnesses and may have **delusional** significance to the patient.

Pressure of speech The speech pattern consequent upon **pressure of thought.** The speech is rapid, difficult to interrupt, and, with increasing severity of illness, the connection between sequential ideas may become increasingly hard to follow. Occurs in manic illness.

Pressure of thought The subjective experience of one's thoughts occurring rapidly, each thought being associated with a wider range of consequent ideas than normal and with inability to remain on one idea for any length of time. Occurs in manic illness.

Priapism A sustained and painful penile erection, not associated with sexual arousal. A rare side-effect of antidepressant medication. If not relieved can cause permanent penile damage.

Pseudocyesis A false pregnancy. May be hysterical or delusional in nature and can occur in both sexes although more commonly in women. The belief in the false pregnancy may be accompanied by abdominal distension, lumbar lordosis, and amenorrhoea.

Pseudodementia A presentation of severe depression in the elderly where the combination of **psychomotor retardation**, apparent cognitive deficits, and functional decline causes diagnostic confusion with **dementia.**

Pseudo-hallucination A false **perception** which is perceived as occurring as part of one's internal experience, not as part of the external world. It may be described as having an 'as if' quality or as being seen with the mind's eye. Additionally, hallucinations experienced as true hallucinations during the active phase of a patient's illness may become perceived as pseudo-hallucinations as they recover. They can occur in all modalities of sensation and are described in psychotic, organic, and drug-induced conditions as well as occasionally in normal individuals. (The hallucinations of deceased spouses commonly described by widows and widowers may have the form of a pseudo-hallucination.)

Pseudologica fantastica The production of convincing false accounts, often with apparent sincere conviction. There may be a grandiose or over-exaggerated flavour to the accounts produced. A feature of Munchausen's disease.

Psychic anxiety See **anxiety**.

Psychogenic polydipsia Excessive fluid intake without organic cause.

Psychological dependence See **Dependence**.

Psychological pillow A **motor symptom** of schizophrenia. The patient holds their head several inches above the bed while lying and can maintain this uncomfortable position for prolonged periods of time.

Psychomotor agitation A combination of **psychic anxiety** and excess and purposeless motor activity. A symptom common to many mental illnesses and found in normal individuals in response to stress.

Psychomotor retardation Decreased spontaneous movement and slowness in instigating and completing voluntary movement. Usually associated with subjective sense of actions being more of an effort and with subjective retardation of thought. Occurs in moderate to severe depressive illness.

Punding A form of stereotyped motor behaviour in which there is apparent fascination with repetitive, mechanical tasks such as arranging items or dismantling and reassembling mechanical objects. It is seen as a side-effect of anti-Parkinsonian medication and in some individuals taking methamfetamine. It bears some similarity to behaviours seen in individuals with autism.

Receptive dysphasia **Dysphasia** affecting the understanding of speech. There is impairment in understanding spoken commands and repeating back speech. There are also significant abnormalities in spontaneous speech with word substitutions, defects in grammar, and syntax and **neologisms**. The abnormal speech so produced is however fluent (cf. **expressive dysphasia**) and the patient may be unconcerned by his deficits.

Reflex hallucination The experience of a real stimulus in one sensory modality triggering a hallucination in another.

Retrograde amnesia The period of **amnesia** between an event (e.g. head injury) and the last continuous memory before the event.

Rumination A **compulsion** to engage in repetitive and pointless consideration of phrases or ideas, usually of a pseudo-philosophical nature. May be resisted for a period with consequent mounting **anxiety**.

'Running commentary' A type of **third-person auditory hallucination** which is a **first-rank symptom** of schizophrenia. The patient hears one or more voices providing a narrative of their current actions, 'he's getting up…now he's going towards the window'.

Russell sign Skin abrasions, small lacerations, and calluses on the dorsum of the hand overlying the metacarpophalangeal and interphalangeal joints found in patients with symptoms of bulimia. Caused by repeated contact between the incisors and the skin of the hand which occurs during self-induced vomiting.

Schizophasia Synonym for **word salad**.

Schizophrenic speech disorder This includes the abnormalities in the form of speech consequent upon **schizophrenic thought disorder**, and those abnormalities in the use of language characteristic of schizophrenia such as use of **neologisms** and **stock words/phrases**.

Schizophrenic thought disorder A group of abnormalities in the subjective description of the form of thought which occurs in schizophrenia. The abnormalities include: **loosening of associations**, **derailment**, **thought blocking**, **fusion**, and **muddling**.

Sensory distortions Changes in the perceived intensity or quality of a real external stimulus. Associated with organic conditions and with drug ingestion or withdrawals. Examples include: hyperacusis (hearing sounds as abnormally loud), micropsia ('wrong end of the telescope effect', perceiving objects which are close as small and far away).

Snapping off Synonym for **thought blocking**.

Somatic anxiety See **Anxiety**.

Somatization The experience of bodily symptoms with no, or no sufficient, physical cause for them, with presumed psychological causation.

Splitting of perception Loss of the ability to simultaneously process complementary information in two modalities of sensation (e.g. sound and pictures on television). Rare symptom of schizophrenia.

Stereotypy A repetitive and bizarre movement which is not goal-directed (in contrast to **mannerism**). The action may have delusional significance to the patient. Seen in schizophrenia.

Stock phrases/stock words Feature of **schizophrenic speech disorder**. The use of particular words and phrases more frequently than in normal speech and with a wider variety of meanings than normal.

Stupor Absence of movement and **mutism** where there is no impairment of consciousness. Functional stupor occurs in a variety of psychiatric illnesses. Organic stupor is caused by lesions in the midbrain (the 'locked-in' syndrome).

Synaesthesia A stimulus in one sensory modality is perceived in a fashion characteristic of an experience in another sensory modality (e.g. 'tasting' sounds or 'hearing' colours). Occurs in hallucinogenic drug intoxication and in epileptic states.

Tangentiality Producing answers which are only very indirectly related to the question asked by the examiner.

Tardive dyskinesia A movement disorder associated with long-term treatment with neuroleptic drugs (although it was described in psychotic patients before the use of these drugs in clinical practice). There is continuous involuntary movement of the tongue and lower face. More severe cases involve the upper face and have choreoathetoid movements of the limbs.

Teleological hallucination Synonym for **command hallucination**.

Terminal insomnia Synonym for **early morning waking**.

Third-person auditory hallucinations Auditory hallucinations characteristic of schizophrenia where voices are heard referring to the patient as 'he' or 'she', rather than 'you'. The **first-rank symptoms** of **'voices heard arguing'** and **'running commentary'** are of this type.

Thought blocking A symptom of **schizophrenic thought disorder**. The patient experiences a sudden break in the chain of thought. It may be explained as due to **thought withdrawal**. In the absence of such **delusional elaboration** it is not a **first-rank symptom**.

Thought broadcasting The delusional belief that one's thoughts are accessible directly to others. A **first-rank symptom** of schizophrenia.

Thought disorder See **Formal thought disorder**.

Thought echo The experience of an auditory **hallucination** in which the content is the individual's current thoughts. A **first-rank symptom** of schizophrenia. Also known as **gedankenlautwerden** or **echo de la pensée**.

Thought insertion The delusional belief that thoughts are being placed in the patient's head from outside. A **first-rank symptom** of schizophrenia.

Tic Sudden twitches of a single muscle or muscle group.

Trichotillomania The **compulsion** to pull one's hair out.

Verbigeration Repetition of words or phrase while unable to articulate the 'next' word in the sentence. Seen in **expressive dysphasia**.

Verschmelzung Synonym for **fusion**.

'Voices heard arguing' A type of auditory **hallucination** which is a **first-rank symptom** of schizophrenia. The patient hears two or more voices debating with one another, sometimes about a matter over which the patient is agonizing (e.g. 'he should take the medication, it's worked before', 'no, not again, he'll not take it this time').

Vorbeigehen Synonym for **Ganser symptom**.

Vorbeireden Synonym for **Ganser symptom**.

Waxy flexibility Synonym for **catalepsy**.

Wernicke's dysphasia A type of **receptive dysphasia** due to cortical lesions in or near the posterior portion of the left first temporal convolution (superior temporal gyrus)—known as the Wernicke area.

Withdrawals The physical sequelae of abstinence from a drug to which one is **dependent**. These are individual to the drug concerned (e.g. sweating, tachycardia, and tremor for alcohol; dilated pupils, piloerection, abdominal pain, and diarrhoea for opiates).

Word salad The most severe degree of **schizophrenic thought disorder** in which no connection of any kind is understandable between sequential words and phrases the patient uses. Also called **schizophasia**.

Evidence-based psychiatry

Introduction

What is evidence-based medicine?

Evidence-based medicine (EBM) is the application of research evidence to medical treatment decisions. Evidence-based practice aims to integrate the best available research evidence with individual clinical experience.

- Best research evidence means the study most likely to yield an accurate and unbiased answer to a question we have about a particular patient or patient group.
- Clinical experience means the skills we have learned during our medical training (e.g. history-taking, bedside examination) and also our ability to elicit our patients' preferences and goals.

Key skills for evidence-based practice

- To be able to ask a clinical question in a way that captures the essence of the 'problem', is structured, and is most likely to yield an answer.
- To be able to search for an answer ('the evidence') to our question in a way that is most efficient.
- To be able to appraise the evidence critically.
- To apply the evidence to the patient.
- To monitor our own progress.

Asking clinical questions

There are generally two types of question we ask about patients: those that we ask them (fact-finding questions) and questions about diagnosis, cause (or harm), treatment, and prognosis (clinical questions). Consider the following patient scenario:

A 29-year-old woman is admitted 6wks post-partum complaining of hearing voices commenting on her actions, and thoughts that her baby is evil. She has never sought help for psychiatric reasons before, although her mother has long-standing bipolar disorder with many previous hospitalizations. She does not wish to be admitted to hospital.

Examples of fact-finding questions include:

- Does she have any wish to harm her baby?
- Is there anyone at home who could support her?
- Does she have any symptoms of affective disorder?
- Is there a history of drug misuse?

Examples of clinical questions include:

- Diagnosis: what is the likelihood that the diagnosis will be schizophrenia given she describes a first-rank symptom of schizophrenia (running commentary)?
- Cause/harm: does a family history of bipolar disorder increase the risk of post-partum psychosis in a relative?
- Treatment: is it likely that this woman would benefit from the administration of ECT?
- Prognosis: what are the chances that the woman will harm her baby?

The ability to tactfully ask fact-finding questions is something taught to us as medical undergraduates and postgraduates. There is no underlying structure to these questions and searching the literature will not provide an answer.

Structuring good clinical questions

Clinical questions, however, follow a standard format which is likely to clarify the question in your own mind, suggest a suitable study type to address the problem, and more likely to yield an answer when you search for one. The general form of a question is as follows (known by the acronym PICO) (See Table 4.1):

P: the patient problem to be addressed. A description of the main characteristics of the patient problem.

I: the intervention being considered (e.g. the treatment or diagnostic test being contemplated). May also be a harmful exposure (e.g. 10yrs of schizophrenia for prognosis, smoking).

C: the comparison intervention (e.g. treatments) is usually compared to placebo or standard therapy; diagnostic tests are usually compared to a gold standard such as post-mortem, although the gold standard test in psychiatry is usually a structured clinical history and examination (e.g. the Structured clinical interview for DSM-IV).

O: the outcome of interest (e.g. improvement in symptoms, accurate diagnosis, side-effects).

Table 4.1 Examples of questions in the PICO format

	P	I	C	O
Diagnosis	In post-partum mothers with psychosis	Do first-rank symptoms	Compared to full clinical examination and follow-up	Suggest a diagnosis of schizophrenia
Cause/harm	In post-partum mothers	Does a family history of bipolar disorder	Compared to no family history of mental illness	Raise the probability of post-partum psychosis
Treatment	In post-partum mothers with psychosis	Does ECT	Compared to antipsychotic drug treatment	Rapidly improve psychotic symptoms
Prognosis*	In post-partum mothers with psychosis	After 1year		What is the chance that the baby will be harmed

*Prognosis questions often have only three parts to their structure, unless two prognostic factors are being compared.

Finding and appraising the evidence

Hierarchy of evidence for therapy questions

After formulating a structured clinical question, the next step is to decide upon the study type best able to provide the answer. For a therapy question, the study types most likely to answer a question in a way that minimizes bias are ranked as follows:

- A systematic review of two or more randomized controlled trials (RCTs)
- A single randomized controlled trial
- A quasi-experimental study without randomization
- Observational studies (e.g. cohort and case control studies)
- Case reports and series
- Expert opinion

Wherever possible, a systematic review of RCTs should be sought because it is less liable to bias than the other studies further down the hierarchy. Many people, when asked 'where would you look for a study to answer your question?', will often suggest 'a textbook' or 'Medline'. However, textbooks are likely to be out of date (especially for therapy) and most doctors have not been trained to use Medline effectively.

Searching Medline (⌘ http://www.PubMed.org)

Medline can be searched by referring to the PICO structure, and by thinking about the hierarchy of evidence. For example, if we wish to ask our question 'in women with post-partum psychosis, does ECT lead to rapid improvement in symptoms when compared to antipsychotic drug treatment?', we might conduct the following search:
1: Post-partum psychosis
2: ECT
3: 1 AND 2
4: random$ (this line will identify most RCTs in any subject)
5: 3 AND 4

Medline is organized by subject headings, but we do not need to know the subject heading to search. Medline will automatically look up a thesaurus and use more effective terms than the ones we specify.

A note on PubMed clinical queries The PubMed website has a feature called 'clinical queries' which searches for articles of a specific design. For example, if you search for 'schizophrenia' AND 'cognitive behavioural therapy' in the clinical queries section of PubMed, you could specify that you are only interested in systematic reviews.

Limitations of Medline Unfortunately, Medline covers only a proportion (<30%) of the psychiatric literature. Embase and PsychINFO cover a greater proportion, but are often not available to health professionals because of their cost. However, many health boards in Scotland and England do have access to both Embase and PsychINFO through Athens (http://www.athens.ac.uk). You should contact your local library for details. Further training on Medline is available on the PubMed website.

Further EBM resources See 📖 pp. 1018–20.

Critical appraisal

Critical appraisal can help us decide if a paper is likely to be valid (i.e. the results are likely to be true) or important (i.e. contain results important for clinical practice). The questions we should ask ourselves in order to address these two areas depend on the study type.

Questions to assess the validity of a systematic review (📖 p. 112)

- Does the review address a clearly focused question?
- Does the review apply suitable quality criteria?
- Does the review search for all relevant articles?
- Are the results consistent from study to study?

Questions to assess the validity of a RCT (📖 p. 114)

- Were patients randomized to two or more treatments and was the allocation of patients to treatments concealed?
- Were patients and investigators blind to the intervention received?
- Were patients treated equally apart from the intervention of interest?
- Was follow-up sufficiently long and complete?
- Were drop-outs accounted for and included in the final results?

Questions to assess the validity of a harm/aetiology study (see Case-control studies 📖 p. 116)

- Was the exposure measured objectively?
- Was the outcome measured objectively and blind to exposure status?
- Was follow-up sufficiently long and complete?
- Did the investigators take into account any potential confounders?

Questions to assess the validity of a diagnostic study (📖 p. 120)

- Were the study patients similar to those on whom the test would be used in clinical practice?
- Were the test and gold standard applied blind to the results of the other?
- Was the test applied irrespective of the results of the gold standard (and vice versa)?

Questions to assess the validity of a prognosis study (see Cohort studies 📖 p. 118)

- Was a representative group of patients assembled at a common, preferably early, point in their illness?
- Were patients followed up prospectively for a sufficiently long period?
- Was the outcome assessed objectively?
- Did the investigators correct for the presence of confounding?

Systematic reviews (SRs) of RCTs[1]

Formulation of questions and protocol Questions should be precise. The research designs, characteristics of participants/interventions, and outcomes should be pre-specified. Research designs (e.g. RCT with inadequate concealment) likely to yield biased results should be excluded, or at least noted and the effects examined in detail.

Search for relevant articles The search should be comprehensive and repeatable. Should include more than Medline, as it is more likely to catalogue English language, positive studies whilst ignoring foreign language, negative studies. Consider grey literature (e.g. abstracts, personal communications, and others) and unpublished articles.

Review of abstracts and retrieval of full text Potentially relevant abstracts should be reviewed by 2+ reviewers with a mechanism for resolving disagreements. The same applies to retrieved articles. Proformas and pre-specified criteria are likely to improve reliability and repeatability.

Summary of included/excluded studies Reasons for exclusion and inclusion should be given to allow scrutiny/repeatability.

Meta-analysis (statistical summary) Study results should be combined statistically, weighted for precision.
- Heterogeneity: results vary from study to study more than expected by chance alone.
- Fixed effects analysis: assumes a single treatment effect, which is estimated by each study in an unbiased manner.
- Random effects analysis: doesn't assume single effect. Produces an average effect across all studies taking heterogeneity into account in the estimate of treatment effect and its confidence interval.
- Publication bias: the tendency for certain studies to be published according to their results. Usually, more positive results are more likely to be published. Measured using a funnel plot (see Fig. 4.1).
- Common statistical tests: χ^2 test for heterogeneity; Q test for heterogeneity; Z test for overall effect.
- Effect size measurements: *dichotomous data* (relative, absolute risks, odds ratios—odds ratios/relative risks preferred because of statistical properties). *Continuous data*: mean difference—for several studies using the same scales. *Standardized effect size* (mean difference/pooled standard deviation)—for several studies using different scales— rescales the results using standard deviation of each scale allowing them to be combined (e.g. 'Cohen's d' and others).

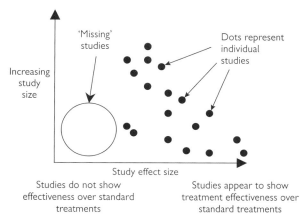

Fig. 4.1 A funnel plot showing how small negative studies appear to be 'missing'.

1 Egger M, Davey Smith G and Altman DG (eds) (2001) *Systematic reviews in healthcare: meta-analysis in context.* London: BMJ Books.

Randomized controlled trials (RCTs)[1]

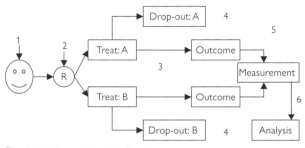

Fig. 4.2 RCTs appraisal criteria flowchart

Appraisal criteria (see Fig. 4.2)

1 **Selection of patients** Are the patients typical of those on whom the drug/therapy will be used in practice (generalizability/external validity)? Do they differ from the average patient in clinical practice such that we would expect (a) the results to not apply at all or (b) there to be a smaller/greater effect in clinical practice?

2 **Randomization** Was the randomization method adequate? Computer generated randomization by a third party on a geographically separated site at the point of entry into the trial is probably 'best'. Would it be possible for patients/clinicians to guess, better than chance, the treatment to which they would eventually be allocated (allocation concealment)? Has randomization succeeded in forming two groups with similar baseline characteristics? Methods of ensuring this are: *minimization* (allocate patients to minimize differences) and *stratification* (stratify randomization by important prognostic/treatment factor).

3 **Performance of interventions** Were patients/clinicians/investigators/ statisticians 'blind' to the treatment? *Note*: There is no universally accepted meaning of blind; authors should explain what they mean.

4 **Drop-out** Was the number of drop-outs in both arms of the trial unequal (differential attrition) or greater than 10–20%? If so, even if the analysis takes this into account, the trial may be biased either to/ against the true effect size.

5 **Measurement** Were all patients analysed in the groups to which they were randomized (intention to treat analysis)? If not, ignoring drop-outs (completer-only analysis) may overestimate effects of treatment.

Methods of intention to treat include:
• Last observation carried forward (assume no change in a score).
• Worst-case scenario (assume drop-outs in active arm have negative outcomes and drop-outs in control arm have positive ones).
• Mean imputation (assume drop-out was average for this group).
• Multiple imputations (model mean and variance taking into account characteristics of the drop-out).

6 Analysis (see Box 4.1) If results are presented as means, typically mean differences are shown, with a t-test or analysis of variance (ANOVA) and 95% confidence interval. If results are 'time to an event', then a Kaplan–Meier curve (survival curve) may be shown with the results of a survival analysis (log rank test, Cox proportional hazards). Often the results are shown as a proportion of people with a good or bad even in both groups (p1 and p2). The number needed to treat (NNT) is given by $1/(p1 - p2)$—see Box 4.1.

Box 4.1 Relative risk, absolute risk, and the number needed to treat

An important value to calculate from RCTs is the number needed to treat (NNT). The NNT arose because of limitations with the terms relative risk (RR) and absolute risk reduction (ARR).

Imagine you have an intervention for schizophrenia: Nopixol. You locate a trial in Medline, which finds the following results: 200 people with schizophrenia were randomized to placebo or Nopixol. 120 people received Nopixol, of which 30 relapsed at 6wks; 80 were randomized to placebo, of which 60 relapsed over the same time. A '2 × 2' table helps to clarify the numbers:

	Relapse	No relapse	
Nopixol	30	90	120
Placebo	60	20	80

- The risk or probability of relapse in the Nopixol group is 30/120 or 0.25. This is called the experimental event rate (**EER**).
- The risk or probability of relapse in the placebo group is 60/80 or 0.75. This is called the control event rate (**CER**).
- The relative risk (**RR**) is the EER/CER = 0.25/0.75, which is 0.33. This means the risk of relapse on Nopixol is 0.33 times the risk on placebo. Another way of saying this would be to say that the relative risk of relapse is reduced by 67% on Nopixol. This is sometimes called the relative risk reduction (**RRR**). This is usually not a good measure of clinical usefulness since if relapse was 100 times less common in both groups, the RR and RRR would stay the same. This would not reflect the fact that clinically the treatment effect had diminished considerably.
- The absolute risk reduction (**ARR**) is the CER − EER = 0.75 − 0.25, which is 0.5. This means that for every person treated with Nopixol, the risk of relapse is reduced by about 50%.
- If the risk for each person is reduced by 50% by Nopixol instead of placebo, then it is intuitive that we need to treat two people to prevent, on average, one relapse. This is called the number needed to treat (**NNT**). More generally, the NNT is equal to 1/ARR, or 1/0.5. In this case the **NNT = 2**.

1 Pocock SJ (1983) *Clinical trials: a practical approach*. Chichester: John Wiley and Sons Ltd.

Case–control studies

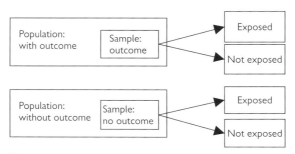

Fig. 4.3 Case–control studies appraisal flowchart

Appraisal criteria (see Fig. 4.3)
- **Exposure** Case–control studies are an alternative to cohort studies when the outcome is rare.
- **Cases** The sample cases (those with the outcome) should ideally be a random sample of all cases from the population. Investigators should say how the sample was selected. You should decide what effect this will have on the sorts of cases included in the study.
- **Controls** The sample controls (those without the outcome) should ideally be a random sample of all controls from the population and be as similar to the cases as possible (except for the exposure of interest). In practice this is difficult.
- **Selection of cases and controls** Ideally should also be independent of exposure. For example, the selection of depressed people from a psychiatric hospital and controls from a community newsletter to assess whether child sexual abuse is associated with depression may introduce bias because people with childhood sexual abuse are possibly more likely to be admitted to hospital in general.
- **Assessment of exposure** Measurement should be conducted objectively and blind to outcome status. In practice this is often difficult to accomplish as raters may be affected by their expectations and those with the outcome may be more likely to recall an exposure in a 'search for meaning' (recall bias).
- **Confounding** Where the controls and cases differ in important respects (apart from the exposure of interest), correction for this may be made in the statistical analysis. Correction should be made only when differences exist in a characteristic which is associated with the exposure and outcome (e.g. age may confound an association between intravenous drug use and depression).

- **Analysis** It is not possible to calculate absolute and relative risks from a case–control study directly since the proportion of people developing the outcome in exposed/non-exposed populations has not been assessed. Odds ratios are often used and may be given, along with a 95% confidence interval. A chi-square test will usually be used. If the investigators have examined to see if increasing levels of exposure are more strongly associated with the outcome, a chi-squared test (for linear trend) or Mantel–Haenszel test may be reported.

Cohort studies

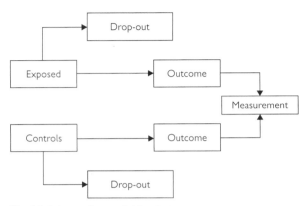

Fig. 4.4 Cohort studies appraisal flowchart

Appraisal criteria (see Fig. 4.4)
- **Exposure** The exposure should be clearly defined and may be stratified into levels of increasing dose. The controls should not be exposed but be similar to the exposed group. Bias will be introduced if controls differ in many ways apart from the exposure (e.g. drug users differ from non-drug users in many respects: employment, criminal record, etc.).
- **Drop-out** Drop-outs are virtually inevitable. The effects may bias the results, especially if drop-outs >20% or unequal. Some studies minimize attrition by consulting several sources, sending reminders, consulting government statistics (e.g. records of hospital admissions), and other methods of tracking people.
- **Measurement** Should be conducted objectively and blind to exposure status. In practice this is sometimes difficult.
- **Retrospective/prospective** Exposure may be ascertained from case notes (retrospectively) or at interview (prospectively). Cohort studies often have retrospective and prospective components.
- **Analysis** $P_{a,b}$—proportion in group a or b who have the outcome, then: $P_a - P_b$ = absolute risk, p_a/p_b = relative risk, NNH = 1/absolute risk. If results are 'time to an event', then a survival analysis may be conducted. Correction for confounding is usually accomplished using ANCOVA, linear regression (outcomes measured on a scale), or logistic regression (where the outcome is an event).

Comparing ways of measuring the importance of an intervention

There are many ways in which the benefit of an intervention can be measured. Cynically, one might expect the authors of an article to present the method which shows their intervention in the best light, so the reader will need to be aware of the main methods by which the utility of an intervention can be measured and their consequent strengths and limitations (see Table 4.2).

Table 4.2 Treatment benefit

Method	Explanation	Advantages	Disadvantages
P-value	Gives the probability that the observed difference between the treatments is due to chance.	Provides a clear test of an investigator's hypothesis and is provided with all major statistical packages.	Clinically insignificant treatments may still be statistically significant. Gives little indication of precision.
Relative risk	Gives the risk of an event in one group divided by the risk in the other group.	Provides a clear indication of how many times better or worse a treatment is compared to another.	May mislead when outcomes are rare, e.g. a relative risk of 10 would be unimpressive if the event occurred only once in 10 000 patients.
Absolute risk	Gives the risk of an event in one group minus the risk in the other group.	Provides a clearer indication of clinical significance. Takes appropriate account of baseline risk.	The figure in itself may not seem very meaningful either to clinicians or to patients.
Number needed to treat (NNT)	States the number of patients required to be treated with the experimental intervention in order to prevent one additional adverse outcome.	Relatively intuitive. Provides a clear indication of how much therapeutic effort is required to bring about one additional 'good' outcome.	In spite of obvious advantages, has not come into universal use. NNTs published in meta-analyses may be misleading unless the patients included in the primary studies are very like your own.

Note: Confidence intervals are a welcome addition to any published figure about treatment benefit because they convey information about precision and statistical significance.

Diagnostic studies

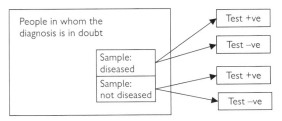

Fig. 4.5 Diagnostic studies appraisal flowchart

Appraisal criteria (see Fig. 4.5 and Table 4.3)
- **Sample** Did the sample consist of people in whom the diagnosis was in doubt and in whom the test would be used in practice?
- **Gold standard** Was a suitable gold standard applied regardless of the test results?
- **Test** Was the test applied blindly without knowledge of the results of the gold standard and vice versa?
- **Reliability** Could the diagnostic test be applied reliably over time or between raters?
- **Diagnostic test performance**
  - What are the sensitivity and specificity? They are portable properties, but less clinically useful than the positive and negative predictive values (PPV and NPV).
  - What are the PPV and NPV? These are useful when you have a test result and you want to know its meaning.
- **Other considerations** Is the test affordable, accurate, and feasible in our setting? What is our patients' post-test probability for a PPV?
  - Post-test odds = Likelihood ratio x Pre-test odds
  - The likelihood ratio (LR) is:

$$LR= \frac{\text{Probability of the test result in someone with the disease}}{\text{Probability of the test result in someone without the diseases}}$$

Table 4.3 Ways of measuring diagnostic utility

Method	Explanation	Advantages	Disadvantages
Sensitivity	Measures the proportion of people with a disorder correctly classified by a test. When sensitivity is very high, a negative test will tend to rule out the disorder (SnNOut).	Easily calculated and intuitive. Usually supplied in published papers. Does not depend on prevalence.	Not very useful in clinical practice unless very high.
Specificity	Measures the proportion of people *without* a disorder correctly classified by a test. When specificity is very high, a positive test will tend to *rule in* the disorder (SpPIn).	Easily calculated and intuitive. Usually supplied in published papers. Does not depend on prevalence.	Not very useful in clinical practice unless very high.
Positive predictive value	Measures the proportion of people with a positive test result who actually have the disorder.	Clinically useful. Easy to understand and communicate to colleagues and patients.	Tends to fall as the prevalence of the disorder falls. May mislead if the prevalence of the disorder in your practice is lower than that of the study.
Likelihood ratio for a positive test	A ratio of the probability of a positive test coming from someone with the disorder compared with one without the disorder.	Does not depend on the prevalence. Can be adapted to a variety of other situations.	More difficult to calculate than the above. May not seem intuitively very meaningful.

Calculating useful values

		Target disorder	
		Present	*Absent*
Diagnostic test result	*Positive*	a	b
	Negative	c	d

Sensitivity = a/(a + c)   Positive predictive value (PPV) = a/(a + b)
Specificity = d/(b + d)   Negative predictive value (NPV) = d/(c + d)
Likelihood ratio for a positive test = Sensitivity/(1 − Specificity)
Likelihood ratio for a negative test = (1 − Sensitivity)/Specificity
Note: Further details on how to calculate these values are provided in several texts[1] and on a number of websites.[2]

1 Lawrie SM, McIntosh AM and Rao S (2000) *Critical appraisal for psychiatry*. Edinburgh: Churchill Livingstone.
2 For example ᔥ http://www.cebm.net.tvt

Qualitative studies

Purpose

Qualitative studies are usually used to measure beliefs or attitudes in situations where quantitative research would be less meaningful or impractical. Results are usually presented as text without numbers or figures in a way that is intended to preserve the richness of the data in its rightful context. For example, 'What are the attitudes of patients with borderline personality disorder to their diagnosis?' might be answered better by describing what the patients actually said than by performing a survey and summarizing attitudes on a scale with medians and inter-quartile ranges.

Appraisal criteria

- **Clear question** Like all studies, the research should address a clear topic or question. Unlike quantitative research, hypotheses may emerge in the course of the study and be tested out.
- **Patient selection** Unlike quantitative research which should address a representative sample, qualitative researchers often 'purposively sample' patients in order to obtain 'typical' or exemplar cases.
- **Information gathering** The gathering and analysis of information is not standardized. Therefore, the study should describe exactly how this was performed.
- **Material engagement** Did investigators make intense contact with their subject material? Did they check reactions? Did investigators seek non-confirming data?
- **Iteration** Did investigators cyclically develop hypotheses and then test them with their sample?
- **Grounding** Were there systematic ways of linking observations with interpretations?
- **Disclosure of investigators' prejudice** Did investigators examine their own attitudes/beliefs/values/preconceptions as they embarked on the study?
- **Coherence** Are the results coherent? Was the interpretation internally consistent?
- **Testimonial validity** Did the study subjects agree with the investigator's interpretations?
- **Reflexive validity** Did the observations change the investigator's understanding of theory?
- **Catalytic validity** Did the investigator reorient, focus, and energize participants?
- **Triangulation** Was there an attempt to confirm the investigations using another method (e.g. by obtaining another sample or by observation of the same sample using a different method)?

Economic studies

Types of studies

- **Cost analysis** Costs only.
- **Effectiveness analysis** Consequences only.
- **Economic analyses** Costs and consequences of ≥2 interventions.

Types of analyses

- **Consequences equal** Cost minimization analysis (find cheapest intervention).
- **Consequences unequal** Outcomes measured in same natural units (e.g. rating scales or admission/readmissions) = cost effectiveness analysis.

If consequences unequal, and benefits measured in different units (e.g. comparing CBT for schizophrenia with ECT for depression) then convert consequences:
- to monetary units = cost–benefit analysis, or
- to patient preferences = cost–utility analysis

Costs and perspective

Costs should be considered from a broad perspective. Interventions which appear to be less expensive and equally effective at a hospital level may shift costs to other areas (e.g. social work, criminal justice system), which were not apparent because of too narrow a perspective.
- **Direct costs** Salaries, drugs, buildings, etc.
- **Indirect costs** Usually gains/losses in productivity.
- **Intangible costs**, e.g. cost of improved health.
- **Incremental cost** Cost of each additional unit of production.
- **Opportunity cost** Benefits forgone by using capital to provide one intervention over another (a concept of economic analysis rather than an actual cost).

Discounting

In order to take into account (1) the preference to pay for things later rather than sooner and (2) the devaluation in currency over time, future costs should be discounted so they appear at current prices. Occasionally economists argue that future *consequences* should also be discounted.

Consequences

The consequences of an intervention should be measured alongside the study used to measure costs (usually a clinical trial). The more rigorous the study design (SRs > RCTs > CTs) and the more valid, the more likely the results of the economic analysis are to be true.

Dominance

If one intervention is more effective and cheaper than an alternative, then choice is easy. In all other situations, consider the incremental cost-effectiveness ratio:

Incremental cost-effectiveness ratio (ICER)=

$$\frac{\text{Differences in costs}}{\text{Differences in consequences}}$$

For example, an intervention causing two extra remissions in schizophrenia at an extra cost of £100 000 has an ICER of £50 000 per additional remission. ICER gives a measure of the extra cost for each additional unit of benefit. There's no cut-off; the ICER should help compare different interventions and come to a decision. Non-parametric statistics are used to give p-values and 95% confidence intervals for the ICER (randomization tests, Monte Carlo analyses).

Sensitivity analysis

Economic analyses make assumptions about costs and consequences of different treatments. To test the robustness of an economic analysis, estimated benefits and costs can be varied one at a time or simultaneously to see if they alter the results of the analysis:

- **One-way** (one variable at a time).
- **Extreme case** (alter a variable to the extremes of its plausible range).
- **Multi-way** (vary two or more variables simultaneously).
- **Monte Carlo analyses** are a way of varying several parameters simultaneously without assuming normality.

Applying the evidence to patients

Having found valid and important new evidence about a particular problem, a couple of further questions need to be asked:

- What is the likely benefit for my patient?
- Does my patient actually want it?

Diagnosis

Diagnostic tests shown to be effective in a research setting may be of little utility in your clinical practice for two main reasons. First, the prevalence of the condition may be different in your setting. If the prevalence of the condition is lower in your setting, the PPV will be lower, although a negative result will actually be more likely to indicate an absence of the condition. Secondly, the test itself may be too costly in terms of the financial, staff, and training resources required.

Patients' values and expectations may also be very important in the context of a disease for which there is no effective intervention (e.g. Huntington's disease) or where the test is itself harmful or unpleasant.

Treatment

Chronic intractable conditions and mild and very benign conditions may fail to show the benefits of therapy demonstrated in clinical trials because the patient's baseline risk differs from those patients initially randomized.

In either situation, it is possible simply to 'guess' what the likely benefit for your patient will be, or one of several numerical methods may be used instead. The simplest numerical method involves an educated guess as to how likely your patient is to benefit compared to the average patient in the trial. If your patient is half as likely to benefit, then the NNT from the trial is doubled. Other techniques are available that are both more accurate and more time-consuming.[1]

Finally, the decision to start a new treatment depends on other things apart from efficacy. First, and most importantly, your patient may actually not want it because of undue side-effects or perhaps the regime (e.g. thrice-daily dosing) may be excessively inconvenient for them.

As well as potential harms, the decision to adopt a treatment or service at a health service level may also take account of economic evaluations.

Note: **Guard against drug company information**! Although drug representatives will extol the virtues of their medication over the competition, often on the basis of efficacy, little evidence exists to suggest, for example, that one antipsychotic is more effective than another.[2] Although doctors do not feel pharmaceutical representatives influence them, evidence from marketing research suggests otherwise.

---

1 Lawrie SM, McIntosh AM, Rao S (2000) *Critical appraisal for psychiatry*. Edinburgh: Churchill Livingstone.
2 Lieberman JA, Stroup TS, McEroy JP, *et al.* (2005) Effectiveness of antipsychotic drugs in patients with chronic schizophrenia. *N Engl J Med* **353**: 1209–23.

Measuring performance and implementing evidence-based practice

In the last few years there has been a proliferation in evidence-based guidelines[1] and attempts to audit our performance against those guidelines.[2]

Guidelines

Guidelines can be thought of as a top-down approach to evidence-based practice. They are particularly useful where there is clear evidence that an intervention is effective in a given condition, but for some reason isn't being given. They can also be useful when there are wide national variations in practice, as is often the case in mental health (e.g. ECT, clozapine).

The process of guideline development is a bit like EBM in miniature. Relevant representatives from all groups (patients, doctors, nurses, pharmacists, etc.) ask key questions which will form the basis for a systematic review. A systematic review is then conducted and the articles are appraised by the guideline group. Articles are graded according to their rigour and members use their clinical judgement in assessing how directly relevant they are to clinical practice in the UK. The group makes recommendations on the evidence, which are then put into a guideline. The adherence to the guideline is then assessed, usually by audit.

Unfortunately, although many good guidelines have been developed, many have not been implemented. This may be because the methodology of guideline development was faulty or, more likely, because the implementation was inadequate.

Strategies for guideline implementation include:[3]
- Educational outreach
- Advertisement
- Local opinion leaders
- Written and computerized reminders
- Reminders at the point of patient care

Audit

Audit is an attempt to measure actual clinical practice against a number of standards of good clinical care. Standards are sometimes drawn from guidelines, where the strength of evidence is overwhelming in a given area. Alternatively, standards of good medical practice are set based on common sense and good medical practice (e.g. we should discuss treatment with patients in a collaborative way).

There is some evidence that audit improves adherence to clinical guidelines and also improves individual patient outcomes. It is a cyclical process, with re-audit every few months/years when standards should be reviewed and changed if necessary.

---

1 E.g. NICE ♒ http:// www.nice.org and SIGN ♒ http://www.sign.ac.uk
2 E.g. CHI ♒ http://www.chi.nhs.uk and CSBS ♒ http://www.nhshealthquality.org/
3 See ♒ http://www.york.ac.uk/inst/crd/ehc51.pdf for further details.

Organic illness

Presentations of organic illness

All psychiatric illnesses are by their nature organic—that is, they involve abnormalities of normal brain structure or function. The term 'organic illness' in modern psychiatric classification, however, refers to those conditions with demonstrable aetiology in central nervous system (CNS) pathology. Organic disorders related to substance misuse are dealt with in Chapter 15. This chapter deals with those disorders that are caused by traumatic, inflammatory, degenerative, infective, and metabolic conditions.

Many psychiatric syndromes can have an organic aetiology. For this reason, every patient who presents with psychiatric symptomatology requires a thorough physical examination (including neurological examination and in some cases special investigations) before a diagnosis of functional illness is made. While psychiatrists do not have to be expert neurologists, a sound knowledge of those conditions that bridge neurology and psychiatry is essential. Historically, these disciplines have not always been separated and, in this era of biological psychiatry, they are once again converging as increasing evidence emerges of brain dysfunction underlying most psychiatric disorders. Having said this, it is important to remember that biological, psychological, and social factors interact in a dynamic two-way process in the generation of psychiatric symptoms.

Listed here (p. 130) are common organic causes of psychiatric syndromes (delirium, dementia, and amnestic disorders are discussed later):

Organic causes of psychosis

- Neurological (epilepsy; head injury; brain tumour; dementia; encephalitis e.g. herpes simplex virus [HSV], human immunodeficiency virus [HIV]; neurosyphilis; brain abscess; CVA).
- Endocrine (hyper/hypothyroidism; Cushing's; hyperparathyroidism; Addison's disease).
- Metabolic (uraemia; sodium imbalance; porphyria).
- Systemic lupus erythematosus (SLE) ('lupus psychosis').
- Medications (steroids; levodopa [L-dopa]; isoniazid; anticholinergics; antihypertensives; anticonvulsants; methylphenidate).
- Drugs of abuse (cocaine; LSD; cannabis; PCP; amfetamines [including mephadrone and 'legal highs']; opioids).
- Toxins.

Organic causes of depression

- Neurological (CVA; epilepsy; Parkinson's disease; brain tumour; dementia; multiple sclerosis [MS]; Huntington's disease; head injury).
- Infectious (HIV; Epstein–Barr virus [EBV]/infectious mononucleosis; brucellosis).
- Endocrine and metabolic (hypothyroidism; Cushing's; Addison's disease; parathyroid disease; vitamin deficiency [B12 and folate]; porphyria).
- Cardiac disease (myocardial infarction [MI]; congestive cardiac failure [CCF]).
- SLE.

- Rheumatoid arthritis.
- Cancer.
- Medications (analgesics; antihypertensives; levodopa [L-dopa]; anticonvulsants; antibiotics; steroids; combined oral contraceptive [OCP]; cytotoxics; cimetidine; salbutamol).
- Drugs of abuse (alcohol; BDZs; cannabis; cocaine; opioids).
- Toxins.

Organic causes of mania

- Neurological (CVA; epilepsy; brain tumour; head injury; MS).
- Endocrine (hyperthyroidism).
- Medications (steroids; antidepressants; mefloquine; interferon, isoniazid; cytotoxics).
- Drugs of abuse (cannabis; cocaine; amfetamines).
- Toxins.

Organic causes of anxiety

- Neurological (epilepsy; dementia; head injury; CVA; brain tumour; MS; Parkinson's disease).
- Pulmonary (chronic obstructive airways disease [COAD]).
- Cardiac (arrhythmias; CCF; angina; mitral valve prolapse).
- Hyperthyroidism.
- Medications (antidepressants; antihypertensives; flumazenil; yohimbine; fenfluramine).
- Drugs of abuse (alcohol; BDZs; caffeine; cannabis; cocaine; LSD; MDMA [ecstasy]; amfetamines).

Dementia: general overview

Essence Dementia is a syndrome characterized by progressive, usually irreversible, global cognitive deficits. Often memory impairment is the first symptom with progression to other deficits including dysphasia, agnosia, apraxia, impaired executive function, and personality disintegration. For a diagnosis to be made there must be significant impairment of normal functioning and other possible diagnoses (see **Differential diagnosis** 🕮 p. 133), particularly delirium or depression, should be excluded.

Common causes Alzheimer's disease (62%), vascular dementia (15%), mixed (10%), Lewy body dementia (4%), fronto-temporal dementia (2%), other (3%).

Reversible causes (15%): subdural haematoma, NPH, vitamin B_{12} deficiency, metabolic causes, hypothyroidism.

Aetiology

- **Parenchymal/degenerative** Alzheimer's disease; vascular dementia; fronto-temporal dementia (including Pick's disease); Parkinson's disease; Huntington's disease; Wilson's disease; MS; motor neurone disease (MND); Lewy body disease; progressive supranuclear palsy; corticobasal degeneration.
- **Intracranial** Tumour; head trauma; subdural haematoma; CVA; normal pressure hydrocephalus (NPH).
- **Infection** Creutzfeldt–Jakob disease (prion disease); neurosyphilis; HIV-associated dementia; tuberculosis (TB); subacute sclerosing panencephalitis (SSPE); other.
- **Endocrine** Hypothyroidism; hyperparathyroidism; Cushing's and Addison's disease.
- **Metabolic** Uraemia; hepatic encephalopathy; hypoglycaemia; calcium imbalance; magnesium imbalance; electrolyte imbalance.
- **Vitamin deficiency** B_{12}; folate; pellagra (niacin); thiamine.
- **Toxins** Prolonged alcohol misuse; heavy metal poisoning.

Clinical features (see Box 5.1)

- Memory impairment: starts with short-term and progresses to long-term.
- History of personality change, forgetfulness, social withdrawal, lability of affect, disinhibition, 'silliness', diminished self-care, apathy, fatigue, deteriorating executive functioning.
- Other specific cognitive deficits are seen in cortical dementias (see 🕮 p. 133).
- Hallucinations and delusions often paranoid (20–40%) and poorly systematized.
- Anxiety and/or depression in 50%.
- Neurological features (e.g. seizures, focal deficits, primitive reflexes, pseudobulbar palsy, long-tract signs).
- Catastrophic reaction, (🕮 p. 88).
- Pathological emotion—spontaneous lability.
- Sundowner syndrome—as evening approaches confusion increases and falls become common.

Differential diagnosis Delirium; depression (pseudodementia 📖 p. 520); amnestic disorders (📖 p. 148); learning disability (LD); psychotic disorders; normal ageing (📖 p. 514).

Investigations Include: FBC; LFT; U&E; glucose; erythrocyte sedimentation rate (ESR); thyroid-stimulating hormone (TSH); calcium; magnesium; phosphate; Venereal Disease Research Laboratory (VDRL) test for syphilis; HIV; vitamin B_{12} and folate; C-reactive protein; blood culture; LP; EEG; chest X-ray (CXR); ECG; CT (optima and axial protocol); MRI; SPECT.

Principles of management

- **Assessment**: diagnostic, functional, and social.
- **Cognitive enhancement**: acetylcholinesterase inhibitors (tacrine; donepezil; rivastigmine); antioxidants (selegiline, vitamin E); ? hormonal (oestrogen; HRT).
- **Treat psychosis/agitation**: consider antipsychotics.
- **Treat depression/insomnia**: SSRIs; hypnotics.
- **Treat medical illness**.
- **Psychological support**: to both patient and care-givers.
- **Functional management**: maximize mobility; encourage independence with self-care, toilet, and feeding; assist with communication.
- **Social management**: accommodation; activities; financial matters; legal matters (power of attorney, wills, and curatorship).

Box 5.1 Clinical syndromes of dementia

Dementias may be classified in terms of primary site of pathology. Since site of pathology in the brain correlates with neuropsychiatric symptomatology, this is a useful system of classification.

1. **Cortical dementias** involve primarily the cortex and are divided into:
   - **Fronto-temporal** e.g. Pick's disease (p. 142). Characterized by prominent personality change which may manifest as a frontal lobe syndrome. A common cause of early-onset dementia, it is often undiagnosed. Language impairments tend to involve reduction in content (semantic anomia). CT shows fronto-temporal atrophy and SPECT shows fronto-temporal metabolism.
   - **Posterior–parietal** e.g. Alzheimer's disease (p. 134). Characterized by early memory loss and focal cognitive deficits. Personality changes are later manifestations. Language impairments involve problems with word-finding (lexical anomia). CT (optima protocol) shows thinning (<12 mm) of the cortex of the medial temporal lobe.

2. **Subcortical dementias** Parkinson's disease (p. 168); Huntington's disease (p. 170); Wilson's disease (p. 171); Binswanger encephalopathy (p. 144); progressive supranuclear palsy (PSNP) (p. 167); HIV-associated dementia (p. 163); NPH (p. 150). *Clinical features:* gross psychomotor slowing; depressed mood; movement disorders; mild amnesia; and personality changes.

3. **Cortical–subcortical dementias** e.g. Lewy body dementia (p. 140). *Clinical features:* cortical and subcortical symptoms.

4. **Multifocal dementias** e.g. CJD (p. 146). *Clinical features:* rapid onset and course; involves cerebellum and subcortical structures.

Alzheimer's disease 1

Also termed 'dementia of the Alzheimer type' (DAT), this is the most common cause (70%) of dementia in older people. It is a degenerative disease of the brain with prominent cognitive and behavioural impairment that is sufficiently severe to interfere significantly with social and occupational function. It affects approximately 500 000 people in the UK and more than 30 million worldwide. A larger number of people have less severe impairments that usually evolve into the full disorder with time. The percentage of the total population aged over 65 is increasing in the developed world, meaning that the burden of DAT-related health care is likely to increase.

Epidemiology Risk of DAT increases with age: 1% at age 60yrs; doubles every 5yrs; 40% of those aged 85yrs. Age-specific incidence is the same for men and women—approximately 50% excess prevalence in women (explained by the greater number of at-risk women given their longer lifespan). Risk factors include: Down's syndrome, previous head injury, or hypothyroidism; family history of Down's syndrome, Parkinson's disease, or DAT.

Possible protective factors Smoking; oestrogen (e.g. hormone replacement therapy [HRT]); non-steroidal anti-inflammatory drugs (NSAIDs); vitamin E; higher level of pre-morbid education.

Pathophysiology

- Amyloid plaques—insoluble β-amyloid peptide deposits as senile plaques or β-pleated sheets in the hippocampus, amygdala, and cerebral cortex. Increased density with advanced disease.
- Neurofibrillary tangles (NFTs)—consist of phosphorylated tau protein and are found in the cortex, hippocampus, and substantia nigra. (NFTs also found in normal ageing, Down's syndrome, dementia pugilistica, and progressive supranuclear palsy.) However, even low densities of NFTs in the cortices of the medial temporal lobes should be considered abnormal.
- The co-occurrence of amyloid plaques and NFTs was described by Alois Alzheimer in his original description of the disorder and is now accepted universally as a hallmark of the disease.
- Up to 50% loss of neurons and synapses in the cortex and hippocampus.
- **Genetics**: 40% have a positive family history of DAT (esp. early onset: <55yrs). Autosomal dominant inheritance—affects <1% of those with dementia.
  - Chromosome 21—the gene for amyloid precursor protein (APP) is found on the long arm. Also implicated in Down's syndrome.
  - Chromosome 19—codes for apolipoprotein E4. Presence of E4 alleles increases risk of DAT; some 15% of Europeans carry the allele.

- Chromosome 14—codes for presenilin 1 (implicated in β-amyloid peptide).
- Chromosome 1—codes for presenilin 11 (implicated in β-amyloid peptide).
- **Cholinergic hypothesis**: the pathological changes lead to degeneration of cholinergic nuclei in the basal forebrain (nucleus basalis of Meynert). This results in ↓cortical acetylcholine (ACh).

Pray, do not mock me: I am a very foolish fond old man,
Fourscore and upward, not an hour more or less;
And, to deal plainly, I fear I am not in my perfect mind.
Methinks I should know you and know this man;
Yet I am doubtful: for I am mainly ignorant what place this is,
and all the skill I have remembers not these garments;
nor I know not where I did lodge last night.
Do not laugh at me;
For as I am a man, I think this lady to be my child Cordelia.

Shakespeare: *King Lear*, Act II Scene 7

Alzheimer's disease 2

Clinical features Symptoms usually start insidiously but first presentation may be related to an identifiable life event.

- **Early symptoms** Failing memory (with disorientation being common, especially for time), muddled efficiency with activities of daily living (ADLs), spatial dysfunction, and changes in behaviour such as wandering and irritability. By the time the patient presents to clinicians, cognitive deficits are usually apparent.
- **Middle symptoms** Intellectual and personality deterioration—aphasia, apraxia (evidenced by awkwardness with the sequence of dressing), and agnosia (inability to recognize parts of the body). Occasionally, a patient may present with Gerstmann syndrome (📖 p. 73), indicating right parietal disease, characterized by finger agnosia, R/L disorientation, acalculia, and dysgraphia), BPSD (behavioural and psychological symptoms in dementia). Impaired visuospatial skills and executive function are common.
- **Late symptoms** Fully dependent. Physical deterioration, incontinence, gait abnormalities, spasticity, seizures (3%), tremor, weight loss, primitive reflexes, extrapyramidal signs.
- **Psychiatric symptoms** Delusions (15%)—usually of a paranoid nature. Auditory and/or visual hallucinations (10–15%)—which may be simple misidentification, and indicate rapid cognitive decline. Depression is common, requiring treatment in up to 20% of patients.
- **Behavioural disturbances** include aggression, wandering, explosive temper, sexual disinhibition, incontinence, excessive eating, and searching behaviour.
- **Personality change** often reflects an exaggeration of premorbid traits with coarsening of affect and egocentricity.

Clinical subtypes and course Mayeux (1985) described four groups:
- The most common presentation is a gradual and progressive decline without distinguishing features.
- A group with early onset (<65), more aphasia and apraxia, a rapid course with severe intellectual decline, and poor survival rate.
- A group with extra-pyramidal signs, severe functional impairment, and associated psychotic symptoms.
- A benign group with little or no progression over a 4-yr follow-up.

Factors associated with poor prognosis
- Greater severity of disease at presentation
- Being male
- Onset <65yrs
- Parietal lobe damage
- Prominent behavioural problems
- Severe focal cognitive deficits such as apraxia
- Observed depression
- Absence of misidentification syndrome

Assessment

- **Detailed history** An informant questionnaire such as the IQCODE can be helpful in this regard).
- **Mental state examination** Noting any clouding of consciousness (delirium), symptoms of depression, psychosis, etc.
- **Cognitive testing** is essential and may begin with a Mini Mental State Examination (MMSE), but later involve specific neuropsychological testing.
- **Physical examination** To detect presence or absence of focal signs, reflexes, and plantar responses, as well as gait disturbance and signs of Parkinson's disease.
- **Blood tests** (📖 p. 133).
- **EEG** useful to exclude delirium, Creutzfeldt–Jakob disease (CJD), etc.—to be considered in atypical cases only.
- **Brain imaging**:
  - CT—cortical atrophy, esp. over parietal and temporal lobes and ventricular enlargement.
  - MRI—(optima protocol) atrophy of grey matter (hippocampus, amygdala, and medial temporal lobe).
  - Single photon emission tomography (SPET)—reduced regional cerebral blood flow (rCBF) in temporal and posterior parietal lobes (also frontal lobes in advanced disease).
  - PET—20–30% reduction in oxygen and glucose metabolism in temporal and posterior parietal lobes.
  - Magnetic resonance spectroscopy (MRS)—↓N-acetylaspartate-typically reserved for use in combination with structural imaging where the diagnosis is in doubt.

Alzheimer's disease 3: pharmacological treatments[1]

Acetylcholinesterase inhibitors (AChEIs) were the first drugs to be licensed for the treatment of DAT. They act by enhancing ACh at cholinergic synapses in the CNS, and in this way may slow progression of the disease, reducing time spent in full nursing care. They have beneficial effects on cognitive, functional, and behavioural symptoms of the disease and are recommended as first-line agents in the treatment of mild–moderate DAT. (See Box 5.2.)

First generation AChEIs

- **Tacrine** Developed in the 1980s; easily absorbed with a short ½ life; liver metabolism; non-linear kinetics; non-selective (also acts at parasympathetic receptors outside the CNS). *Problems*: Gastrointestinal tract (GIT) side-effects; ↑liver enzymes/hepatotoxicity; wide dose range, therefore unpredictable kinetics; 4× daily dosage.

Second generation AChEIs

Similar efficacy over 6mths; long-term efficacy unknown. Switching between agents is acceptable.

- **Donepezil** Piperidine derivative, developed in 1996; GIT absorbed with liver metabolism; long ½ life (70hrs); highly selective (acts centrally only); linear kinetics. *Problems*: GIT side-effects at high dose; bradycardia; GIT bleed (rare); contraindicated in asthma. *Benefits*: selective therefore ↓side-effects; no liver toxicity; predictable kinetics; narrow dose range; 1× daily dosage. Dose: 5–10mg/day.
- **Rivastigmine** Developed in 1998; short ½ life (12hrs); inhibits AChE and butyrylcholinesterase in CNS. *Problems*: GIT side-effects; 2× daily dosage. *Benefits*: Not metabolized by the liver and least likely to cause drug–drug interactions. *Dose*: start with 1.5mg twice daily (BD); increase to 3–6mg BD—now available in a modified release once daily (OD) form or 24hr patch (thought to be helpful in reducing GI side-effects).
- **Galantamine** Selectively inhibits AChE and acts as an allosteric ligand at nicotinic ACh receptors; metabolized in liver; ½ life (5hrs); selective. *Problems*: 2× daily dosage. Dose: 4–12mg BD.

NMDA-receptor partial antagonist The NMDA receptor binds excitatory glutamate in the CNS and has a role in LTP and learning/memory function.

- **Memantine** In Feb 2002, this new agent was approved in Europe for the treatment of moderately severe to severe DAT (MMSE 3–14). It is a non-competitive, PCP-site, *N*-methyl-*D*-aspartate (NMDA) antagonist that may protect neurons from glutamate-mediated excitotoxicity. Trials show benefits of memantine augmentation of donepezil. Cochrane review indicates use in DAT, vascular, and mixed dementia.

Other (possible) treatment strategies Although only at experimental stages, there is some evidence for other approaches to DAT.

These include: antioxidants (vitamin E; selegiline); anti-inflammatories; secretase inhibitors; metal chelators; amyloid-B-peptide vaccination; cholesterol-lowering drugs; red wine (!). There is ongoing work looking at possible neuroprotective effects of lithium.

Box 5.2 NICE guidance on drug treatment for Alzheimer's disease—donepezil, rivastigmine, and galantamine (No 19)

The three drugs—donepezil, rivastigmine, and galantamine—should be made available in the NHS as one component of the management of those people with mild and moderate Alzheimer's disease (AD) whose MMSE score is above 12 points, under the following conditions:

- Diagnosis that the form of dementia is AD must be made in a specialist clinic according to standard diagnostic criteria.
- Assessment in a specialist clinic, including tests of cognitive, global, and behavioural functioning and of activities of daily living, should be made before the drug is prescribed.
- Clinicians should also exercise judgement about the likelihood of compliance; in general, a carer or care-worker who is in sufficient contact with the patient to ensure compliance should be a minimum requirement.
- Only specialists (including old age psychiatrists, neurologists, and care of the elderly physicians) should initiate treatment. Carers' views of the patient's condition at baseline and follow-up should be sought. If GPs are to take over prescribing, it is recommended that they should do so under an agreed shared-care protocol with clear treatment end points.
- A further assessment should be made, usually 2–4 months after reaching maintenance dose of the drug. Following this assessment, the drug should be continued only where there has been an improvement or no deterioration in MMSE score, together with evidence of global improvement on the basis of behavioural and/or functional assessment.
- Patients who continue on the drug should be reviewed by MMSE score and global, functional, and behavioural assessment every 6 months.
  - The drug should normally only be continued while their MMSE score remains above 12 points, and their global, functional, and behavioural condition remains at a level where the drug is considered to be having a worthwhile effect.
  - When the MMSE score falls below 12 points, patients should not normally be prescribed any of these three drugs.
  - Any review involving MMSE assessment should be undertaken by an appropriate specialist team, unless there are locally agreed protocols for shared care.

1 Scarpini E, Scheltens P, Feldman H (2003) Treatment of Alzheimer's disease: current status and new perspectives. *Lancet (Neurol)* **2**: 539–47.

Dementia with Lewy bodies (DLB)

Common form of senile dementia (~15–20% of cases in hospital[1] and community-based samples[2]) that shares clinical and pathological features of both DAT and Parkinson's disease.

Epidemiology Age of onset: 50–83yrs. Age at death: 68–92yrs. 4>5.

Clinical features Dementia (relative sparing of STM); Parkinsonism (~70%: bradykinesia, limb rigidity, gait disorder); fluctuating cognitive performance and level of consciousness; complex hallucinations—visual (~60%: often people and animals, auditory (~20%)—with associated emotional responses; significant depressive episode (~40%); recurrent falls/syncope (~30%: due to autonomic dysfunction), transient disturbances of consciousness (mute and unresponsive for several minutes); antipsychotic sensitivity (~60%). The mean survival time/rate of cognitive decline is similar to Alzheimer's disease (but rapid deterioration over 1–2yrs does occur). Worsening of Parkinsonism is similar in rate to Parkinson's disease (10% decline per year). See Box 5.3 for a summary of diagnostic criteria.

Pathological features Typically 'mixed' picture. **Lewy bodies** Eosinophilic intracytoplasmic neuronal inclusions of abnormally phosphory-lated neurofilament proteins aggregated with ubiquitin and A-synuclein, found in brainstem nuclei (esp. basal ganglia), paralimbic, and neocortical structures. Associated neuronal loss (esp. brain-stem and basal forebrain cholinergic projection neurones—with associated ↓ACh transmission in neocortex). **Lewy neurites** Distinctive pattern of ubiquitin and A-synuclein immunoreactive neuritic degeneration—in substantia nigra, hippocampal region (CA2/3), dorsal vagal nucleus, basal nucleus basilis of Meynert, and transtentorial cortex (may be more relevant to neuropsychiatric symptom formation than cortical Lewy bodies). **Alzheimer-type changes** Senile plaques present in a similar density and distribution, fewer neurofibrillary tangles, less tau pathology. **Vascular disease** occurs in ~30% with unknown clinical significance.

Differential diagnosis Other dementia syndromes (esp. DAT), delirium, neurological causes (e.g. Parkinson's disease, progressive supranuclear palsy, multiple system atrophy, CJD), psychiatric disorders (e.g. late-onset delusional disorder, depressive psychosis, mania).

Investigations
- **CT/MRI**: relative sparing of medial temporal lobes in most cases. Moderate increases in deep white-matter lesions, frequent periventricular lucencies on MRI.
- **SPECT HMPAO scan** (blood flow): global (esp. occipital), medial temporal lobes relatively preserved.
- **SPECT FP-CIT** (presynaptic dopamine transporter): reduced in putamen (like Parkinson's disease).
- **ApoE genotype**: ↑frequency of ε4 allele.

Management
- **Antipsychotics** Avoid/use with great caution: severe sensitivity reactions (40–50%)—e.g. irreversible Parkinsonism, impairment of

consciousness, neuroleptic malignant syndrome (NMS)-like autonomic disturbances—with 2–3-fold increase in mortality.
- **AChEIs** Not yet recommended by National Guidelines, substantial provisional evidence suggests AChEIs effective in some DLB cases (↑cognitive function, ↓apathy/psychosis/agitation).
- **Other** No clear evidence for antidepressants, anticonvulsants, or BDZs for psychiatric and behavioural symptoms. Clonazepam may be useful for sleep disturbance (vivid dreams, muscle atonia, excessive jerking, and other complex movements). Anti-Parkinsonian medication—use cautiously for clinically significant motor symptoms (risk of exacerbating psychotic symptoms).

Box 5.3 Consensus criteria for the clinical diagnosis of probable and possible dementia with Lewy bodies[3]

- The central feature required for a diagnosis of DLB is progressive cognitive decline of sufficient magnitude to interfere with normal social or occupational function. Prominent or persistent memory impairment may not necessarily occur in the early stages but is usually evident with progression. Deficits on tests of attention and of fronto-subcortical skills and visuospatial ability may be especially prominent.
- Two of the following core features are essential for a diagnosis of probable DLB; one is essential for possible DLB.
  - Fluctuating cognition with pronounced variations in attention and alertness.
  - Recurrent visual hallucinations, which are typically well-formed and detailed.
  - Spontaneous motor features of Parkinsonism.
- Features supportive of the diagnosis are:
  - Repeated falls; syncope; transient loss of consciousness; neuroleptic sensitivity; systematized delusions; hallucinations in other modalities.
- A diagnosis of DLB is less likely in the presence of:
  - Stroke, evident as focal neurological signs or on brain imaging.
  - Evidence on physical examination and investigation of any physical illness, or other brain disorder, sufficient to account for the clinical picture.

---

1 Weiner M (1999) Dementia associated with Lewy bodies: dilemmas and directions. *Arch Neurol* **56**: 1441.

2 Holmes C, Cairns N, Lantos P, *et al.* (1999) Validity of current clinical criteria for Alzheimer's disease, vascular dementia and dementia with Lewy bodies. *Br J Psych* **174**: 45–50.

3 McKeith I, Del Ser T, Spano P, *et al.* (2000) Efficacy of rivastigmine in dementia with Lewy bodies: a randomized, double-blind, placebo-controlled international study. *Lancet* **356**: 2031–6.

Fronto-temporal dementia (FTD) (Pick's disease)[1,2]

A form of dementia, characterized by preferential atrophy of fronto-temporal regions, with usually early onset (accounts for ~20% of presenile cases). Early symptoms include personality change and social disinhibition, preceding memory or other cognitive impairment (Box 5.4).

Clinical features Profound alteration in character/social conduct, relative preservation of perception, spatial skills, praxis, memory. **Decline/ impaired regulation of social conduct**: (e.g. breaches of etiquette, tactlessness, disinhibition, changes in usual behaviour, passivity, inertia, overactivity, pacing, and wandering). **Emotional blunting**: e.g. primary emotions (happiness, sadness, fear) and social emotions (embarrassment, sympathy, empathy). **Impaired insight**: of symptoms and expression of distress. **Dietary changes**: overeating, preference for sweet foods. **Perseverative behaviours** (e.g. drinking from an empty cup). Speech: echolalia, perseveration, verbal stereotypies, mutism. **Cognitive**: frontal lobe dysfunction: impaired attention, ineffective retrieval strategies, poor organization, lack of self-monitoring and concern for accuracy. **Neurological**: no early signs; primitive reflexes and Parkinsonism (with progression); MND signs (in a minority). Onset usually 45–65yrs, can occur before age 30 and in the over 65s. ♂=♀. Mean time to death 8yrs (range 2–20yrs). Family history (FHx) in 50%.

Clinical subtypes Disinhibited form: orbito-medial frontal and anterior temporal regional pathology. **Apathetic form**: extensive frontal (esp. dorsolateral) lobe pathology. **Stereotypic form**: marked striatal/variable cortical involvement (often temporal>frontal). *Note*: changes in social behaviour often related to right-hemispheric pathology. Repetitive/compulsive behaviours may be associated with striatal pathology and the disinhibited form, suggesting temporal lobe pathology (unlike OCD, anxiety is not experienced).

Pathological features Macroscopic: bilateral atrophy of frontal and anterior temporal lobes, degeneration of the striatum. **Microscopic**: 3 subtypes (similar distribution of changes within frontal/temporal lobes): Common (*microvacuolar*) type (60%)—loss of large cortical nerve cells, spongiform degeneration (microvacuolation) of the superficial neurophil, minimal gliosis, and no swellings or inclusions in remaining nerve cells; *Pick type* (25%)—loss of large cortical nerve cells, widespread gliosis, minimal or no spongiform (microvacuolar) change, swollen neurons and inclusions positive for tau and ubiquitin (in most cases); limbic system and striatum more seriously damaged; *Associated with MND* (15%) demonstrating microvacuolar (rarely Pick-type) histological features like MND.

Differential diagnosis DAT, cerebrovascular dementia, rare forms of fronto-temporal lobar degeneration (e.g. 'semantic' dementia, progressive non-fluent aphasia, progressive apraxia).

Investigations Neuropsychology: Impaired frontal lobe function, relatively spared memory, speech, and perceptuospatial functions. **EEG**:

usually normal. **CT/MRI**: bilateral (asymmetrical) abnormalities of frontal/temporal lobes. **SPECT**: frontal and/or temporal lobe abnormalities. A significant proportion of patients will have normal structural imaging. **Genetics**: associations with: 17q21–22 (familial inheritance) and mutations in the tau gene; 3; 9q21–22 (familial amyotrophic lateral sclerosis).

Management Currently, no specific treatments. **AChEIs**: unlikely to be beneficial (no specific abnormality of the cholinergic system). **SSRIs**: of limited benefit for behavioural symptoms (disinhibition, overeating, and compulsions).

Box 5.4 Behavioural features of FTD specified in diagnostic criteria

Core features
- Insidious onset and gradual progression.
- Early decline in social interpersonal conduct.
- Early impairment in regulation of personal conduct.
- Early emotional blunting.
- Early loss of insight.

Supportive features
- Behavioural disorder:
  - Decline in personal hygiene and grooming.
  - Mental rigidity and inflexibility.
  - Distractibility and impersistence.
  - Hyperorality and dietary changes.
  - Perseverative and stereotyped behaviour.
  - Utilization behaviour.
- Speech and language:
  - Altered speech output (aspontaneity and economy of speech/ pressured speech).
  - Stereotypy of speech.
  - Echolalia.
  - Perseveration.
  - Mutism.
- Physical signs:
  - Primitive reflexes.
  - Incontinence.
  - Akinesia, rigidity, and tremor.
  - Low and labile blood pressure.
- Investigations:
  - **Neuropsychological**: significant impairment on frontal lobe tests; absence of severe amnesia, aphasia, or perceptuospatial disorder.
  - **EEG**: normal on conventional EEG, despite clinically evident dementia.
  - **Brain imaging** (structural and/or functional): predominant frontal and/or temporal abnormality.

1 Neary D, Snowden JS, Gustafson L, *et al.* (1998) Frontotemporal lobar degeneration: a consensus on clinical diagnostic criteria. *Neurology* **51**: 1546–54.
2 Snowden JS, Neary D, Mann DM (2002) Frontotemporal dementia. *Br J Psychiat* **180**: 140–3.

Vascular dementia

Vascular dementia is the second most common cause of dementia after DAT, accounting for 20% of cases. It can coexist with DAT and results from thromboembolic or hypertensive infarction of small and medium-size vessels. Features that suggest vascular dementia include: sudden onset; stepwise deterioration; and risk factors for cardiovascular disease. Its presentation is variable and three syndromes are commonly recognized.[1]

1. *Cognitive deficits following a single stroke* Not all strokes result in cognitive impairment, but when they do the deficits depend upon the site of the infarct. Cognitive deficits tend to be particularly severe with certain mid-brain and thalamic strokes. Cognitive deficits may remain fixed or recover, either partially or completely.

2. *Multi-infarct dementia (MID)* Multiple strokes lead to stepwise deterioration in cognitive function. Between strokes there are periods of relative stability. There are often risk factors for cardiovascular disease.

3. *Progressive small-vessel disease (Binswanger disease)* Multiple microvascular infarcts of perforating vessels lead to progressive lacunae formation and white matter leukoariosis on MRI. This is a subcortical dementia with a clinical course characterized by gradual intellectual decline, generalized slowing, and motor problems (e.g. gait disturbance and dysarthria). Depression and pseudobulbar palsy are not uncommon.

Epidemiology Most common in the 60–70yrs age group. ♂>♀. Other risk factors include: family or personal history of cardiovascular disease, smoking, diabetes mellitus, hypertension, hyperlipidaemia, polycythaemia, coagulopathies, sickle cell anaemia, valvular disease, atrial myxoma, and carotid artery disease. There are rare familial cases with onset in the 40s—cerebral autosomal dominant arteriopathy with subcortical infarcts and leukoencephalopathy (CADASIL).

Clinical features[2] Onset may follow a CVA and is more acute than DAT. **Emotional and personality changes** are typically early, followed by **cognitive deficits** (including memory deficits) that are often fluctuating in severity. **Depression** with episodes of **affective lability** and **confusion** are common, especially at night. **Behavioural slowing, anxiety**, and occasional episodes of cerebral ischaemia occur frequently. Physical signs include features of arteriovascular disease together with neurological impairments (e.g. rigidity, akinesia, brisk reflexes, pseudobulbar palsy). 10% have **seizures** at some point. Course is stepwise, with periods of intervening stability. Prognosis is poorer than in DAT with average lifespan of 5yrs from onset. Cause of death is usually ischaemic heart disease (50%), CVA, or renal failure.

Investigations
- Routine 'dementia screen' (📖 p. 133).
- Serum cholesterol, clotting screen, vasculitis screen (ESR; C-reactive protein [CRP]; complement; anti-nuclear factor [ANF]; rheumatoid factor; anti-DNA antibodies; antiphospholipid antibodies; etc.), and

syphilis serology are additional tests in unusual cases (e.g. 'young strokes').
- ECG, CXR, CT, and MRI are essential.
- Other investigations may include: echocardiography (for cardiac/valvular defects or disease); carotid artery Doppler ultrasound.

Management
- Establish causative factors.
- Medical or surgical diseases that are contributory need to be treated early.
- Daily aspirin may delay course of disease.
- General health interventions include changing diet, stopping smoking, managing hypertension, optimizing diabetic control, and increasing exercise.

1 Rossor M, Brown J (1998) Vascular and other dementias. In: R Butler and B Pitt, eds, *Seminars in old age psychiatry*. London, Gaskell.
2 Gelder M, Gath D, Mayou R, *et al.* (1996) *Oxford textbook of psychiatry*, 3rd edn. Oxford: Oxford University Press.

Prion diseases

Prion diseases are rapid, aggressive, dementing illnesses caused by deposits of prion proteins throughout the brain. They are rare and are best considered as slow virus infections. Prions spread throughout the brain by causing irreversible change in neighbouring tissue. The typical pathological finding is a spongy encephalopathy, and in terms of the nosology of the dementias, prion disease is considered a multifocal dementia. While prion diseases tend to respect the species barrier (e.g. 'scrapie' is a prion disease limited to sheep), there is emerging evidence that this is not always the case (e.g. vCJD). Three diseases are recognized in humans.

Creutzfeldt–Jakob disease (CJD)

A rare disease (approximately 50 cases/year in UK) of 50–70yrs-olds with equal sex distribution. 85% cases are spontaneous or sporadic; 10% result from genetic mutation; 5% result from iatrogenic transmission during transplant surgery of dura, corneal grafts, and pituitary growth hormone. The clinical picture is one of rapidly deteriorating dementia, cerebellar and extra-pyramidal signs, myoclonus, and death within a year. EEG shows periodic complexes. CT atrophy of cortex and cerebellum.

New variant CJD (vCJD): BSE

The rise of vCJD followed an epidemic of bovine spongiform encephalopathy (BSE) in cattle. BSE is a prion disease of cows that is thought to have been spread by cattle feeds that contained CNS material from infected cows. The disease in humans affects mainly young people in their 20s and is characterized by early anxiety and depressive symptoms, followed by personality changes, and finally a progressive dementia. Ataxia and myoclonus are prominent and the typical course is 1–2yrs until death. EEG and CT changes are similar to CJD.

Kuru

This was a rare disease of New Guinea cannibals who ate the brains of their deceased relatives. The incubation period was prolonged—up to 40yrs before disease onset, then progression was rapid and fatal (Box 5.5).

Box 5.5 Recent research reveals 'cannibalism genotype'

Researchers at University College London have recently suggested that cannibalism was common and widespread in human ancestors. They analyzed DNA from 30 elderly Fore women from Papua New Guinea who had participated in many cannibalistic feasts before they were banned by the Australian government in the 1950s. It was the practice of the Fore for women and children to consume the brains of dead kin in the belief that this act would 'recycle' the spirit of the dead within the living. At the peak of the epidemic (1920–1950) kuru killed 1% of the population annually. Most of the women survivors tested by researchers had a particular genotype that was much less common in the younger population, indicating that it conferred substantial protection against the disease. Interestingly, none of the patients who have to date contracted new variant CJD in Britain carry the protective genotype. This suggests that this genotype is protective against prion diseases in humans. The researchers then examined DNA from various ethnic groups around the world and found that all, except the Japanese, carried the protective genotype to a similar degree. Genetic tests showed that this gene could not be there by chance, but was a result of natural selection. This implies that ancestral human populations were exposed to some form of prion disease. Researchers conclude that frequent epidemics of prion disease caused by cannibalism in human ancestors would explain the worldwide existence of the protective genotype in modern humans.

From Mead S, Stumpf MP, Whitfield J, *et al.* (2003) Balancing selection at the prion protein gene consistent with prehistoric kurulike epidemics.

Science **300**: 640–3.

Amnestic disorders

The amnestic disorders are syndromes characterized by memory impairment (anterograde and/or retrograde amnesia), which are caused by a general medical condition or substance use, and where delirium and dementia have been excluded as causative of the amnesia. Amnestic disorders may be transient or chronic (< or >1mth). Amnestic conditions usually involve some or all of the following neuroanatomical structures: frontal cortex; hippocampus and amygdala; dorsomedial thalamus; mamillary bodies; and the periaqueductal grey matter (PAG). In terms of neurochemistry, glutamate transmission at the NMDA receptor is often implicated in amnesia, mainly due to its role in memory storage in the limbic system: long-term potentiation (LTP). A number of amnestic disorders are recognized:

Wernicke's encephalopathy (📖 p. 572)

An acute syndrome, with a classic tetrad of symptoms (ataxia, ophthalmoplegia, nystagmus, and acute confusional state), caused by thiamine depletion, usually related to alcohol abuse, and associated with pathological lesions in the mamillary bodies, PAG, thalamic nuclei, and the walls of the third ventricle.

Korsakoff psychosis (📖 p. 572)

Amnesia and confabulation associated with atrophy of the mamillary bodies, usually following Wernicke's encephalopathy (rarer causes include: head injury; hypoxia brain injury; basal/temporal lobe encephalitis; and vascular insult).

Vascular disease

Insults to the hippocampus (especially involving the posterior cerebral artery or basilar artery) may result in an amnestic disorder. Other regions implicated include: parietal–occipital junction; bilateral medio-dorsal thalamus; basal forebrain nuclei (e.g. aneurysm of the anterior communicating artery).

Head injury

An open or closed head injury involving acceleration or deceleration forces may result in injury to the anterior temporal poles (as this structure collides with the temporal bone). Anterograde or post-traumatic amnesia (PTA) is prominent with retrograde amnesia relatively absent. Prognosis is related to length of PTA—better prognosis associated with PTA of less than 1wk.

HSV encephalitis

Affects medial temporal lobes and results in deficits in short-term memory (STM) storage.

Temporal lobe surgery

Bilateral damage or surgery to the medial temporal lobes results in an inability to store new short-term memories (e.g. 'patient HM') (see Box 5.6).

Hypoxic brain damage

Hypoxia following asphyxia from CO poisoning, near drowning, etc., may damage sensitive CA1 and CA3 neurons in the hippocampus. This results in problems with STM storage.

MS

40% of patients have some amnesia due to plaques in the temporal lobes and diencephalon resulting in difficulty with recall.

Alcohol blackouts ('palimpsest')

Significant alcohol intoxication may lead to amnesia for the period of intoxication. This usually only occurs in the context of chronic alcohol misuse.

ECT

There may be a period of mild anterograde and/or retrograde amnesia for several hours following administration of ECT. More rarely there may be ongoing patchy memory loss for up to 6–9mths.

Transient global amnesia (TGA)

This is a syndrome of amnesia lasting 6–24hrs caused by transient ischaemia of the temporal lobes and/or diencephalon. It is more common over 50yrs and may occur in the context of hypertension or migraine. Differential diagnosis includes dissociative disorders and malingering, and diagnosis is often unclear.

Other causes of amnesia

Substances (BDZs, anticholinergics); space-occupying lesions (e.g. tumours); hypoglycaemia.

Box 5.6 Patient HM

On 23 August 1953, patient HM underwent a bilateral medial temporal lobe resection in an attempt to control his epileptic seizures. This resulted in a severe anterograde memory impairment that has made HM one of the most studied patients in the history of cognitive psychology.

HM's syndrome is surprisingly isolated, with impairment mostly limited to his inability to register new facts into long-term memory, despite immediate memory being preserved for both verbal and non-verbal tasks. Although his operation was performed when he was 27, his memories are intact until age 16, with an 11-year retrograde amnesia.

His IQ is above average, with almost normal language production and comprehension—he can understand and produce complex verbal material (but is impaired on tests of semantic and symbolic verbal fluency). His perceptual abilities are normal except for his sense of smell (2° to damage of the olfactory tracts). Despite the fact that some of his spatial abilities are compromised, he does not have any attentional deficit.

Normal pressure hydrocephalus (NPH)

Essence A syndrome where there is dilatation of cerebral ventricles (especially third ventricle) and normal cerebrospinal fluid (CSF) pressure at lumbar puncture. It typically presents with the triad of: dementia, gait ataxia, and urinary incontinence. Importantly, the dementia is potentially reversible if NPH is treated promptly.

Aetiology 50% cases are idiopathic. 50% are secondary to mechanical obstruction of CSF flow across the meninges (e.g. meningitis; subarachnoid haemorrhage; trauma; radiotherapy).

Clinical features There is progressive slowing of cognitive and motor functioning consistent with a pattern of subcortical dementia. Ataxia is due to pyramidal upper motor neuron paraparesis. Urinary incontinence is a late symptom.

Investigations CT scan shows ↑size of the lateral ventricles and thinning of the cortex. 24-hr intracranial pressure monitoring shows typical 'β' pattern.

Treatment Those cases where NPH is secondary to an identified cause are the best candidates for ventriculo-peritoneal shunt.

Chronic subdural haematoma (SDH)

Essence An insidious and fluctuating organic syndrome may result from an undetected chronic subdural haematoma. An SDH results from rupture of the bridging veins between the dura and arachnoid mater and tends to occur over the frontal and/or parietal cortices. In 30% of cases there is bilateral SDH. SDH should be suspected where there is a changing pattern in cognitive function, especially if risk factors for SDH exist: post trauma; elderly after a fall; infancy; cerebral atrophy (e.g. chronic alcoholism); clotting disorders.

Clinical features An SDH may only manifest with symptoms months after it develops, therefore there may be no history of recent trauma. Headache, altered level of consciousness, and amnesia may all occur, often with fluctuations in severity. Typically, the mental state may be variable on different occasions and there may be periods of unusual drowsiness as well as both cognitive and physical slowness and sluggishness. Minor focal signs are sometimes detected. The general trend is towards a dementia picture, which is characteristically of a subcortical nature.

Investigations CT scan during the first 3wks may not show the SDH as it is isodense during the early phase. Therefore, contrast should be used. Later on, as the SDH liquefies, a low-density convexity may be detected over the fronto-parietal cortex.

Treatment Surgical drainage of SDH via burr holes. Steroids for conservative treatment.

Psychiatric sequelae of CVA

A range of psychiatric problems may occur following stroke. These include:

Cognitive disorders
- Vascular dementia (see 📖 p. 144).
- Subcortical dementia (see 📖 p. 133).
- Amnestic disorder (see 📖 p. 148).

Personality changes
These tend to involve a constriction in the range of interests and a loss of intellectual flexibility. Irritability is common and 'catastrophic reactions' may occur in response to stress or change in routine. Emotional flexibility may be reduced and affective responses often become shallow and stereotyped.

Pathological emotionalism
May occur 4–6wks post-CVA, especially following left frontal infarcts. Presentation involves outbursts of unprovoked and uncontrollable emotion and distress, with disinhibition a major feature.

Post-stroke depression
Depressive illness after stroke is extremely common, occurring in up to 60% of cases. Its onset is usually between 3 and 24mths following the stroke. It was a neglected phenomenon until recently. Many cases are mis- or under-diagnosed with symptoms being attributed to the cognitive insult.

Aetiology *Biological factors*—direct physiological effects of the brain injury, with location (e.g. left anterior frontal), large size, increased age, and female gender being risk factors. *Psychological factors*—sudden dependency; disability; premorbid personality traits (especially neurotic or highly independent individuals). *Social risk factors*—being alone; lack of social support; financial worries.

Treatment Antidepressants: SSRIs and mianserin are considered safe following stroke but some evidence suggests that TCAs are more efficacious.

Psychoses
Manic, hypomanic, and paranoid psychoses may result from a CVA, especially right hemisphere infarcts. Peduncular hallucinosis is an uncommon psychosis characterized by visual and auditory hallucinations and is associated with infarcts involving the pons and midbrain.

Korsakoff psychosis (📖 p. 572)
A rare chronic complication of subarachnoid haemorrhage.

Psychiatric aspects of head injury[1]

Head injuries are unfortunately common in a world where there is mass use of motor vehicles and widely misused alcohol. The peak incidence of head injury is in individuals between the ages of 15 and 24yrs and improved medical care has resulted in larger numbers of individuals surviving with neuropsychiatric consequences. Most head injury survivors who present to psychiatric services have emotional symptoms and personality changes ranging from subtle to severe. A smaller number manifest serious and lasting cognitive sequelae, such as apathy, disinhibition, and amnesia. There are also important acute psychiatric effects.

Acute psychological effects of head injury

Most significant head injuries are closed and involve a period of loss of consciousness (which may extend from brief concussion to prolonged coma). Often amnesia follows recovery of consciousness:

- **Post-traumatic amnesia (PTA)** extends from the time of the injury until normal memory resumes. Apparently normal behaviour often occurs during this period. PTA may end abruptly.
- **Retrograde amnesia (RA)** includes the period between the last clearly recalled memory prior to the injury and the injury itself. It is usually a dense amnesia that is brief, lasting seconds or minutes, and shrinks with time.

Acute post-traumatic delirium (PTD)

A state that may follow severe head injury and occurs as the individual begins to regain consciousness. This is sometimes also called 'post-traumatic psychosis' and is characterized by prolonged and variable confusion, with or without behavioural symptoms, anxiety, affective lability, paranoia, delusional misinterpretation, and hallucinations.

Factors associated with increased psychiatric morbidity following head injury

- Increased duration of loss of consciousness
- Increased duration of PTA
- Increased duration of PTD
- Increased age, arteriosclerosis, and alcoholism
- Increased area of damage
- Increased neurological sequelae (focal deficits, epilepsy, etc.)
- Dominant or bilateral hemisphere involvement

Chronic psychiatric syndromes following head injury

A number of chronic syndromes are recognized following head injury:

- **Cognitive impairment** Especially after closed head injuries with PTA lasting >24hr. There may be focal cognitive deficits such as amnesia, or diffuse problems including slowing, apathy, affective blunting, decreased concentration, executive difficulties, amnesia, and affective lability. Catastrophic reactions and emotional incontinence may occur. In its severest form the cognitive impairment may present as a dementia (post-traumatic dementia). If symptoms are severe, it is particularly important to exclude NPH, SDH, or co-existing DAT. *Treatment:* antipsychotics; stimulants.

- **Personality/behavioural changes** Personality changes are most likely after head injury to the orbito-frontal lobe or anterior temporal lobe. 'Frontal lobe syndrome' is characterized by disinhibition, impulsivity, irritability, and aggressive outbursts. *Treatment:* may include β-blockers (e.g. atenolol), carbamazepine.
- **Psychoses** A schizophrenia-like psychosis with prominent paranoia is associated with left temporal injury, while affective psychoses (esp. mania in 9% patients) are associated with right temporal or orbito-frontal injury. There is also an increased prevalence of schizophrenia post-head injury (2.5% develop the disorder). *Treatment:* cautious use of antipsychotics (risk of seizure), anticonvulsants.
- **Neurotic disorders** Depressive illness is most common but anxiety states (including PTSD) are common sequelae. Persistent depression and anxiety occur in roughly 1/4 of head injury survivors. Suicide risk is also higher post head injury. *Treatment:* SSRIs, ECT.
- **'Punch-drunk syndrome'** Boxers may develop diffuse injury to the cortex, basal ganglia, and cerebellum, giving rise to extra-pyramidal symptoms or a subcortical dementia. Pathology shows cerebral atrophy and neurofibrillary tangles.
- **'Post-traumatic syndrome'** Also called 'post-concussional syndrome'. This is a common phenomenon after head injury. The main symptoms are: headache; dizziness; insomnia; irritability; emotional lability; increased sensitivity to noise, light, etc.; fatigue; poor concentration; anxiety; and depression. Although this syndrome was previously thought to be a purely psychological phenomenon (since in many cases the injury was minor), it is now recognized that it probably involves a complex interplay of both organic and non-organic factors.

Factors influencing psychiatric disability and prognosis

- Mental constitution—i.e. vulnerability due to genetics, temperament (premorbid personality: increased risk in histrionic, hypochondriacal and dependent personalities), IQ (cerebral reserve), age.
- Emotional impact of injury—i.e. extent of psychological trauma.
- Setting, circumstances, and repercussions of injury.
- Iatrogenic factors.
- Home and social environment (including secondary gain issues).
- Compensation and litigation issues (including secondary gain issues).
- Post-traumatic epilepsy (PTE)—occurs in 5% closed and 30% open head injuries (usually during first year) and worsens prognosis.
- Size and location of brain damage: frontal, temporal, dominant side worse.

Sequelae in children

Less psychopathology after head injury due to increased brain plasticity. Recovery may continue for up to 5yrs after injury (as opposed to ~2yrs in adults). Problems are generally behavioural in nature and include aggression, delinquency and attention deficit hyperactivity disorder (ADHD)-like syndromes.

1 Rao V, Lyketsos C (2000) Neuropsychiatric sequelae of traumatic brain injury. *Psychosomatics* **41**: 95–103.

Psychiatric aspects of epilepsy 1

The lifetime prevalence of experiencing a 'seizure' is approximately 5%, while the prevalence of epilepsy (recurrent seizures) is 0.5–1%. Most (~60%) cases of epilepsy have unknown aetiology. Seizures may be *generalized* or *focal*. Generalized seizures involve the whole cortex and lead to loss of consciousness (LOC). Focal seizures begin in one area of the cortex and may become *secondarily generalized*. Focal seizures are sub-classified as *simple partial* (i.e. localized motor/sensory features without LOC or memory loss); *complex partial* (i.e. with or without aura/automatism, and associated changes in conscious level). Between 10% and 50% of patients with epilepsy have psychiatric symptoms.

Psychiatric aspects of epilepsy may be related to:
- Psychosocial consequences of diagnosis (e.g. unemployment, stigma and ostracism, restricted activities, dependency).
- Psychiatric syndromes directly attributed to epilepsy.
- Neuropsychiatric effects of medication.

Psychiatric syndromes attributed to epilepsy are best considered by their temporal relationship to seizures (pre-ictal, ictal, post-ictal, inter-ictal).

Pre-ictal
- Patients may experience a variety of vague symptoms during the days and hours leading up to the seizure. These are termed **prodromal symptoms** and include feelings of tension, dysphoria, and insomnia.
- An **aura** may occur immediately prior to seizure onset. This is most common in complex partial seizures (CPSs)—temporal lobe epilepsy or extra-temporal epilepsy (e.g. frontal CPSs). Auras are typically stereotyped, e.g. autonomic or visceral aura (epigastric sensation); derealization and depersonalization experiences; cognitive symptoms (dysphasia, 'forced thinking', ideomotor aura, déjà vu, jamais vu, fugue and twilight states); affective symptoms (anxiety, euphoria); perceptual experiences (auditory, visual, sensory, and olfactory hallucinations or illusions).

Ictal
- **Automatisms** May occur during the seizure and suggest a focal origin for the seizure such as medial temporal lobe. There is LOC during the ictus and amnesia for the automatism, which usually lasts <5mins. There are simple or complex stereotyped movements that tend to be disorganized and purposeless (although complex actions may be carried out). At this time the individual seems 'out of touch'. Automatisms may be the basis of twilight and fugue states (EEG may aid differential diagnosis).
- **Epilepsy partialis continuans (EPC)** A condition of prolonged CPSs, lasting hours–days (may be confused with delirium or psychosis) (e.g. temporal, frontal, or cingulate seizures). There are variable behavioural, cognitive, and perceptual symptoms and periods of amnesia.
- **Bizarre aggressive behaviour.**

Post-ictal

- **Post-ictal delirium** A very common (10%) confusional state following a seizure with disorientation, inattention, variable levels of consciousness, and sometimes paranoia. Tends to last hours to days and shows a trend towards improvement and normal consciousness. If prolonged, suspect EPC.
- **Post-ictal psychosis**[1] Usually follows a cluster of seizures or an increase in the frequency of seizures; may follow withdrawal of anticonvulsant therapy. Thought to result from sub-threshold kindling activity. It usually only occurs in individuals with epilepsy for >10yrs (particularly associated with a left temporal lobe focus). Clinically, there is an initial non-psychotic interval (lasting hours to weeks) following a seizure. Thereafter, the individual develops a brief psychotic episode with variable psychotic and affective symptoms. The episode resolves after a period of days to 1mth. It may recur 2 or 3 times in a year. EEG shows marked changes during the psychotic episode.

Inter-ictal

- **Brief inter-ictal psychosis** occurs unrelated to a seizure, when there is good control of epilepsy. In this way seizures are antagonistic to the psychosis in that the EEG normalizes during the psychosis. This is called *forced normalization*. A seizure may end the psychotic episode. This form of psychosis has been termed *alternating psychosis* (i.e. there is an inverse relationship between severity of epilepsy and severity of psychosis). There may be premonitory symptoms such as anxiety and insomnia while the psychosis is characterized by hallucinations and paranoia. Notably the antagonistic relationship between seizures and psychosis is demonstrated where anticonvulsants may aggravate psychosis, and where antipsychotics may reduce the seizure threshold.
- **Chronic inter-ictal 'schizophrenia-like' psychosis** A chronic schizophrenia-like psychotic illness is 6–12 times more common in epileptics than in the general population. It is particularly associated with left temporal lobe epilepsy and is more common in early onset severe epilepsy and in women with epilepsy. There is often a period of 10–15yrs that elapses between diagnosis of epilepsy and onset of the psychotic illness. Clinically the illness is very similar to idiopathic schizophrenia, although there tends to be a prominent affective component. The chronic course is likewise similar. There is typically no family history of schizophrenia and an absence of premorbid schizotypal traits. Pathologically, it may represent the cumulative effects of chronic kindling due to a temporal lobe focus, e.g. in temporal lobe epilepsy (TLE).

1 Sachdev P (1998) Schizophrenia-like psychosis and epilepsy: the status of the association. *Am J Psychol* **155**: 325–36.

Psychiatric aspects of epilepsy 2

Other presentations

Cognitive deterioration is a common outcome of chronic epilepsy and is caused by a number of factors, including repeated seizures with cerebral hypoxia as well as the neurological effects of chronic anticonvulsant therapy.

Neuroses Epilepsy is associated with a 50% risk of a major depressive episode. Suicide risk is also increased ×25 over non-epileptics. There is an increased prevalence of conversion disorder in epileptics, including an increased risk of 'pseudoseizures'.

Mania Flor-Henry first described the association between right-side TLE and manic illness.

Epileptic personality syndrome Also named the Waxman–Geshwind syndrome, this is a controversial phenomenon traditionally associated with chronic TLE. The classic traits include: religiosity; hyposexuality; hypergraphia; and 'viscosity of personality'.

Violence Also a controversial issue. There does seem to be an increased risk of violence and aggression in people with TLE or frontal lobe epilepsy. 'Episodic dyscontrol' is believed to be the result of sub-threshold kindling in these regions of the brain and anticonvulsants are often effective in reducing aggressive outbursts.

The ecstatic seizures of Prince Myshkin

He was thinking, incidentally, that there was a moment or two in his epileptic condition almost before the fit itself (if it occurred in waking hours) when suddenly amid the sadness, spiritual darkness and depression, his brain seemed to catch fire at brief moments…His sensation of being alive and his awareness increased tenfold at those moments which flashed by like lightning. His mind and heart were flooded by a dazzling light. All his agitation, doubts and worries, seemed composed in a twinkling, culminating in a great calm, full of understanding…but these moments, these glimmerings were still but a premonition of that final second (never more than a second) with which the seizure itself began. That second was, of course, unbearable.

Dostoevsky: *The Idiot*

HIV/AIDS and psychiatry 1

The HIV/AIDS epidemic means that, increasingly, psychiatrists are encountering individuals with psychological and neuropsychiatric complications of HIV infection. In some developing countries, rates of infection are as high as 20–30% (with rates in hospitals as high as 70–80%). Both diagnosis with the disease and the mortality associated with it have major consequences for the psychological and social functioning of individuals and their communities. In areas where large numbers of young adults are dying from the disease, there are even larger numbers of children becoming orphans, with all the developmental, emotional, and social problems associated with the loss of parental care and support. In other communities people with HIV/AIDS are subject to stresses related to their lifestyle choices (e.g. prejudice related to sexual orientation or directed at those with addictions). Stigma also contributes to the psychological burden of infected individuals and their families.

Improved outcome for patients on anti-retroviral therapy brings additional stresses related to living with uncertainty about the future. The responsibility of carers working with patients with HIV/AIDS goes far beyond treating immediate physical problems. Holistic practice requires the health care professional to adopt a true biopsychosocial approach with appreciation of the emotional state of the patient as well as the host of social, economic, spiritual, and ethical challenges accompanying diagnosis with the disease.

Contexts in which psychiatric problems may arise

There are a number of contexts in which psychiatric problems may arise in relation to HIV/AIDS:

- The 'worried well' (i.e. HIV -ve people may be concerned about being infected due to contact with HIV +ve sources/individuals).
- Pre-test anxiety.
- Post-test stress may precipitate a psychiatric illness such as adjustment disorder, major depressive episode, and suicidality.
- Living with HIV/AIDS often results in stressful life events (e.g. losing a job, becoming economically disadvantaged, experiencing social alienation).
- In some cases, individuals with psychiatric needs (e.g. victims of abuse; LD patients) may be more vulnerable to becoming infected with the virus.
- HIV directly infects neurons in the brain causing neuropsychiatric symptoms.
- HIV +ve individuals are susceptible to 2° opportunistic infections and/or tumours of the CNS, which may manifest as neuropsychiatric symptoms.
- Anti-retroviral medications may cause psychiatric symptoms (e.g. zidovudine [AZT (azidothymidine)] may precipitate a major depressive episode, while isoniazid prophylaxis has been known to [AET (azidothymidine)] precipitate a psychotic illness).

Counselling HIV/AIDS patients

- **Pre-test counselling** Consider: meaning of a +ve result; what actions the individual will take; confidentiality issues; fears of individual; high-risk behaviours; reactions to stress; social and other implications of +ve result.
- **Post-test counselling** Clarify distortions; assess emotions; decide who to tell; discuss prevention of transmission; offer support to individual and family.

Ethical issues

- **HIV testing**: issues of informed consent; only test without consent if a test result will significantly alter clinical management.
- **Confidentiality**: encourage individual to tell sexual partner and other medical personnel; if individual refuses, one may be obliged to inform without consent.
- **Resource allocation**: e.g. availability of anti-retroviral drugs.

HIV/AIDS and psychiatry 2: clinical presentations

Depression
At least 30–50% of individuals suffer a major depressive episode at some time following diagnosis. Clearly depression in this context has multiple causes and the challenge is to identify all the contributory factors. Depressive illness should be differentiated from physical effects of HIV (weight loss, loss of energy, etc.) as well as from HIV-associated dementia.

Treatment: SSRIs, but problems of weight loss and headache; newer compounds such as nefazodone and venlafaxine may be indicated.

Suicide
There is a 30x increased risk of suicide in individuals who are HIV +ve. High-risk times include: at diagnosis; at the death of an HIV +ve friend; as the individual experiences deterioration in physical health.

Mania
Manic symptoms may develop in the context of HIV psychosis or as a result of treatment with anti-retroviral agents such as zidovudine (AZT). *Treatment*: Lithium is preferable (beware risk of toxicity) since there is some evidence suggesting that sodium valproate may increase viral replication and reduce white cell count (WCC).

Anxiety
Infection with the virus is associated with increased risk of generalized anxiety disorder (GAD), panic disorder, PTSD, and OCD.

Chronic pain
Up to 80% of patients experience chronic pain at some point, in particular chronic headache. This may lead some individuals to self-medicate, putting them at risk of substance dependence.

Delirium
Delirium occurs in up to 30% of infected patients and is sometimes irreversible. It is caused either by direct infection of the brain by the virus or by 2° infections and/or tumours. Delirium may be the initial manifestation of HIV-associated dementia.

Psychosis
A psychotic illness characterized by fluctuating symptoms that may alter over hours to days may occur in the context of HIV infection. Atypical bizarre psychotic symptoms may give way to prominent mixed affective symptoms, which in turn may change to a withdrawn apathetic state.

Aetiological factors include the effects of stress, medications, and 2° infections/tumours superimposed on the effects of direct infection of the brain by the virus. Thus psychosis is a common early manifestation of subsequent HIV-associated dementia and it is likely that mild cognitive deficits co-exist with the psychotic illness.

Preferred treatment includes low-dose haloperidol or an atypical antipsychotic (e.g. olanzapine, quetiapine)—due to increased sensitivity to extra-pyramidal side-effects. Anti-retroviral agents such as zidovudine (AZT) may also reduce psychotic symptoms.

HIV-associated dementia (HAD)

Previously termed AIDS dementia, HAD is a relatively common outcome in full-blown AIDS.

Epidemiology 90% of AIDS patients have CNS changes post-mortem. 70–80% develop a cognitive disorder. 30% develop HAD. Mean survival after diagnosis with HAD is 6 months.

Pathology
(a) Direct CNS infection: HIV is neurotropic, entering the brain through endothelial gaps; the virus attaches to group 120 on CD4 +ve sites of microglial cells; a cascade opens calcium channels leading to glutamate and nitrous oxide excitotoxicity; this results in neuronal death and increased apoptosis. Sites include basal ganglia and subcortical and limbic white matter.
(b) Opportunistic infections/tumours: toxoplasmosis, papovavirus, cytomegalovirus (CMV), HSV, non-Hodgkin's lymphoma, and Kaposi sarcoma give rise to variable neuropathology including encephalitis and focal necrosis.

Clinical presentation
- *Early 'minor' cognitive disorder:* asymptomatic HIV +ve patients may have very early CNS infection that is often discounted as stress. Symptoms include cognitive slowing and memory deficits as well as motor slowing and subtle incoordination.
- *HIV-associated dementia (HAD):* with worsening of symptoms, the clinical picture constitutes a dementia syndrome and is an AIDS-defining disorder. Clinical features are classified as cognitive (subcortical dementia, focal cognitive deficits, amnesia, mutism), motor (movement disorders, e.g. tremor, ataxia, choreo-athetosis, spasticity, myoclonus), and affective (depression, apathy, agitation, disinhibition, mania). Cognitive decline can be assessed using the *HIV Dementia Scale and the Global Deterioration Scale of Reisberg* (functional measure).

Investigations CT/MRI: atrophy, ↑T2 signal. CSF: opportunistic infection, cytology, enzyme-linked immunosorbent assay (ELISA) +ve. EEG: generalized slowing.

Treatment Reverse transcriptase inhibitors (zidovudine [AZT]) delay HAD progression, while protease inhibitors reduce HIV load.

Neuropsychiatric aspects of CNS infections

Viral encephalitis

- **Mumps, varicella-zoster, arbovirus, rubella**—may result in behavioural problems, learning difficulties, and ADHD-like symptoms in children.
- **HSV 1**—involves inferior frontal and anterior temporal lobes, resulting—in the acute phase—in delirium, hallucinations, and TLE. Chronic outcomes include Korsakoff psychosis, dementia, and Kluwer–Bucy syndrome. *EEG*: slowing with bursts of increased slow-wave in the temporal region.
- **Influenza**—a rare chronic outcome is *encephalitis lethargica* (see 📖 p. 167), characterized by Parkinsonism, oculogyric crises, and psychosis.
- **Epstein–Barr virus/infectious mononucleosis**—may result in myalgic encephalitis or chronic fatigue syndrome.
- **Measles**—rarely gives rise to subacute sclerosing panencephalitis, a slow virus infection. *Features*: behavioural problems, deteriorating intellectual function, movement disorders (ataxia, myoclonus), seizures, and, finally, dementia in a child. *Pathology*: white and grey matter changes to occiput, cerebellum and basal ganglia. *EEG*: periodic complexes.

Tuberculosis

- **TB meningitis**—especially in children and young adults; caseating exudate covers the base of the skull leading to vascular infarcts and hydrocephalus; cranial nerves may become involved. *Psychiatric symptoms*: apathy; withdrawal; insidious personality changes; delirium; hallucinations; chronic behavioural problems.
- **Tuberculoma**—presents with focal signs, seizures, raised intracranial pressure (ICP).

Neurosyphilis

Historically known as **general paresis of the insane** or **Cupid's disease**, neurosyphilis is a chronic outcome of direct spirochaetal infection of the brain parenchyma. It manifests more commonly in men in their 40s–50s, roughly 15–20yrs after infection. The spirochaetes have a predilection for frontal and parietal lobes and the disease typically presents as a progressive frontal dementia.

Classic symptoms Grandiosity, euphoria, and mania with mood-congruent delusions. Disinhibition, personality change, and memory impairment are also common.

Neurological features Argyll–Robertson pupils; 'trombone tongue'; tremor; ataxia; dysarthria; myoclonus; hyperreflexia; spasticity; and extrapyramidal signs.

Megalomania in general paralysis

Gentlemen,—You have before you today a merchant, aged forty-three, who sits down with a polite greeting, and answers questions fluently and easily…His illness began about two years ago. He became absent-minded and forgetful, to such an extent at last that he was dismissed by the firm for whom he had worked. Then, a year ago, he became excited, made extensive purchases and plans, weeping now and then in the deepest despair, so that he had to be taken into the hospital. On admission, he felt full of energy…and intended to write verses here, where he was particularly comfortable. He could write better than Goethe, Schiller, and Heine. The most fabulous megalomania quickly developed. He proposed to invent an enormous number of new machines, rebuild the hospital, build a cathedral higher than that at Cologne, and put a glass case over the asylum. He was a genius, spoke all the languages in the world, would cast a church of cast-steel, get us the highest order of merit from the Emperor, find a means of taming the madmen, and present the asylum library with 1000 volumes, principally philosophical works. He had quite godly thoughts…When at its height, the disease may present a great resemblance to maniacal states, but the physical examination and proof of the defective memory will save us from confusing it with them. So also will the senseless nature of the plans and the possibility of influencing them, and the feebleness and yielding character of the manifestations of the will, which are all greater in general paralysis.

Kraepelin E (1913) *Lectures on Clinical Psychiatry*,
3rd English edn. London: Baillière, Tindall and Cox.

Autoimmune disorders and psychiatry

Systemic lupus erythematosus (SLE)

This multi-system autoimmune vasculitis is most common in women in their 30s and neuropsychiatric symptoms occur in 75% of individuals with the disease. CNS changes include microvasculitis with infarction, inflammation, and coagulopathy. Seizures, cranial nerve palsies, peripheral neuropathy, 'spinal stroke', and other focal signs may occur in addition to dermatological, rheumatological, haematological, and cardiovascular complications of the disorder. Importantly, drugs used to treat the condition may have psychiatric side-effects (e.g. steroids; isoniazid; hydralazine). Psychiatric symptoms occur in 60% of cases and syndromes include:

- **Lupus psychosis**—transient psychotic episodes with a recurrent and fluctuating course. Relapses are frequent and symptoms are variable with auditory and visual hallucinations as well as paranoia, affective instability, and disturbed sensorium characteristic of the illness. Severe and prolonged psychosis due to SLE may result in vascular dementia.
- **Depression**—up to 30% of SLE patients experience clinically significant depressive illness.
- **Schizophrenia-like psychosis**—a rare finding in SLE.

Polyarteritis nodosa (PAN)

Most common in young men, PAN is an immune-mediated necrotizing vasculitis characterized by saccular aneurysms and infarction. Neuropsychiatric findings include: stroke; focal signs; seizures; 'spinal stroke'; delirium; auditory and visual hallucinations.

Movement disorders in psychiatry

Movement disorders occur in three contexts within psychiatry:

- **Extra-pyramidal diseases with psychiatric symptoms** (e.g. Parkinson's disease)
- **Psychiatric disorders with abnormal movements** (e.g. stereotypies; tics)
- **Medication-induced movement disorders** (e.g. EPSEs)

Pathophysiology Movement disorders commonly involve a disequilibrium of neurotransmitters such as dopamine (DA), acetylcholine (ACh), and gamma-aminobutyric acid (GABA) within the circuits of the basal ganglia. Levels of DA and ACh tend to be inversely related. For example, in Parkinsonism, there is ↓DA with ↑ACh; conversely, chorea is characterized by ↑DA and ↓ACh.

Core symptoms in extra-pyramidal disease:

- **Negative symptoms**—bradykinesia, postural abnormalities, etc.
- **Positive symptoms**—rigidity and involuntary movements (resting tremor, chorea, athetosis, hemiballismus, dystonia)

Parkinsonism This is a syndrome characterized by 4 core symptoms: slow 'pill-rolling' tremor (4Hz); rigidity; bradykinesia; postural abnormalities.

Aetiology:

- Degenerative diseases—idiopathic Parkinson's disease (PD) (85% cases); progressive supranuclear palsy (PSNP); multiple system atrophy (MSA); corticobasal degeneration (CBD); ALS–dementia–Parkinson complex of Guam (ADPG)
- Medication—neuroleptics; antidepressants
- Toxins—cobalt; manganese; magnesium; organophosphates
- Infections—encephalitis lethargica (post-influenza); CJD
- Miscellaneous—CVA of the basal ganglia; trauma of the basal ganglia; NPH; neoplasia of the basal ganglia; dementia pugilistica (punch-drunk syndrome); Lewy body dementia

Multiple system atrophy (MSA) 3 syndromes: striatonigral degeneration; Shy–Drager syndrome; olivopontocerebellar degeneration. Characterized by: Parkinsonism; ataxia; vertical gaze palsies; pyramidal signs; autonomic abnormalities.

Progressive supranuclear palsy (PSNP) Also known as Steele–Richardson–Olszewski syndrome, PSNP has its onset in the 50s and 60s and is characterized by a tetrad of clinical findings: subcortical dementia; pseudobulbar palsy; supranuclear palsy; dystonia (of the head and neck).

Encephalitis lethargica Roughly 20yrs after the great influenza epidemic of the 1920s, large numbers of patients who had suffered influenza encephalitis during the epidemic developed this disorder (also called post-encephalitic Parkinsonism). **Clinical findings**: Parkinsonism; oculogyric crises; pupillary abnormalities; psychosis). The disorder was the subject of the book (and film) by Oliver Sacks entitled *Awakenings*.

Parkinson's disease (PD) and psychiatry

Parkinson's disease results in progressive impairment of voluntary initiation of movement, associated with a dementia of variable severity, as well as psychiatric morbidity. It is caused by gradual loss of dopaminergic neurons in the substantia nigra (pars compacta). This results in reduced DA and increased ACh in the basal ganglia. The remaining cells of the substantia nigra contain Lewy bodies.

Epidemiology Occurs in 20:100 000 people; typically has its onset in the 50s and peaks during the 70s; ♂:♀ = 3:2; 5% of cases are familial; 25% patients are disabled or die within 5yrs and ~60% within 10yrs; rare survival ~20yrs.

Symptoms and signs of PD
- **Tremor**—resting, 'pill-rolling' tremor of 4Hz; this is an early sign that may start unilaterally and may be asymmetrical in intensity; tremor increases with excitement or fatigue and diminishes during sleep.
- **Rigidity**—'lead-pipe' or 'cog-wheel' rigidity, especially in flexor muscles.
- **Bradykinesia**—slowness; difficulty initiating movement; reduced facial expression and blinking; 'mask facies'; reduced arm swing; 'festinating gait'; reduced voluntary speech; micrographia; 'freezing' episodes.
- **Postural abnormalities**—flexed posture; postural instability with frequent falls.
- **Autonomic instability**—postural hypotension; constipation; urinary retention; sweaty, greasy, seborrhoeic skin; hypersalivation with drooling.
- **Fatiguability**.
- **+ve glabellar tap**.
- **'Air pillow sign'**.

Dementia in PD

20–30% of patients develop some cognitive deterioration. Risk of dementia in patients with PD is increased 2–3-fold. Risk of dementia increases with increasing age, increasing severity of symptoms, and coexistent cardiovascular disease.

Clinically Usually a subcortical dementia with slowing, impaired executive function, personality change, and memory impairment. Some patients merely develop subtle cognitive deficits (difficulties with shifting and sequence).

Pathology Due to reduced DA in the frontal lobes; there is some evidence of overlap with DLB (📖 p. 140), while some patients have coexisting DAT.

Depression in PD

Very common finding with 40–70% patients affected. While depression may be partly reactive to receiving the diagnosis or experiencing a worsening of PD symptoms, the depressive illness may be due to the actual disease process itself. Specifically, reduced levels of monoamines (DA, NE, 5HT) may lead to depression. Mood fluctuations are often noted in association with changes in plasma DA levels. Depression in PD is more common in women and in left-sided disease and is often atypical in nature.

Treatment SSRIs; ECT (improves the depressive illness but can precipitate delirium).

Psychosis/delirium in PD

Psychotic depression is most common. Psychosis is commonly due to medications used in PD such as:

- Anticholinergics—delirium; agitation; hallucinations; etc.
- Levodopa (L-dopa) and DA agonists—10–50% have psychiatric complications including delirium, psychosis, and mania.

Treatment Use atypical antipsychotics with a lower risk of EPSEs.

Huntington's disease (HD)

A genetic disease characterized by a combination of progressive dementia and worsening chorea. There is autosomal dominant inheritance with
100% penetrance; thus 50% of a patient's offspring will be affected. Onset
of symptoms and diagnosis is usually after the patient has reproduced. A
diagnostic test has become available which allows presymptomatic diagnosis, but as no treatment is available, there are major ethical issues surrounding screening.

Pathology The genetic defect is a trinucleotide repeat of CAG—
between 37 and 120 repeats on chromosome 4. ↓↓GABA neurons in the
basal ganglia; this leads to increased stimulation of the thalamus and cortex
by the globus pallidus. Also increase in DA transmission.

Clinical features Classic triad of chorea, dementia, and a family history
of HD. Chorea is a movement disorder characterized by initial jerks, tics,
gross involuntary movements of all parts of the body, grimacing, and dysarthria. There is increased tone with rigidity and stiffness, positive primitive
reflexes, and abnormal eye movements.

Clinical course Onset usually during 30s and 40s; a small number of
juvenile onset cases; deteriorating course to death within 10–12yrs.

Psychiatric syndromes Occur in 60–75% of patients with HD.
• Anxiety and depression are common
• Psychosis occurs early and paranoia is common—'schizophrenia-like'
• Aggression and violence
• Subcortical dementia—slowing, apathy, and amnesia

Investigations EEG: slowing. CT/MRI: atrophy of basal ganglia with
'boxing' of the caudate and dilation of ventricles. PET: ↓metabolism in
the basal ganglia.

Treatment No treatment arrests the course of the disease. However,
haloperidol (or other antipsychotics) may help reduce abnormal
movements.

Wilson's disease (WD)

A rare genetic disease mapped to the long arm of chromosome 13 that involves an abnormality of copper metabolism. Copper deposits in the liver cause cirrhosis and in the basal ganglia, resulting in degeneration of the lentiform nucleus (hepato-lenticular degeneration).

Clinical features Onset in childhood/adolescence or early adulthood. Liver cirrhosis. Extra-pyramidal (E/P) signs include: tremor; dystonia; increased tone; flapping tremor of wrists; wing-beating tremor of shoulders; risus sardonicus of face; bulbar signs (dysphagia, dysarthria); Kayser–Fleisher rings (green-brown corneal deposits).

Psychiatric syndromes
- Mood disturbances—common
- Subcortical dementia—25%
- Psychosis—rare

Investigations ↑serum/urine copper; ↓caeruloplasmin.

Treatment Penicillamine.

Other movement disorders

Tics

Tics are spontaneous, stereotyped movements that can be motor or vocal and usually involve ↑DA in the basal ganglia. Tics are classified as 1° or 2°.

1° tics

A spectrum with genetic overlap with each other and with ADHD and OCD (📖 p. 376):
- Tourette's syndrome
- Transient tic disorder
- Chronic motor or vocal tic disorder

2° tics

- Infection—CJD; Sydenham's chorea; encephalitis
- Drugs—levodopa (L-dopa); methylphenidate; cocaine; amfetamines
- Other—toxic carbon monoxide (CO); CVA; trauma

Tremor

- **Exaggerated physiological tremor**—(8–12Hz); occurs at rest and with action; causes: stress; anxiety; caffeine; medications.
- **Essential tremor**—(6–12Hz); at rest, with action and postural; most noticeable symmetrically in upper limbs.
- **Extrapyramidal tremor**—(4Hz); resting tremor; e.g. Parkinsonism.
- **Cerebellar, midbrain, or red nucleus**—(4–6Hz); intention tremor; causes: trauma; vascular; MS; neoplasia; etc.

Catatonia (📖 p. 992)

A motor syndrome that has several causes and is diagnosed (DSM-IV) by the presence of 2 or more of the following:
- Motor immobility—catalepsy ('waxy flexibility'); stupor
- Motor excitement
- Negativism or mutism
- Posturing, stereotypies, or mannerisms
- Echolalia or echopraxia

Schizophrenia and related psychoses

Introduction

Schizophrenia and the related psychotic illnesses belong to a group of disorders traditionally called the 'functional psychoses'. 'Functional' in this context means a disorder of brain *function* with no corresponding *structural* abnormality. Despite improvements in our understanding of the pathology of these disorders, their aetiology is currently unknown and there is no definitive diagnostic test available. For this reason, diagnosis is made clinically, using operationally defined criteria (characteristic symptoms and signs) and specific exclusion criteria (e.g. absence of primary organic disorder).

The cardinal feature of schizophrenia and the related psychotic illnesses is the presence of psychotic symptoms—hallucinations and/or delusions. These symptoms are *qualitatively* different from normal experiences rather than the *quantitatively* abnormal responses of the neurotic and affective disorders and because of this they are regarded—by patients and other health professionals—as *more* serious and needing *immediate* psychiatric attention. However, when an individual experiences hallucinations or becomes paranoid that people are talking about them, for example, it does not mean they necessarily have a severe and enduring mental disorder. They could be experiencing a reaction to drugs (prescribed or recreational), be experiencing severe anxiety, be acutely confused, or have early signs of dementia. The differential diagnosis encompasses almost all psychiatric diagnoses (see 🔲 p. 180) as well as some 'normal experiences'. Careful history-taking and appropriate investigations (see 🔲 p. 187) are essential.

Of the psychoses, schizophrenia has received the greatest attention in terms of research. This is almost certainly because of the dramatic and devastating effects the disorder can have on an individual's quality of life and their prospects for employment, marriage, and parenthood. Schizophrenia affects about 1 in 100 individuals, usually beginning in late adolescence or early adulthood. Untreated, it runs a chronic, deteriorating course. In addition to the personal tragedy, schizophrenia creates a substantial public health burden due to the cost of lifelong health care needs and lost productivity.

The symptoms of schizophrenia are conventionally divided into positive symptoms (an excess or a distortion of normal functioning) and negative symptoms (a decrease or loss of functioning):

- **Positive symptoms** Delusions (commonly persecutory, thought interference, or passivity delusions). Hallucinations (usually auditory hallucinations commenting on the subject or referring to them in the third person e.g. 'he looks like a fool'). Formal thought disorder (a loss of the normal flow of thinking usually shown in the subject's speech or writing).
- **Negative symptoms** Impairment or loss of volition, motivation, and spontaneous behaviour. Loss of awareness of socially appropriate behaviour and social withdrawal. Flattening of mood, blunting of affect and anhedonia. Poverty of thought and speech.

Fortunately, there are effective interventions that can benefit individuals and help them to lead more normal lives. Current research is directed towards establishing the cause(s) of schizophrenia and investigating the possibility of *early* interventions in those identified at high risk for the disorder or with prodromal symptoms (possible early signs of the disorder). Other psychoses with more specific symptoms, e.g. delusional misidentification syndromes (see 📖 p. 230), may even help us understand how we normally perceive the world and help solve the mystery of the true nature of conscious experience.

Why are there so few famous people with schizophrenia?

Often there is a history of declining social and educational function which precludes significant achievements (sometimes in spite of early promise). The chronic course of the condition and the major disruptions caused by periods of more severe symptoms also make it less likely that a person with schizophrenia will achieve as much as their peers. Until relatively recently there have been few specific treatments for the disorder, and even today prognosis is at best guarded.

Nonetheless, there are notable exceptions to the rule: people who have battled with the disorder and achieved greatness in their chosen fields—in the arts, Vaslov Fomich Nijinski (1891–1950), the God of the Dance, whose personal account is to be found in his autobiography *The Diary of Vaslov Nijinksy* (1999); in sport, Lionel Aldridge (1941–1998), a member of Vince Lombardi's legendary Green Bay Packers of the 1960s, who played in two Super Bowls, and, until his death, gave inspirational talks on his battle against paranoid schizophrenia; and, in popular music, Roger (Syd) Barrett (1946–2006) of Pink Floyd and Peter Green (1946–) of Fleetwood Mac. Perhaps the most famous, due to a recent academy award-winning dramatization of his life, is the mathematician John Forbes Nash Jr (1928–), who was awarded (jointly with Harsanyi and Selten) the 1994 Nobel Prize in Economic Science for his work on game theory. His life story (upon which the film was based) is recorded by Sylvia Nasar in the book *A Beautiful Mind* (1998).

Historical views of schizophrenia

In 1856, Morel coined the term *Démence Précoce* to describe a once bright and active adolescent patient who had gradually become silent and withdrawn. Other clinical descriptions included Kahlbaum's *Katatonie* (1868), Griesinger's *primare Verrücktheit* (1868), Hecker's *Hebephrenie* (1869), and Sommer's inclusion of deteriorating paranoid syndromes in the concept of dementia (1894).

In 1896 Emil Kraepelin described and separated the two major forms of insanity on the basis of different symptoms, course, and outcome. The first, **manic-depressive insanity**, had a relapsing and remitting course, with full recovery after each episode. The second grouped together catatonia, hebephrenia, and the paranoid psychoses under the term **dementia praecox**, which had a progressive deteriorating course, where any improvement was only partial.

Over the next two decades (and further revisions of his textbook), Kraepelin's ideas were gradually accepted. Later the influence of Freud's psychoanalytical ideas shifted the focus from Kraepelin's 'disease of the brain' to a 'splitting of the mind' (schizophrenia), as proposed by Eugen Bleuler in his book *Dementia praecox or the group of schizophrenias* (1911). He believed the disorder to be due to a 'loosening of associations' between psychic functions, with fundamental symptoms being thought disorder, blunting/incongruity of affect, autism, and ambivalence. He added 'simple schizophrenia' to Kraepelin's subtypes and did not consider hallucinations, delusions, and catatonic symptoms to be necessary for the diagnosis. This view of schizophrenia was to have a profound influence on clinical practice, particularly in the USA.

European psychiatrists, particularly in Germany, continued to regard schizophrenia as a disease of the brain. Detailed classification systems were developed based on symptomatology, culminating in the teachings of Kurt Schneider, who described 'symptoms of first rank' in the acute phase of the illness (see 📖 p. 95) and 'second-rank symptoms' which, although highly suggestive of schizophrenia, could also occur in other psychoses (e.g. emotional blunting, perplexity, and other kinds of delusions and hallucinations).

The differences in diagnostic practices were highlighted in the 1970s. In 1972, Cooper found identical symptomatology in psychiatric admissions in New York and London, but higher rates of schizophrenia diagnosed in New York. Similarly, in 1973, the WHO's *International pilot study of schizophrenia* found the incidence of schizophrenia, using agreed diagnostic criteria, to be 0.7–1.4 per 10 000 aged 15–54 across all countries studied, but with much higher rates of diagnosis evident in the USA and the USSR. This was explained by broader syndrome definition, related in the USA to considering many milder abnormalities as part of the schizophrenia spectrum, and in the USSR to the political pressure to declare dissidents insane.

This led to an international push towards operationally defined criteria (based on symptoms and course), with various systems proposed. The St Louis Criteria (Feighner *et al.* 1972) require the patient to have been continuously ill for 6mths, with no prominent affective symptoms, the presence of delusions, hallucinations, or thought disorder, and for personal and family history to be taken into account (marital status, age under 40, premorbid social adjustment). Other systems adopt the Schneiderian concept of schizophrenia, including Catego (Wing *et al.* 1974)—a computer program that uses the Present State Examination (PSE) to generate diagnoses; Spitzer *et al.*'s (1975) research diagnostic criteria (RDC)—requiring at least 2wks duration, lack of affective symptoms, presence of thought disorder, and hallucinations and delusions similar to Schneiderian first-rank symptoms; as well as our current versions of the ICD-10 (WHO 1992) and the American Psychiatric Association's DSM-IV (1994) (see 📖 p. 178).

With the advent of neuroimaging, the biological substrate of schizophrenia could be investigated in the living brain. In 1974 Ingvar and Franzén showed, with the aid of radiolabelled xenon gas, that blood flow was reduced in the frontal lobes. In 1976 Johnstone *et al.* published the first controlled CT brain study which found enlarged ventricles associated with poorer cognitive performance. In the absence of an aetiological model of schizophrenia, pathophysiological models were developed to describe and explain the varieties of presentations found within the disease. In 1980 Crow described his 'Two syndrome hypothesis', dividing schizophrenia into *type 1* (predominant positive symptoms, acute onset, good premorbid adjustment, good treatment response, normal cognition and brain structure, reversible neurochemical disturbance) and *type 2* (predominant negative symptoms, insidious onset, poor premorbid adjustment, poor treatment response, impaired cognition, structural brain abnormalities—ventricular enlargement—underlying irreversible neuronal loss). The first quantitative MRI study by Andreasen *et al.* in 1986 also demonstrated smaller frontal lobes, and reduced intracranial and cerebral volume, providing further evidence for schizophrenia as a neurodevelopmental disorder.

Based upon examination of symptomatology and functional brain imaging Liddle (1992) identified three syndromes in schizophrenia disease processes with associated perfusion patterns. This 'Three syndrome hypothesis of schizophrenia' consists of: (1) *Psychomotor poverty syndrome*—poverty of speech, flattened affect, and decreased spontaneous movement; hypoperfusion of left dorsal prefrontal cortex, extending to the medial prefrontal cortex and the cingulate cortex and hypoperfusion in the head of caudate; reduced ability to generate action; (2) *Disorganization syndrome*—disorders of form of thought and inappropriate affect; hypoperfusion of right ventral prefrontal cortex and increased activity in anterior cingulate and dorsomedial thalamic nuclei projecting to the prefrontal cortex; relative hypoperfusion of Broca's area and bilateral hypoperfusion of parietal association cortex; reduced ability to inhibit inappropriate mental activity; and (3) *Reality distortion syndrome*—delusions and hallucinations; increased activity in left parahippocampal region and left striatum; disorder of internal monitoring.

Schizophrenia research in the last two decades has focused more on finding fundamental neuronal, neurochemical, or cognitive mechanisms than on localizing specific symptoms (see 📖 p. 182). It is hoped that this approach may provide workable hypotheses that can facilitate the search for molecular mechanisms and lead to new treatment approaches.

The diagnosis of schizophrenia

The diagnosis of schizophrenia is made on the basis of the patient's symptoms, and currently no confirmatory test is available. DSM-IIIR (and its successor DSM-IV) and ICD-10 set out operational criteria against which a clinical diagnosis can be confirmed (see Table 6.1). Both give greater weight to certain types of delusions or hallucinations formerly referred to as first-rank (see 📖 p. 95).

ICD-10 schizophrenia

1. At least one of the following:
- Thought echo, insertion, withdrawal, or broadcasting.
- Delusions of control, influence, or passivity; clearly referred to body or limb movements or specific thoughts, actions, or sensations; and delusional perception.
- Hallucinatory voices giving a running commentary on the patient's behaviour or discussing him/her between themselves, or other types of hallucinatory voices coming from some part of the body.
- Persistent delusions of other kinds that are culturally inappropriate or implausible (e.g. religious/political identity, superhuman powers and ability).

2. Or, at least two of the following:
- Persistent hallucinations in any modality, when accompanied by fleeting or half-formed delusions without clear affective content, persistent over-valued ideas, or occurring every day for weeks or months on end.
- Breaks of interpolations in the train of thought, resulting in incoherence or irrelevant speech or neologisms.
- Catatonic behaviour such as excitement, posturing, or waxy flexibility, negativism, mutism, and stupor.
- Negative symptoms such as marked apathy, paucity of speech, and blunting or incongruity of emotional responses.
- A significant and consistent change in the overall quality of some aspects of personal behaviour, manifest as loss of interest, aimlessness, idleness, a self-absorbed attitude, and social withdrawal.

3. Duration of ≥ 1mth.

DSM-IV schizophrenia

A. Characteristics of symptoms: two or more of the following, each present for a significant portion of time during a 1-mth period (or less if successfully treated):
- Delusions
- Hallucinations
- Disorganized speech
- Grossly disorganized or catatonic behaviour
- Negative symptoms (i.e. affective flattening, alogia, or avolition)

Note: Only one 'A' symptom is required if delusions are bizarre or hallucinations consist of a voice keeping up a running commentary on the person's behaviour or thoughts, or two or more voices conversing with each other.

B. Social/occupational dysfunction
C. Duration: continuous signs of the disturbance persist for at least 6mths. This 6-mth period must include at least 1mth of symptoms that meet criterion A.

Note: DSM-IV also allows for course specifiers: *episodic*—with (no) inter-episode residual symptoms (with negative symptoms); *continuous* (with prominent negative symptoms); *single episode in partial remission* (with prominent negative symptoms); *single episode in full remission*; *other or unspecified pattern*.

Table 6.1 Categories

ICD-10	DSM-IV	Key symptoms
Paranoid schizophrenia	Paranoid type	Delusions and hallucinations
Hebephrenic schizophrenia	Disorganized type	Disorganized speech behaviour (often silly/shallow) and flat or inappropriate affect
Catatonic schizophrenia	Catatonic type	Psychomotor disturbance (see p. 992)
Undifferentiated schizophrenia	Undifferentiated type	Meeting general criteria, but no specific symptom subtype predominates
Post-schizophrenic depression		Some residual symptoms, but depressive picture predominates
Residual schizophrenia	Residual type	Previous 'positive symptoms' less marked; prominent 'negative' symptoms
Simple schizophrenia		No delusions or hallucinations—a 'defect state' (negative symptoms) gradually arises without an acute episode

Differential diagnosis of schizophrenia

The differential diagnosis of schizophrenia is wide. Early in the course of the illness there may be significant uncertainty as to the true diagnosis. In general, compared to other disorders with psychotic symptoms, in schizophrenia there is a broader range of psychotic symptoms (e.g. other than relatively circumscribed delusions) and greater functional impairment.

Substance-induced psychotic disorder
(e.g., alcohol, stimulants, hallucinogens, steroids, antihistamines, sympathomimetics). Careful history-taking may reveal onset, persistence, and cessation of symptoms to be related to drug use or withdrawal.

Psychotic disorder due to a general medical condition
Focused history, examination, and investigations should help exclude other disorders including brain disease (e.g. head injury, CNS infection, CNS tumor, TLE, post-epileptic states, vCJD), metabolic (hypernatraemia, hypocalcaemia) or endocrine disturbance (hyperthyroidism, Cushing's syndrome).

Mood disorders with psychotic features
Mood and related biological symptoms are usually more severe and precede psychosis. The psychotic features will usually be *mood congruent* (📖 p. 236). There may be a personal or family history of affective disorder.

Acute/transient (brief) psychotic disorder and schizophreniform disorder
Diagnosed only after the psychotic symptoms have resolved based on the time course (see 📖 p. 226).

Sleep-related disorders
When symptoms characteristically only occur whilst falling asleep or on waking up (hypnagogic/hypnopompic hallucinations—see 📖 p. 57). If there is excessive daytime tiredness due to lack of sleep or side-effects of medication symptoms may occur at any time of the day.

Delusional disorder
Presence of at least one non-bizarre delusion with a lack of thought disorder, prominent hallucinations, mood disorder, and flattening of affect (see 📖 p. 220).

Dementia and delirium
Evidence of cognitive impairment or altered/fluctuating level of consciousness, respectively. Delirium characteristically has a waxing and waning course. *Note*: also consider 'late paraphrenia' which has an extensive literature and is thought to be distinct from delusional disorder and schizophrenia, associated with social isolation, ageing, medical problems/treatments, and sensory loss (see 📖 p. 522).

Body dysmorphic disorder
Significant overlap with delusional disorder, few significant differentiating factors exist (see 📖 p. 810).

Post-traumatic stress disorder
Evidence of a past, life-threatening trauma (see 📖 p. 390).

Pervasive developmental disorder
Evidence of impairment in functioning from the pre-school years.

Obsessive–compulsive disorder
Significant overlap with delusional disorder and, if reality testing regarding obsessions or compulsions is lost, delusional disorder is often diagnosed (see 📖 p. 376).

Hypochondriasis
Health concerns generally are more amenable to reality testing and are less fixed than in delusional disorder.

Paranoid personality disorder
Absence of clearly circumscribed delusions, presence of a pervasive, stable pattern of suspiciousness or distrust (see 📖 p. 495).

Schizotypal personality disorder
Odd or eccentric behavior, absence of clearly circumscribed delusions (see 📖 p. 495).

Misidentification syndromes
Easily confused with delusional disorder, may be associated with other CNS abnormalities (see 📖 p. 230).

Induced/shared psychotic disorder
Evidence that relatives or close friends share similar delusional beliefs (see 📖 p. 228).

Anxiety disorder
Sometimes patients use 'paranoia' or 'feeling paranoid' to describe over-concern, hypersensitivity, anxiety, agoraphobia, or social phobia—clarification is all that is required when terminology has acquired common parlance.

Factitious disorder
Rarely psychotic symptoms may be feigned, usually to avoid responsibilities and/or to maintain a sick role (see 📖 p. 814).

Aetiological theories

Neurochemical abnormality hypotheses

It seems unlikely that the aetiology of schizophrenia can be fully attributed to a single neurotransmitter abnormality (although there are precedents, notably Parkinson's disease). In the study of models for psychosis, particularly with the psychotomimetic (psychosis-mimicking) effects of certain drugs, there is evidence for the involvement of multiple neurotransmitters in the genesis of psychotic symptoms. Some of the evidence implicating different neurotransmitters is outlined here (📖 p. 182).:

Dopaminergic overactivity

- The fact that all known effective antipsychotics are DA antagonists.
- Positive correlation between the antipsychotic efficacy of a drug and its potency as a DA receptor antagonist.
- Induction of psychotic symptoms by dopaminergic agents (e.g. amfetamine, cocaine, phencyclidine [PCP], levodopa [L-dopa], bromocriptine).
- Imaging studies showing that amfetamine induces a greater displacement of radiolabelled-ligand bound to D_2 receptors in the striatum in never-treated schizophrenia patients (suggesting a predisposition to increased DA release).
- Evidence of a correlation between the DA metabolite homovanillic acid (HVA) plasma levels and both severity of psychotic symptoms and treatment response to antipsychotics.

Glutaminergic hypoactivity

- NMDA receptor antagonists, (e.g. ketamine, PCP) have been shown to induce both positive and negative symptoms of schizophrenia in healthy volunteers (possibly via modulation of the DA system) and exacerbate symptoms of patients with schizophrenia.
- The effects of ketamine (in both animals and humans) are attenuated by antipsychotic medication (notably clozapine).
- Facilitation of NMDA receptor function by glycine (which binds to a modulatory site on NMDA receptors) and D-cycloserine (a selective partial agonist at the glycine modulatory site) may lead to symptomatic improvement.

Serotonergic (5-HT) overactivity

- The primary mode of action of LSD is through partial 5-HT agonism, associated with sensory distortions and hallucinations.
- The efficacy of clozapine in treatment-resistant schizophrenia is thought to be due to its combined dopaminergic and serotonergic antagonism.

α-adrenergic overactivity

- Some antipsychotics also have clear adrenergic antagonism.
- Increased levels of noradrenaline (NE) have been found in the CSF of patients with acute psychotic symptoms.
- Chronic treatment with antipsychotic drugs leads to decreased firing rates in the locus coeruleus (the origin of the noradrenergic system).

γ-aminobutyric acid (GABA) hypoactivity
- Loss of GABA inhibition has been shown to lead to overactivity in other neurotransmitter systems (e.g. DA, 5-HT, NE).
- There is some evidence to support loss of GABAergic neurons in the hippocampus of patients with schizophrenia.
- Use of benzodiazepines may augment the therapeutic effects of antipsychotics by their GABA facilitation.

The neurodevelopmental hypothesis

Some authors hypothesize that schizophrenia may be a disorder of neurodevelopment based on the following:
- There is an excess of obstetric complications in those who develop the disorder.
- Affected subjects have motor and cognitive problems which precede the onset of illness.
- Schizophrenic subjects have abnormalities of cerebral structure at first presentation.
- Schizophrenic subjects have dermatoglyphic and dysmorphic features.
- Although the brain is abnormal, gliosis is absent—suggesting that differences are possibly acquired *in utero*.

The disconnection hypothesis

Neuropsychological, neuroanatomical, and functional investigations (SPET, PET, fMRI) have revealed:
- Widespread reductions in grey matter in schizophrenia (particularly temporal lobe).
- Disorders of memory and frontal lobe function occurring in a background of widespread cognitive abnormalities.
- Reduced correlation between frontal and temporal blood flow on specific cognitive tasks.
- A reduction in white matter integrity in tracts connecting the frontal and temporal lobes.

These findings have led to speculation that frontal–temporal/parietal connectivity may be the final common pathway for the development of schizophrenia.

Other theories

In the 1960s social theories of schizophrenia (e.g. schizophrenogenic mother, marital skew and schism) were common. They are now of historical interest only, not having withstood scientific scrutiny. A number of other theories exist, including those which postulate that schizophrenia is an abnormality of information processing (Braff, 1993), a problem of working memory (Goldman-Rakic, 1994), caused by cognitive dysmetria (Andreasen et al., 1999), an inability to think in 'meta-representations' or grasp 'theory of mind' (Pickup & Frith, 2001), a neurodegenerative disorder (Weiberger & McClure, 2002), a disorder of language (Berlim & Crow, 2003), or due to abnormal neuronal migration and the DISC1 gene (Johnstone et al., 2011).

Epidemiology of schizophrenia

Incidence

The incidence of schizophrenia worldwide is relatively similar when restricted, operational diagnostic criteria are used to establish the diagnosis. The incidence in the UK and US is around 15 new cases per 100 000 population. ♂ = ♀, although males tend to have an earlier onset than females (23 vs. 26yrs) and develop more severe illnesses. A few studies have reported a falling incidence over time, although this may be due to changing diagnostic practices/criteria.

Prevalence

The lifetime risk of schizophrenia is between 15 and 19 per 1000 population. The point prevalence is between 2 and 7 per 1000. There are some differences between countries, although these differences are minimized when a restrictive definition of schizophrenia based on first-rank symptoms is used.

Fertility

Early studies reported low fertility in both men and women with schizophrenia. More recent studies suggest that although men are reproductively disadvantaged, the fertility of women with schizophrenia has increased probably due to deinstitutionalization.

Mortality

The diagnosis of schizophrenia carries around a 20% reduction in life expectancy. Suicide is the most common cause of premature death in schizophrenia. It accounts for 10–38% of all deaths in schizophrenia. Risk is probably highest in the year after first presentation and is greater in men.

Morbidity

There is significant comorbidity in patients with schizophrenia:
- Common medical problems that occur more frequently, e.g. communicable diseases (HIV, HepC, TB), epilepsy, diabetes, arteriosclerosis, IHD.
- Rare conditions that co-occur with schizophrenia, e.g. metachromic leukodystrophy, acute intermittent porphyria, coeliac disease, dysmorphic features (high-arched palate, low-set ears, minor physical abnormalities).
- Substance misuse—cannabis, stimulants, and nicotine in particular.

Inheritance

Genetic factors account for the majority of liability to schizophrenia. Heritability estimates range from 60–80%. The risk of developing schizophrenia when one has an affected relative is shown in Table 6.2. Molecular genetic studies have implicated certain genes—most evidence is for:
- *Neuregulin*: NRG1 on chromosome 8p21-22—has multiple roles in brain development, synaptic plasticity and glutamate signalling.
- *Dysbindin*: DTNBP1 on chromosome 6p22.3—helps regulate glutamate release.

- *DISC1* (Disrupted In SChizophrenia): a balanced chromosomal translocation (1,11)(q42;q14.3)—has multiple roles in synaptic signalling and cell functioning.
- *Catecholamine O-methyl transferase* (COMT) polymorphism (e.g. valine to methionine substitution at codon 158—Val158Met): helps regulate dopamine function in the frontal cortex.

It is likely that an individual needs to have several genes 'of small effect' that interact with each other and with time-specific exposure to other environmental risk factors.

Environmental factors

The following have been associated with an increased risk of schizophrenia:

- Complications of pregnancy, delivery, and the neonatal period.
- Delayed walking and neurodevelopmental difficulties.
- Early social services contact and disturbed childhood behaviour.
- Severe maternal malnutrition.
- Maternal influenza in pregnancy and winter births.
- Degree of urbanization at birth.
- Use of cannabis, especially during adolescence.

Table 6.2 Schizophrenia liability based on affected relatives

Family member(s) affected	Risk (approximate)
Identical twin	46%
One sibling/fraternal twin	12–15%
Both parents	40%
One parent	12–15%
One grandparent	6%
No relatives affected	0.5–1%

Examination of the patient with psychotic symptoms

A thorough medical history, including a systematic review and thorough physical examination, is important is the assessment of all patients presenting with psychotic symptoms. It is all too easy to focus on the psychiatric aspects of the assessment to the exclusion of medical aspects which may inform the diagnosis and aid treatment planning.

Key features in systematic review
- Neurological—headache, head injury, abnormal movements of the mouth or tongue, diplopia, hearing or visual impairment (delusional disorder is more common when there is sensory impairment), fits/faints/blackouts/dizzy spells, altered consciousness or memory problems, stroke, coordination problems, marked tremor or muscle stiffness.
- Respiratory—dyspnoea, orthopnea.
- Cardiovascular—chest pain, palpitations.
- Gastrointestinal—constipation (can be side-effect of anticholinergic psychotropic drugs), nausea, vomiting.
- Genitourinary—urinary hesitancy (retention related to anticholinergic drugs); in women, a menstrual history; for both: sexual problems (which may be secondary to medication).

Mental state examination
- Aside from the more obvious psychotic features, a comprehensive assessment includes asking about mood, sleep, symptoms of anxiety, and cognitive function.
- Be sure to check orientation, attention, concentration, and anterograde/retrograde memory at a minimum—always consider underlying neurological condition when disorientation is present or if memory problems are severe or persistent in spite of adequate treatment.

Diagnostic formulation
Even in the absence of a specific cause, the aetiology of schizophrenia is predominantly influenced by factors affecting the brain. However, the following areas might be considered as a guide to the assessment of predisposing, precipitating, and perpetuating factors:
- **Biological** Consider family history of psychiatric illness, recent substance misuse, drug non-compliance, history of obstetric complications, brain injury, and comorbid medical illness.
- **Psychosocial** Consider recent stressful life events, family cohesion/friction, living conditions, attitude and knowledge of illness.

Physical examination
- Full physical examination is essential for all inpatients.
- The need for a complete physical examination in an outpatient setting tends to be based on presenting complaints and/or the availability of adequate facilities/time constraints.

- There really can be no excuse for overlooking systemic comorbidities—at the very least arrange for the primary care physician to review the patient or reschedule a longer appointment somewhere where facilities are available.
- A full neurological examination may be the most important investigation, and should focus on gait inspection; examination of the extremities for weakness and/or altered sensation; examination of hand–eye coordination; examination of smooth ocular pursuit; and examination of the cranial nerves. Scales, such as the Abnormal Involuntary Movement Scale (AIMS), may be useful to record and monitor potential movement side-effects of medication.

Investigations

Blood tests
- *Routine*: U&Es, LFT, calcium, FBC, glucose.
- *When suggested by history/examination*: VDRLs, TFTs, parathyroid hormone (PTH), cortisol, tumour markers.

Radiological
- CT or MRI in the presence of suggested neurological abnormality or persistent cognitive impairment.
- CXR only where examination/history suggests comorbid respiratory/cardiovascular condition.

Urine
- Urinary drugs screen (particularly stimulants and cannabis).
- Microscopy and culture (where history suggestive).

Other
- EEG rarely necessary unless history of seizure or symptoms suggest TLE.

Special investigations
- 24-hr collection for cortisol (if Cushing's disease suggested from history/examination).
- 24-hr catecholamine/5-HIAA collection for suspected phaeochromocytoma/carcinoid syndrome respectively.

Presentations of psychotic illness

When discussing the management of schizophrenia in particular, and the psychotic illnesses more generally, it is helpful to consider two distinct but related phases: the *acute psychotic episode* and the *maintenance phase*. An acute psychotic episode may represent a first episode or a relapse of schizophrenia or may represent another illness within the differential diagnosis (📖 p. 180). The aim of treatment in an acute episode is to abolish psychotic symptoms while minimizing distress and ensuring patient safety. Treatment of acute episodes is similar whatever the underlying diagnosis.

Once psychotic symptoms have been abolished (or improved as far as possible), one enters the maintenance phase. Here the concern shifts to prophylaxis (which often includes maintenance medication), rehabilitation, and maximization of function. Unfortunately acute psychotic relapse is possible in schizophrenia despite optimum maintenance treatment.

Prodromal schizophrenia

'Prodrome' is a retrospective concept relating to evidence of premorbid change in an individual who later develops a condition. In schizophrenia, there is evidence of prodromal symptoms in 80–90% of cases (10–20% have acute onset). The typical presentation is of non-specific or negative symptoms (early prodrome) followed by attenuated, mild, positive symptoms (late prodrome).[1] The main problem in detecting attenuated or subthreshold symptoms is that the rate of conversion to schizophrenia is low. Use of specific screening tools such as the PACE (Personal Assessment and Crisis Evaluation Clinic), COPS (Criteria of Prodromal Syndromes), or SIPS (Structured Interview for Prodromal Syndromes), raises detection rates to 20–40%.[2] These populations are perhaps better termed as having an 'at-risk' mental state (ARMS) for psychosis, or being at 'ultra high risk' (UHR) of psychosis. Whether treatment is indicated at this stage remains controversial (see 📖 p. 195).

The first schizophrenic episode

The first episode of schizophrenia in an individual generally occurs in late adolescence or early adult life. Many people experiencing their first episode will have no personal or family experience of mental ill-health and some will lack insight that their symptoms are a result of mental illness. As a result many patients will present in crisis and not directly complaining of psychotic symptoms. The range of possible presentations is very wide, however the following presentations (or their variants) are commonly seen:

- A spouse or relative noticing withdrawn or bizarre behaviour.
- Failure to achieve educational potential with referral by school or student health services.
- Onset of personality change, social withdrawal and 'odd' behaviour.
- Presentation via criminal justice system (see section on schizophrenia and offending, 📖 p. 690).
- Presentation following deliberate self-harm or suicide attempt.
- Complaining to council/police etc. on basis of delusional symptoms (e.g. hearing voices of neighbours throughout the night).

- Occasionally the first sign may be symptoms more typically characteristic of another disorder (e.g. depression, mania, OCD, panic disorder).

The first episode of schizophrenia is often a time of diagnostic uncertainty (and occasionally the diagnosis may take months/years to become clear). Frequently, the clinical picture includes comorbid substance misuse, personality difficulties, recent stressful life events, or a combination of all three. It is usually necessary to admit people suspected of first schizophrenic episodes in order to assess the extent of their psychopathology, to provide a time for education of both the patient and their family, and to provide pharmacological and psychological treatments in an environment where compliance can be carefully assessed. Inpatient admission is always necessary where the patient poses a significant danger to themselves or others.

Subsequent episodes

Subsequent presentations may be due to relapse of psychotic symptoms after remission, a deterioration in or a change in the quality of partially treated psychotic symptoms, or a crisis relating to life events in a patient who, as a result of their illness, has an impaired ability to manage stress.

Relapses can occur spontaneously in the absence of causative factors and in spite of good compliance with anti-psychotic treatment. However, very often relapses relate to medication non-compliance, drug or alcohol misuse or life stresses (or a combination of these).

Often in an individual patient the time course, prodromal features and symptomatology of a relapse are characteristic—the so-called 'relapse signature'. Educating patient and carers about these warning signs, and awareness of and documentation of these features within the treating team, are important parts of relapse prevention.

1 Yung AR, Phillips LJ, McGorry PD, *et al.* (1998) Prediction of psychosis: a step towards indicated prevention of schizophrenia. *Br J Psychiat* Suppl **172**: 14–20.
2 Miller TJ, McGlashan TH, Rosen JL, *et al.* (2002) Prospective diagnosis of the initial prodrome for schizophrenia based on the Structured Interview for Prodromal Syndromes: preliminary evidence of interrater reliability and predictive validity. *Am J Psychiat* **159**: 863–5.

Initial assessment of acute psychosis

Issues affecting initial management decisions

In view of the range and variety of presentations and the broad differential (💷 p. 180), it is difficult to be prescriptive in dealing with a patient who presents with psychotic symptoms. Symptoms may range from mild para-noid ideas to elaborate and firmly held delusions with associated auditory hallucinations urging the patient to violence. Often it is difficult to estab-lish a clear history initially, and assessment is focused on the immediate concerns:

- The risk they currently pose to themselves—not just the possibility of acts of self-harm or suicide, but also because of other aspects of their behaviour (e.g. police becoming involved, family relationships, work, continued driving, etc.).
- Risk of violence—the nature of risk (💷 p. 692) and any association with current symptoms (e.g. delusions about a specific person or group of individuals; what the 'voices' are telling them to do).
- The degree of insight retained by the patient and the likelihood of them cooperating with medical management.
- Whether hospital admission or transfer to a psychiatric ward is warranted to assess and manage the acute symptoms (with or without the use of the Mental Health Act).
- Whether their current behaviour is so disturbed as to require urgent treatment (💷 p. 990) to allow further assessment, including physical examination and other routine investigations (💷 p. 187).
- The person's current social circumstances and the level of support available to them (partner, relatives, friends, community psychiatric nurse [CPN], etc.) that may allow some flexibility in management (as well as being a source of third-party information).

The greatest influence on your course of action will often be the reason why the person has been referred in the first place (e.g. brought up by a concerned relative, no longer able to be managed at home, breach of the peace, self-referral because of own concerns, attempted suicide).

When there is a good account of the history of the presenting complaint(s), it may be possible to establish the most likely diagnosis and proceed accordingly, e.g. a drug- or alcohol-related disorder, acute confu-sional state (💷 p. 790), first episode of schizophrenia (💷 p. 188), relapse of known schizophrenia (💷 p. 189), delusional disorder (💷 p. 220), acute psychotic disorder (💷 p. 226).

During initial assessment, particularly with *unmedicated* patients, record (verbatim if possible) specific aspects of the patient's psychopathology (nature and content of delusions and hallucinations), before they become modified by the necessary use of medication. This information is important as it will influence later decisions regarding, for example, assessment of treatment response and need for continued use of the Mental Health Act (MHA).

Many patients with a psychotic presentation will have comorbid drug and/or alcohol problems. The fact that the psychotic episode is suspected to be wholly or partially attributable to comorbid substance use should not be allowed to affect the treatment offered acutely, which should be planned on the basis of the nature and severity of the psychotic symptoms and the associated risk. On recovery from the acute episode the comorbid substance use should become a focus for clinical attention.

The need for hospital admission

As noted in Issues affecting initial management decisions, 📖 p. 190, certain clinical features and situations will determine whether hospital admission (or transfer to psychiatric ward) is necessary:

- High risk of suicide or homicide.
- Other illness-related behaviour that endangers relationships, reputation, or assets.
- Severe psychotic, depressive, or catatonic symptoms.
- Lack of capacity to cooperate with treatment.
- Lack or loss of appropriate psychosocial supports.
- Failure of outpatient treatment.
- Non-compliance with treatment plan (e.g. depot medication) for patients detained under the MHA.
- Significant changes in medication for patient at high risk of relapse (including clozapine 'red' result—📖 p. 213).
- Need to address comorbid conditions (e.g. inpatient detoxication, physical problems, serious medication side-effects).

Suitability of the ward environment

A busy psychiatric ward may not be an ideal environment for a patient experiencing acute psychotic symptoms. As far as possible the person should be nursed in calm surroundings (a single room, if possible), with minimal stimulation (e.g. unfamiliar people, TV, radio). A balance should be struck between the need for regular observation and the likelihood that this may reinforce persecutory delusions. If behaviour becomes unmanageable, despite regular medication, it may be necessary to consider referral of the patient to a more secure environment, e.g. an intensive psychiatric care unit (IPCU).

Early review

Regular review is critical in the first 72hrs to assess any improvement in mental state, response to medication, level of observation needed, and carry out statutory duties under the MHA (including the need for continued detention, if emergency powers have been used). This is also a time for information-gathering from friends, family, GP, other agencies, etc. and organizing any investigations, including physical examination and routine blood tests that may not have been possible initially.

Initial treatment of acute psychosis

The management of psychotic patients should include, wherever possible, the usual features of good medical practice: undertaking a comprehensive assessment of medical, social, and psychological needs; involving patients and their relatives in decisions about medical care; and providing patients and carers with clear verbal and, if necessary, written information (see NICE guidelines, Box 6.1).

Emergency treatment of behavioural disturbance

Follow guidance as detailed for the management of acute behavioural disturbance (🕮 p. 990).

Points to note

- Attempts to defuse the situation should be attempted, whenever possible.
- Reassurance and the offer of voluntary oral/intramuscular medication is often successful.
- The content of delusions and hallucinations is of poor diagnostic value, but may better predict violence/behavioural disturbance.
- Act decisively and with sufficient support to ensure restraint and forcible administration of medication proceeds without unnecessary delay or undue risk to the patient or staff.
- Do not attempt to manage severe violence on an open ward when secure facilities with appropriately trained staff are available elsewhere.

Instigation of antipsychotic treatment

In the treatment of psychotic symptoms, antipsychotic medication has the strongest evidence base. Although little evidence exists to support the choice of one drug over the other, the following may be used as a guide to treatment.

Option 1

- Commence an SGA (e.g. olanzapine, amisulpride, risperidone, quetiapine—see p. 202) at an effective dose (see the *British National Formulary* [BNF]).
- Use long-acting BDZ (e.g. diazepam) to control non-acute anxiety/behavioural disturbance.

Option 2

- Prescribe a low potency FGA (such as chlorpromazine, initially in the range 75–200mg/day in divided doses) for a first episode.
- Increase the dose according to clinical effect and the need for sedation.
- Previous episodes and the response/side-effects experienced should inform the management of subsequent episodes.
- No additional antipsychotic benefit is likely when doses of 400–600mg chlorpromazine (or equivalent) are exceeded; however, sedation may be a useful effect of increasing the dose above this level.

Extra-pyramidal side-effects (EPSEs)

Extra-pyramidal side-effects including dystonias, Parkinsonism and akathisia are common side-effects of treatment with antipsychotic medication, and are a frequent cause of non-compliance.

- EPSEs are less likely with option 1, although the tolerability of both options overall is approximately equal.
- Prescribe procyclidine (or alternative) orally as required for Parkinsonian side-effects.
- Review regularly, since requirement for procyclidine may diminish over time and the drug may contribute to non-response and tardive dyskinesia.

Box 6.1 Updated NICE guidelines (CG82[1]) advice on second generation antipsychotics (SGAs)

Although previous guidelines (2002) had advocated use of 'atypical' drugs as first line choice, this is no longer the case. Instead, for people with newly diagnosed schizophrenia, NICE advises:

- Offering oral antipsychotic medication.
- Providing information and discuss the benefits and side-effect profile of each drug with the service user.
- The choice of drug should be made by the service user and health care professional together, considering: the relative potential of individual antipsychotic drugs to cause extra-pyramidal side-effects (including akathisia), metabolic side-effects (including weight gain) and other side-effects (including unpleasant subjective experiences); the views of the carer where the service user agrees.
- Not initiating regular combined antipsychotic medication, except for short periods (e.g. when changing medication).
- Offering clozapine to people with schizophrenia whose illness has not responded adequately to treatment despite the sequential use of adequate doses of at least two different antipsychotic drugs, at least one of which should be a non-clozapine second generation antipsychotic.

1 NICE clinical guideline 82 (Mar 2009) Schizophrenia: core interventions in the treatment and management of schizophrenia in adults in primary and secondary care. http://www.nice.org.uk/nicemedia/live/11786/43608/43608.pdf

Maintenance phase

The post-acute phase

With the emergence of 'stability' (i.e. less active psychotic symptoms, less behavioural disturbance), treatment shifts towards the gradual simplification of medication regimes and maximization of tolerability. The patient may be more able to engage actively with other therapeutic modalities available in the hospital environment. Time to remission of symptoms is very variable and may take 3–9mths or more. It is important the patient and their family/friends have realistic expectations.

Continuing treatment

A more considered view of management may be taken once maximal improvements are considered to have occurred. This is the time to establish the *minimal effective dose of medication* and maintenance regimes can often be significantly lower than those needed for management of the acute phase of the illness. A secondary goal is the minimization of side-effects with the aim of establishing compliance with medication. Finally, there is the more complex goal of rehabilitation: returning the patient to their highest possible level of social and occupational functioning. The final steps in this process may require the input, where available, of better resourced multidisciplinary rehabilitation units or community teams over many months with the ultimate aims of successful discharge (📖 p. 196) and outpatient follow-up (📖 p. 198).

Comorbid depression

Depression can affect up to 70% of patients in the acute phase but tends to remit along with the psychosis. In the maintenance phase, post-psychotic or post-schizophrenic depression occurs in up to 1/3 of patients and there is some evidence that TCAs (e.g. imipramine) may be effective. Surprisingly, despite it being common clinical practice, there are few studies supporting other interventions such as SSRIs.

Managing negative symptoms

Specific interventions may help to mitigate the impact of persistent negative symptoms:
- Ensure EPSEs (esp. bradykinesia) are detected and treated by anticholinergics, amantadine, reducing antipsychotics, or switching to lower potency/SGA agent.
- If there is evidence of dysphoric mood consider treating with antidepressants, anxiolytics, reducing antipsychotic dose, supportive management, or switching to SGA.
- Address the contribution of the environment (e.g. institutionalization, lack of stimulation) by resocialization and/or rehabilitation.
- If patient is on long-term medication consider reduction to minimal reasonable maintenance dose, switching to SGA, or clozapine.
- If clozapine is prescribed, consider augmentation with antidepressant, lamotrigine, or a suitable second antipsychotic (see 📖 p. 208).

Addressing comorbid substance use

As previously noted there is significant comorbidity of substance abuse in patients with schizophrenia. Whilst this may complicate and exacerbate positive and negative symptoms, sometimes patients believe they are self-medicating and may be reluctant to give up a 'useful' treatment. Elements of a pragmatic approach include:

- A comprehensive assessment, including why and how substances are taken, as well as routine testing for substance misuse.
- Optimization of antipsychotic medication and consideration of clozapine for patients with persisting substance misuse.
- The offer of specific treatment for substance misuse and possibly referral to local drug and alcohol services—whilst psychosocial approaches will be the mainstay (including relapse prevention), the possible benefits of pharmacotherapy should not be ignored e.g. nicotine substitution/withdrawal, alcohol detoxification, opiate substitution.

Box 6.2 A note on prodromal interventions

Before an individual fulfils DSM-IV/ICD-10 criteria for schizophrenia, there may be an intervening period of disturbed behaviour and partial psychotic symptoms that suggest, especially in the presence of other risk factors, that schizophrenia is imminent and inevitable (see p. 188). This observation has led some to propose early interventions for schizophrenia which aim to prevent a schizophrenic episode by treating these prodromal symptoms. Preliminary evidence suggests that low-dose antipsychotics, CBT, and antidepressants can improve presenting symptoms[1]. However, there is no convincing evidence yet that any intervention can delay, prevent, or reduce the severity of the onset of a psychotic illness. Neither is there evidence that the mean duration of untreated psychosis (DUP) in patients who develop psychosis improves the long-term outcome. Recent guidance (e.g. BAP Schizophrenia Consensus Group) recommends[2]:

- Develop a therapeutic relationship to allow for further assessment, review, 'watchful waiting', and monitoring of symptoms.
- Assess the nature and impact of any substance use.
- Any use of antipsychotic medication should be treated as an off-label, short-term, individual trial using the lowest possible dose and with careful monitoring of symptom response and side-effects.
- Individual CBT is an acceptable alternative to drug treatment.

The resource implications necessitate a specific early intervention service which may not be economically justified.

---

1 Ruhrmann S, Bechdolf A, Kühn K-U, *et al.* (2007) Acute effects of treatment for prodromal symptoms for people putatively in a late initial prodromal state of psychosis. *Br J Psychiat* **191** (Suppl. 51): 88–95.

2 www.bap.org.uk/pdfs/Schizophrenia_Consensus_Guideline_Document.pdf

Discharge planning

Good communication between members of the multidisciplinary team (psychiatry, community nurse, GP, social worker, etc.) is essential for good overall care. This may be formalized using the care programme approach (CPA), when patients are detained under the MHA, although many of the components are useful in everyday practice:

Components of CPA (as implemented in Edinburgh):
- Assess clinical and other needs.
- Formulate a care plan.
- Arrange discharge planning meeting where patient, carer(s), and key clinical staff are invited.
- Appoint a care manager who should be contacted in case of concern.
- Maintain contact with the patient.
- Decide on criteria for recall and/or other interventions.
- Document the people involved in the care package and their responsibilities.
- Arrange to meet again as a group.

Medication

Continue antipsychotic medication at minimum necessary dose. Possible regimes include:
- An SGA antipsychotic (e.g. amisulpride, olanzapine, risperidone, quetiapine).
- A preferably non-sedating, FGA antipsychotic (e.g. trifluoperazine, flupentixol, haloperidol).
- Depot antipsychotic medication, particularly where use of oral medication has resulted in relapse due to non-compliance. Depot medication is slightly more effective[1] than oral antipsychotic treatment.
- High-potency FGA antipsychotics (trifluoperazine, haloperidol) and olanzapine may be given once daily. This may be an advantage in non-compliant, institutionalized, or cognitively impaired patients.
- In patients with complicated drug regimes, cognitive impairment, or dubious compliance, consider a compliance aid such as a multicompartment compliance aid (e.g. Dosette® box).

Psychological[2]
- Family therapy and psychoeducation are effective in reducing relapse.
- Less convincing evidence also exists for CBT.
- Compliance therapy may be helpful.

Social/community
- Social work and housing involvement are often necessary.
- Community psychiatric nurses (CPNs) may help to provide information/education and monitor for early signs of relapse.
- For patients on depot, non-attendance at GP surgery/CPN appointment may act as an early warning system.

Service provision

- Community mental health teams provide effective treatment.
- Assertive community treatment may provide additional benefits.
- CPA may reduce the risk of losing contact.
- Day hospitals can provide an alternative to inpatient care in some situations.

1 Adams CE, Fenton MK, Quraishi S, and David AS (2001) Systematic meta-review of depot antipsychotic drugs for people with schizophrenia. *Br J Psychiat* **179**: 290–9.
2 Nadeem Z, McIntosh A and Lawrie S (2003) Schizophrenia. *Clin Evidence* **9**: 1103–33.

Outpatient treatment and follow-up

Medical
- Conduct a MSE at every appointment.
- Enquire about side-effects and attitude to medication.
- Record any recent life events or current stresses.
- Enquire about suicidal ideas and, if appropriate, homicidal ideas.
- When symptoms appear unresponsive to treatment, review the history and provide additional investigations/interventions as appropriate (e.g. clozapine).
- Conduct appropriate investigations where complications of illness or its treatment arise (e.g. LFTs, FBC, U&Es, glucose), or where monitoring is indicated (e.g. high-dose guidelines ⬚ p. 209, ECG— when cardiac complications are common).

Psychological
- Above all, try to provide supportive and collaborative treatment wherever possible.
- Provide education about schizophrenia and its treatment.
- Do not dismiss concerns, even if apparently based on delusional content.[1]
- Offer to meet family members or carers where appropriate.
- Be aware that following an acute episode, post-psychotic depression (see ⬚ p. 194) is particularly common but also treatable.[2]

Social
- Remember statutory obligations (e.g. review of compulsory powers).
- Consider referral to social work where there are housing, benefit, or other problems.
- Drop-in community centres and other support provided by non-statutory or voluntary organizations are often helpful.
- Consider interventions offered by other professions (e.g. occupational therapy, physiotherapy) when particular problems arise (e.g. poor sleep, hygiene, anxiety management, etc.).
- Some patients and their carers find user organizations helpful (e.g. SANE or Rethink—see useful addresses ⬚ p. 1017).

There is usually a large degree of uncertainty regarding the course and prognosis in first-episode patients, regardless of their presenting symptoms or demographic/personal history.

Box 6.3 Outcome in schizophrenia

Approximate guide to course and prognosis at 13yrs' follow-up:[1]
- Approximately 15–20% of first episodes will not recur.
- Few people will remain in employment.
- 52% are without psychotic symptoms in the last 2yrs.
- 52% are without negative symptoms.
- 55% show good/fair social functioning

Prognostic factors

Poor prognostic factors
- poor premorbid adjustment
- insidious onset
- onset in childhood or adolescence
- cognitive impairment
- enlarged ventricles
- symptoms fulfil more restrictive criteria (e.g. DSM-IV)

Good prognostic factors
- marked mood disturbance, especially elation, during initial presentation
- family history of affective disorder
- female sex
- living in a developing country

1 Mason P, Harrison G, Glazebrook C, *et al.* (1995) Characteristics of outcome in schizophrenia at 13 years. *BJP*, **167**: 596–603.

1 McCabe R, Heath C, Burns T, and Priebe S (2002) Engagement of patients with psychosis in the consultation: conversation analytic study. *BMJ* **325:** 1148–51.
2 Whitehead C, Moss S, Cardno A, and Lewis G (2003) Antidepressants for the treatment of depression in people with schizophrenia: a systematic review. *Psychol Med* **33:** 589–99.

First generation antipsychotics (FGAs)

Group 1—aliphatic phenothiazines

Chlorpromazine-like drugs with mainly anti-adrenergic and antihistaminergic side-effects including pronounced sedation, moderate antimuscarinic effects and moderate EPSEs (for drug doses equivalent to 100mg chlorpromazine—see Table 6.3).

Chlorpromazine (non-proprietary and Largactil®)
- 75–300mg daily in divided doses (or at night)—max 1g daily
- Available as I/M injection (25–50mg every 6–8hrs)
- Also available as 25mg or 100mg suppositories

Promazine
- 400–800mg daily in divided doses
- Rarely causes haemolytic anaemia
- Usually used for agitation and restlessness, e.g. 100mg qds (25–50mg for elderly)

Group 2—piperidine phenothiazines

Thioridazine-like drugs with mainly antimuscarinic side-effects and fewer EPSEs than groups 1 and 3

Pericyazine (Neulactil®)
- 75–300mg daily in divided doses
- In behavioural management: 15–30mg daily in divided doses

Group 3—piperazine phenothiazines and others

Trifluoperazine-like drugs with mainly anti-dopaminergic side-effects. These drugs are potent antipsychotics but tend to produce troublesome EPSEs, particularly at higher doses. They have limited sedative properties.

Trifluoperazine (non-proprietary and Stelazine®)
- No stated maximum dose
- For psychosis or behavioural management—5mg bd increased by 5mg after 1wk then every 3 days according to response

Fluphenazine (Prolixin)
- Available in decanoate (long-acting) form

Perphenazine (Fentazin®)
- 12–24mg daily
- For behavioural management usually 4mg tds
- Rarely causes SLE

Flupentixol (Depixol®)
- 3–9mg twice daily (max 18mg daily)
- Also available as depot (see 🕮 p. 216)

Zuclopenthixol (Clopixol®)
- 20–30mg daily in divided doses, max 150mg daily
- Available in injectable forms as *acetate*—for management of acute behavioural disturbance (Clopixol acuphase®) and *decanoate*—for depot injection (Clopixol Conc®)—see 🕮 p. 216

Haloperidol (non-proprietary and Haldol®)
- 1.5–5mg 2–3 times daily in divided doses (max 30mg daily)
- Available as IM injection (2–10mg every 4–8 hrs, max 18mg daily)

Pimozide (Orap®)
- 2–20mg daily
- Increase slowly by 2–4mg at intervals not less than 1wk
- May be more effective for monodelusional states, e.g. hypochondriasis, delusional jealousy

Sulpiride (non-proprietary and Dolmatil®)
- 200–400mg twice daily
- Lower max dose for negative symptoms (800mg daily) than for positive symptoms (2.4g daily)

Table 6.3 Antipsychotic dose equivalents

Drug	Equivalent dose
ORAL	
1st generation	
Benperidol	2mg
Chlorpromazine	100mg
Flupentixol	2mg
Haloperidol	3mg
Pericyazine	24mg
Perphenazine	8mg
Pimozide	2mg
Promazine	100mg
Sulpiride	200mg
Trifluoperazine	5mg
Zuclopenthixol	25mg
2nd generation	
Amisulpride	100mg
Aripiprazole*	10mg
Clozapine	100mg
Olanzapine	5mg
Paliperidone*	0.75–1.5mg
Quetiapine*	50–75mg
Risperidone	0.5–1mg
DEPOT	
Flupentixol decanoate	10mg/wk
Fluphenazine decanoate	5–10mg/wk
Haloperiol decanoate	15mg/wk
Olanzapine pamoate*	37.5mg/wk
Paliperidone*	7.5mg/wk
Pipothiazine palmitate	10mg/wk
Risperidone depot	12.5mg/wk
Zuclopenthixol decanoate	100mg/wk

*based on efficacy data

Second generation antipsychotics (SGAs[1])

Although not a separate class of antipsychotics, the newer 'atypical' drugs do have a slightly different pharmacokinetic profile. They have a wider therapeutic range and are generally less likely to cause EPSEs and raise serum prolactin levels (for completeness, additional SGAs are listed in Box 6.4).

Olanzapine (Zyprexa®)
- Receptor antagonism: $5\text{-}HT_{2A} = H_1 = M_1 > 5\text{-}HT_{2C} > D_2 > \alpha_1 > D_1$.
- Optimum dose 5–20mg per day.
- Available as an orodispersible tablet, a short-acting intramuscular (IM) injection and depot (olanzapine embonate/olanzapine pamoate or ZypAdhera® see 📖 p. 217).
- EPSEs similar to placebo in clinical doses with less increase in prolactin than haloperidol or risperidone.
- Side-effects of sedation, weight gain, dizziness, dry mouth, constipation, and possible glucose dysregulation.

Risperidone (Risperdal®)
- Receptor antagonism: $5\text{-}HT_2 > D_2 = \alpha_1 = \alpha_2$; little histamine H_1 affinity; minimal D_1, $5\text{-}HT_1$ affinity.
- Available as orodispersible tablet and depot preparation (Risperdal Consta® see 📖 p. 217).
- Dosage 4–6mg daily given in 1–2 doses (max 16mg daily).
- Less EPSEs than conventional antipsychotics at lower doses, but dystonias and akathisia can occur (esp. if dose >6mg or in elderly) and can raise prolaction (PL) and cause weight gain.

Paliperidone (Invega®)
- Paliperidone (9-OH risperidone) is the major active metabolite of risperidone.
- Receptor antagonism: as for risperidone.
- Available as modified release tablet or depot preparation (Xeplion® see 📖 p. 217).
- Dosage 6mg in the morning, adjusted in increments of 3mg over at least 5 days; usual range 3–12mg daily.
- Low potential for EPSEs and, due to limited hepatic metabolism, reduced drug interactions.

Quetiapine (Seroquel®)
- Receptor antagonism: $H_1 > \alpha_1 > 5\text{-}HT_2 > \alpha_2 > D_2$.
- Usual dose 300–450mg daily in two divided doses (max 750mg daily).
- EPSEs = placebo with no increase in prolactin.
- Can cause sedation, dizziness (postural hypotension), constipation, dry mouth, weight gain, and alterations in triglycerides and cholesterol.

Clozapine (Clozaril®, Denzapine®, Zaponex®)

See 📖 pp. 210–15.

Amisulpride (non-proprietary and Solian®)

- Selective and equipotent antagonism for D_2 and D_3 with negligible affinity for other receptors.
- Similar efficacy to haloperidol for acute and chronic schizophrenia.
- Optimum dose 400–800 mg (max 1.2g) per day in two divided doses.
- Lower dose (50–300 mg) may be more effective for patients with mainly negative symptoms.
- EPSEs similar to placebo at lower doses but dose-dependent EPSEs and prolactinaemia at higher doses.
- Less weight gain compared with risperidone or olanzapine.

Aripiprazole (Abilify®)

- D_2 receptor partial agonist; partial agonist at 5-HT$_{1A}$ receptors; high-affinity antagonist at 5-HT$_{2A}$ receptors; low/moderate affinity antagonist at H_1 and α_1 receptors; no anticholinergic effect.
- Dosage 10–30mg once daily, optimum dose 10–20mg once daily.
- Low EPSEs similar to placebo at all doses (akathisia-like symptoms can occur in the first 2–3wks of treatment with associated insomnia—use of additional hypnotic may be clinically necessary).
- Does not increase plasma prolactin levels (and may decrease levels) and weight gain is less likely.

---

1 In deference to the BNF and in light of recent controversies over classification of antipsychotics, we have adopted the abbreviations & FGA and SGA for consistency only. It may in fact be better to simply call them all 'antipsychotics'. For further discussion see Kendall T (2011) The rise and fall of the atypical antipsychotics *Br J Psychiat* **199**: 266–8.

Box 6.4 Other SGAs (not currently listed in BNF)

Zotepine (Zoleptil®)

Discontinued by Healthcare Logistics from the UK market from Jan 2011 for commercial reasons.

- High affinity for D_1 and D_2 receptors, also 5-HT$_2$, 5-HT$_6$, and 5-HT$_7$ receptors, 25–100mg tds
- Inhibits NE re-uptake
- Effective against positive and negative symptoms of schizophrenia but controlled trial data limited
- EPSEs less than FGAs
- Increased risk of seizures at higher doses (above 300mg)
- Weight gain, sedation, constipation, asthenia, dry mouth, akathisia
- Raised hepatic enzymes

Sertindole (Serdolect®)

Voluntarily withdrawn by Lundbeck in Dec 1998 due to concerns about arrhythmias associated with increase in QTc. Limited reintroduction in Jun 2002 in Europe under strict monitoring for patients in clinical trials and who are intolerant of at least one other antipsychotic.

- D_2, 5-HT$_2$, and α_1 antagonist with D_2 limbic selectivity
- Effective against positive and negative symptoms of schizophrenia
- 12–20mg single daily dose (max 24mg daily)
- EPSEs = placebo
- Increase in QTc—needs ECG monitoring
- Other side-effects include: nasal congestion, decreased ejaculatory volume, postural hypotension and dry mouth and raised liver enzymes

Approximate guide to course and prognosis at 13 years' follow-up:[1]

- Approximately 15–20% of first episodes will not recur.
- Few people will remain in employment.
- 52% are without psychotic symptoms in the last two years.
- 52% are without negative symptoms.
- 55% show good/fair social functioning

Prognostic factors

Poor prognostic factors

- poor premorbid adjustment
- insidious onset
- onset in childhood or adolescence
- cognitive impairment
- enlarged ventricles
- symptoms fulfill more restrictive criteria (e.g. DSM-IV)

Good prognostic factors

- marked mood disturbance, especially elation, during initial presentation
- family history of affective disorder
- female sex
- living in a developing country

Antipsychotic side-effects

Tolerability

No single antipsychotic is substantially better tolerated than another at daily doses of <12mg haloperidol or equivalent. However, FGAs prescribed above this range are less well tolerated and probably also less effective than SGA drugs (Box 6.5). The choice of antipsychotic therefore depends substantially on the profile of side-effects and which ones are more important to avoid.

- **Sedation** *Avoid* chlorpromazine/promazine. *Prescribe* high-potency antipsychotics (e.g. haloperidol) or non-sedating SGA (risperidone, amisulpride).
- **Weight gain** *Avoid* phenothiazines, olanzapine and clozapine. *Prescribe* haloperidol, fluphenazine.
- **EPSEs** *Avoid* high-dose FGAs. *Prescribe* SGA.
- **Postural hypotension** *Avoid* phenothiazines. *Prescribe* haloperidol, amisulpride, trifluoperazine.

Extra-pyramidal side-effects (EPSEs)

- *Acute dystonia* Contraction of muscle group to maximal limit, typically sternocleidomastoid and tongue, although can be widespread (e.g. opisthoclonus); eye muscle involvement (e.g. oculogyric crisis) may occur. Virtually always distressing and preceded by increasing agitation. *Treatment* Parenteral antimuscarinic (e.g. procyclidine 10mg intravenously [IV])—see 🕮 p. 954 for more detail.
- *Parkinsonism* Tremor, rigidity, and bradykinesia occurring >1wk after administration. *Treatment* Consider dose reduction/use of oral antimuscarinic (e.g. procyclidine 5mg three times daily [tds])—see 🕮 p. 944 for more detail.
- *Akathisia* Restlessness, usually of lower limbs, and a drive to move. Occurs usually >1mth after initiation of antipsychotic drug. *Treatment* Propranolol and benzodiazepines may be helpful. Symptoms can be notoriously difficult to treat—see 🕮 p. 946 for more detail.
- *Tardive dyskinesia (TD)* Continuous slow writhing movements (i.e. athetosis) and sudden involuntary movements, typically of the oral–lingual region (chorea). Symptoms of TD tend to be irreversible. *Treatment*[1] Although a consequence of antipsychotic treatment, there is little evidence that a reduction in the dose of antipsychotic improves symptoms in the short or long term. Vitamin E may prevent deterioration but does not improve established symptoms—see 🕮 p. 950.

Anticholinergic side-effects

Dry mouth, blurred vision, difficulty passing urine, urinary retention, constipation, rarely: ileus, glaucoma.

Anti-adrenergic side-effects

Postural hypotension, tachycardia (sometimes bradycardia), sexual dysfunction (particularly erectile dysfunction—see 🕮 p. 938).

Antihistaminic side-effects

Sedation, weight gain (although precise mechanism unclear—see
📖 p. 930).

Idiosyncratic

Cholestatic jaundice, altered glucose tolerance, hypersensitivity reactions, skin photosensitivity (sun block important in sunny weather), yellow pigmentation to skin (chlorpromazine), neuroleptic malignant syndrome (rigidity, fluctuating consciousness, and pyrexia)—may be fatal, requires immediate transfer to general medical care and usually ICU/anaesthetic support/dantrolene may be helpful—see 📖 p. 956 for more detail.

Box 6.5 SGAs vs. FGAs?

Recent effectiveness studies such as the Clinical Antipsychotic Trials of Intervention Effectiveness (CATIE),[1] the Cost Utility of the Latest Antipsychotic drugs in Schizophrenia Study (CUtLASS),[2] and the European First-Episode Schizophrenia Trial (EUFEST)[3] have been interpreted as showing no differences between FGAs and SGAs (with the possible exception of clozapine and perhaps olanzapine). Although this may be true in terms of overall effectiveness, most clinicians (and patients) would agree there are many real differences among drugs, particularly when it comes to side-effects. Whilst guidelines from NICE or the BAP may provide helpful frameworks for rational prescribing, treatment ought to be individualized through a shared decision-making process. Tolerability is a huge factor in adherence (see 📖 p. 924) and it ought to be remembered that the best antipsychotic in the world will not work if the patient does not actually take it.

1 Lieberman JA, Stroup TS, McEvoy JP, et al. (2005) Effectiveness of antipsychotic drugs in patients with chronic schizophrenia. *NEJM* **353**: 1209–1223.
2 Jones PB, Barnes TRE, Davies L, et al. (2006) Randomized controlled trial of the effect on quality of life of second- vs. first-generation antipsychotic drugs in schizophrenia: Cost Utility of the Latest Antipsychotic Drugs in Schizophrenia Study (CUtLASS 1). *Arch Gen Psychiatry* **63**: 1079–87.
3 Kahn RS, Fleischhacker WW, Boter H, et al. (2008) Effectiveness of antipsychotic drugs in first-episode schizophrenia and schizophreniform disorder: an open randomised clinical trial. *Lancet* **371**: 1085–97.

1 Soares-Weiser KV and Joy C (2003) Miscellaneous treatments for neuroleptic-induced tardive dyskinesia. *Cochrane Database Syst Rev* **3**: CD000208.

An approach to treatment-resistant schizophrenia (TRS)

Definition
Treatment resistance is the failure to respond to two or more antipsychotic medications given in therapeutic doses for 6wks or more. Patients with refractory symptoms generally have more severe functional impairments and are more likely to have abnormalities of cerebral structure and neuropsychology. See Box 6.6 for guidelines.

Prevalence
Approximately 30% of patients respond poorly to antipsychotic medication, and the number of people who show 'total non-response' is ~7%.

Aetiology
The aetiology is uncertain. However, the following factors may be important:
- Neurodevelopmental factors: soft signs, history of obstetric complications, cognitive impairment.
- Drug non-compliance.
- Lack of adequate treatment: poor drug administration/absorption. However, over-treatment (>12mg haloperidol or equivalent) may also lead to poor tolerability/response.
- Aggravating factors *despite* adequate treatment: concurrent drug or alcohol misuse, anticholinergic effects of anti-Parkinsonian medication or antidepressants.

Management
- *Clarify diagnosis* The clinical history and presentation should always be re-inspected to ensure the correct diagnosis has been reached.
- *Address comorbidity* Comorbid substance misuse is common in schizophrenia and worsens outcome.
- *Non-compliance* Consider interventions such as psychoeducation, compliance therapy, or family therapy to improve compliance with prescribed medication.
- *Pharmacological interventions* Clozapine is the intervention most strongly supported by the evidence, and there is evidence that depot antipsychotic medication may convey a small advantage over an oral dose.
- *Clozapine resistance* Switching from clozapine to a previously untried SGA (e.g. olanzapine, risperidone, quetiapine) might be of benefit in partial treatment resistance. In more difficult cases, augmentation of clozapine with benzamides (sulpiride, amisulpride) and anti-epileptics (lamotrigine) shows some success[1].
- *Rehabilitation* Consider the role of NHS /non-NHS rehab facilities in maximizing function, maintaining quality of life, and supporting those who remain symptomatic despite treatment—best evidence supports combination of medication with psychosocial treatments.

Box 6.6 Guidelines for the use of high-dose antipsychotics

Where a patient has failed to respond to, or has only partially responded to, antipsychotic medication, some practitioners advocate high-dose prescribing. High-dose prescribing refers either to the prescription of a single antipsychotic at doses greater than the BNF maximum, or the prescription of two or more antipsychotics with a combined chlorpromazine equivalent dose of >1g daily (see the table on 📖 p. 201). Although there may be a therapeutic response to this approach in some individual patients *there is no evidence* that high-dose prescribing confers any therapeutic advantage. The Royal College of Psychiatrists[1] suggest the following guidelines for high-dose prescribing:

- High-dose antipsychotic prescribing (>1g chlorpromazine or equivalent) should be avoided wherever possible.
- Consider alternative approaches including adjuvant therapy and newer or SGA antipsychotics such as clozapine.
- Bear in mind risk factors, including obesity—particular caution is indicated in older patients, especially those over 70.
- Consider potential for drug interactions.
- Where patients receive one or more antipsychotics at high dose, regular physical examination, ECG, LFTs, U&Es, FBC should be performed.
- Carry out ECG to exclude abnormalities such as prolonged QT interval; repeat ECG periodically and reduce dose if prolonged QT interval or other adverse abnormality develops.
- Increase dose slowly and not more often than weekly.
- Carry out regular pulse, blood pressure, and temperature checks; ensure that patient maintains adequate fluid intake.
- Consider high-dose therapy to be for a limited period and review regularly; abandon if no improvement after 3 months (return to standard dosage).
- A local protocol should exist for the purpose of informing good medical practice.

1 Royal College of Psychiatrists London, Council Report CR138 (May 2006) *Consensus statement on high-dose antipsychotic medication.* 🕸 http://www.rcpsych.ac.uk/files/pdfversion/CR138.pdf

1 Kerwin, RW and Bolonna, A (2005) Management of clozapine-resistant schizophrenia. *Adv Psychiat Treat* **11**: 101–6.

Clozapine 1: general guidelines

Clozapine, an SGA antipsychotic, is a dibenzodiazepine derivative. Shortly after its introduction to clinical practice in the mid-1970s it was withdrawn from use because of several episodes of fatal agranulocytosis in patients on treatment. It was thought to have special efficacy in treatment-resistant schizophrenia, and this clinical belief was supported by an important trial by Kane *et al.* (1988), leading to its reintroduction in psychiatric practice, albeit with strict limitations to its prescription. Patients on clozapine and doctors prescribing the drug must be registered with a central monitoring agency and have regular, initially weekly, full blood counts with discontinuation of the drug where there is evidence of neutropenia.

Evidence from a Cochrane systematic review[1] has shown clozapine to be more effective than FGA medication in the management of acute schizophrenia (NNT 6) in both the short- and long-term and of even greater benefit in those patients resistant to FGAs (NNT 5). Clozapine is also more acceptable in long-term treatment than FGA antipsychotic drugs (usually haloperidol or chlorpromazine: NNT 6).

In the CATIE trial (McEvoy *et al.* 2006),[2] clozapine was demonstrated to be superior in both treatment response (positive and negative symptoms) and compliance for patients who failed to improve on an SGA and who were randomized to receive either another SGA or clozapine.

NICE guideline[3] (CG82 Schizophrenia (update) Mar 2009)

NICE recommends: *'Offer clozapine to people with schizophrenia whose illness has not responded adequately to treatment despite the sequential use of adequate doses of at least two different antipsychotic drugs. At least one of the drugs should be a non-clozapine second-generation antipsychotic.'*

Mode of action

Clozapine mainly blocks D_1 and D_4 receptors; its effects on D_2 receptors are relatively less than traditional FGAs. The lower affinity of clozapine for D_2 receptors may partially explain its lack of EPSEs and hyperprolactinaemia. Clozapine does have significant anticholinergic, antihistaminergic, and anti-adrenergic activity, which accounts for its common side-effects (see p. 214).

The superior efficacy of clozapine in treating resistant schizophrenic patients may be due to its additional blockade of $5HT_2$ receptors. Antipsychotic activity also may be due to an increased turnover of GABA in the nucleus accumbens, which inhibits dopaminergic neurons.

Pharmacokinetics

Rapidly absorbed when taken orally (unaffected by food). Extensive first-pass metabolism means only 27–50% of a dose reaches the systemic circulation unchanged, with wide interindividual variations in the resulting plasma concentrations (influenced by factors such as smoking, hepatic metabolism, gastric absorption, age, and possibly gender). Steady-state plasma concentrations take 7–10 days of treatment. Mean terminal elimination half-life ranges from 6–33hrs. Onset of antipsychotic effect may take several weeks, but maximal effects can require several months (and improvement may continue for up to 2yrs).

Interactions (see Table 6.4 for summary)

- Lithium can increase the risk of developing seizures, confusion, dyskinesia, and possibly neuroleptic malignant syndrome (NMS).
- May interfere with the action of AChEIs (e.g. donepezil and tacrine).
- Smoking cigarettes increases the clearance of clozapine and may result in a substantial reduction in clozapine plasma concentrations.
- Plasma concentrations of clozapine are increased by caffeine (caffeinism is surprisingly common in this population), hence dose changes will be necessary when there is a change in caffeine-drinking habits.

Contraindications

Previous/current neutropenia or other blood dyscrasias; previous myocarditis, pericarditis and cardiomyopathy; severe renal or cardiac disorders; active or progressive liver disease/hepatic failure. (See BNF for a complete list.)

Table 6.4 Clozapine interactions

Effect	Examples
Increased drowsiness, sedation, dizziness, and the possibility of respiratory depression	Ethanol, H_1-blockers, opiate agonists, anxiolytics, sedatives/hypnotics, tramadol, and TCAs
Increased possibility of developing myelosuppressive effects	Use of clozapine with other drugs known to cause bone marrow depression (e.g. chemotherapy agents)
Drugs known to induce CYP1A2 activity may reduce efficacy	Carbamazepine, phenobarbital, phenytoin, rifabutin, and rifampicin
Drugs known to inhibit the activity of CYP1A2 may increase clozapine serum levels	Cimetidine, clarithromycin, ciprofloxacin, diltiazem, enoxacin, erythromycin, or fluvoxamine
Drugs known to inhibit the activity of CYP2D6 may increase clozapine serum levels	Amiodarone, cimetidine, clomipramine, desipramine, fluoxetine, fluphenazine, haloperidol, paroxetine, quinidine, ritonavir, sertraline, and thioridazine
Highly protein-bound drugs (may increase serum concentrations)	Digoxin, heparin, phenytoin, or warfarin
Worsening of anticholinergic effects	H_1-blockers; phenothiazines; TCAs; and other drugs with antimuscarinic properties
Increased risk of hypotension	Antihypertensive agents

1 Wahlbeck K, Cheine M and Essali MA (2003) Clozapine versus typical neuroleptic medication for schizophrenia. *Cochrane Database Syst Rev* **3**: CD000059.
2 McEvoy JP, Lieberman JA, Stroup TS, *et al.*, and CATIE Investigators (2006) Effectiveness of clozapine versus olanzapine, quetiapine, and risperidone in patients with chronic schizophrenia who did not respond to prior atypical antipsychotic treatment. *Am J Psychiat* **163**: 600–10.
3 ⟳ http://guidance.nice.org.uk/CG82/NICEGuidance/pdf/English.

Clozapine 2: starting and stopping

Initiation of treatment and monitoring

This is best done as either an inpatient or where appropriate facilities exist for monitoring (e.g. at a day-patient facility). All patients must be registered with a monitoring service (see Table 6.5). A normal leukocyte (WBC > 3500/mm^3, neutrophils > 2000/mm^3) count must precede treatment initiation. FBCs must be repeated (and sent to monitoring service) at weekly intervals for 18wks and then fortnightly until 1 year. Blood monitoring should continue monthly indefinitely thereafter. If there are concerns about compliance, serum blood levels may also be checked (see 📖 p. 928 for reference range).

Table 6.5 Clozapine monitoring services

Brand (manufacturer)	Formulation	Monitoring
Clozaril® (Novartis)	T: 25mg (scored), 100mg	Clozaril Patient Monitoring Service (CPMS) Login: https://www.clozaril.co.uk/
Denzapine® (Merz)	T: 25mg (scored), 50mg, 100mg	Denzapine Monitoring Service (DMS) Login: https://www.denzapine.co.uk/
	S: 50mg/mL	Support: http://www.denzapinesupport.co.uk/
Zaponex® (TEVA UK)	T: 25mg (scored), 100mg	Zaponex Treatment Access System (ZTAS) Login: http://www.ztas.co.uk/

Key: T=tablets; S=suspension

Dose (see Table 6.6)

- Starting regime: 12.5mg once or twice on first day, then 25–50mg on second day, then increased gradually (if well tolerated) in steps of 25–50mg daily over 14–21 days up to 300mg daily in divided doses (larger dose at night; up to 200mg daily may be taken as a single dose at bedtime).
- May be further increased in steps of 50–100mg once or twice weekly.
- Usual dose 200–450mg daily (max 900mg daily).
- *Note:* increase in seizure frequency occurs above 600mg/day.

'Traffic light' notification

Telephone (urgent action)

- *No sample received* Send another sample to CPMS/DMS/ZTAS and the local haematology laboratory so that the next supply of medication may be dispensed.
- *Sample non-suitable for analysis* As for 'no sample received'.
- *Abnormal haematological results* (e.g. neutrophil count). Either repeat the blood count or STOP clozapine with advice regarding further monitoring (i.e. *Red light* situation—see **Written reports**, 📖 p. 213).

Written reports

- *Green light* Normal—clozapine may be administered to the patient.
- *Amber light* Caution—further sampling advised. If either WCC falls to 3000–3500/mm^3 or the absolute neutrophil count falls to 1500–2000/mm^3, blood monitoring must be performed at least twice weekly until the WCC and absolute neutrophil count stabilize within the range 3000–3500/mm^3 and 1500–2000/mm^3, respectively, or higher.
- *Red light* STOP clozapine immediately. If the WCC < 3000/mm^3 or the absolute neutrophil count < 1500/mm^3, discontinue treatment with clozapine. Take blood samples daily until abnormality is resolved. Seek specialist advice from a haematologist. Monitor patients closely for symptoms suggestive of infection. Do not administer other antipsychotic drugs.

Discontinuation

Abrupt discontinuation of clozapine is not recommended, unless required by the patient's medical condition (e.g. leukopenia). *Gradually discontinue* over 1–2wks (like the initiation schedule in reverse). Patients should be carefully observed for the recurrence of psychotic symptoms during drug discontinuation. Symptoms related to cholinergic rebound, such as profuse sweating, headache, nausea, vomiting, and diarrhoea may also occur.

Table 6.6 Clozapine dosing guidelines

Day	Morning dose (mg)	Night-time dose (mg)
1	–	12.5
2	12.5	12.5
3	25	25
4	25	25
5	25	50
6	25	50
7	50	50
8	50	75
9	75	75
10	75	100
11	100	100
12	100	125
13	125	125
14	125	150
15	150	150
18	150	200
21	200	200
28	200	250

Note: Gradually increase by 50–100 mg/week (max dose should not exceed 900 mg/day). Routine blood level monitoring is not recommended; however, increasing dose until a plasma level of 350mcg/L is achieved is sometimes recommended. If adverse effects are noted, reduce dose until side-effects settle, then increase again more slowly. Lower doses may be required for elderly, female, or non-smoking patients, and if the patient is on other medication that may affect the metabolism of clozapine. Where there has been a break in treatment of more than 48 hr, treatment should be re-initiated with 12.5mg once or twice on the first day, and re-escalated.

Clozapine 3: side-effects

(See Table 6.7 for management)

Common side-effects
- *Anticholinergic* Constipation, dry mouth, blurred vision, difficulty passing urine.
- *Anti-adrenergic* Hypotension, sexual dysfunction.
- *Other* Sedation, weight gain, nausea, vomiting, ECG changes, headache, fatigue, hypersalivation, tachycardia, hypertension, drowsiness, dizziness.

Less common
- Fainting spells.
- Gastric discomfort.
- Small involuntary muscle contractions.
- Periodic catalepsy (reduced responsiveness and prolonged lack of movement).
- Enuresis.

Rarer or potentially life-threatening
- Impaired temperature regulation, fever, hepatitis, cholestatic jaundice, pancreatitis.
- *Agranulocytosis:* leukopenia, eosinophilia, leukocytosis. (*Note:* the risk of **fatal agranulocytosis**[1] is estimated to be 1:4250 patients treated.)
- Thrombocytopenia (discontinuation of clozapine is recommended if platelet count falls below 50 000/mm^3).
- Dysphagia.
- Circulatory collapse, arrhythmias, myocarditis, cardiomyopathy, pericarditis, pericardial effusion, thromboembolism. Discontinue if persistent tachycardia occurs in the first 2mths of treatment. *Note:* The risk of **fatal myocarditis** or **cardiomyopathy** is estimated to be up to 1:1300 patients treated, although there is wide variation in data (e.g. USA—1:67 000 patients treated).
- Pulmonary embolism (*Note:* The risk of **fatal pulmonary embolism** is estimated to be 1:4500 patients treated.)
- Confusion, delirium, restlessness, agitation.
- Diabetes mellitus, hypertriglyceridaemia, intestinal obstruction, paralytic ileus, enlarged parotid gland, fulminant hepatic necrosis.
- Interstitial nephritis, priapism, skin reactions.
- Neuroleptic malignant syndrome.

Of note: clozapine actually *reduces* mortality in schizophrenia, mainly due to a lower risk of suicide.

Table 6.7 Dealing with clozapine side-effects

Problem	Possible solution
Constipation	Encourage high-fibre diet, adequate fluid intake, use of aperients if persistent
Fever	Symptomatic relief, check FBC and look for sources of infection
Hypersalivation	Consider use of hyoscine hydrobromide (up to 300 micrograms tds)
Hypertension	Monitor closely, slow rate or halt dose increase, if persistent consider use of hypotensive agent (e.g. atenolol)
Hypotension	Advise caution when getting up quickly, monitor closely, slow or halt dose increase
Nausea	Consider use of anti-emetic (avoid metoclopramide and prochlorperazine if previous problems with EPSEs)
Neutropenia/ agranulocytosis	Stop clozapine, if outpatient admit to hospital
Nocturnal enuresis	Avoid fluids in the evening, alter dose scheduling, if severe consider use of desmopressin
Sedation	Reschedule dosing to give smaller morning or total dose
Seizures	Withhold clozapine for 24 hr, recommence at lower dose, consider prophylactic anticonvulsant (e.g. valproate)
Weight gain	Dietary and exercise counselling (see 🕮 p. 930)

1 A report of data from the Clozaril® National Registry revealed that agranulocytosis occurred in 400 (0.6%) of 67 600 patients during the period of 1990–95. 12 of these 400 patients died; 340 of these 400 developed agranulocytosis in the first 6mths of therapy. The incidence rate of 0.6% is similar to earlier data published in 1993. The risk of developing agranulocytosis increased with age and was higher in women.

Antipsychotic depot injections

Antipsychotics may be given as a long-acting depot injection (the active drug in an oily suspension) injected into a large muscle (usually gluteus maximus), allowing for sustained release over 1–4wks. Previously, only FGAs were available, but now a number of SGA preparations have been developed and are finding their place in clinical practice. Dose for dose, the efficacy of these preparations is not greater than oral medication, but they do increase likelihood of compliance.

Indications Poor compliance with oral treatment, failure to respond to oral medication, memory problems or other factors interfering with ability to take medication regularly, clinical need to ensure patient compliance (e.g. due to treatment order for patients detained on MHA).

Administration (see Table 6.8 Dosing schedules, and dose equivalents 📖 p. 201) Test dose: as undesirable side-effects can be prolonged. Not more than 2–3mL of oily injection should be administered at any one site. Correct injection technique (including the use of z-track technique) and rotation of injection sites are essential. If the dose needs to be reduced to alleviate side-effects, remember plasma-drug concentration may not fall for some time after reducing the dose and it may be many weeks before side-effects subside.

Specific side-effects Pain/swelling at injection site, rarely abscesses, nerve palsies. Side-effects as for oral medication but may take 2–3 days to emerge and persist for weeks after discontinuation. May be more likely to cause EPSEs than oral preparations (good evidence is lacking).

⚠**Post-injection syndrome** Depot olanzapine pamoate carries an unpredictable risk (1.4% of patients or 1:1500 injections) of idiosyncratic excessive sedative akin to olanzapine overdose between 1–6hrs post-injection. It is recommended that after injection the patient should be observed for at least 3hrs for any signs of this syndrome (e.g. sedation, acute confusion/aggression, EPSEs, dysarthria/ataxia, or seizure, see Box 6.7).

Box 6.7 Depot dosing

Olanzapine
- Olanzapine 10mg/day (oral): start 210mg/2 weeks or 405mg/4 weeks, maintenance after 2 months treatment, 150 mg/2 weeks or 300 mg/4 weeks.
- Olanzapine 15mg/day (oral): start 300mg/2 weeks, maintenance after 2 months, 210mg every 2 weeks or 405mg every 4 weeks.
- Olanzapine 20mg/day (oral): start 300mg/2 weeks, maintenance after 2mths, 300mg/2 weeks.
- Adjust dose according to response; max 300mg every 2 weeks.

Risperidone depot dosing
- Risperidone up to 4mg/day (oral), start 25mg/2 weeks.
- Over 4mg/day risperidone (oral), start 37.5mg/2 weeks.
- Dose adjusted at intervals of at least 4 weeks in steps of 12.5mg to max 50mg/2 weeks.
- During initiation oral risperidone should be continued for 4–6 weeks; oral dosing may also be used during dose adjustment of depot.

ANTIPSYCHOTIC DEPOT INJECTIONS **217**

Table 6.8 Dosing schedules for depot antipsychotics

Generic name	Brand name	t½	Peak dose	Time to steady state	Test dose	Test to treatment interval	Starting dose	Dose interval	Max. dose
Flupentixol decanoate	Depixol®	8d (sd); 17d (md)	3–7d	10–12wks	20mg	7d	20–40mg	2–4wks	400mg/wk
Fluphenazine decanoate	Modecate®	6–10d (sd); 14–100d (md)	6–48h	6–12wks	12.5mg	4–7d	12.5–100mg	14–35d	
Haloperidol decanoate	Haldol®	18–21d	3–9d	10–12wks	50mg	4wks	50mg	4wks	300mg/4wks
Olanzapine pamoate	ZypAdhera®	23–42d	2–4d	12wks	See 📖 p. 216. For patients taking oral olanzapine; risk of post-injection syndrome.				
Paliperidone	Xeplion®	25–49d	13d	10–16wks	150mg	8d	100mg	4wks	150mg/4wks
Pipotiazine palmitate	Piportil®	14–21d	9–10d	8–12wks	25mg	4–7d	25–50mg	4wks	200mg/4wks
Risperidone	Risperdal Consta®	3–6d	4–6wks	6–8wks	See 📖 p. 216. Release of drug starts 3wks after injection and subsides by 7wk.				
Zuclopenthixol decanoate	Clopixol®	17–21d	4–9d	10–12wks	100mg	7d	200–500mg	1–4wks	600mg/wk

t½ = elimination half-life; d = days; h(s) = hour(s); wk(s) = week(s); sd=single dose; md=multiple dose; supp = supplementation

Disorders related to schizophrenia

Both ICD-10 and DSM-IV describe a number of disorders which show significant symptomatic overlap with schizophrenia. It is currently unclear whether these disorders represent distinct disorders, or (as seems more likely) they share some degree of common aetiology with schizophrenia.

Schizoaffective disorder

This disorder has features of both affective disorder and schizophrenia which are present in approximately equal proportion. Its nosological status is uncertain since some believe it to be a variant of schizophrenia; others, bipolar disorder; and some believe it represents a point on a continuum of 'unitary psychosis' lying between schizophrenia and mood disorders.[1] Lifetime prevalence is 0.5–0.8% with limited data available on gender and age differences.

ICD-10 criteria

- Schizophrenic and affective symptoms simultaneously present and both are equally prominent.
- Excludes patients with separate episodes of schizophrenia and affective disorders and when episodes are in the context of substance use or other medical disorder.

DSM-IV criteria

- Major depressive, manic, or mixed episode concurrent with symptoms that meet criterion A for schizophrenia.
- ≥2wks of delusions and/or hallucinations without prominent mood symptoms.
- Symptoms meeting criteria for a mood episode are present for a substantial portion of the active and residual periods.
- The disturbance is not due to the direct physiological effects of a drug of abuse or medication or a general medical condition.

Treatment

As for schizophrenia but treat manic or depressive symptoms as outlined in bipolar disorder (see 📖 pp. 326–31).

Prognosis

Depressive symptoms are more likely to signal a chronic course compared to manic presentations. Good/poor prognostic factors are the same as for schizophrenia. Overall, prognosis is better than schizophrenia (as there is usually a non-deteriorating course) and worse than primary mood disorder.

Schizotypal disorder

Schizotypal disorder is classified along with schizophrenia and related disorders in ICD-10, but along with cluster A/'odd-eccentric' personality disorders in DSM-IV. It shares some of the clinical features of schizophrenia, but not the delusions or hallucinations. It is seen in approximately 3% of the general population and approximately 4.1% of psychiatric inpatients. The disorder tends to run a stable course.

It is currently viewed as representing 'partial expression' of the schizophrenia phenotype—although the underlying mechanism for this is unclear. Evidence for this view includes the fact that monozygotic (MZ) twin studies have shown an increased risk of schizotypy in the unaffected relative, that schizotypy is more common in the other first-degree relatives of schizophrenic subjects than in the general population, and that relatives of schizotypal subjects have an increased risk of schizophrenia.

Symptoms (DSM-IV criteria)
Ideas of reference. Excessive social anxiety. Odd beliefs or magical thinking. Unusual perceptions (e.g. illusions). Odd/eccentric behaviour or appearance. No close friends/confidants. Odd speech. Inappropriate or constricted affect. Suspiciousness or paranoid ideas.

Differential diagnosis
Autism, Asperger syndrome, expressive/mixed receptive–expressive language disorder, chronic substance misuse, other personality disorders (especially borderline, schizoid, and paranoid).

Treatment
Risperidone ($\leq$2mg/day)[2] has some support from an RCT. Other antipsychotics may also be helpful. There is little evidence in support of other interventions but highly structured supportive CBT may be best.

Schizophreniform disorder
(Included under 'other schizophrenia' in ICD-10)
The original term referred to patients with schizophrenic symptoms with a good prognosis[3] and now refers to a schizophrenia-like psychosis that fails to fulfil duration criterion for schizophrenia in DSM-IV. The treatment is the same as for an acute episode of schizophrenia. It is most common in adolescence and young adults and is much less common than schizophrenia with a lifetime prevalence of 0.2%.

DSM-IV
- Criteria A, D, and E of schizophrenia are met.
- An episode of the disorder (including prodromal, active, and residual phases) lasts at least 1mth but less than 6mths.
- Specified as with good prognostic features (as evidenced by 2+ of: onset of prominent psychotic symptoms within 4wks of the first noticeable change in usual behavior or functioning; confusion or perplexity at the height of the psychotic episode; good premorbid social and occupational functioning; no evidence of premorbid personality disorder; absence of blunted or flat affect).

Course and prognosis
Psychosis lasting for more than 1mth but less than 6mths. Patients return to baseline functioning once the disorder has resolved. Progression to schizophrenia is estimated to be between 60–80%. Some patients have 2 or 3 recurrent episodes.

Treatment
Antipsychotics ± a mood stabilizer and psychotherapy.

1 Mellor C (2007) Schizoaffective, paranoid and other psychoses. In: Stein G and Wilkinson G, eds, *Seminars in general adult psychiatry*, 2nd rev edn, pp. 187–201. London: Rcpssych Publications.
2 Koenigsberg HW, Reynolds D, Goodman M, *et al.* (2003) Risperidone in the treatment of schizotypal personality disorder. *J Clin Psychiat* **64**: 628–34.
3 Langfeldt G (1982) Definition of 'schizophreniform psychoses'. *Am J Psychol* **139**: 703.

Delusional disorder 1: clinical features

Essence Delusional disorder is an uncommon condition in which patients present with circumscribed symptoms of non-bizarre delusions, but with absence of prominent hallucinations and no thought disorder, mood disorder, or significant flattening of affect. Symptoms should have been present for at least 1mth (DSM-IV). ICD-10 specifies at least 3mths for *delusional disorder* but, if it is less than this, allows diagnosis under *other persistent delusional disorder*. DSM-IV specifies particular subtypes (see Box 6.8).

Points to note
- Patients rarely present directly to psychiatrists. More often they may be seen by other physicians due to somatic complaints, lawyers due to paranoid ideas, or the police when they act on or complain about their delusions.
- Careful assessment and diagnosis is vital, because delusions are the final common pathway of many illnesses (see 🕮 p. 222). When delusional disorder is discovered, treatment can be fraught with difficulty because of the reticent nature of such patients. With persistence, a combination of biopsychosocial treatments can be effective.

Diagnosing pathological delusions—key points[1]
Clinical judgement is necessary to distinguish delusions from over-valued ideas, particularly when the ideas expressed are not necessarily bizarre or culturally abnormal (and may actually have some basis in reality). Such judgements may be informed by:
- The degree of plausibility.
- Evidence of systemization, complexity, and persistence.
- The impact of the beliefs on behaviour.
- Allowing for the possibility that they might be culturally sanctioned beliefs different from one's own.
- Observation of associated characteristics, including hallucinations.
- History of 'morbid change'.
- Evidence of other risk factors (see **Risk factors**, 🕮 p. 221).

Clinical features Level of consciousness is unimpaired; observed behaviour, speech, and mood may be affected by the emotional tone of delusional content (e.g. hyperalertness with persecutory delusions); thought process is generally unimpaired, but thought content reflects preoccupation with circumscribed (usually single theme), non-bizarre delusions; hallucinations may occur, but generally are not prominent and reflect delusional ideas (more commonly olfactory/tactile than visual/auditory); cognition and memory are generally intact; insight and judgement are impaired to the degree that the delusions influence thought and behaviour; risk should be formally assessed (e.g. potential for violence to self and others and past history of previous behaviour influence by delusions)—persistent anger and fear are risk factors for aggressive 'acting-out' behaviours.

Epidemiology Relatively uncommon, but not rare—prevalence estimated at 0.025–0.03% (may account for 1–2% of hospital admissions); age range 18–90yrs (mean 40–49yrs); ♂ = ♀ but delusional jealousy more common in men and erotomania more common in women; 50% of patients are in employment; 80% are married.

Risk factors Advanced age, social isolation, group delusions, low socio-economic status, premorbid personality disorder, sensory impairment (particularly deafness), recent immigration, family history, and history of head injury or substance abuse disorders.

Course and prognosis Onset may be acute or insidious. Course is very variable—with treatment: remission (33–50%), improvement (10%), persisting symptoms (33–50%). Better prognosis in acute subtypes, where stress is a factor, and for jealous or persecutory subtypes. If symptoms have persisted for >6mths outcome is worse.

Box 6.8 DSM-IV subtypes[1]

- **Erotomanic (De Clérambault syndrome)** Patients present with the belief that some important person is secretly in love with them. Clinical samples are often female and forensic samples contain a preponderance of males. Patients may make efforts to contact this person, and some cases are associated with dangerous or assaultive behaviour.
- **Grandiose** Patients believe they fill some special role, have some special relationship, or possess some special ability(ies).They may be involved with social or religious organizations.
- **Jealous[2] (Othello syndrome)** Patients possess the fixed belief that their spouse or partner has been unfaithful. Often patients try to collect evidence and/or attempt to restrict their partner's activities. This type of delusional disorder has been associated with forensic cases involving murder.
- **Persecutory** This is the most common presentation of delusional disorder. Patients are convinced that others are attempting to do them harm. Often they attempt to obtain legal recourse (litigious or 'querulous paranoia'), and they sometimes may resort to violence.
- **Somatic** Varying presentation, from those who have repeat contact with physicians requesting various forms of medical or surgical treatment to patients who are delusionally concerned with bodily infestation, deformity (see dysmorphophobia 📖 p. 810), or odour.
- **Mixed** Presence of one or more of the above themes; no single theme predominating.
- **Unspecified** The theme cannot be determined or does not fit the listed categories.

1 ICD-10 subtypes are similar: Erotomanic, Grandiose, Jealous, Persecutory, Litigious, Hypochondriacal, and Self-referential.

2 Shepherd M (1961) Morbid jealousy: some clinical and social aspects of a psychiatric symptom. *Journal of Mental Science* **107**: 607–753. (The 'classic' paper.)

1 Manschreck T (1996) Delusional disorder: the recognition and management of paranoia. *J Clin Psychiat* **57**(Suppl. 3): 8.

Delusional disorder 2: differential diagnosis and aetiology

Differential diagnoses

- **Substance-induced delusional disorders** (e.g. alcohol, stimulants, hallucinogens, steroids, antihistamines, sympathomimetics). Careful history-taking may reveal onset, persistence, and cessation of symptoms to be related to drug use.
- **Other physical disorders** Focused history, examination, and investigations should help exclude other disorders (e.g. head injury, CNS infection, epilepsy).
- **Mood disorders with delusions (manic and depressive types)** Mood and related biological symptoms are usually more severe and precede delusions.
- **Schizophrenia** Presence of psychotic symptoms other than relatively circumscribed delusions, greater functional impairment.
- **Dementia and delirium** Evidence of cognitive impairment or altered/fluctuating level of consciousness.
- **Elderly patients (late paraphrenia)** Thought to be distinct from delusional disorder (see 📖 p. 522) and schizophrenia, associated with social isolation, ageing, medical problems/treatments, and sensory loss.
- **Dysmorphophobia/body dysmorphic disorder** (see 📖 p. 810) Significant overlap with delusional disorder, few significant differentiating factors exist.
- **Obsessive–compulsive disorder** (see 📖 p. 376) Significant overlap with delusional disorder and, if reality testing regarding obsessions or compulsions is lost, delusional disorder often is diagnosed.
- **Hypochondriasis** (see 📖 p. 808) Health concerns generally are more amenable to reality testing and are less fixed than in delusional disorder.
- **Paranoid personality disorder** (see 📖 p. 495) Absence of clearly circumscribed delusions, presence of a pervasive, stable pattern of suspiciousness or distrust.
- **Misidentification syndromes** (see 📖 p. 230) Easily confused with delusional disorder, may be associated with other CNS abnormalities.
- **Induced/shared psychotic disorder** (see 📖 p. 228) Evidence that relatives/close friends share similar delusional beliefs.

Aetiology

Delusional disorders represent a heterogeneous group of conditions that appear distinct from mood disorders and schizophrenia, although there is significant diagnostic (and genetic) overlap with paranoid personality traits/disorder. Data suggest that among patients diagnosed with delusional disorder, 3–22% are later reclassified as schizophrenic and fewer than 10% are later diagnosed with a mood disorder.

Biological
- Delusions can be a feature of a number of biological conditions, suggesting possible biologic underpinnings for the disorder.
- Most commonly, neurological lesions associated with the temporal lobe, limbic system, and basal ganglia are implicated in delusional syndromes.
- Neurological observations indicate that delusional content is influenced by the extent and location of brain injury.
- Prominent cortical damage often leads to simple, poorly formed, persecutory delusions.
- Lesions of the basal ganglia elicit less cognitive disturbance and more complex delusional content.
- Excessive dopaminergic and reduced acetylcholinergic activity have been linked to the formation of delusional symptoms.

Psychological/psychodynamic
- Freud proposed that delusions served a defensive function, protecting the patient from intrapsychically unacceptable impulses through reaction formation, projection, and denial.
- Cognitive psychology regards delusions as the result of cognitive defects where patients accept ideas with too little evidence for their conclusions; delusions as the result of attempting to find a rational basis for abnormal perceptual experiences.

Social/other
Certain social situations may increase the chances of developing delusional disorder, e.g.:
- distrust and suspicion
- social isolation
- jealousy
- lowered self-esteem
- people seeing their own defects in others
- rumination over meaning and motivation

Delusional disorder 3: assessment and management

Assessment

Patients with delusional disorder are exceptionally difficult to assess. At interview they may be evasive, guarded, and suspicious. Often they become irritated, angry, or hostile. They may be overly sensitive to some lines of questioning, even to the point of threatening legal action. Assessment should include:

- A thorough history and MSE.
- Information-gathering (third party and other sources).
- Exclusion of underlying causation (including physical investigations) to rule out other conditions that commonly present with delusions (see *differential diagnosis*, 📖 p. 222).
- Clearly documented risk assessment (especially aggression/self-harm).

Where there is significant risk to another person/partner, duty of care may override patient confidentiality and allow warning of that individual and/or informing the police (see 📖 p. 900).

Management

Typical obstacles to the treatment of delusional disorder:

- The patient's denial of the illness which causes difficulties in establishing a therapeutic alliance.
- The patient's experiences of significant social and interpersonal problems (which may confirm their firmly held beliefs).
- The fact that antipsychotic medication is often of limited efficacy.

Admission to hospital ought to be considered if there is a clear risk of harm to self or violence towards others. Otherwise, outpatient treatment is preferred. Approaches to management include:

- **Separation** From source or focus of delusional ideas (if possible).
- **Pharmacological**[1]
  - Data for the pharmacotherapy are limited to case reports or small open-label interventions.
  - Given the symptomatic overlap with psychotic disorders, antipsychotics have some utility.
  - There was a widely held anecdotal view supporting the preferential use of pimozide. However, although there are no full-scale clinical trials, what evidence there is suggests that no antipsychotic is preferentially effective; that response rates are around 50%, with 90% of patients seeing some improvement; and that somatic delusions are the most likely to respond.
  - The evidence also favours the use of SSRIs given the overlap with OCD, body dysmorphic disorder, and mood disorder.
  - Benzodiazepines may be useful when there are marked anxiety symptoms.
  - Data for the use of anticonvulsant agents and mood stabilizers are even more limited.

- **Psychological/psychotherapeutic**
  - *Individual therapy* requires persistence in establishing a therapeutic alliance without validating or overtly confronting the patient's delusional system.
  - *Supportive therapy* may help with isolation and distress stemming from the delusional beliefs (reframing problems due to delusional beliefs as symptoms).
  - *Cognitive techniques*: reality testing and reframing. Insight-orientated therapy to develop a sense of 'creative doubt' in the internal perception of the world through empathy with the patient's defensive position.
  - *Educational and social interventions* Social skills training (e.g. not discussing delusional beliefs in social settings) and minimizing risk factors (e.g. sensory impairment, isolation, stress, and precipitants of violence).
- **Post-psychotic depression**
  - 10% or more of delusional disorder patients who respond to antipsychotics may develop severe depression with risk of suicide.
  - Withdrawal of antipsychotic may improve mood but worsen delusions; hence, the addition of an antidepressant may be indicated whilst maintaining the lowest effective dose of antipsychotic. Later the antidepressant may be gradually withdrawn.

1 Manschreck TC (2006) Recent advances in the treatment of delusional disorder. *Can J Psychiatry* **51**: 114–19.

Acute and transient psychotic disorders

(referred to as 'Brief psychotic disorder' in DSM-IV)

Clinical features Sudden onset, variable presentation (including perplexity, inattention, formal thought disorder, delusions or hallucinations, disorganized or catatonic behaviour), usually resolving within less than 1mth (DSM-IV) or 3mths (ICD-10).

Aetiology Sometimes these disorders occur in the context of an acute stressor (both ICD-10 and DSM-IV allow for specifying 'with or without' marked stressor(s)/acute stress), e.g. life events such as bereavement, marriage, unemployment, imprisonment, accident, childbirth, or migration and social isolation (with language and cultural factors).

Epidemiology Associated with certain personality types (e.g. paranoid, borderline, histrionic); more prevalent in developing nations where there is a strong emphasis on traditional values (may demonstrate culture-specific features, 🔲 p. 910). Age of onset is later in industrialized nations. More common in women.

Differential diagnosis
- Organic disorders—dementia/delirium
- Bipolar affective disorder (BAD)/depression—delusions of guilt and persecution
- Drug and alcohol disorders
- Personality disorder—paranoid/borderline/histrionic
- Culture-specific disorders (see 🔲 p. 910)
- Factitious disorder/malingering
- Schizophrenia (if it persists for more than 1mth)

Management (cf. 🔲 p. 224)
- Assessment is vital to make the appropriate diagnosis.
- Short-term admission may be necessary to prevent any suicidal or aggressive tendencies, to provide support, nursing care, and specific assistance with psychosocial stressors.
- Where medication is considered, short-term use of antipsychotics/ BDZs may be helpful (as for acute behavioural disturbance, 🔲 p. 988).
- Antidepressants/mood stabilizers may be useful to prevent relapse/ further episodes.
- Address specific social issues and consider reality-orientated, adaptive, supportive psychotherapy.

Course and prognosis
- By definition these disorders are brief and resolve within days, weeks, or months.
- Prognosis is better if there is a short interval between onset and full-blown symptoms (DSM-IV: within 4wks). Also better if there is confusion and perplexity, good premorbid social and occupational functioning, and absence of blunted or flat affect.
- Outcome is better than schizophrenia (both socially and symptomatically).

- Relapse is common, with increased mortality and suicide rates compared with the general population.
- The chances of recurrence are high and follow-up/low-dose pharmacotherapy is recommended to continue for at least 1–2yrs (and withdrawn cautiously with close clinical review).

Box 6.9 ICD-10 subtypes

ICD-10 allows for these disorders to occur with or without the presence of an acute stressor, and outlines the following subtypes:
- **Acute polymorphic psychotic disorder with or without symptoms of schizophrenia**
  - Variable and changeable psychotic symptoms (from day to day, or hour to hour) with frequent intense emotional turmoil.
  - Includes Perris's (1974) 'cycloid psychosis' after Karl Leonard's description for which the treatment of choice is lithium (Perris 1978).
  - Also 'bouffée délirante' (Magnan 1895), the concept of which was reviewed by Allodi (1982) who stressed the avoidance of long-term medication, highlighting sociocultural factors, especially migration and language.
- **Acute schizophrenia-like psychotic disorder** Also referred to as 'brief schizophreniform psychosis' or 'schizophrenic reaction' where the psychotic symptoms are relatively stable but have not lasted more than a month (ICD-10, DSM-IV brief psychotic disorder), or have lasted between 1mth and 6mths (DSM-IV schizophreniform disorder).
- **Other acute predominantly delusional psychotic disorder**.
  - Onset is acute (2wks or less), delusions or hallucinations present most of the time. If delusions persist for longer than 3 mths, then the diagnosis is that of *persistent delusional disorder* (see 📖 p. 220).
  - Includes the Scandinavian concept of 'psychogenic/reactive psychosis' for which the prognosis is good and the treatment of choice is supportive psychotherapy and the short-term use of medication (Stromgren 1989).
  - 'Hysterical psychosis' (Hirsch and Hollander 1969), which includes 3 subtypes: culturally sanctioned behaviour (like culture-specific disorders); appropriation of psychotic behaviour (conversion process); true psychosis ('failure of repression when faced with acute stress in a vulnerable ego', in e.g. histrionic personality)—in USA this is used as a diagnostic label for 'reactive psychosis'.
  - 'Ganser syndrome'—characterized by approximate answers, disorientation, clouding of consciousness, hallucinations, motor disturbance, anxiety or apathy, normal activities of daily living (ADLs), sudden resolution with amnesia for the period of illness. Proposed mechanisms read much like the differential diagnosis for acute and transient psychotic disorders (see 📖 p. 226): hysterical conversion, organic confusion, psychosis, or malingering.

Induced delusional disorder

(referred to as 'Shared delusional disorder' in DSM-IV)
Also known as '**folie à deux**' (or even '**folie à trois**' or '**folie à familie**'!),
this disorder was recognized and described by Harvey as early as 1651,
and recently reviewed as a concept by Howard in 1994. Silveira and
Seeman (1995) also reviewed the literature and found equal sex ratio;
broad range of ages; 90% couples, siblings, or parent/child; comorbidity
with depression, dementia, and mental retardation; 2/3 socially isolated;
and a common association with hallucinations. Without intervention the
course is usually chronic. The content of the shared belief depends upon
the delusions of the individual with the primary illness. Examples may
include: persecutory beliefs ('them': the paranoid pseudocommunity[1]—
Cameron, 1949), delusional parasitosis, delusional belief in a place being
haunted, belief in having a child who does not exist, other misdenficiation
delusions, or apocalyptical beliefs in cults and quasi-religions (with the
serious risk of altruistic mass suicide).

Subtypes

- *Folie imposée*—the delusions of an individual with a primary psychotic
  illness are adopted by another healthy individual (separation alone
  usually cures the normally healthy individual).
- *Folie simultanée*—when two persons with primary psychotic illness
  develop the same delusions at the same time.
- *Folie communiqué*—after a period of resistance, a healthy individual
  adopts the delusions of a person with primary psychotic illness
  (separation is less successful without other interventions).
- *Folie induite*—pre-existing primary psychosis in both patients, but one
  patient has adopted their fellow patient's delusions.

Aetiology

Psychodynamic theories

These include the fear of losing an important relationship in an otherwise isolated individual with little scope for reality testing; or the passive
acceptor has repressed oedipal fantasies that are released by the psychotic
partner causing identification of dominant partner with a parent.

Learning theory

Psychotic thinking is learned through 'observational learning'.

Social isolation

Isolation due to language, geographical barriers, and personality may also
play a part in the development of the illness.

Management

- Separation—may lead to complete remission in up to 40% of cases.
- Psychological—aimed at giving up delusional beliefs (equivalent to
  rejecting a close relationship).
- Pharmacological—for the active *not* the passive partner (except in the
  case of *folie simultanée* when both patients require treatment).

1 Cameron N (1949) The paranoid pseudo-community. *American Journal of Sociology* **49**: 32–8.

Delusional misidentification syndromes

Usually manifest as symptoms of an underlying disorder (e.g. schizophrenia, mood disorder, delusional disorder, organic disorder), these syndromes rarely occur in isolation and hence are not included separately in ICD-10 or DSM-IV. Recently, interest has been focused on these rare (and bizarre) symptoms because of the insight they may give into the normal functioning of the brain (a 'lesion' paradigm). Examples include:

Capgras delusion (l'illusion de sosies)—the patient believes others have been replaced by identical or near identical imposters. Can apply to animals and other objects, and often associated with aggressive behaviour.

Frégoli delusion (l'illusion de Frégoli)—an individual, most often unknown to the patient, is actually someone they know 'in disguise'. The individual is often thought to be pursuing or persecuting the patient.

Intermetamorphosis delusion—the patient believes they can see others change (usually temporarily) into someone else (both external appearance and internal personality).

Subjective doubles delusion—the patient believes there is a double ('doppelgänger') who exists and functions independently.

Autoscopic syndrome—the patient sees a double of themselves projected onto other people or objects nearby.

Reverse subjective double syndrome—the patient believes that they are an imposter in the process of being physically and psychologically replaced.

Reverse Frégoli syndrome—the patient believes others have completely misidentified them.

Aetiology

Psychodynamic Views include seeing these syndromes as the extremes of normal misidentification due to intense focusing on particular details; the effects of beliefs/emotions on perception; the effects of vivid imagination in a person experiencing a disorder of mood, judgement, and coenesthesia; manifestations of the defence mechanisms of projection, splitting, or regression with loss of identity and flawed reconstruction.

Biological There may be evidence of underlying right hemisphere dysfunction, anterior cortical atrophy, temporal lobe pathology, bifrontal disconnectivity—with resultant impaired facial recognition, dissociation of sensory information from normal affect, and failure to suppress inappropriate, repetitive behaviour.

Management

- Full physical and psychiatric assessment.
- Interventions should be directed towards any underlying problem.
- Antipsychotics/anticonvulsants may also treat clearly organic cases.

Depressive illness

Introduction

Depressive disorders are common, with a prevalence of 5–10% in primary care settings. They rank fourth as causes of disability worldwide, and it has been projected that they may rank second by the year 2020. The prevalence of *depressive symptoms* may be as high as 30% in the general population with women being twice as likely to be affected as men.

Although effective treatments are available, depression often goes undiagnosed and undertreated. Symptoms often are regarded by both patients and physicians as *understandable* given current social circumstances and/or background. Although in many cases this may be true, people should not be denied interventions that may help relieve some of the disabling symptoms of the disorder, allowing them to cope better with any current social problems.

It should be borne in mind that depressive disorder has significant potential morbidity and mortality. Suicide is the second leading cause of death in persons aged 20–35yrs and depressive disorder is a major factor in around 50% of these deaths. Depressive disorder also contributes to higher morbidity and mortality when associated with other physical disorders (e.g. myocardial infarction [MI]) and its successful diagnosis and treatment has been shown to improve both medical and surgical outcomes. It is also associated with high rates of comorbid alcohol and substance misuse, and has a considerable social impact on relationships, families, and productivity (through time off work).

The majority of patients will present to primary care, often with problems other than low mood (see 📖 p. 240). Physicians ought to remain alert to this possibility as early interventions may be critical in the prevention of major morbidity and comorbidity.

There remains an innate reluctance to consider *pharmacological* interventions for *emotional* problems, despite overwhelming evidence of efficacy. There is also a widespread concern that drugs which improve mood *must* be addictive, despite evidence to the contrary. While medication is not the only possible treatment for mild to moderate depression, when antidepressants are prescribed the onus is on the physician to give a *therapeutic* dose for an *adequate* length of time. Treatment failure is often due to patient non-compliance, particularly when the patient feels that their problems have not been taken seriously and they have been 'fobbed off'. In a group of patients who generally have feelings of low self-worth or guilt, it is critical that they understand the rationale behind any treatment, and that their progress is regularly reviewed, at least in the early stages.

Depression amongst the famous

As depression is common it is not surprising that many famous people have had a depressive illness (see Box 7.1). However, there still remains a stigma attached to psychiatric illness and it is only recently that people have become more willing to discuss their illnesses publicly. A recent study examined the lives of almost 300 world-famous men and found that over 40% had experienced some type of depression during their lives.[1] Highest rates (72%) were found in writers, but the incidence was also high in artists (42%), politicians (41%), intellectuals (36%), composers (35%), and scientists (33%).

Box 7.1 Famous people who have publicly stated they have had a depressive illness include:

Alanis Morissette, musician, composer
Anthony Hopkins, actor
Barbara Bush, former First Lady (US)
Billy Joel, musician, composer
Courtney Love, musician, actor
Donny Osmond, musician
Ellen DeGeneres, comedienne, actor
Elton John, musician, composer
Germaine Greer, writer
Halle Berry, actress
Harrison Ford, actor
Janet Jackson, musician
Jessica Lange, actress
Jim Carrey, actor, comedian
Joan Rivers, comedienne, TV host
John Cleese, comedian, actor, writer
Leonard Cohen, musician, writer
Lou Reed, musician
Marie Osmond, musician
Marlon Brando, actor
Monica Seles, athlete (tennis)
Ozzy Osbourne, musician
Paul Gascoigne, professional footballer
Paul Merton, comedian
Paul Simon, composer, musician
Roseanne Barr, actress, writer, comedienne
Sheryl Crow, musician
Sinead O'Connor, musician
S.P. Morrissey, musician
Stephen Hawking, scientist, writer
Winona Ryder, actress

Other famous people (deceased) known to have had a depressive illness: Samuel Beckett, Menachem Begin, Kurt Cobain, Michel Foucault, Judy Garland, Ernest Hemingway, Audrey Hepburn, William James, Franz Kafka, Claude Monet, Richard M. Nixon, Laurence Olivier, Wilfred Owen, George S. Patton, Sylvia Plath, Jackson Pollock, Cole Porter, Mark Rothko, Dmitri Shostakovich, Tennessee Williams, Yves Saint Laurent.

1 Post F (1994) Creativity and psychopathology. A study of 291 world-famous men. *Br J Psychiat* **165**: 22–34.

Historical perspective

The changing face of depression[1]

Current ideas of what constitutes depression date from the mid-18th century. Earlier, the illness was understood in terms of 'melancholia', from classical humoural theories (melancholia derived from the Greek *melaina kole*—black bile), reflecting 'intensity of idea' (Haslam 1809), i.e. the presence of few, rather than many, delusions. Sadness or low mood were not primary symptoms. The 'melancholic' symptoms we now regard as part of depressive disorder would have been called 'vapours', 'hypochondria', or 'neuroses'. 'Depression', a term used to mean 'reduced functioning' in other medical disciplines, came to be associated with 'mental depression', adopted because it implied a physiological change, defined as 'a condition characterized by a sinking of the spirits, lack of courage or initiative, and a tendency to gloomy thoughts' (Jastrow 1901).

The concept was enlarged and legitimized by Kraepelin (1921) who used the term 'depressive states' in his description of the unitary concept of 'manic-depressive illness', encompassing melancholia simplex and gravis, stupor, fantastical melancholia, delirious melancholia, and involutional melancholia. A number of assumptions surrounded the affective disorders; they involved the primary pathology of affect, and had stable psychopathology and brain pathology, were periodic in nature, had a genetic basis, occurred in persons with certain personality traits, and were 'endogenous' (unrelated to precipitants).

In 1917 Freud published *Mourning and melancholia*, influencing more than a generation of practitioners in emphasizing cognitive and psychic factors in the aetiology of depression, and shifting clinical descriptions from *objective* behavioural signs to *subjective* symptoms.

Over the intervening years there has been much debate as to whether a 'biological' type of depression exists separate from a 'neurotic' type. Terminology has fluctuated around endogenous, vital, autonomous, endomorphic, and melancholic depression, characterized by distinctive symptoms and signs, a genetic basis, and running an independent course unrelated to psychosocial factors. In contrast, 'neurotic' or 'reactive' depression could manifest in multiple forms, showed clear responsiveness to the environment, and ran a more variable course. Both ICD-10 and DSM-IV fudge the issue somewhat by using severity specifiers (i.e. mild, moderate, severe), as well as symptom specifiers (i.e. somatic symptoms, psychotic symptoms).

The advent of antidepressant drugs in the 1950s introduced a further complication into the mix. Although ECT was widely accepted as a treatment for 'vital' depression, the idea of a drug treatment for 'reactive' depressive disorders ran counter to the received wisdom of the psychological basis to these conditions and the need for psychological treatment.

The antidepressants and beyond

The antidepressant effects of isoniazid were first observed in 1952 by Lurie and Salzer in patients being treated for TB. Similar effects were noted for reserpine by Shepherd and Davies, who conducted the first RCT in psychiatry, clearly demonstrating efficacy in anxious depression in 1955. The psychiatric community was initially reluctant to accept the idea of chemical 'cures' for mental disorders. It was not until iproniazid was promoted by Kline in 1957 as a 'psychic energizer', capable of treating 'nervous' conditions, that the tide began to turn.

In 1956, Kuhn demonstrated the antidepressant effects of imipramine, the tricyclic antidepressant (TCA), marketed worldwide in 1958, closely followed by amitriptyline in 1960. At the same time new anxiolytics were also emerging, with meprobamate in 1955, and the first benzodiazepine—chlordiazepoxide—in 1960. The search for greater dissociation of anxiolytic and sedative properties led to the introduction of diazepam in 1963.

The downside of this new psychopharmacology was the over-prescription in the 1960s and '70s of these drugs to help with 'the problems of living' and evidence of dependence, particularly in the case of the benzodiazepines. As a result, *non-pharmacological* treatments flourished, in the form of 're-branded' psychotherapies.

Behind the scenes, biological psychiatrists and psychopharmacologists developed the monoamine theories of depression, based upon the discovery of the neuropharmacological action of the antidepressants. This led to the development of more *selective* antidepressants—in the first instance, the SSRIs, with zimelidine patented in 1971, and indalpine marketed in 1978.

The emphasis on safety and side-effect issues when comparing the SSRIs with TCAs, and the decline of the benzodiazepines, opened the floodgates in the 1980s and '90s for the promotion of SSRIs (e.g. fluoxetine [1989]) not only in the treatment of depression, but also for anxiety disorders. Advances in monoamine theories also allowed the development of 'dual-action' agents (e.g. SNRIs—venlafaxine [1995]; NaSSAs—nefazodone [1995]/mirtazapine [1997]; DNRIs—bupropion [2000]) and other *selective* agents (e.g. NARIs—reboxetine [1997]).

Current theories of depression attempt to integrate biological models of stress (involving the hypothalamic–pituitary–adrenal [HPA] axis) with evidence from biological psychology, genetics, neuropharmacology, and functional neuropathology. A multifactorial biopsychosocial model (see p. 245) emerged, which helped to unite the divergent ideas of depression.

Clinical symptoms and signs are seen as the final common pathway in a complex interaction between genes and the environment in determining *predisposition* or *biological vulnerability*, which *may* subsequently lead to *biological variations* in functioning necessary for behavioural and emotional change. This may be due to further psychosocial stressors or genetically predetermined factors, which give rise to alterations in *brain functioning*. Research into these interdependent factors may well lead to greater understanding of the aetiology of depressive disorder, as well as allowing the development of diagnostic tests and *individualized* treatments.

1 For an exhaustive critique of conceptual ideas see: Jackson SW (1987) *Melancholia and depression: from Hippocratic times to modern times*. New Haven: Yale University Press.

Diagnosis 1: symptoms

Although the terminology is slightly different between ICD-10 and DSM-IV (see Table 7.1), the core symptoms are almost identical and, for a positive diagnosis, should fulfil the following criteria:

- Present for at least 2 wks and represent a change from normal.
- Are not secondary to the effects of drug/alcohol misuse, medication, a medical disorder, or bereavement (see 📖 p. 393).
- May cause significant distress and/or impairment of social, occupational, or general functioning.

Core symptoms

- *Depressed mood:* present most of the day, nearly every day, with little variation, and often lack of responsiveness to changes in circumstances. There may be diurnal variation in mood with mood being worse in the morning and improving as the day goes on.
- *Anhedonia:* markedly diminished interest or pleasure in all, or almost all, activities most of the day, nearly every day (as indicated by either subjective account or observation made by others).
- *Weight change:* loss of weight when not dieting or weight gain (e.g. a change of more than 5% of body weight in a month), associated with decreased or increased appetite.
- *Disturbed sleep:* insomnia (with early morning wakening 2–3 hr sooner than usual) or hypersomnia (especially in atypical depression, see 📖 p. 462).
- *Psychomotor agitation or retardation:* observable by others, not just subjective feelings of restlessness or being slowed down.
- Fatigue or loss of energy.
- Reduced libido.
- *Feelings of worthlessness or excessive or inappropriate guilt (which may be delusional):* not just self-reproach or guilt about being ill.
- Diminished ability to think or concentrate or indecisiveness.
- *Recurrent thoughts of death or suicide* (not 'fear of dying'), which may or may not have been acted upon.

Somatic symptoms

Also called biological, melancholic (DSM-IV), or vital. Include:

- Loss of emotional reactivity.
- Diurnal mood variation.
- Anhedonia.
- Early morning wakening.
- Psychomotor agitation or retardation.
- Loss of appetite and weight.
- Loss of libido.

Psychotic symptoms/features

- *Delusions:* e.g.
  - poverty;
  - personal inadequacy;
  - guilt over presumed misdeeds;

- responsibility for world events—accidents, natural disasters, war;
- deserving of punishment;
- other nihilistic delusions.
- *Hallucinations:* e.g.
  - *auditory*—defamatory or accusatory voices, cries for help or screaming;
  - *olfactory*—bad smells, such as rotting food, faeces, decomposing flesh;
  - *visual*—tormentors, demons, the Devil, dead bodies, scenes of death or torture.
  Note: These examples are *mood-congruent*. However, other *mood-incongruent* psychotic symptoms are also possible (i.e. persecutory delusions, thought insertion/withdrawal, delusions of control—not of a clearly depressive nature).
- Catatonic symptoms or *marked psychomotor retardation* (depressive stupor).

Table 7.1 ICD-10 and DSM-IV terminology

ICD-10	DSM-IV
Depressive episode	*Depressive disorders*
Mild depressive episode:	major depressive disorder, single episode; major depressive disorder, recurrent
without somatic symptoms; with somatic symptoms	
Moderate depressive episode:	*Severity specifiers*
without somatic symptoms; with somatic symptoms	mild, moderate, severe (with/without psychotic features), partial/full remission
Severe depressive episode:	*Special syndrome specifiers*
without psychotic symptoms; with psychotic symptoms	with catatonic, melancholic, or atypical features; with post-partum onset
Other depressive episode	
Depressive episode unspecified	
Recurrent depressive episode	*Longitudinal course specifiers*
	with/without full inter-episode recovery; with seasonal pattern; with rapid cycling
	Depressive disorder, not otherwise stated
	premenstrual dysphoric disorder; minor depressive disorder; recurrent brief depressive disorder; post-psychotic depressive disorder of schizophrenia; major depressive disorder; superimposed on delusional disorder; psychotic disorder NOS; active phase of schizophrenia; uncertain aetiology
	Dysthymic disorder

Diagnosis 2: caseness and subtypes

Clinically significant depressive episode (minimum criteria)
- ICD-10 specifies the presence of at least 2 *typical symptoms* (depressed mood, anhedonia, or fatigue), *plus* at least 2 others from the *core symptoms* list.
- DSM-IV requires the presence of 5 or more symptoms from the core symptoms list (at least one of which must be *depressed mood* or *anhedonia*).

Severity criteria
- Both ICD-10 and DSM-IV distinguish *mild*, *moderate*, and *severe episodes* on the basis of symptomatology (see Table 7.2).

Subtypes
- *Non-melancholic (DSM-IV) or without somatic symptoms (ICD-10):* essentially, defined as absence of psychotic or marked somatic symptoms, this subtype captures the clinical picture historically described by 'neurotic depression' (in those with certain premorbid personality traits and/or high levels of anxiety) and 'reactive depression' (due to a severely stressful life event—see 🕮 p. 384). Counter-intuitively, there is little need to subdivide on the basis of there being a clear precipitant. Life events appear to be provoking factors, but only in those with a predisposition to depression, and treatment should focus on the underlying disorder, as well as coming to terms with any significant provoking factors. Recent research[1] also supports the long-held clinical impression of two different presentations:
  - *Irritable/hostile depression*—younger, anxiety expressed as irritability, history of 'acting out' behaviours in response to stress (e.g. yelling, smashing things up, recklessness, impulsiveness, deliberate self-harm [DSH]). Poor response to antidepressants.
  - *'Anxious' depression*—shy and withdrawn, highly anxious ('always a worrier'), usually early onset depression, with a recurrent, persistent course, increased likelihood of drug/alcohol dependency, and frequent DSH/attempted suicide. Better response to antidepressants (e.g. SSRIs).
- *Melancholic (DSM-IV) or with somatic symptoms (ICD-10):* the presence of 'somatic symptoms' (see 🕮 p. 236) defines what is regarded as a more 'biological' or 'endogenous' depressive episode, which is more severe (and more amenable to antidepressant treatment). DSM-IV also includes 'excessive or inappropriate guilt', although this may often be difficult to distinguish from delusional guilt. In clinical studies, the best distinguishing factor from 'non-melancholic' disorders is actually the presence of psychomotor disturbance (an *objective sign* manifest by motor retardation, periodic agitation, and reduced/slowed cognitive functioning).
- *With psychotic symptoms (ICD-10) or features (DSM-IV):* usually there is pervasive depressed mood (no reactivity) and marked psychomotor

disturbance (sometimes to the point of depressive stupor/catatonia) accompanying delusions (commonly) and hallucinations (10–20%). Constipation is often a feature (~30%), unrelated to medication, and may have a delusional interpretation (e.g. presence of cancer, bowels having been sewn up).

Table 7.2 Severity criteria

	ICD-10	DSM-IV
Mild	2 typical symptoms + 2 other core symptoms	5 core symptoms + minor social/occupational impairment
Moderate	2 typical symptoms + 3+ other core symptoms	5+ core symptoms + variable degree of social/occupational impairment
Severe	3 typical symptoms + 4+ other core symptoms	5+ core symptoms + significant social/occupational impairment

1 Parker G, Hadzi-Pavlovic D, Roussos J, et al. (1998) Non-melancholic depression: the contribution of personality, anxiety and life events to subclassification. *Psychol Med* **28**: 1209–19.

Diagnosis 3: other clinical presentations

There may be marked individual variation in the clinical presentation. Sometimes anxiety may also be prominent (*mixed anxiety and depressive disorder*—ICD-10). Patients with a depressive disorder may not present complaining of low mood, but may consult with other primary problems. The possibility of a depressive disorder should be borne in mind, particularly in the primary care setting, where many of these patients first seek treatment.

Indirect presentations may include:

• Insomnia, fatigue, or other somatic complaints (e.g. headache, GI upset, change in weight). On further questioning patients may describe irritability or anhedonia, but attribute this as secondary to what they regard as the primary problem (see ⌨ p. 428, ⌨ p. 816, ⌨ p. 806).

• Elderly persons presenting with agitation, confusion, or a decline in normal functioning (pseudodementia)—see ⌨ p. 524.

• Children presenting with symptoms such as irritability, decline in school performance, or social withdrawal—see ⌨ p. 656.

• Persons from a different cultural background presenting with culture-specific symptoms—see ⌨ p. 914.

Other symptoms that may hinder diagnosis

• Presence of a physical disorder whose 2° symptoms (e.g. anorexia, fatigue, insomnia) may mask symptoms of depression.

• Histrionic behaviour (making assessment of severity difficult).

• Exacerbation of other underlying disorders (phobias, OCD—especially when there are depressive ruminations).

• Hypochondriacal ideas (which may have been long-standing).

• The presence of self-harming behaviours (e.g. cutting, frequent overdose) which may represent underlying borderline traits (usually individuals will say they have *never* felt happy, or describe chronic feelings of 'emptiness').

• Cognitive impairment or LD (which may mask depressive symptoms, or appear more severe because of depression and hence improve with antidepressants).

• Alcohol and drug misuse (primary or secondary).

Other subtypes of depressive disorder

These are formally recognized in DSM-IV, but are subsumed under the rubric 'other depressive episodes' in ICD-10. They include:

• Atypical depression (⌨ p. 262)

• Postnatal depression (⌨ p. 474)

• Seasonal affective disorder (⌨ p. 263)

• Premenstrual dysphoric disorder (⌨ p. 470)

As a description of the experience of the symptoms of depression, the following has never been bettered:

I have of late but wherefore I know not lost all my mirth, forgone all custom of exercises; and indeed it goes so heavily with my disposition that this goodly frame, the earth, seems to me a sterile promontory, this most excellent canopy, the air, look you, this brave o'erhanging firmament, this majestical roof fretted with golden fire, why, it appears no other thing to me than a foul and pestilent congregation of vapours. What a piece of work is a man! how noble in reason! how infinite in faculty! in form and moving how express and admirable! in action how like an angel! in apprehension how like a god! the beauty of the world! the paragon of animals! And yet, to me, what is this quintessence of dust? man delights not me: no, nor woman neither.

Shakespeare: *Hamlet,* Act II Scene 2

Epidemiology

Prevalence 6-mth prevalence range: 2.2% (ECA)—5.3% (NCS)—6.7% (NCS-R; note 2% prevalence of severe episodes) in the general population.

Lifetime rates Wide range: 4.4% (ECA)—16.5% (NCS-R)—30% (Virginia Twin Study); most authorities agree the true rate in the general population is probably 10–20%. There is also evidence that rates are increasing among younger adults.

Sex ratio ♂:♀ = 1:2.

Risk factors (see also 📖 p. 244)
- *Genetic* (see Box 7.2): heritability estimates range from 17 to 75% (mean 37%) and families also have high rates of anxiety disorders and neuroticism suggesting a shared genetic basis.
- *Childhood experiences:* loss of a parent (inconsistent across studies), lack of parental care, parental alcoholism/antisocial traits, childhood sexual abuse. *Note:* cumulative childhood disadvantage confers a greater risk than any single variable. High intelligence and one good adult relationship are protective and increase resilience.
- *Personality traits:* anxiety, impulsivity, obsessionality (i.e. high neuroticism scores).
- *Social circumstances:*
  - *Marital status*—men, low rates associated with marriage, high rates with separation or divorce; women, probably similar, but less clear-cut).
  - Brown and Harris[1] found that, for women, having 3 or more children under the age of 11, lack of paid employment, and lack of a confiding relationship were associated with increased risk of depression (recent studies support the lack of a confiding relationship, but not the other factors).
  - *Adverse life events*—particularly 'loss' events (increased risk 2–3mths after event) in vulnerable individuals.
- *Physical illness:* especially if chronic, severe, or painful. Neurological disorders (e.g. Parkinson's disease, MS, stroke, epilepsy) have higher risk (perhaps due to 'shared' pathology). Higher rates also noted in post-MI, diabetic, and cancer patients, although family or personal histories of depression are important determinants of occurrence.

Comorbidity About two-thirds of patients will also meet criteria for another psychiatric disorder (e.g. anxiety disorders, substance misuse, alcohol dependency, personality disorders).

Box 7.2 Genetic factors

While the existence of genetic vulnerability to depression is well-established in family and twin studies, progress in the identification of its molecular basis has been slow. Functional candidate gene studies have identified few replicable associations, and genome-wide linkage studies have yielded suggestive rather than conclusive results. Genome-wide association studies (GWAS) have detected suggestive evidence for a role of genetic variants in the piccolo (*PCLO*) gene (which encodes a presynaptic cytomatrix protein that influences monoamine neurotransmitter release and regulation of the HPA axis) and neuroligin-1 (*NLGN1*, which has a role in formation and remodelling of CNS synapses). However, the general findings of these studies indicate that the genetic liability to depression is likely to involve multiple genetic variants of weak effects.[1]

Similarly, GWAS of antidepressant treatment outcome which hope ultimately to help match medications with patients have been disappointing. Three independent samples—The Sequenced Treatment Alternatives to Relieve Depression sample (STAR*D) (*n* = 1953), the Munich Antidepressant Response Signature (MARS) sample (*n* = 339) and the Genome-based Therapeutic Drugs for Depression (GENDEP) sample (*n* = 706)—fail to report any results that achieved genome-wide significance, suggesting that larger samples and better outcome measures will be needed.[2]

1 Lewis CM, Ng MY, Butler AW, *et al.* (2010) Genome-wide association study of major recurrent depression in the U.K. population. *Am J Psychiat* **167**: 949–57.
2 Laje G, McMahon FJ (2011) Genome-wide association studies of antidepressant outcome: a brief review. *Progr Neuro-Psychopharmacol Biolog Psychiat* **35**: 1553–7.

1 Brown GW, Harris TO (1978) *Social origins of depression: a study of psychiatric disorders in women.* London: Tavistock Publications.

Aetiology 1

The aetiology of depression has yet to be fully understood, however it is likely to be due to the interplay of biological, psychological, and social factors in the lifespan of an individual. Psychosocial stressors may play a role both as *precipitants* and *perpetuating factors*, increasing the risk of chronicity and recurrence; while individuals with established depression are at higher risk of further stressors of many kinds. One attempt to integrate these factors is the biopsychosocial model (see Fig. 7.1).

Early adverse experience

Developmental or social effects have previously been viewed as not being biological in nature. The modern view is that the foetal environment and later environmental stressors do have neurobiological consequences mediated through the HPA axis. These changes in stress regulation may contribute to the expression of psychiatric disorder. More research is needed in this area as data from human studies is limited.

Personality/temperament factors

These are enduring traits with a biological basis, influenced over the lifespan by inherited factors, experience, and maturation. They mediate the level and nature of response to sensory experience, regulated by context, and manifest as subjective emotions and objective behaviours. Certain temperaments (e.g. neuroticism or high 'N') may increase vulnerability to depression, perhaps due to the presence of autonomic hyperarousal (heightened responses to emotional stimuli), lability (unpredictable responses to emotional stimuli), or negative biases in attention, processing and memory for emotional material.

Psychological factors

Disruption of normal social, marital, parental, or familial relationships is correlated with high rates of depression, and is a risk factor for recurrence. An aetiological role has yet to be demonstrated, but adverse childhood experiences/chronic stressors may influence the sensitivity of individuals to later stressful events. Low self-esteem (negative view of self, the past, current events, and the future) is proposed as a vulnerability factor—it remains debatable whether this is a *causal* factor or merely a *symptom* of depression.

Gender

Although the increased prevalence of depression in women is a robust finding, explanations of why this may be so are various. These include: restricting social and occupational roles, being over- or under-occupied, ruminative response styles, and endocrine factors (suggested by increased risk of depression in the premenstrual and post-partum periods). There is little supportive evidence for these theories. One popular hypothesis is that women are more likely to admit to depressive symptoms, whereas men are not and tend to express their symptoms differently (e.g. through alcohol abuse and antisocial behaviour).

Social factors

In explaining why people of low socio-economic status (i.e. low levels of income, employment, and education) are at demonstrably higher risk of depression, two main arguments exist: *social causation*—stress associated with such problems leads to depression (i.e. an environmental argument); and *social selection*—predisposed individuals drift down to lower social positions, or fail to rise from them (i.e. a genetic argument).

Note: There is stronger evidence for the social causation argument, as *social isolation* has been shown to be a key risk factor.

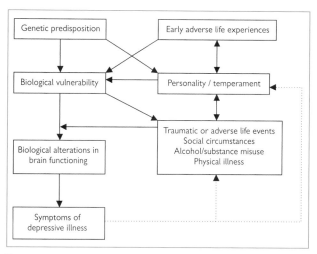

Fig. 7.1 The biopsychosocial model of depression.

Aetiology 2

Brain pathology

Structural brain changes Severe depression is associated with ventricular enlargement and sulcal prominence. Increased rate of white matter lesions in older patients (perhaps related to vascular disease). Refractory cases associated with reduced grey matter in left hippocampus (correlating with verbal memory), basal ganglia and thalamus. Other studies find reduced cortical volumes in the left parietal and frontal association areas.

Post-mortem findings Reduced GABA function, abnormal synaptic density or neuronal plasticity in the hippocampus; glial cell abnormalities; reduced expression of SERT mRNA in dorsal raphe nucleus.[1]

Functional imaging (see Box 7.3) Studies report hypoperfusion in frontal, temporal, and parietal areas (esp. older patients) and increased perfusion in frontal and cingulate cortex (in younger patients, associated with good treatment response). Activation, lesioning, and brain stimulation studies in humans[2] all point to 2 functionally segregated areas of the prefrontal cortex as being critical neural substrates for depression: the ventromedial prefrontal cortex (vmPFC)—associated with negative affect, physiological symptoms, self-awareness/insight; and the dorsolateral prefrontal cortex (dlPFC)—associated with cognitive/executive functioning, (re)-appraisal of affect states, suppression of emotional responses.

Neurotransmitter abnormalities

The discovery that all antidepressants increase monoamine (i.e. 5-HT, NE, DA) release and/or reduce their reuptake in the synaptic cleft, led to development of the *monoamine theory of depression*, which suggests that reduced monoamine function may cause depression. Blunted neuroendocrine responses and symptom induction by tryptophan depletion (5-HT precursor) suggest an important role for 5-HT.

Neuroendocrine challenge tests

Blunted prolactin and growth hormone (GH) responses to tryptophan/citalopram (5-HT system), blunted GH responses to clonidine (NE system) and apomorphine (DA system), increased GH response to physostigmine (ACh system) suggest reduced monoamine functioning and increased cholinergic functioning in depression. Increased cortisol seen in ~50% of patients (particularly 'endogenous' subtype), associated with adrenal hypertrophy, and dexamethasone non-suppression of cortisol (also in other psychiatric conditions, hence not a sensitive test, despite apparent specificity of ~96%).

Thyroid abnormalities

Abnormalities in the thyrotropin (TSH) response to TRH have been found—both blunting and enhancement—despite normal thyroid hormone levels, suggesting further research necessary esp. when T_3 shown to have utility in treatment resistant cases (see 🕮 p. 260).

Changes in sleep pattern

Early morning wakening is most typical in endogenous or melancholic depression; initial insomnia, frequent waking, and unsatisfactory sleep are also commonly seen in depression. Causal relationship of sleep to depression currently unknown. In severe depression there is reduced total SWS and shortened REM latency (secondary to increased cholinergic [REM-on], and/or reduced serotonergic/noradrenergic [REM-off] drive.) Sleep changes resolve with recovery from depression and sleep disturbance may be an early predictor of impending relapse.

Box 7.3 Endophenotypes, imaging, and genetic correlates in the aetiology of depression

Imaging studies identify traits or 'endophenotypes' that are heritable, intermediate phenotypes associated with depression. These presumably have a simpler genetic basis than the full syndrome (or even individual symptoms), making them more amenable to genetic analysis, and enabling the generation of testable hypotheses. Examples include:

- Mood-congruent phenomenon of increased activity of the amygdala in response to negative stimuli, which is likely moderated by the 5-HT transporter gene (SLC6A4) promoter polymorphism (5-HTTLPR).
- Hippocampal volume loss esp. in elderly or chronically ill samples related to val66met brain-derived neurotrophic factor (BDNF) gene variant and 5-HTTLPR SLC6A4 polymorphism.
- White matter pathology in elderly and more severely ill samples (allowing for complications of cerebrovascular disease).
- Increased blood flow or metabolism of the subgenual anterior cingulate cortex (sgACC) and associated grey matter loss.
- Attenuation of the usual pattern of fronto-limbic connectivity, particularly a decreased temporal correlation in amygdala–anterior cingulate cortex (ACC) activity.
- Decreased 5-HT1A binding in the raphe, medial temporal lobe, and medial prefrontal cortex (mPFC), and a functional polymorphism in the promoter region of the 5-HT1A gene.
- Alterations in the binding potential of the 5-HT transporter.

Hopefully, it will not be long before we begin to see further advances in these areas as epigenetic, copy-number variant, gene–gene interaction, and **GWAs** (see p. 243) approaches are brought to bear on imaging data.

See review: Savitz JB and Drevets WC (2009) Imaging phenotypes of major depressive disorder: genetic correlates. Neuroscience 164: 300–30.

---

1 Arango V, Underwood MD, Boldrini M, et al. (2001) Serotonin 1A receptors, serotonin transporter binding and serotonin transporter mRNA expression in the brainstem of depressed suicide victims. Neuropsychopharmacol 25: 892–903. Note: If replicated, this has profound implications for those who have taken MDMA and other methamfetamines.

2 Steele JD and Lawrie SM (2004) Segregation of cognitive and emotional function in the prefrontal cortex: a stereotactic meta-analysis. Neuroimage 21: 868–75.

Differential diagnosis

- *Other psychiatric disorders:* dysthymia, stress-related disorders (adjustment disorders/bereavement, PTSD), bipolar disorder, anxiety disorders (OCD, panic disorder, phobias), eating disorders, schizoaffective disorders, schizophrenia (negative symptoms), personality disorders (esp. borderline personality disorder [BPD]).
- *Neurological disorders:* dementia, Parkinson's disease, Huntington's disease, MS, stroke, epilepsy, tumours, head injury.
- *Endocrine disorders:* Addison's disease, Cushing's disease, hyper/hypothyroidism, perimenstrual syndromes, menopausal symptoms, prolactinoma, hyperparathyroidism, hypopituitarism.
- *Metabolic disorders:* hypoglycaemia, hypercalcaemia, porphyria.
- *Haematological disorders:* anaemia.
- *Inflammatory conditions:* SLE.
- *Infections:* syphilis, Lyme disease, and HIV encephalopathy.
- *Sleep disorders:* esp. sleep apnoea.
- *Medication-related:* antihypertensives (beta-blockers, reserpine, methyldopa, and calcium channel blockers); steroids; H2 blockers (e.g., ranitidine, cimetidine); sedatives; muscle relaxants; chemotherapy agents (e.g. vincristine, procarbazine, L-asparaginase, interferon, amphotericin B, vinblastine); medications that affect sex hormones (oestrogen, progesterone, testosterone, gonadotrophin-releasing hormone [GnRH] antagonists); cholesterol-lowering agents; and psychiatric medication (esp. antipsychotics)
- *Substance misuse:* alcohol, BDZs, opiates, marijuana, cocaine, amfetamines, and derivatives.

Diagnosis and investigations

Diagnosis

- The diagnosis of depression is primarily based on a good psychiatric history and physical examination (see **Why don't psychiatrists look at the brain?** 📖 p. 10).
- In addition to focused questioning on mood (see 📖 pp. 49–51; 📖 p. 236), it is useful to administer a standardized rating scale such as the Hamilton Depression Rating Scale (HAM-D), the Beck Depression Inventory (BDI) or the Zung Self-Rating Depression Scale[1] as a baseline measure prior to any change to management plans.
- Given the significant comorbidity with anxiety, some clinicians will also rate anxiety symptoms separately, e.g. the Hamilton Anxiety Rating Scale (HAM-A), the Beck Anxiety Inventory (BAI), or the Zung Self-Rating Anxiety Scale.[2]
- Patients with depression often complain of poor memory or concentration. In these cases it is also worth administering the MMSE (see 📖 p. 70). If cognitive impairment is significant, further more detailed neuropsychological testing may be indicated (e.g. ACE-R).

Investigations

There are no specific tests for depression. Investigations focus on the exclusion of treatable causes (see **Differential diagnosis** 📖 p. 248), or other secondary problems (e.g. loss of appetite, alcohol misuse).

- *Standard tests:* FBC, ESR, B_{12}/folate, U&Es, LFTs, TFTs, glucose, Ca^{2+}.
- *Focused investigations:* only if indicated by history and/or physical signs:
  - urine or blood toxicology;
  - breath or blood alcohol;
  - arterial blood gas (ABG);
  - thyroid antibodies;
  - antinuclear antibody;
  - syphilis serology;
  - additional electrolytes—e.g. phosphate, magnesium, zinc;
  - dexamethasone suppression test (Cushing's disease);
  - cosyntropin stimulation test (Addison's disease);
  - lumbar puncture (VDRL, Lyme antibody, cell count, chemistry, protein electrophoresis);
  - CT/MRI, EEG.

---

1 The Zung Self-Rating Depression Scale is copyright © free and one version can be found at: ℘ http://healthnet.umassmed.edu/mhealth/ZungSelfRatedDepressionScale.pdf
2 The Zung Self-Rating Anxiety Scale is also copyright © free and can be found at: ℘ http://healthnet.umassmed.edu/mhealth/ZungSelfRatedAnxietyScale.pdf

Course and prognosis

Points to note
- Depression may occur at any age, although late onset depression may be milder, more chronic, more likely to be associated with life events, and more likely to have a subclinical prodrome.
- Depressive episodes vary from 4–30wks for mild–moderate cases, to an average of about 6mths for severe cases (25% will last up to 1yr).
- Episodes of recurrent depression tend to be shorter (4–16wks).
- 10–20% of patients will have a chronic course, with persistent symptoms lasting over 2yrs.
- The majority of patients experiencing a depressive episode will have further episodes later in life (risk of recurrence is ~30% at 10yrs, ~60% at 20yrs), but inter-individual variation makes it impossible to predict the likely period of time before future episodes, although, as with bipolar disorder, the greater the number of recurrences, the shorter the time between episodes.
- Risk of recurrence is greater when there are residual symptoms after remission (about a third of cases), e.g. low mood, anxiety, sleep disturbance, reduced libido, and physical symptoms (headache, fatigue, GI upset).
- There is good evidence that modern antidepressant treatments impact significantly upon all these quoted figures, reducing the length of depressive episodes; and if treatment is given long term, the incidence of residual symptoms is less, there are fewer recurrent episodes, and chronicity may be as low as 4%.

Mortality
- Suicide rates for severe depressive episodes vary, but may be up to 13% (i.e. up to 20 times more likely than the general population), with a slightly higher rate for those who have required hospital admission (12–19%). For less severe episodes rates are much lower.
- The overall death rate for patients with depression is higher than the general population (SMR 1.37–2.49) with the cause of death usually due to suicide, drug and alcohol problems, accidents, cardiovascular disease, respiratory infections, and thyroid disorders.

Prognostic factors
- *Good outcome:* acute onset, endogenous depression, earlier age of onset.
- *Poor outcome:* insidious onset, neurotic depression, elderly, residual symptoms, neuroticism, low self-confidence, comorbidity (alcohol or drug problems, personality disorders, physical illness), lack of social supports.

Management principles and outpatient treatment

Initial assessment
- *History:* key areas of enquiry include:
  - any clear psychosocial precipitants;
  - current social situation;
  - use of drugs/alcohol;
  - past history of previous mood symptoms (including 'subclinical' periods of low or elevated mood, previous DSH/suicide attempts);
  - previous effective treatments;
  - premorbid personality;
  - family history of mood disorder;
  - physical illnesses;
  - current medication.
- *MSE* (see 📖 p. 249): focused enquiry about subjective mood symptoms, somatic symptoms, psychotic symptoms, symptoms of anxiety, thoughts of suicide. Objective assessment of psychomotor retardation/agitation, evidence of DSH, cognitive functioning (MMSE).
- *Physical examination:* focused on possible differential diagnoses (see 📖 p. 248).
- *Baseline investigations* (see 📖 p. 249).

Questions of severity and initial treatment options[1]
- When depressive symptoms are mild, of recent onset, and there is no previous history of more severe mood disorder, most guidelines suggest refraining from use of antidepressants. Close, active monitoring is advised and, depending on patient preference, the use of individual guided self-help (based on CBT principles), computerized cognitive behavioural therapy (CCBT), or structured group physical activity programmes.
- Antidepressants may be considered where there is:
  - a past history of moderate or severe depression;
  - an initial presentation of subthreshold depressive symptoms that have been present for a long period (typically at least 2yrs);
  - subthreshold depressive symptoms or mild depression that persist(s) after other interventions.
- Treatment for moderate or severe depression combines antidepressant medication (see 📖 pp. 256–9) and a high-intensity psychological intervention (e.g. CBT or IPT—see 📖 p. 256).
- Usually pharmacological treatment can be initiated on an outpatient basis (severe cases may require admission—see 📖 p. 254).
  - Choice of antidepressant is guided by anticipated safety and tolerability, physician familiarity (which allows for better patient education in anticipation of adverse effects), presenting symptoms, and history of prior treatments (see 📖 p. 266).

- Initially follow-up will usually be fairly frequent (1–4wks) to monitor treatment response and assess for any unwanted side-effects.
- Once treatment is established (and is effective) the time between appointments may be increased (see 📖 p. 255 and 📖 pp. 256–9 for further guidance).

1 See NICE (2009) *Depression: the treatment and management of depression in adults.* Clinical Guideline CG90 (this is a partial update of NICE clinical guideline 23). ℘ http://www.nice.org.uk/nicemedia/live/12329/45888/45888.pdf

Hospital admission

Sometimes acute episodes of depressive disorder are severe enough to require hospital admission (which may be on a compulsory basis). As for all psychiatric disorders, issues of safety and the provision of effective treatment will govern the decisions about whether a patient can remain in the community.

Points to note

- Due to symptoms of low self-esteem or guilt, some patients may refuse admission to hospital because they feel unworthy or they are 'using up a valuable bed'. Sympathetic reassurance that this is not the case and that the clinician believes they are sufficiently ill to benefit from hospital admission may avoid unnecessary detention.
- Some patients (or relatives) may demand admission to hospital. Although this usually is due to personality factors, it may also be due to (sometimes erroneous) ideas of what may be reasonably achieved in a hospital setting (e.g. intensive psychotherapy for one specific issue), or reflect undisclosed factors that have created a social crisis. A non-confrontational approach in eliciting the reasons behind such demands may reveal other important issues that may help the decision-making process (including those which may be dealt with by other agencies, e.g. emergency accommodation/refuge).

Common reasons for hospital admission

- Serious risk of suicide (see 📖 p. 51).
- Serious risk of harm to others (esp. children—see 📖 p. 663).
- Significant self-neglect (esp. weight loss).
- Severe depressive symptoms.
- Severe psychotic symptoms.
- Lack or breakdown of social supports.
- Initiation of ECT.
- Treatment-resistant depression (where inpatient monitoring may be helpful).
- A need to address comorbid conditions (e.g. physical problems, other psychiatric conditions, inpatient detoxification).

Suitable environment?

Where there is significant risk of harm to self (or others), admission should be to a ward where close observation and monitoring are possible. Observation levels ought to be regularly reviewed. The ward environment is often not the quiet sanctuary patients hope for and this may lead to difficult decisions in balancing the risk of self-harm against the use of compulsory admission. Careful assessment of a patient's insight into their illness, issues of comorbid substance misuse, and clear evidence of their ability to seek additional support when symptoms are worse, may allow for a more flexible approach in permitting time out from the ward environment (perhaps in the company of a responsible relative or friend).

Aftercare following discharge

Following hospital discharge, or for outpatients started on antidepressant treatment, initial follow-up should be regular (2–4 wks) to monitor progress, ensure treatment response is maintained, and to allow time for other supports (e.g. CPN services, crisis/home treatment services, day hospitals, specific psychotherapies) to become established.

⚠ **Risk of suicide is increased at this time** as energy and motivation improve and the patient struggles with the consequences of being unwell.

Key aims for follow-up

- Establishing and maintaining a therapeutic alliance.
- Monitoring the patient's psychiatric status.
- Providing education regarding depressive disorder and the treatment options.
- Enhancing treatment compliance.
- Monitoring side-effects of medication.
- Identifying and addressing any significant comorbidity.
- Promoting regular patterns of activity and rest.
- Identifying unmet needs for specific (practical) support, counselling, (bereavement, stress management), or psychotherapy.
- Promoting understanding of and adaptation to the psychosocial effects of symptoms.
- Identifying new episodes early.
- Reducing the morbidity and sequelae of depressive disorder.

The ultimate aim is a return to normal activities (academic, employment, home life, social activities), usually in a graded way as the resolution of symptoms allows, using a collaborative approach.

Maintenance treatment (see 📖 pp. 255–9) will usually be monitored in the primary care setting, with specific advice about continuation of medication and what to do should symptoms recur.

Treating depressive illness (without psychotic features)

First-line treatment
- Antidepressant drugs are effective in 65–75% of patients.
- For mild–moderate episodes, or where antidepressants are contraindicated (e.g. recent MI), CBT or other psychotherapies may have a role (see 📖 p. 252 for NICE recommendations CG90).
- The combination of psychological approaches and pharmacotherapy may be synergistic, but in severe cases treatment—at least initially—is almost exclusively pharmacological or physical (e.g. ECT).

Choosing an antidepressant
The decision about *which* antidepressant to choose will depend upon:
- *Patient factors:* age, sex, comorbid physical illness (cardiac, renal, liver, neurological)—see 📖 pp. 972–7), previous response to antidepressants.
- *Issues of tolerability:* see 📖 p. 266.
- *Symptomatology:* sleep problems (more sedative agent), lack of energy/hypersomnia (more adrenergic/stimulatory agent), mixed (e.g. with anxiety/panic—SSRI/imipramine), OCD symptoms (clomipramine/SSRI), risk of suicide (avoid TCAs).

Adequate trial
Generally an adequate trial of an antidepressant is defined as at least 4wks of the highest tolerated dose (up to BNF maximum).

⚠ Suicide risk
The risk of suicide may actually be *increased* in the early stages of antidepressant treatment. Often patients with previous marked psychomotor retardation have been unable to act upon their thoughts of self-harm. Partial treatment response may 'free' them to do this, hence careful monitoring is critical (and admission to hospital may be indicated).

Treatment failure—second-line treatment
Failure of an adequate trial of an antidepressant may occur in ~25% of cases. A similar number of patients will experience unacceptable side-effects, leading to the withdrawal of the agent without completing an adequate trial. For these patients, second-line treatment is with an alternative agent usually from a different class of antidepressant, or from the same class but with a different side-effect profile.

Partial responders (see also 📖 p. 260)
~50% of patients who have only partially responded to a TCA, SSRI, or MAOI may benefit from the addition of lithium (usual dose 600–900mg/d). Treatment response is generally observed within 2wks. Alternative 'augmentative' strategies include the use of triiodothyronine (T_3, or L-tryptophan.

ECT[1] (see 📖 p. 284)

- ECT may be considered as a first-line therapy when there are severe biological features (e.g. significant weight loss/reduced appetite) or marked psychomotor retardation.
- It is sometimes used when the patient is at high risk of harming themselves or others (where there is clear evidence of repeated suicide attempts or significantly aggressive behaviour) or where psychotic features are prominent (see 📖 p. 258). Under these circumstances issues of consent to treatment must be considered (see 📖 p. 284).
- It may also be considered as a second- or third-line treatment for non-responders to pharmacotherapy.

Maintenance therapy

First episode

- A collaborative approach with the patient should emphasize compliance (even when feeling 'better') with advice to continue the effective treatment for 6mths to 1yr after remission (particularly if there are residual symptoms).
- Discontinuation should be gradual and if there is recurrence of symptoms revert to effective dose with further attempt at withdrawal after at least a further 4–6mths.
- Often patients wish to continue medication indefinitely (particularly after a severe episode) and reassurance should be given that there is no evidence of any specific long-term problems with such a course of action.

Recurrent episodes

- If period between episodes is less than 3yrs, or with severe episodes (esp. with marked suicidal thought/actions) prophylactic treatment should be maintained for at least 5yrs (often indefinitely—risk of relapse if medication stopped is 70–90% within 5yrs).
- Otherwise treat as for *first episode*.

ECT

- If ECT has been used as a first-line therapy, and remission maintained with medication, treat as for 'First episode'.
- If ECT has been used successfully as second- or third-line treatment, consider *maintenance* ECT as an option (*note:* not recommended in recent NICE guidelines—see 📖 p. 292) where there is evidence that ECT effectively treats relapse of symptoms. There is some evidence that ECT every 2wks may be an effective prophylactic (this does not preclude further trials of pharmacotherapy).

---

1 Recently published NICE guidelines (see 📖 p. 285) do not allow for some of these uses of ECT. However, NICE guidance does not override the individual responsibility of health professionals to make decisions appropriate to the circumstances of a specific patient (such action should be discussed, documented in the notes, and, where appropriate, validated by a second opinion).

Treating depressive illness (with psychotic features)

ECT (see 📖 p. 284)

- For depression with psychotic features, ECT should be considered as first-line therapy, as evidence supports the superior efficacy of ECT to pharmacotherapy in this patient group, with significant benefit in 80–90% of cases (note: current NICE guidelines do not support this practice—see 📖 p. 285).
- Often issues of consent or relative contraindications may preclude the immediate use of ECT and its role is often that of a second-line treatment after partial response or failure of pharmacotherapy.

Combination treatment (antidepressant plus antipsychotic)

- It is usual to commence treatment with an antipsychotic agent (as for an acute psychotic episode, see 📖 p. 192) for a few days before commencing an antidepressant. This allows for a period of assessment (to exclude a primary *psychotic* disorder), may improve compliance (when psychotic symptoms clearly improve with medication), avoids potential *worsening* of psychotic symptoms with an antidepressant (in some predisposed individuals), and may help identify the 30–50% of patients who do respond to an antipsychotic alone. This approach is effective in 70–80% of patients.
- There is no clear evidence for any *particular* combination of medication being more efficacious, but the available evidence supports use of an atypical (SGA).[1] However, it is not unusual for low doses of older antipsychotics (FGAs) to be used, e.g. chlorpromazine (25–100mg at night). The most studied is olanzapine–fluoxetine combination, mainly due to the fact that it is available as a single capsule (OFC—Symbyax®) in the USA.[2]
- A recent meta-analysis suggests that starting an antidepressant first and adding the antipsychotic if necessary may be a better strategy as far as cost–benefit to the patient.[3]

Additional practice points

- Symptoms ought to be carefully monitored, as antipsychotic side-effects may mask improvement in depressive symptoms—hence use of lowest effective dose is advocated (e.g. around 2–4mg haloperidol or equivalent).
- Combinations of antidepressant/antipsychotic may worsen side-effects common to both (e.g. sedation, anticholinergic effects) and careful dose titration is necessary.
- Once acute psychotic symptoms have resolved, a lower dose of antipsychotic (or withdrawal) may be indicated, particularly when patients begin to manifest side-effects (which were not seen in the acute stages, even with higher doses)—with careful monitoring for recurrence of psychotic symptoms.

Dual-action agents

There is some evidence that single agents with dual actions, such as amoxapine (a tetracyclic antidepressant with significant D_2 antagonism), or antipsychotics, such as aripiprazole, clozapine, olanzapine, quetiapine, or risperidone may be effective in treating both aspects of depression with psychotic symptoms. To date, evidence does not exist to support use of these agents for *long-term* treatment: where there are issues of compliance/tolerability the utility of using a *single* agent is attractive, but should be considered carefully.[3]

Maintenance therapy

- When ECT has been used, maintenance usually involves the treatment of the underlying depressive symptoms with an antidepressant (as in episodes *without* psychotic symptoms, see 📖 p. 256).
- When combination treatment has been successful, maintenance often involves a clinically effective antidepressant with the lowest effective antipsychotic dose. As for dual-action agents, evidence is lacking with regard to long-term treatment and this tends to be pragmatic, on the basis of continued symptomatology.
- In view of the *severity* of the disorder, prophylactic use of an antidepressant and/or antipsychotic is prudent (often indefinitely, as for recurrent depressive episodes, see 📖 p. 257).

1 Nelson JC, Papakostas GI (2009) Atypical antipsychotic augmentation in major depressive disorder: a meta-analysis of placebo-controlled randomized trials. *Am J Psychiat* **166**: 980–91.

2 Recent RCT evidence actually suggests a combination approach is superior to antipsychotic alone for olanzapine vs. olanzapine/fluoxetine: (Rothschild AJ, Williamson DJ, Tohen MF, *et al.* (2004) A double-blind, randomized study of olanzapine and olanzapine/fluoxetine combination for major depression with psychotic features. *J Clin Psychopharmacol* **24**: 365–73), olanzapine/sertraline vs. olanzapine/placebo (Meyers BS, Flint AJ, Rothschild AJ, *et al.* (2009) A double-blind randomized controlled trial of olanzapine plus sertraline vs. olanzapine plus placebo for psychotic depression: the study of pharmacotherapy of psychotic depression (STOP-PD). *Arch Gen Psychiat* **66**: 838–47), and for OFC (olanzapine–fluoxetine) vs. olanzapine or fluoxetine alone (Trivedi MH, Thase ME, Osuntokun O, *et al.* (2009) An integrated analysis of olanzapine/fluoxetine combination in clinical trials of treatment resistant depression. *J Clin Psychiatry* **70**: 387–96).

3 Wijkstra J, Lijmer J, Balk FJ, *et al.* (2006) Pharmacological treatment for unipolar psychotic depression: systematic review and meta-analysis. *Br J Psychiat* **188**: 410–15.

An approach to treatment-resistant depression

Commonly defined as 'failure to respond to adequate (dose and dura-tion—i.e. max BNF dose for at least 4 wks) courses of 2 antidepressants, or 1 antidepressant and ECT'. The consequences of resistant depression include reduced quality of life, excessive strain on relationships (which may lead to break-up of families), significant personal economic impact, increased physical comorbidity (e.g. malignancy, cardiovascular disease, even premature death), increased risk of suicide, therapeutic aliena-tion (making further interventions difficult due to difficulties forming a therapeutic alliance), and high use of psychiatric services (without clear benefit).

Differentiating treatment resistance

It is important to distinguish actual treatment resistance from chronicity of symptoms. Apparent treatment failure may also occur due to: incorrect initial diagnosis (i.e. not depressive disorder in the first place), inadequate initial treatment, poor compliance, incomplete formulation (esp. role of maintaining factors), and issues of comorbidity (both physical and other psychiatric disorders).

Risk factors for treatment resistance

Concurrent physical illness, drug/alcohol abuse, personality disorder, high premorbid neuroticism, long period of illness prior to treatment.

Management[1]

- *Review diagnostic formulation:* is diagnosis correct? Are there any unaddressed maintaining factors (e.g. social, physical, psychological)? *Note:* a proportion of individuals with chronic, refractory depression will have unrecognized bipolar disorder.
- *Check patient understanding/compliance:* serum levels may help.
- *Continue monotherapy at maximum tolerable dose:* may mean exceeding BNF guidelines (esp. if there has been partial benefit).
- *Consider change in antidepressant:* try different class of antidepressant.
- *Consider augmentation with a mood stabilizer:* e.g. lithium.
- *Consider additional augmentative agents:* e.g. T_3, tryptophan (see Box 7.4).
- *Consider combining antidepressants from different classes:* caution is advised, due to possible serious adverse reactions (e.g. 📖 p. 960).
- *Consider use of ECT:* see 📖 p. 284 (esp. if severe biological features or psychotic symptoms).
- *Consider possibility of psychosurgery or other advanced intervention:* see 📖 pp. 296–9.

---

1 Useful guidance and assessment tools for treatment-resistant depression including advice regard-ing criteria for 'adequate treatment' can be found on the Dundee Advanced Intervention Service website: 🔗 http://www.advancedinterventions.org.uk/library_tools.htm

Points to note

- There is little definitive evidence to support any specific augmentative regime (see Box 7.5).
- Spontaneous remission is possible: 'regression to the mean' suggests that symptoms will improve; bear in mind that the natural life of depression is 6–18mths, even when untreated.
- Psychological and social interventions, particularly when psychosocial factors appear paramount, may be important (often overlooked or undisclosed) aspects of management.

Box 7.4 Tryptophan (L-Tryptophan, Optimax®)

- *Mode of action:* precursor for serotonin.
- *Indications:* restricted specialist use as an adjunct for treatment-resistant depression (lasting more than 2yrs).
- *Usual dose:* 1g tds, increased to max 6g/day.
- *Common adverse effects:* drowsiness, headache, nausea, dizziness, eosinophilia–myalgia syndrome (rare, monitoring of FBC necessary).

Box 7.5 STAR*D trial

The Sequenced Treatment Alternatives to Relieve Depression (STAR*D) trial is one of the largest independent studies undertaken by the NIMH to examine the effectiveness of a variety of treatments for non-psychotic major depression. The initial report was published in the *American Journal of Psychiatry* in Nov. 2006.[1]

- A fairly representative outpatient sample ($n = 3671$) underwent 4 steps:
  - *Level 1*—citalopram;
  - *Level 2*—switch (to bupropion, sertraline, venlafaxine XR, or cognitive therapy) or combine (bupropion, buspirone, cognitive therapy);
  - *Level 2a*—if cognitive therapy alone or plus citalopram add or switch to bupropion or venlafaxine XR;
  - *Level 3*—switch (to nortriptyline or mirtazapine) or augment (with lithium or T_3);
  - *Level 4*—switch (to tranylcypromine) or combine (venlafaxine XR plus mirtazapine).
- Remission rates were 37%, 31%, 14%, and 13% for each level, with an overall cumulative remission rate of 67%.
- The trial highlighted patient preference for combinations/augmentations and provided some evidence to support certain strategies: e.g. lithium or T_3 augmentation; combining citalopram plus bupropion, buspirone, or venlafaxine plus mirtazapine.

1 Rush AJ, Trivedi MH, Wisniewski SR, *et al.* (2006) Acute and longer-term outcomes in depressed outpatients requiring one or several treatment steps: a STAR*D report. *Am J Psychiat* **163**: 1905–17.

Atypical depressive episode

Regarded as a subtype of depressive disorder, rather than a separate entity. Atypical features coded in DSM-IV as an 'episode specifier' (like melancholic, post-partum, catatonic). Listed under 'other depressive episodes' in ICD-10.

Clinical features
- Mood is depressed, but remains reactive (able to enjoy certain experiences but not to 'normal' levels).
- Hypersomnia (sleeping more than 10hrs/day, at least 3 days/wk, for at least 3mths).
- Hyperphagia (excessive eating with weight gain of over 3kg in 3mths).
- 'Leaden paralysis' (feeling of heaviness in the limbs, present for at least 1hr/day, 3 days/wk, for at least 3mths).
- Over-sensitivity to perceived rejection.[1]
- Other infrequent symptoms may include: initial insomnia rather than early morning wakening (EMW); reversed diurnal mood variation (better in the morning); severe motor retardation; absence of feelings of guilt.

Epidemiology Onset usually in late teens and early twenties, often (up to 30%) family history of affective disorders.

Comorbidity Higher rates of anxiety (esp. panic disorder and social phobia), somatization disorder (see p. 802), alcohol and drug misuse than in other depressive disorders.

Management
- Best evidence is for the use of phenelzine (15mg/day increased gradually to 60–90mg/day in divided doses—continue for 8–12wks to assess benefit) or another monoamine oxidase inhibitor (MAOI) (see p. 272 for guidance on prescribing/dietary advice). RIMAs theoretically ought to be as effective and safer (but evidence is lacking).
- Alternatives include SSRIs (e.g. fluoxetine or sertraline), or possibly a NARI (e.g. reboxetine).
- TCAs have traditionally been regarded as less effective. However, some individuals may respond well, and the best evidence is for the use of imipramine.
- Where there is failure to respond to an adequate trial of an antidepressant, follow management principles outlined at pp. 256–9 and p. 260).

---

1 'Rejection sensitivity' (to both *real* and *imagined* rejection) adds to the difficulty of managing atypical depression, as the patient may have had adverse experiences with doctors in the past, been labelled as 'personality disordered', and may find the idea of a therapeutic alliance alien.

Seasonal affective disorder (SAD)

Somewhat controversial concept, both in terms of diagnosis (see **clinical features**) and treatment (using light therapy—📖 p. 298). In DSM-IV *seasonal pattern* is included in specifiers describing the course of recurrent depressive episodes of both depressive and bipolar disorder. Included under 'recurrent depressive disorder' in ICD-10.

Clinical features There must be a clear seasonal pattern to recurrent depressive episodes (i.e. they have occurred at the same time of year each time and fully remit once the season is over). In the northern hemisphere this is said to be usually around January/February ('winter depression'). Symptoms are generally mild to moderate with low self-esteem, hypersomnia, fatigue, increased appetite (including carbohydrate craving), weight gain, and decreased social and occupational functioning.

Aetiology It is unclear whether this constitutes a separate subtype of depressive disorder, or whether it is simply a manifestation of atypical depression (see 📖 p. 262). The speculated mechanism involving melatonin synthesis has not been confirmed in controlled studies, and some authors suggest that seasonal psychosocial factors may be more important in determining the timing of recurrent depressive episodes (e.g. increased work demands over the Christmas and New Year periods for shopworkers).

Epidemiology In the US, prevalence of SAD is estimated at ~5%, ♂:♀ = 1:5.

Management

- *Light therapy* (see 📖 p. 298): initially, 2hrs of 2500lux (or equivalent) on waking (response seen within 5 days and full response in 1–2 wks). Maintenance therapy should be given all winter (30min of 2500lux every 1–2 days). Patients should avoid exposure to bright light during night-time. *Good prognostic factors*—patients with clear hypersomnia, carbohydrate craving, reduced energy in the afternoon.
- *Pharmacological:* best evidence for bupropion XL (licensed in the USA not UK), SSRIs (sertraline, citalopram, escitalopram, fluoxetine). Alternatives include pre-sunrise propranolol (60mg/day) to suppress morning melatonin; melatonin/agomelatine at night; or other antidepressants (e.g. mirtazapine, reboxetine, duloxetine, moclobemide).

Dysthymia (ICD-10)/dysthymic disorder (DSM-IV)

Previously considered a subtype of personality disorder. Essentially, the presence of chronic, low-grade depressive symptoms. These may be long-standing, but careful history-taking reveals a time when the person *did* feel 'well'. It is possible to have superimposed depressive episodes (double depression), when care is needed in assessing treatment response, as baseline may be dysthymic, rather than euthymic.

Clinical features
- Depressed mood (>2yrs).
- Reduced/increased appetite.
- Insomnia/hypersomnia.
- Reduced energy/fatigue.
- Low self-esteem.
- Poor concentration.
- Difficulties making decisions.
- Thoughts of hopelessness.

Aetiology Findings suggest dysthymia is biologically related to depressive disorder, e.g. family history suggesting shared genetics; shortened REM latencies in sleep studies; diurnality of symptoms; TRH/TSH challenge test abnormalities; low testosterone and adrenal-gonadal steroid levels; lowered IL-1-β; small genual corpus callosum volume; enlarged amygdala; s-allele polymorphism of 5-HT transporter gene.

Epidemiology Prevalence 3–5%, ♂:♀ 1:2, usually early onset (<20yrs), but late-onset subtype seen (>50yrs).

Course Less severe. More chronic than depression. Community studies show low spontaneous remission rate (2–20yrs, median 5yrs).

Management
- *Pharmacological:* SSRIs are probably the treatment of choice with best evidence for citalopram (40mg/day) and fluoxetine (20–40mg/day). Alternatives include moclobemide, TCAs (e.g. amitriptyline, desipramine, imipramine), MAOIs, or low dose amisulpiride (25–50mg/day). Drug therapy may take several months to show benefit[1] and should be regarded as a long-term treatment.
- *Psychological:* although evidence is lacking, CBT may be useful (usually in combination with an antidepressant).

Prognosis
Variable: spontaneous recovery reported as 13% over 1yr in community samples; outpatient studies suggest 10–20% of treated patients achieve remission within 1yr; ~25% suffer chronic symptoms.

1 Silva de Lima M, Moncrieff J, Soares B (2000) Drugs versus placebo for dysthymia. *Cochrane Database System Rev* **9**: CD001130.

Antidepressants

Assumed mode of action

All currently available antidepressants appear to exert antidepressant action by increasing the availability of monoamines (5-HT, NE, and DA) via one or more of the following:

- Presynaptic inhibition of reuptake of 5-HT, NE, or DA.
- Antagonist activity at presynaptic inhibitory 5-HT or NE receptor sites, which enhances neurotransmitter release.
- Inhibition of monoamine oxidase, reducing neurotransmitter breakdown.
- Increasing the availability of neurotransmitter precursors.

Although this net increase happens almost immediately following administration, initial resolution of depressive symptoms generally takes 10–20 days, implying therapeutic effect involves mechanisms possibly related to receptor regulation over time/changes in intracellular signalling.

Selectivity vs. specificity

Although the newer antidepressants are more *selective* than the TCAs and MAOIs in their pharmacological effects, this should not be confused with them being more *specific* for any particular type of depressive symptoms. All antidepressants have unwanted and often unpleasant side-effects. A balance needs to be struck between efficacy in treating psychiatric symptoms and the possibility of iatrogenic problems. Patients may not be able to tolerate the anticholinergic side-effects of TCAs, or will be unable to achieve a therapeutic level because of side-effects. Similarly, nausea or GI upset may limit the usefulness of SSRIs in some individuals. Sometimes side-effects may be useful (e.g. sedation for patients with insomnia) or combinations of antidepressants may be more efficacious than one alone (or may offset side-effects) (e.g. mirtazapine + SSRIs/SNRIs for sexual side-effects; SSRI + trazodone combination for those troubled by insomnia, but who have responded well to the antidepressant effects of the SSRI).

Cautionary notes

Particular caution is necessary in prescribing for certain patient groups (see 🕮 pp. 968–79) such as those with renal or hepatic impairment, cardiac problems, epilepsy; pregnant or breast-feeding women; the elderly; children; and those on other medications which may interact with antidepressants. There are also well-recognized problems such as weight gain (🕮 p. 930), hyponatraemia (🕮 p. 966), sexual dysfunction (🕮 p. 938), and discontinuation syndromes (🕮 p. 964).

Combining/switching antidepressants (see Table 7.3)

An adequate 'washout' period is required when switching to or from the MAOIs, whereas it is usual to cross-taper between other antidepressants (i.e. gradually reducing the dose of one, whilst slowly increasing the dose of the other). During this process, or when combining antidepressants, side-effects may be enhanced (due to pharmacokinetic effects) and it is possible to induce the serotonin syndrome (see 🕮 p. 960).

The following pages outline the main groups of antidepressants. This information should be used as a guide and the clinician is always advised to consult manufacturers' data sheets, or more detailed formularies, for less common problems or specific details of administration.

Table 7.3 Swapping or stopping antidepressants

FROM \ TO	TCAs	Hydrazines	Tranylcypromine	Moclobemide	Citalopram/Escitalopram	Fluoxetien	Fluvoxamine	Paroxetine	Sertraline	Venlafaxine	Duloxetine	Mianserin	Trazodone	Mirtazapine	Reboxetine	Bupropion	Agomelatine
TCAs	NRP	1 wk	1 wk	1 wk Care	Care	Great care	Great care	Great care	Care	Care	SS	NRP	NRP	NRP	NRP	NRP	NRP
Hydrazines	1–2 wks	2 wks	2 wks	NRP DR 2 wks	2 wks	2 wks	2 wks	2 wks	2 wks	2 wks	2 wks	2 wks	2 wks Care	2 wks	2 wks	1 wk	NRP
Tranylcypromine	2 wks	2 wks		NRP DR 2 wks	2 wks	2 wks	2 wks	2 wks	2 wks	2 wks	2 wks	2 wks	2 wks	2 wks	2 wks	1 wk	NRP
Moclobemide	OccP	NRP	NRP		NRP	2 wks	NRP	NRP	NRP	NRP	SS	NRP	NRP	NRP	NRP	NRP	NRP
Citalopram/Escitalopram	Care	1 wk	NRP	1 wk		SS	SS	SS	SS	NRP	SS	NRP	Care	NRP	NRP	NRP	NRP
Fluoxetine	Great care	5 wks	5 wks	3 wks	SS		SS	SS	SS	Care	SS	NRP	Care	NRP	NRP	NRP	NRP
Fluvoxamine	Great care	4–5 days	1–2 wks	3 days	SS	SS		SS	SS	Care	SS Care	NRP	Care	NRP	NRP	NRP	Care

Paroxetine	Great care	2 wks	2 wks	5 days	SS	SS	SS		SS	Care	SS	NRP	Care	NRP	NRP	NRP	NRP
Sertraline	Care	1–2 wks	1–2 wks	7–13 days	SS	SS	SS	SS		Care	SS	NRP	Care	NRP	NRP	NRP	NRP
Venlafaxine	NRP	1 wk	1 wk	NRP	Care	Care	Care	Care	Care		SS	NRP	Care	NRP	NRP	NRP	NRP
Duloxetine	SS	5 days	5 days	SS	SS Care	SS	SS	SS	SS	SS		NRP	SS	NRP	NRP	SS	NRP
Mianserin	NRP	2 wks	2 wks	NRP	NRP	NRP	NRP	NRP	NRP	NRP	NRP		NRP	NRP	NRP	NRP	NRP
Trazodone	OccP	2 wks	2 wks	NRP	Care	Care	Care	Care	Care	Care	SS	NRP		NRP	NRP	NRP	NRP
Mirtazapine	NRP	1 wk	1 wk	NRP	NRP	NRP	NRP	NRP	NRP	NRP	NRP	NRP	NRP		NRP	NRP	NRP
Reboxetine	NRP	1 wk	1 wk	NRP	NRP	NRP	NRP	NRP	NRP	NRP	NRP	NRP	NRP	NRP		NRP	NRP
Bupropion	Care	1 wk	1 wk	NRP	NRP	NRP	NRP	NRP	NRP	NRP	NRP	NRP	NRP	NRP	NRP		NRP
Agomelatine	NRP	NRP	NRP	NRP	NRP	NRP	Care	NRP	NRP	NRP	NRP	NRP	NRP	NRP	NRP	NRP	
Just stopping	Over 4 wks	Over 4 wks	Over 4 wks	Over 4 wks	Over 4 wks	Reduce to 20mg then stop	Over 4 wks	Slowly over at least 4 wks	Over 4 wks	Slowly over at least 4 wks	Slowly over at least 4 wks	Over 4 wks	Over 4 wks	Over 4 wks	Over 4 wks	Over 4 wks	NRP

Key: NRP, no reported problems; SS, risk of serotonin syndrome; OccP, occasional problems; DR, dietary restrictions should continue

Tricyclic antidepressants (TCAs)

- See Table 7.4.
- *Common mode of action and effects/side-effects:*
  - *Serotonin/noradrenaline (and dopamine) reuptake inhibition*—antidepressant effects.
  - *Anticholinergic (antimuscarinic—M1)*—dry mouth, blurred vision, constipation, urinary retention, drowsiness, confusion/memory problems (particularly in the elderly), palpitations/tachycardia.
  - *Adrenergic antagonism (α1)*—drowsiness, postural hypotension (occasionally syncope), tachycardia, sexual dysfunction.
  - *5-HT$_2$ antagonism*—anxiolytic, reduced sexual dysfunction, sedation.
  - *Antihistaminergic (H1)*—drowsiness, weight gain.
- *Advantages:* well-established efficacy and large literature (in all varieties of patient groups); possibly more effective in severe depression; low cost.
- *Disadvantages:* toxicity in overdose; may be less well tolerated than SSRIs; all TCAs may slow cardiac conduction and lower seizure threshold.
- *Contraindications:* acute MI, heart block, arrhythmias, IHD, severe liver disease, pregnancy and lactation (see 📖 pp. 968–79).
- *Cautions* (also see 📖 p. 266): cardiovascular, liver, renal disease; endocrine disorders (hyperthyroidism, adrenal tumours, diabetes); urinary retention/prostatic hypertrophy; constipation; glaucoma; epilepsy; psychotic disorders; patients with thoughts of suicide; elderly (use lower doses).
- *Significant interactions (variable for different agents—always check data sheets):* alcohol, anticoagulants, anticonvulsants, antihypertensives, antipsychotics, barbiturates, BDZs (rare), cimetidine, digoxin, MAOIs (rare), methylphenidate, morphine, SSRIs, smoking.
- *Monitoring:* it is good practice to monitor cardiac and liver function, U&Es, FBC, and weight during long-term therapy.

Table 7.4 Tricyclic antidepressants (TCAs)

Drug	Half-life (hr)	Formulations	Usual starting dose	Usual maintenance dose	Max daily dose	Notes	Indications
Amitriptyline	8–24	T 10/25/50mg C 25/50mg S25 or 50mg/5mL	75mg/day (divided or just at night)	100–150mg	150mg	Metabolized to nortriptyline	Depression, nocturnal enuresis, chronic pain, migraine, insomnia
Clomipramine (Anafranil®)	17–28	C 10/25/50mg SR 75mg Inj 12.5mg/mL	10mg/day	30–150mg/day (divided or just at night)	250mg	Most SSRI-like of the TCAs. Can be given IV/IM	Depression, OCD & phobic disorders, adjunctive treatment of cataplexy (in narcolepsy)
Dosulepin (Prothiaden®)	14–40	C/T 25mg	75–150mg/day	75–150mg/day	225mg (hospital)		Depression (with anxiety)
Doxepin (Sinepin®)	8–24	C 10/25/50/75mg	75mg/day	Up to 300mg/ day (divided if <100mg/d)	300mg		Depression (esp. if sedation needed)
Imipramine	4–18	T 10/25mg S25mg/5mL	25mg up to tds	50–100mg/day	200mg	Metabolized to desipramine	Depression, nocturnal enuresis
Lofepramine (Gamanil®)	1.6–5	T 70mg S 70mg/5mL	70mg/day	70–210mg/day	210mg	May be safer in over-dose. Least proconvulsant. Metabolized to desipramine	Depression
Nortriptyline (Allegron®)	18–96	T 10/25mg	25mg tds	75–100mg	150mg	Manufacturer recommends plasma monitoring in doses <100mg/d (therapeutic window 50–150ng/mL)	Depression, nocturnal enuresis
Trimipramine (Surmontil®)	7–23	T 10/25mg C 50mg	75mg/day	150–300mg/day	300mg	May be very sedating	Depression (with anxiety)

Key: T = tablets; C = capsules; S = oral suspension/solution; SR = modified release capsules; Inj = injectable form

Monoamine oxidase inhibitors (MAOIs) and reversible monoamine oxidase inhibitors (RIMAs)

- *Mode of action:*
  - *MAOIs:* irreversible inhibition of MAO-A (acts on NE, DA, 5-HT, and tyramine) and MAO-B (acts on DA, tyramine, phenylethylamine, benzylamine), leading to accumulation of monoamines in synaptic cleft (Table 7.5).
  - *RIMAs:* act by reversible inhibition of MAO-A (Table 7.5).
- *Side-effects:*
  - *Risk of hypertensive crisis* due to inhibition of intestinal MAO, allowing pressor amines to enter the bloodstream (hence foods high in tyramine and certain medications should be avoided).
  - *Sources of dietary tyramine:* cheese (except cottage and cream cheese), meat extracts and yeast extracts (including Bovril®, Marmite®, Oxo®, and other fermented soya bean extracts), alcohol—including low-alcohol drinks (especially chianti and fortified wines and beers), non-fresh fish, non-fresh poultry, offal, avocado, banana skins, broad-bean pods, caviar, herring (pickled or smoked).
  - *Medications:* indirect sympathomimetics (amfetamine, fenfluramine, ephedrine, phenylephrine, phenylpropanolamine), cough mixtures containing sympathomimetics, nasal decongestants with sympathomimetics, levodopa (L-dopa), pethidine, antidepressants (TCAs, SSRIs/SNRIs, mirtazapine, bupropion, St John's wort [Box 7.6]). These effects may be less with RIMAs. However, large amounts of tyramine-rich food should be avoided.
  - *Other side-effects:* antimuscarinic actions, hepatotoxicity, insomnia, anxiety, appetite suppression, weight gain, postural hypotension, ankle oedema, sexual dysfunction, possible dependency.
- *Indications:* usually used as second-line therapy for treatment-resistant depression (particularly atypical symptoms)/anxiety disorders (with or without panic attacks).
- *Cautions:* cardiovascular disease, hepatic failure, poorly controlled hypertension, hyperthyroidism, porphyria, phaeochromocytoma.
- *Advantages:* well-established efficacy in a broad range of affective and anxiety disorders.

Table 7.5 MAOIs and RIMAs

Drug	Class	Half-life (hr)	Formulations	Usual starting dose	Usual maintenance dose	Max daily dose	Notes
Isocarboxazid	MAOI	36	T 10mg	30mg/day (divided or single daily dose)	10–40mg/day	60mg/day	Hydrazine derivative—less stimulating
Moclobemide (Manerix®)	RIMA	1–2	T 150mg	150mg bd	150–600mg/day	600mg/day	May be used for social phobia. Possible hyponatraemia. 'Cheese reaction' least likely
Phenelzine (Nardil®)	MAOI	1.5	T 15mg	15mg tds	15mg every other day to 15mg qds	60mg/day (hospital 90mg/day)	Hydrazine derivative—less stimulating
Tranylcypromine	MAOI	2.5	T 10mg	10mg bd	10mg/day	30mg/day (or greater if supervised)	Most stimulant of MAOIs (amfetamine-related). Do not give after 3p.m. Increased risk of significant interactions

Key: T = tablets

- *Disadvantages:* dietary restrictions and drug interactions (less so with RIMAs).
- *Other significant drug interactions (variable for MAOIs vs. RIMAs—always check data sheets):* antidiabetics, anti-epileptics, antihypertensives, antipsychotics, barbiturates, BDZs, β-blockers, buspirone, cimetidine, dopaminergics (selegiline), dextromethorphan, mazindol, pethidine, morphine, 5-HT$_1$ agonists (rizatriptan, sumatriptan), tetrabenazine.

Selective serotonin reuptake inhibitors (SSRIs)

- *Common mode of action and effects/side-effects:* serotonin reuptake inhibition (leads to ↑5-HT in synaptic cleft; see Table 7.6).
  - *5-HT$_{1A}$ agonism*—antidepressant, anxiolytic, anti-obsessive, anti-bulimic effects.
  - *5-HT$_2$ agonism*—agitation, akathisia, anxiety/panic, insomnia, sexual dysfunction.
  - *5-HT$_3$ agonism*—nausea, GI upset, diarrhoea, headache.
- *Advantages:* ease of dosing; may be better tolerated than TCAs—less cardiotoxic; fewer anticholinergic side-effects; low toxicity in overdose.
- *Disadvantages:* commonly cause nausea and GI upset, headache, restlessness, and insomnia; may be less effective for severe depressive episodes; problems on discontinuation (see 🕮 p. 964).
- *Contraindications:* manic episode, concomitant use of MAOIs.
- *Cautions* (also see 🕮 p. 266): variable and significant inhibitory effects on hepatic P450 (particularly CYP2D6) enzymes. Hence, take care when co-prescribing with drugs that undergo extensive liver metabolism and have a narrow therapeutic range.
- *Significant interactions (variable for different agents—always check data sheets):* alcohol, anticoagulants, anticonvulsants, antipsychotics, BDZs, β-blockers, bupropion, buspirone, cimetidine, cyproheptadine, hypoglycaemics, lithium, methadone, MAOIs, morphine, smoking, TCAs, theophylline, warfarin.

Box 7.6 St. John's wort (SJW, Hypericum perforatum)

Considered a first-line antidepressant in many European countries (and recently becoming popular in the US); not yet in the UK. May be effective for mild–moderate depressive symptoms.[1]
- *Mode of action:* recent research suggests it may act as a weak SSRI (and/or NARI/MAOI).
- *Usual dose:* 300mg tds (with food to prevent GI upset).
- *Notable interactions:* anticoagulants (esp. warfarin), antidepressants (risk of serotonin syndrome—🕮 p. 960), anti-epileptics, antivirals, barbiturates, ciclosporin, digoxin, 5-HT$_1$ agonists (rizatriptan, sumatriptan), oral contraceptives, theophylline.

1 Linde K, Berner MM, Kriston L. (2008) St John's wort for major depression. *Cochrane Database System Rev* **4**: CD000448.

Table 7.6 Selective serotonin reuptake inhibitors (SSRIs)

Drug	Half-life (hr)	Formulations	Usual starting dose	Usual maintenance dose	Max daily dose	Notes	Indications
Citalopram (Cipramil®)	33	T 10/20/40mg S 40mg/mL	20mg od (10mg for panic, increase slowly)	20–60mg od	60mg	Least likely to interact with other drugs. Less likely to reduce seizure threshold (caution)	Depression, panic disorder (with or without agoraphobia)
Escitalopram (Cipralex®)	30	T 5/10/20mg S 10mg/mL	10mg od (5mg for panic, increase slowly)	5–20mg od	20mg	The active enantiomer of citalopram	Depression, panic disorder (with or without agoraphobia), social anxiety
Fluoxetine (Prozac®)	24–140	C 20/60mg S 20mg/5mL	20mg od	20–60mg od	60mg	Most alerting. May cause weight loss	Depression (with or without anxiety symptoms), OCD, bulimia nervosa, PMDD
Fluvoxamine (Faverin®)	13–22	T 50/100mg	50–100mg od	100–300mg (if <150mg, in divided doses)	300mg	Moderately sedating	Depression, OCD
Paroxetine (Seroxat®)	10–24	T 20/30mg S 20mg/10mL	20mg od (10mg for panic, increase slowly)	20–50mg od	50mg	Most anticholinergic. Withdrawal syndrome may be more frequent. May be sedating	Depression (with or without anxiety), OCD, panic disorder (with or without agoraphobia), social phobia, PTSD, GAD
Sertraline (Lustral®)	25–36	T 50/100mg	50mg (25mg for PTSD, increase slowly)	50–200mg od	200mg	Moderately alerting. Fewer drug interactions, but caution still necessary	Depression (with or without anxiety), OCD, PTSD

Key: T = tablets; C = capsules; S = oral suspension/solution

Other antidepressants 1

- *Mode of action:* 5-HT and NE reuptake inhibition.
- *Common adverse effects:* nausea, GI upset, constipation, loss of appetite, dry mouth, dizziness, agitation, insomnia, sexual dysfunction, headache, nervousness, sweating, weakness.

Venlafaxine (Efexor®, Efexor XL® plus many other brand names)
- *Half-life:* 1–2hrs; peak plasma conc. 5hrs (10hrs for metabolite: desmethylvenlafaxine [Pristiqs® US licence for depression, anxiety, and menopausal symptoms, 2008—not licensed in UK yet]).
- *Formulations:* 37.5/75mg tabs (MR 75/150mg caps; 75/150/225mg tabs).
- *Indications:* depression, GAD, social anxiety.
- *Usual dose:* depression, 37.5mg bd (or 75mg od of MR form), increased if necessary after at least 2wks to max 375mg/day. Severe depression, begin at 150mg/day, increasing by 75mg every few days to max dose 375mg/day. For GAD and social anxiety, 75mg od (increased 2-weekly to max 225mg/day).
- *Advantages:* variable pharmacological profile over dose range; possibly more rapid onset of action than other antidepressants; available in controlled release form allowing od administration.
- *Disadvantages:* moderate to high doses less well tolerated; need to monitor blood pressure (BP) at doses over 200mg; troublesome side-effects; discontinuation effects common.

Duloxetine (Cymbalta®, Yentreve®)
- *Half-life:* 8–17hrs; peak plasma conc. 6hrs.
- *Formulations:* 30/60mg capsules.
- *Cautions:* potential hepatotoxicity (i.e. cases of severe elevations of liver enzymes or liver injury with a hepatocellular, cholestatic, or mixed pattern have been reported); also caution in glaucoma secondary to mydriasis.
- *Indications:* depression, GAD, diabetic neuropathy, stress urinary incontinence.
- *Usual dose:* depression 60mg od; GAD start with 30mg od, increasing as necessary to max 120mg/day; diabetic neuropathy 60–120mg/day (divided doses); stress urinary incontinence 20–40mg bd.
- *Advantages:* as for venlafaxine, but no controlled release form available. May have utility in treating chronic pain and urinary incontinence.
- *Disadvantages:* dose-dependent elevations in BP require monitoring; discontinuation effects common (*note*: little evidence that doses greater than 60mg/day confer any additional benefit in depression).

Mianserin
- *Mode of action:* similar to TCAs, but with less anticholinergic side-effects.
- *Half-life* 12–29hrs; peak plasma conc. 1-3hrs.
- *Formulations:* 10/30mg tabs.
- *Indications:* depression, particularly if sedation required.

- *Common adverse effects:* as for TCAs, but less cardiovascular problems, blood dyscrasias more common (esp. elderly—FBC recommended 4-wkly for first 3mths of treatment, therafter 3–6-monthly; stop treatment and check FBC if fever, sore throat, stomatitis, or other signs of infection develop), jaundice, arthritis, arthralgia.
- *Usual dose:* 30–40mg (elderly 30mg) daily in divided doses or as a single night-time dose, increased gradually as necessary; usual range 30–90mg/day.
- *Advantages:* better side-effect profile than some TCAs (e.g. cardiotoxicity), sedating (which may be a desirable effect).
- *Disadvantages:* idiosyncratic adverse effects.

Serotonin antagonist/reuptake inhibitors (SARIs)

Trazodone (Molipaxin®)
- *Mode of action:*
  - *5-HT$_{1A/1C/2A}$ antagonism*—sedating/anxiolytic, less sexual dysfunction;
  - *5-HT agonism through the active metabolite (m-chlorophenylpiperazine)*—antidepressant effect;
  - *α_1 antagonism*—orthostatic hypotension;
  - *H_1 antagonism*—sedation and weight gain.
- *Common adverse effects:* sedation; orthostatic hypotension; otherwise similar to TCAs (but less anticholinergic and cardiotoxic); rarely priapism (discontinue immediately: see 📖 p. 942).
- *Half-life:* 3–7hrs; peak plasma conc. 0.5–2hrs.
- *Formulations:* 50/100mg caps; 150mg tabs; liquid 50mg/5mL.
- *Indications:* depression (esp. with insomnia), anxiety disorders.
- *Usual dose:* 150mg/day (as divided dose or just at night), increased to 300mg/day (max dose 600mg/day in divided doses—in hospital). For anxiety, start at 75mg/day—max 300mg/day.
- *Advantages:* sedation (may be used in low doses as an adjunct to other less sedating antidepressants or to counter sexual dysfunction), safer in epilepsy than TCAs.
- *Disadvantages:* the higher doses necessary for antidepressant effects may not be tolerated.

Other antidepressants 2

Noradrenergic and specific serotonergic antidepressant
(NaSSA)

Mirtazapine (Zispin SolTab®)

- *Mode of action:*
  - α_2 *antagonism*—increases 5-HT and NE release (antidepressant)
  - α_1 *antagonism*—orthostatic hypotension
  - M_1 *antagonism*—anticholinergic side-effects
  - 5-HT$_{2A/C}$ *antagonism*—sedating/anxiolytic, less sexual dysfunction
  - 5-HT$_3$ *antagonism*—reduced nausea/GI upset
  - H_1 *antagonism*—sedation and weight gain
- *Common adverse effects:* sedation (greater at lower doses), increased appetite, weight gain. *Less common:* transaminase elevation, jaundice, oedema, orthostatic hypotension, tremor, myoclonus, blood dyscrasias (rare agranulocytosis—if a patient develops a sore throat, fever, stomatitis or signs of infection accompanied by neutropenia, discontinue medication and closely monitor patient).
- *Half-life:* 20–40hrs; peak plasma conc. 1–3hrs.
- *Formulations:* 15/30/45mg tabs/orodispersible tabs; oral solution 15mg/mL.
- *Indications:* depression (with anxiety, agitation, insomnia, weight loss).
- *Usual dose:* 15–30mg nocte, increased if necessary to max 45mg/day (divided dose or just at night).
- *Advantages:* low toxicity in overdose, less sexual dysfunction and GI upset.
- *Disadvantages:* weight gain, sedating effects may be lost at higher doses (may be used to advantage).

Noradrenaline reuptake inhibitor (NARI)

Reboxetine (Edronax®)

- *Mode of action:* NE reuptake inhibition.
- *Common adverse effects:* insomnia, sweating, postural hypotension/dizziness, tachycardia, sexual dysfunction, dysuria, urinary retention, dry mouth, constipation, hypokalaemia if used long term in the elderly.
- *Half-life:* 13hrs; peak plasma conc. 2hrs.
- *Formulations:* 4mg tabs (scored).
- *Indications:* depression (particularly with atypical features).
- *Usual dose:* 4mg bd, increased after 3–4 wks to 10mg/day in divided doses (max 12mg/day).
- *Advantages:* novel mode of action; alerting effects may be useful for patients with symptoms of fatigue or hypersomnia; may improve social functioning; relatively safe in overdose.
- *Disadvantages:* mainly due to adverse effects.

Noradrenergic and dopaminergic reuptake inhibitor (NDRI)

Bupropion (Zyban®)

- *Mode of action:* NE and DA reuptake inhibition.
- *Common adverse effects:* agitation/insomnia, dry mouth, GI upset (nausea, vomiting, abdominal pain, constipation), hypertension (esp. if also using nicotine patches), risk of seizures (0.4%), taste disturbance.
- *Half-life:* 3–16hrs (12–38hrs active metabolite hydroxybupropion); peak plasma conc. 4hrs.
- *Formulations:* 150mg MR.
- *Indications:* depression (with marked psychomotor retardation or hypersomnia), but only licensed in UK for treatment of nicotine dependence (and possibly withdrawal from other stimulants); may be useful in adult/child ADHD (unlicensed).
- *Usual dose:* 150mg od, increased after 6 days to 150mg bd max 300mg/day max single dose 150mg, min 8h between doses (max duration of treatment for nicotine dependence 7–9 wks).
- *Advantages:* unusual mode of action, alerting effects may be useful for patients with symptoms of fatigue or hypersomnia, may help treat impulse disorders/addictions when used primarily as an antidepressant.
- *Disadvantages:* possible seizure induction, hypersensitivity reactions (rare, but may be severe).

Melatonin agonist and specific serotonin antagonist (MaSSA)

Agomelatine (Valdoxan®)

- *Mode of action:*
  - MT_1/MT_2 melatonin agonism—may promote sleep;
  - $5\text{-}HT_{2C}$ antagonism—may increase NE and DA in frontal cortex.
- *Common adverse effects:* nausea, dizziness, headache, somnolence, insomnia, migraine, diarrhoea, constipation, upper abdominal pain, sweating, back pain, fatigue, anxiety, raised serum transaminases; *less commonly*: paraesthesia, blurred vision, eczema; *rarely*: hepatitis, rash, suicidal behaviour.
- *Half-life:* 1–2hrs (no major active metabolites); peak plasma conc. 1–2hrs.
- *Formulations:* 25mg coated tablet.
- *Indications:* depression (with initial insomnia).
- *Usual dose:* 25mg nocte increased if necessary after 2wks to 50mg nocte.
- *Advantages:* unusual mode of action, possibly useful if there is significant sleep–wake disturbance, well tolerated: no known discontinuation symptoms, sexual side-effects, weight gain, or cardiac effects.
- *Disadvantages:* need to check liver function before starting and afterwards (recommended: 6, 12, 24 wks). Therapeutic role remains to be established as just launched in UK in 2009.

ECT 1: background

Electroconvulsive therapy (ECT)

A highly effective (if controversial) treatment for depression (particularly with psychotic symptoms). May act more rapidly than antidepressant medication. Advances in brief anaesthesia and neuromuscular paralysis, introduction of brief pulse ECT machines, and the use of EEG monitoring, have led to improved safety and tolerability. Decline in the use of ECT reflects the influence of non-evidence-based factors, rather than being an indicator of its efficacy (see Box 7.7). Over the last 20yrs, there have been active efforts to improve standards of delivery, education, and training. These are set out clearly in recent APA and RCPsych publications.[1,2] ECT clinics in England and Wales, Northern Ireland, and the Republic of Ireland are accredited by ECTAS.[3] In Scotland the equivalent body is SEAN.[4]

Does ECT actually work ?

- A recent meta-analysis of all ECT studies in depression[5] found:
  - ECT vs. all placebo (n = 523) OR 4.77 (95% CI: 2.39–9.49).
  - ECT vs. sham ECT (n = 245) OR 2.83 (95% CI: 1.30–6.17).
  - ECT vs. pill placebo (n = 266) OR 11.08 (95% CI 3.10–39.65).
  - ECT vs. antidepressants (RCTs) (n = 892) OR 3.72 (95% CI 2.60–5.32).

Mode of action

Controversial therapy needs a sound evidence-base. Presuming ignorance ('we don't really know how it works, but it does…') ignores real progress in our understanding of ECT.

- *Rejected theories: psychoanalytical views* of ECT efficacy incorporating 'fear', 'regression', or 'punishment' have been largely discredited; *brain injury theory* (see 🕮 p. 295); *amnestic theory:* ECT has some effects on cognitive function (see 🕮 p. 294), but this is not the 1° mode of action.
- *Anticonvulsant/altered functional activity theory:* ECT acts as a powerful anticonvulsant (increases seizure threshold, delta activity, and inhibitory transmitters, e.g. GABA and opioids) causing a reduction in functional activity in specific brain regions related to the therapeutic response (rCBF/glucose metabolism shows reduction in anterior frontal regions post-ictally and for weeks to months after, associated with better outcomes and correlating with raised seizure threshold).
- *Antidelirium/restorative sleep theory:* ECT does lead to EEG changes (e.g. increased delta activity with greater amplitude and reduced frequency) similar to those seen in normal sleep and correlated with clinical improvement. Whether this is a therapeutic action or an (albeit important) epiphenomenon is not certain.
- *Neurochemical theories:* despite the fact that neurochemical explanations have been advocated for explaining how ECT works, supporting evidence comes from pre-clinical and animal work. Preliminary human studies support a role for DA and GABA/glutamate.
- *Neuroendocrine theory:* it is proposed that ECT works by correcting a dysregulation of neuropeptides through diencephalic stimulation.

Studies have found ECT enhances production and release of several neuropeptides (e.g. TRH, prolactin, corticotropin, cortisol, oxytocin, vasopressin, beta-endorphin and, less consistently, GH). However, these changes could be non-specific effects of stress/seizure and not necessarily the therapeutic effect of ECT.

• *Other (speculative): neurogenesis:* the animal model of ECT has been shown to promote neurogenesis in non-human primates; *gene transcription:* the likelihood of remission with ECT in patients with treatment-resistant depression has been associated with two polymorphisms related to dopamine metabolism in the prefrontal cortex; *brain derived neurotrophic factor (BDNF):* preliminary evidence suggests serum BDNF concentrations increase after ECT.

Further reading

Shorter E and Healy D (2007) *Shock therapy: a history of electroconvulsive treatment in mental illness.* Piscataway Township: Rutgers University Press.

Box 7.7 ECT: an historical perspective

The use of convulsive treatments for psychiatric disorders originated with the clinical observation of apparent antagonism between schizo-phrenia (then *dementia praecox*) and epilepsy. Patients who had a seizure were relieved of their psychotic symptoms and Meduna noted increased glial cells in the brains of patients with epilepsy compared with reduced numbers in those with schizophrenia. In 1934, he induced a seizure with an injection of camphor-in-oil in a patient with catatonic schizophrenia, and continued this treatment every 3 days. After the fifth seizure the patient was able to talk spontaneously, and began to eat and care for himself for the first time in 4yrs, making a full recovery with 3 further treatments. Chemically-induced convulsive treatments using camphor or metrazol (pentylenetetrazol) became accepted for the treatment of schizophrenia, but had problems. Cerletti and Bini introduced the use of 'electric shock' to induce seizures in 1938, a method that became the standard. Initially, ECT was unmodified (i.e. without anaesthetic or muscle relaxant), but because of frequent injury, curare was first used as a muscle relaxant in the 1940s followed by succinylcholine in the 1950s. Advances in brief anaesthesia mean the current procedure is much safer and recovery more rapid. *Indications* have also changed, with the major-ity of patients receiving ECT for severe depressive illness, although it is also effective in other conditions (see 📖 p. 284).

1 American Psychiatric Association (2001) *The practice of electroconvulsive therapy: recommendations for treatment, training and privileging,* 2nd edn. Washington, DC: APA.

2 Royal College of Psychiatrists (2005) *The ECT handbook,* 2nd edn. The third report of the Royal College of Psychiatrists' Special Committee on ECT (Council Report CR128). London: Royal College of Psychiatrists.

3 ECTAS is the Royal College of Psychiatrists' ECT Accreditation Service. 🖰 http://www.rcpsych.ac.uk/quality/qualityandaccreditation/ectclinics/ectas.aspx

4 SEAN is the Scottish ECT Accreditation Network. 🖰 http://www.sean.org.uk/

5 Pagnin D, de Queiroz V, Pini S, *et al.* (2004) Efficacy of ECT in depression: a meta-analytic review. *J ECT* **20**: 13–20.

ECT 2: indications, contraindications, and considerations

Indications (see Box 7.8)

- *Depressive episode:* severe episodes, need for rapid antidepressant response (e.g. due to failure to eat or drink in depressive stupor; high suicide risk), failure of drug treatments, patients who are unable to tolerate side-effects of drug treatment (e.g. puerperal depressive disorder—see 📖 p. 470), previous history of good response to ECT, patient preference.
- *Other indications:* treatment-resistant psychosis and mania (50–60% effective), schizoaffective disorder (see 📖 p. 218), catatonia (see 📖 p. 992), neuroleptic malignant syndrome (see 📖 p. 956), neurological crises (e.g. extreme Parkinsonian symptoms: on–off phenomena), intractable seizure disorders (acts to raise seizure threshold).

Contraindications There are no *absolute* contraindications. Where possible, use of ECT should be limited for patients with cerebral aneurysm, recent MI, cardiac arrhythmias, intracerebral haemorrhage, acute/impending retinal detachment, phaeochromocytoma, high anaesthetic risk, and unstable vascular aneurysm or malformation (see 📖 p. 292).

Other considerations

- *Time-limited action:* benefit from ECT tends to dissipate after a couple of weeks. There is a need for a clear maintenance plan to be in place before the course of ECT finishes. ECT should not be considered the only treatment—except in very rare cases when continuation/maintenance treatment is indicated (see 📖 p. 292).
- *Consent* (📖 p. 794): guidelines on ECT vary between legislatures concerning use of capacity legislation/Mental Health Act. Decisions rest on assessment of capacity, informal/formal status, active (or advance statement) refusal, potential as a life-saving intervention.
- *Side-effects:* ECT does cause potential side-effects (see 📖 p. 294) and the administration of ECT will always be a balance of risk and benefit. Of particular note is the potential to cause cognitive problems (see 📖 p. 294) and this may dictate electrode positioning (see 📖 p. 289). Fig. 7.2. (See Table 7.7 for effects of psychiatric drugs on ECT).

Box 7.8 NICE Technology Appraisal 59

Guidance on the use of electroconvulsive therapy (May 2003)
ECT is used only to achieve rapid and short-term improvement of severe symptoms after an adequate trial of other treatment options has proven ineffective and/or when the condition is considered to be life-threatening, in individuals with severe depressive illness, catatonia, prolonged or severe manic episode…The current state of the evidence did not allow the general use of ECT in the management of schizophrenia to be recommended…ECT is not recommended as a maintenance therapy in depressive illness because the longer-term benefits and risks of ECT have not been clearly established…The decision as to whether ECT is clinically indicated should be based on a documented assessment of the risks and potential benefits to the individual, including: the risks associated with the anaesthetic, contemporaneous comorbidities, anticipated adverse events, particularly cognitive impairment, and the risks of not having the treatment.

ECT 3: work-up and administration

ECT work-up
- Ensure full medical history and current medication noted on ECT recording sheet.
- Also note any relevant findings from physical examination.
- Ensure recent routine blood results available (FBC, U&Es, any other relevant investigations).
- If indicated, arrange pre-ECT CXR and/or ECG.
- Ensure consent form has been signed.
- Ensure ECT prescribed correctly.
- Inform anaesthetic team of proposed ECT.
- Inform ECT service of proposed ECT.
- Ensure patient is aware of the usual procedure and when treatment is scheduled.

Pre-ECT checks
- Check patient's identity.
- Check patient is fasted (for 8hrs) and has emptied their bowels and bladder prior to coming to treatment room.
- Check patient is not wearing restrictive clothing and jewellery/ dentures have been removed.
- Consult ECT record of previous treatments (including anaesthetic problems).
- Ensure consent form is signed appropriately.
- Check no medication that might increase or reduce seizure threshold has been recently given.
- Check ECT machine is functioning correctly.
- Ensure dose settings are correct for specific patient.

Administration of anaesthetic
- Establish IV access.
- Attach monitoring (heart rate [HR], BP, EEG, electromyograph [EMG]).
- Ventilate patient with pure oxygen via face mask.
- Give muscle relaxant, followed by short-acting anaesthetic.
- Hyperventilation with oxygen is sometimes used to augment seizure activity.
- Insert bite-block between patient's teeth to protect tongue and teeth from jaw clenching (due to direct stimulation of masseter muscles).

Administration of ECT
- Apply electrodes to scalp (see Fig. 7.2 for positioning).
- Test for adequate contact between the electrodes and the scalp prior to treatment ('self-test' function on the ECT machine).
- Administer dose.
- Monitor length of seizure (see 📖 p. 290).
- Record dose, seizure duration, and any problems on ECT record (and ensure anaesthetic administration also recorded).
- Transfer patient to recovery.

Table 7.7 Psychiatric drugs and ECT. *Note:* Ensure anaesthetist is fully informed of all medications the patient is currently taking

Drug class	Notes	Considerations	Recommendations
Benzodiazepines	May reduce antidepressant efficacy of ECT. Make seizures less likely	Avoid if possible. Consider non-BDZ hypnotics. Do not suddenly stop if well established	Lowest dose possible. Do not give immediately before ECT (rule of thumb at least 3hrs pre-ECT for last dose)
Antidepressants	May augment antidepressant effect of ECT. Reported prolongation of seizures. Reported tardive seizure	Use low initial stimulus (dose titration methods). Problems reported more for SSRIs	Do not suddenly stop—need for safe reduction to min. dose. Prophylaxis may necessitate addition of antidepressant towards end of ECT course (inform ECT team of this)
Lithium	Reduces seizure threshold. May prolong seizures. May increase post-ictal confusion (case reports only)	Use low initial stimulus (dose titration methods)	Not contraindicated during ECT
Anticonvulsants	Raise seizure threshold	Clarify if drug is for treatment of epilepsy or as a mood stabilizer. Higher doses of ECT may be necessary	If prescribed for epilepsy continue—don't stop. If a mood stabilizer continue initially and only reduce if seizure induction is problematic
Antipsychotics	All tend to reduce seizure threshold. Concerns about clozapine due to case reports of prolonged and tardive seizures may be overstated	Use low initial stimulus (dose titration methods)	Clozapine should be withheld 12hrs before any anaesthetic and restarted once fully recovered

Recovery
- Ensure that there is an adequate airway.
- Monitor the patient's pulse and BP until stable.
- There should be continuous nursing presence and observation until the patient is fully orientated.
- Maintain IV access until able to leave recovery.

Bilateral or unilateral eletrode placement?[1]
The balance of the evidence points to bilateral electrode placement being preferable in terms of speed of action and effectiveness. In the past UECT was associated with substantially less memory impairment commonly associated with the old sine wave stimulation in BECT. Local ECT policy may vary, but the usual reasons for using unilateral/bilateral electrode placement are:
- *BECT*: when speed of response is a priority, previous failure of UECT, previous good response without significant memory problems to BECT.
- *UECT*: speed of response less important, previous good response to UECT, where minimizing memory problems is a priority, e.g. cognitive impairment already present.

1 Kellner CH, Knapp R, Husain MM, et al. (2010) Bifrontal, bitemperal and right unilateral electrode placement in ECT: randomised trial. Br J Psychiatry **196**: 226–34.

Fig. 7.2 ECT Electrode placement.

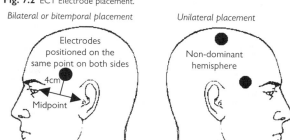

Bilateral or bitemporal placement

Electrodes positioned on the same point on both sides

4cm

Midpoint

Unilateral placement

Non-dominant hemisphere

- *Bilateral ECT (BECT)*: one electrode is applied to each side of the head. This positioning is also referred to as bitemporal ECT or bi-frontotemporal ECT. The centre of the electrode on the left (L) and the right (R1) should be 4cm above, and perpendicular to, the midpoint of a line between the lateral angle of the eye and the external auditory meatus.
- *Unilateral ECT (UECT)*: the electrodes are applied to the same 'non-dominant' hemisphere (which is usually the right-hand side). The first electrode (R1) is in the same position as before, but the second electrode (R2) is applied over the parietal surface of the scalp. The exact position on the parietal arc is not crucial; the aims are to maximize the distance between the electrodes to reduce shunting of electrical current and to choose a site on the arc where the electrode can be applied firmly and flat against the scalp. The position illustrated in the figure is also known as the 'temporo-parietal' or 'd'Elia' positioning.

ECT 4: notes on treatment

► Ensure you have had adequate training and supervision before administering ECT.[1]

Energy dosing

Because the higher the stimulus used, the greater the likelihood of transient cognitive disturbance, and because once the current is above seizure threshold, further increases only contribute to post-ECT confusion, there are a number of dosing strategies used. *Local policy and the type of ECT machine used will dictate which method is preferred.* For example:

- *Dose titration:* the most accurate method, delivering the minimum stimulus necessary to produce an adequate seizure, and therefore to be preferred. Treatment begins with a low stimulus, with the dose increased gradually until an adequate seizure is induced. Once the approximate seizure threshold is known, the next treatment dose is increased to about 50–100% (for BECT) or 100–200% (for UECT—some protocols 500–800%) above the threshold. The dose is only increased further if later treatments are sub-therapeutic, and the amount of dose increase will be governed by local policy.
- *Age dosing:* selection of a predetermined dose calculated on the basis of the patient's age (and the ECT machine used). The main advantage is that this is a less complex regime. However, there is the possibility of 'overdosing' (i.e. inducing excessive cognitive side-effects) because seizure threshold is not determined.

As ECT itself raises the seizure threshold, the dose is likely to rise by an average of 80% over the length of a treatment course. Higher (or lower) doses will also be needed when the patient is taking drugs that raise (or lower) the seizure threshold (see 📖 p. 287, Table 7.7).

Effective treatment

When a subtherapeutic treatment is judged to have occurred, the treatment is repeated at different energy settings (see **Energy dosing**).

- *EEG monitoring*: the gold standard with an ictal EEG having typical phases (see Fig. 7.3). Presence of these features (RCPsych ECT *Handbook* 'new' [2005] criteria), no matter how short the seizure activity, is deemed to constitute a therapeutic treatment. Usually the ictal EEG activity lasts 25–130s (motor seizure 720% less).
- *Timing of convulsion:* where EEG monitoring is not used, the less reliable measure of length of observable motor seizure is used, with an effective treatment defined as a motor seizure lasting at least 15s from end of ECT dose to end of observable motor activity (RCPsych *ECT Handbook* 'old' [1995] criteria: 15+s visible motor seizure or 25+s on EEG).
- *Cuff technique:* often under-used technique involving isolation of a forearm or leg from the effects of muscle relaxant, by inflation of a BP cuff to above systolic pressure. As the isolated limb does not become paralysed, the motor seizure can be more easily observed.

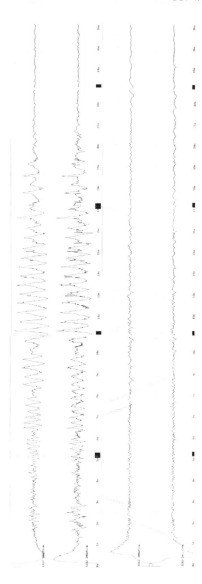

Fig. 7.3 EEG monitoring of ECT.

'Real world' examples of EEG traces for: (A) a short 'therapeutic' seizure (20s visual and 22s EEG) and (B) a subthreshold 'non-therapeutic' stimulation. In example (A) typical features are seen: 1. End of electrical stimulation; 2. Latent phase—low voltage polyspike activity (no visible convulsion); 3. Increasing amplitude of polyspike activity and slowing of frequency (associated with clonic phase of convulsion); 4. Classic 3Hz 'spike and wave' (delta) activity; 5. Gradual loss of 3Hz pattern; 6. Endpoint with lower amplitude and frequency than baseline ('post-ictal suppression').

1 www.rcpsych.ac.uk/pdf/ECT%20competencies%20for%20web.pdf

ECT 5: further notes on treatment

Other physiological effects of ECT

- *Musculoskeletal—direct stimulation:* tonic contraction—opisthotonus, supraphysiological bite (not blocked by relaxants; may cause dental injury; bite block essential); generalized (tonic–clonic) seizure—risk of fractures (vertebral, long-bone, avulsion).
- *Cardiovascular* (cf. 📖 p. 284): cerebrovascular: increased metabolic requirements due to seizure—increased CBF; increase cerebral blood volume; raised ICP. Autonomic effects: increased vagal tone— bradycardia, risk of asystole/AF, salivation; adrenaline release (peak during seizure, resolve over 10–20mins)—tachycardia, hypertension (post-ECT monitoring essential).
- *Neuroendocrine* (see 📖 p. 282): increase in ACTH, cortisol, glucagon may lead to insulin resistance (closely monitor diabetic patients).
- *Other:* increased intra-gastric pressure—possible risk of aspiration (appropriate pre-ECT fasting/premed). Raised intraocular pressure (risk in narrow angle glaucoma, recent ophthalmic surgery).

A course of ECT

- Rarely will a single treatment be effective to relieve the underlying disorder (but this does occasionally occur).
- ECT is usually given twice a week, sometimes reducing to once a week once symptoms begin to respond. This limits cognitive problems, and there is no evidence that treatments of greater frequency enhance treatment response.
- Treatment of depression usually consists of 6–12 treatments; treatment-resistant psychosis and mania up to (or sometimes more than) 20 treatments; and catatonia usually resolves in 3–5 treatments.

Continuation or maintenance ECT[1]

Continuation ECT (C-ECT)

Refers to the provision of additional treatments during the 6-mth period after remission for the primary purpose of preventing relapse.

Maintenance ECT (M-ECT)

Refers to the prophylactic use of ECT for periods longer than 6mths past the index episode for the purposes of mitigating recurrence.

- Although not recommended in NICE guidelines (see 📖 p. 285, Box 7.8), the most recent RCPsych *ECT Handbook* (2005) accepts the lack of evidence-base but recognizes there are likely to be some patients in the UK who will be prescribed continuation ECT and recommends the guidelines of the APA (2001):
  - there is clear evidence of a previous good response to ECT;
  - evidence for resistance or intolerance to pharmacotherapy;
  - the patient is able to provide informed consent;
  - evidence that the patient's cognitive function and physical condition do not preclude the ongoing administration of ECT;

  • the patient's attitude, circumstances, and level of social support
    are conducive to ensuring treatment compliance and safety after
    treatment.
• There is no specific or universally supported treatment schedule for
  C-ECT; however, after completing a course of conventional bi-weekly
  ECT, a common strategy is: weekly for 1mth; fortnightly for 1mth;
  monthly for up to 6mths after remission.
• Only in exceptional circumstances should M-ECT (i.e. > 6mths after
  remission) be considered as a treatment option, in close consultation
  with the patient, and a formal review by another consultant, preferably
  with specific ECT experience.
• Usually patients are aware of how effective ECT has been for them
  and a collaborative approach can be established (balancing frequency
  of ECT against return of symptoms and side-effects, esp. memory
  problems).

Outpatient ECT
ECT is given to outpatients in exceptional circumstances only:
• Mild to moderate illness as defined by a psychiatrist (e.g. CGI 2–4).
• Availability of 24hr supervision to ensure safety and observation.
• The patient should not have active thoughts of suicide.
• Regular (weekly) assessment by the consultant (or deputy).

ECT in pregnancy
• ECT may be the preferred treatment choice due to its rapid action.
• ECT in the second or third trimesters may present more technical
  difficulties for the anaesthetist as the risk of aspiration of stomach
  contents increases.
• The patient's obstetrician and the anaesthetist should be involved
  before a decision is taken to proceed to treatment.
• Preparation for ECT should be as per routine with the addition of any
  instructions from the anaesthetist, for example the administration of
  antacids on the morning of treatment.
• Any concerns should be reported urgently to the obstetrician.

ECT in children and adolescents
An exceptionally rare circumstance—hence, special provisions apply:
• The Royal College of Psychiatrists recommends that for those under
  16yrs two further opinions are sought in addition to the treating
  consultant: one from a child and adolescent psychiatrist, and one from
  another psychiatrist from a different clinical unit.
• Adolescents aged 16–18 are able to consent and refuse treatment in
  the same way as an adult, but parental approval is advised. In Scotland
  those under 16 can consent *if* they understand the process but again
  parental approval is advised.
• For compulsory treatment it should be noted that the provisions of
  legislation governing ECT have no lower age limit.

1 Trevino BA, McClintock SM, and Husain MM (2010) A review of Continuation Eloctroconvulsive
Therapy: application, safety, and efficacy. *Journal of ECT* **26**: 186–95.

ECT 6: side-effects and other specific problems

Side-effects
- *Early:* some loss of short-term memory see **ECT and memory loss**. retrograde amnesia—usually resolves completely (64%), headache (48%—if recurrent, use simple analgesia), temporary confusion (10–27%, nausea/vomiting (9%), clumsiness (5%), muscular aches.
- *Late:* loss of long-term memory (rare—see **ECT and memory loss**).
- *Mortality:* no greater than for general anaesthesia in minor surgery (2:100 000)—usually due to cardiac complications in patients with known cardiac disease (hence need for close monitoring).

Specific problems
- *Persistent ineffective seizures:* check use of drugs that may raise seizure threshold, consider use of IV caffeine or theophylline.
- *Prolonged seizures* (i.e. over 150–180s): administer IV diazemuls (5mg) repeated every 30s until seizure stops (alternative—midazolam). Lower energy dosing for next treatment.
- *Post-seizure confusion:* reassurance, nurse in a calm environment, ensure safety of patient, if necessary consider sedation (e.g. diazemuls/ midazolam). If a recurrent problem, use a low dose of a BDZ prophylactically during recovery, immediately after ECT.

ECT and memory loss
- Research has focused on retrograde amnesia because of (highly publicized) claims that ECT causes more enduring deficits in past memories (esp. autobiographical) than new memories.
- These studies show that the period closest to receiving ECT is least well remembered and can be permanently lost.
- Recent systematic reviews of the evidence for loss of past memories[1] highlight the difficulties in interpreting the literature, e.g. unknown sensitivity of autobiographical memory measures, need for premorbid measures of cognitive status. Nevertheless, they find:
  - autobiographical memory loss does occur;
  - it is related to how ECT is administered.
- Specific recommendations to minimize memory loss include: use of right UECT; brief pulse rather than sine wave ECT; dose titration; limited number and frequency of ECT sessions.

Does ECT damage the brain?
- Psychiatrists—such as Peter Breggin, author of 'Toxic Psychiatry' (1993) and 'Brain-Disabling Treatments in Psychiatry' (2007)—have been very vocal opponents of ECT, believing official reports have deliberately ignored evidence of negative effects.
- Even proponents of ECT in early writings suggested they believed that a degree of cerebral damage (akin to a concussion) was necessary for ECT to work—the rejected *brain injury theory*.

- Strong evidence against ECT causing damage comes from a primate study comparing ECT, MCT, or anaesthesia alone which reports no histological lesions after 6wks of daily treatment.[2]
- There are few post-mortem reports, but one study found no histopathological evidence of brain injury in the brain of a 92-year-old lady with major depression who had received 91 sessions of ECT during the last 22yrs of her life.[3]
- Most mental health associations and colleges including the APA and RCPsych have concluded there is no evidence that ECT causes structural brain damage (see Box 7.9).

Box 7.9 Structural brain damage from ECT

'Prospective CT and MRI studies show no evidence of ECT-induced structural changes. Some early human autopsy case reports from the unmodified ECT era reported cerebrovascular lesions that were due to agonal changes or undiagnosed disease. In animal ECS studies that used a stimulus intensity and frequency comparable to human ECT, no neuronal loss was seen when appropriate control animals, blind ratings, and perfusion fixation techniques were employed. Controlled studies using quantitative cell counts have failed to show neuronal loss even after prolonged courses of ECS. Several well-controlled studies have demonstrated that neuronal loss occurs only after 1.5 to 2 hours of continuous seizure activity in primates, and adequate muscle paralysis and oxygenation further delay these changes. These conditions are not approached during ECT.'

Devanand DP, Dwork AJ, Hutchinson ER, *et al.* (1994) Does ECT alter brain structure? *Am J Psychiat* **151**: 957–70.

'It is more dangerous to drive to the hospital than to have the treatment. The unfair stigma against ECT is denying a remarkably effective medical treatment to patients who need it.'

Charles Kellner, Professor of Psychiatry, Mount Sinai Hospital, New York City quoted in *USA Today* (Dec. 6, 1995) whilst editor of Convulsive Therapy (now *Journal of ECT*).

1 Fraser LM, O'Carroll RE, Ebmeier KP (2008) The effect of electroconvulsive therapy on autobiographical memory: a systematic review. *J ECT* **24**: 10–17.
2 Dwork AJ, Arango V, Underwood M, *et al.* (2004) Absence of histological lesions in primate models of ECT and magnetic seizure therapy. *Am J Psychiat* **161**: 576–8.
3 Scalia J, Lisanby SH, Dwork AJ, *et al.* (2007) Neuropathological examination after 91 ECT treatments in a 92-year-old woman with late-onset depression. *J ECT* **23**: 96–8.

Neurosurgery for mental disorder (NMD)

Despite the controversial nature of irreversible neurosurgery for mental disorders, it is surprising that patients—rather than psychiatrists—often raise the issue, particularly when they retain insight into the chronic, intractable nature of their illness. Neurosurgery is only performed in exceptional cases (see Box 7.10) when all other treatments have failed, and its use is governed by specific mental health legislation. It is still possible, however, to encounter patients who have had surgical procedures performed in the past, and this may complicate the diagnosis of current problems (e.g. depression, OCD, dementia, esp. frontal lobe symptoms) when there is demonstrable damage to key brain structures on CT/MRI.

Current criteria for NMD[1]
- Severe mood disorders, OCD, severe anxiety disorders.
- The patient must want the operation.
- All other reasonable treatments have repeatedly failed (i.e. pharmacological, ECT, psychological).
- The patient remains ill, but has capacity to provide informed consent.

Current surgical techniques
These employ stereotactic methods, using pre-operative MRI to establish target coordinates and a fixed stereotactic frame (or new 'frameless' stereotactic instruments utilizing infrared positioning). Lesioning may be effected by implantation of yttrium rods or radio-frequency lesioning. Lesions are localized to the orbito-frontal and anterior cingulate loop (the 'limbic' loop), which is strongly implicated in the regulation of emotion and mood,[2] e.g.:
- Stereotactic subcaudate tractotomy (SST).
- Anterior cingulotomy (ACING).
- Stereotactic limbic leucotomy (SLL) (combining subcaudate tractotomy and anterior cingulotomy).
- Anterior capsulotomy (ACAPS).

Adverse effects
Older techniques were associated with severe amotivational syndromes (up to 24%), marked personality change (up to 60%), and epilepsy (up to 15%). Stereotactic techniques report minimal post-operative problems with confusion (3–10%), incontinence (1–9%), apathy, weight gain, and seizures (dependent on the type of surgery). More significant personality change and impaired social or cognitive functioning are infrequent and there is more likely to be improvement.

Outcome
Given the treatment-resistant nature of the patients receiving surgery, reports of good outcome are surprisingly high (e.g. depression: 34–68%; OCD: 27–67%), although results should be cautiously interpreted in view of the obvious lack of any control data. ACAPS and SLL appear better for OCD, and ACING and SST for severe mood disorder.

Box 7.10 Psychosurgery—an historical perspective

In 1935, Egas Moniz and Almeida Lima carried out the first 'prefrontal leucotomy' (based on the work of Fulton and Jacobsen in bilateral ablation of prefrontal cortices in chimpanzees, 1934). At the time this was viewed with great enthusiasm (culminating in Moniz being awarded a Nobel Prize for his work in 1949) and other practitioners adapted the early procedures, with Freeman and Watts introducing the standard 'prefrontal leucotomy' (the notorious lobotomy) in 1936, publishing a standard textbook *Psychosurgery* in 1942, and Freeman pioneering 'transorbital leucotomy' in 1946.

The impact of surgical treatment at a time when there were few other physical treatments should not be underestimated, and around 12 000 procedures were performed between 1936 and 1961 in the UK alone (over 40 000 in the US). Techniques were refined (e.g. open cingulotomy, bimedial leucotomy, orbital undercut) from earlier blind, freehand procedures. However, the advent of effective psychopharmacological treatments and changes in the social climate led to a marked decline in practice from the 1960s onwards.

Nowadays, the term 'psychosurgery' has been abandoned, and replaced with the more accurate 'neurosurgery for mental disorder'. Modern techniques could not be further removed from older procedures and utilize neuroimaging and neurosurgical techniques to lesion clearly defined neuroanatomical targets (see 🕮 p. 296). Between 1984 and 1994 there were a total of only 20 operations per year performed in the UK,[1] and since then the number has diminished further. Available data for England and Wales report 5 procedures in 2005–7 and 2 procedures in 2007–9.[2] In Scotland the Dundee Advanced Intervention Service reported only 5 procedures for 2010/11.[3]

1 CRAG Working Group (1996) *Neurosurgery for mental disorder*. Scotland: HMSO (J2318 7/96).
2 The Mental Health Act Commission (2009) *Thirteenth Biennial Report (2007–2009)*. 🕸 http://www.cqc.org.uk/sites/default/files/media/documents/mhac_biennial_report_0709_final.pdf
3 🕸 http://www.advancedinterventions.org.uk/pdf/Reports/AIS_Annual_Report_2011.pdf

1 For current criteria in UK see Dundee Advanced Intervention Service website: 🕸 http://www.advancedinterventions.org.uk/referrals_criteria_NMD.htm
2 Alexander GE, Crutcher MD, DeLong MR (1990) Basal ganglia-thalamocortical circuits: parallel substrates for motor, oculomotor, 'prefrontal' and 'limbic' functions. *Progr Brain Res* **85**: 119–46.

Other physical treatments

Light therapy (phototherapy)

First introduced for the treatment of SAD (a proposed new syndrome at the time) by Rosenthal,[1] on the basis that bright light therapy might ameliorate symptoms of winter depression, due to effects on circadian and seasonal rhythms mediated by melatonin. Recent research has suggested that the effects of phototherapy may be independent of melatonin and produce a 'phase advance' in circadian rhythms (hence, treatment may be best given first thing in the morning). It is usually administered by use of a light box (alternatives include light visors) producing 2500–10 000 lux. Treatment duration is for 2hrs (with 2500 lux) or 30min (with 10 000 lux) a day, with a course lasting 1–3wks (treatment response is usually noticeable within 5 days). If no response within 3wks, discontinue. When effective, continue until time of natural remission to prevent relapse. Dawn-stimulating alarm clocks that gradually illuminate the bedroom over 2hrs to around 250 lux at the point of waking may also be effective.

Adverse effects Particularly with 10 000 lux: headache, visual problems—e.g. eye strain, blurred vision—usually settle; if persistent, reduce duration or intensity of exposure; increased irritability; rarely: manic episodes, increased thoughts of suicide (possibly due to alerting effect and increased energy).

Indications SAD (see 🕮 p. 263), circadian rhythm disorders (see 🕮 p. 436), possibly other depressive disorders and dysthymia.

Contraindications Agitation, insomnia, history of hypomania/mania.

Repetitive transcranial magnetic stimulation (rTMS)

Currently being researched. However, the difference in stimulation parameters used across reported studies makes comparisons difficult. The rationale for treatment is either to increase activity in the left dorsolateral prefrontal cortex (using high-frequency stimulation, e.g. 20Hz) or to reduce activity in the right dorsolateral prefrontal cortex (using low-frequency stimulation, e.g. 1Hz). Initial results in treatment-resistant depression ought to be viewed with caution (see Cochrane review[2]), although this mode of therapy presents an attractive alternative to ECT, without the accompanying risks and adverse effects. NICE recommendations suggest rTMS ought to be used only in research.[3]

Adverse effects Minimal, but patients often report headache or facial discomfort; rarely seizure induction.

Indications Experimental treatment for treatment-resistant depression; possible use in treatment of treatment-resistant auditory hallucinations; negative symptoms of schizophrenia; OCD; panic disorder.

Contraindications History of stroke, brain tumour, or epilepsy.

Magneto-convulsive therapy (MCT)

Another experimental treatment that utilizes the potential problem of seizure induction by rTMS. A varying magnetic field is used to induce seizures in a more controlled way than is possible with ECT. The potential advantages include targeting of brain structures essential for treatment response, and reduction in side-effects (particularly memory impairment).[4]

Vagus nerve stimulation (VNS)

Vagus stimulation by implanted pacemaker (first used as a treatment for epilepsy) has been tested as a treatment of depression since 1998. Stimulation is of the left cervical vagus nerve using bipolar electrodes, attached below the cardiac branch (usually 0.5ms pulse-width, at 20–30Hz, with 30s stimulation periods alternating with 5min breaks). Response rates of 31–40% (short-term)[5] and 27–58% (long-term) have been quoted for treatment-resistant depressive disorder, but the quality of this evidence is low and further research is required. NICE recommends special arrangements.[6]

Adverse effects May include voice alteration (e.g. hoarseness), pain, coughing, and dysphagia.

Deep brain stimulation (DBS)

Best regarded as an experimental treatment for OCD and depression. Has been used in the treatment of neurological disorders including: Parkinson's disease, tremor, dystonia, refractory pain syndromes, and epilepsy. Involves implantation of bilateral electrodes under stereotactic guidance and MRI confirmation. Targets for DBS in OCD include the anterior limb of the internal capsule (like ACAPS NMD) and for depression the subgenual cingulate gyrus (like ACING NMD). Initial reports of long-term outcomes are promising.[7]

Adverse effects Reported problems include throbbing/buzzing sensations, nausea, jaw tingling, and unexpected battery failure resulting in rebound depression with marked suicidal ideation.

1 Rosenthal NE, Sack DA, Gillin JC, et al. (1984) Seasonal affective disorder. A description of the syndrome and preliminary findings with light therapy. Arch Gen Psychiat 41: 72–80.
2 Rodriguez-Martin JL, Barbanoj JM, Schlaepfer T, et al. (2002) Transcranial magnetic stimulation for treating depression. Cochrane Database System Rev 2: CD00393.
3 NICE (2007) Transcranial magnetic stimulation for depression. Interventional procedure guidance IPG242. http://www.nice.org.uk/nicemedia/live/11327/38391/38391.pdf
4 Lisanby SH, Schlaepfer TE, Fisch HU, et al. (2001) Magnetic seizure therapy of major depression. Arch Gen Psychiat 58: 303–5.
5 George MS, Sackeim HA, Rush AJ, et al. (2000) Vagus nerve stimulation: a new tool for brain research and therapy. Biol Psychiat 47: 287–95.
6 NICE (2009) Vagal nerve stimulation for treatment-resistant depression. Interventional procedure guidance IPG330. http://www.nice.org.uk/nicemedia/live/12149/46667/46667.pdf
7 Kennedy SH, Giacobbe P, Rizvi SJ, et al. (2011) Deep brain stimulation for treatment-resistant depression: follow-up after 3 to 6 years. Am J Psychiat 168: 502–10.

Bipolar illness

Introduction

Bipolar affective disorder (commonly known as manic depression) is one of the most common, severe, and persistent psychiatric illnesses. In the public mind it is associated with notions of 'creative madness', and indeed it has affected many creative people—both past and present (see Box 8.1). Appealing as such notions are, most people who battle with the effects of the disorder would rather live a normal life, free from the unpredictability of mood swings, which most of us take for granted.

Chameleon-like in its presentation, the symptoms may vary from one patient to the next, and from one episode to the next within the same patient. The variety of presentations make this one of the most difficult conditions to diagnose. More than other psychiatric disorders, the clinician needs to pay attention to the life history of the patient, and to third-party information from family and friends.

Classically, periods of prolonged and profound depression alternate with periods of excessively elevated and/or irritable mood, known as mania. The symptoms of mania characteristically include a decreased need for sleep, pressured speech, increased libido, reckless behaviour without regard for consequences, and grandiosity (see 📖 p. 306). In severe cases, there may be severe thought disturbances and even psychotic symptoms. Between these highs and lows, patients usually experience periods of full remission.

This classic presentation appears, however, to be one pole of a spectrum of mood disorders (see 📖 p. 312). A milder form of mania (hypomania), associated with episodes of depression, may also occur (see 📖 p. 310). There is also a subclinical presentation—cyclothymia—in which an individual may experience oscillating high and low moods, without ever having a significant manic or depressive episode (see 📖 p. 334). Equally, it may be difficult to distinguish a manic episode with psychotic symptoms from schizoaffective disorder (see 📖 p. 218) on the basis of a single episode.

Full assessment should consider: the number of previous episodes (which may have been subclinical); the average length of previous episodes; the average time between episodes; the level of psychosocial functioning between episodes; previous responses to treatment (especially treatment of early depressive episodes); family history of psychiatric problems; and current (and past) use of alcohol and drugs.

Although at the present time there is no cure for bipolar disorder, for most cases effective treatment is possible and can substantially decrease the associated morbidity and mortality (the suicide rate is high). Some patients do develop severe or chronic impairments and may need specific rehabilitative services. In general, however, the specific aims of treatment are to decrease the frequency, severity, and psychosocial consequences of episodes, and to improve psychosocial functioning between episodes.

Box 8.1 Famous people and bipolar disorder

Famous people who have publicly stated they have bipolar disorder

Buzz Aldrin, astronaut
Tim Burton, artist, movie director
Francis Ford Coppola, director
Patricia Cornwell, writer
Ray Davies, musician
Robert Downey Jr, actor
Carrie Fisher, writer, actor
Larry Flynt, magazine publisher
Connie Francis, actor, musician
Stephen Fry, actor, author, comedian
Stuart Goddard (Adam Ant), musician
Linda Hamilton, actor
Kay Redfield Jamison, psychologist, writer
Ilie Nastase, athlete (tennis), politician
Axl Rose, musician
Ben Stiller, actor, comedian
Gordon Sumner (Sting), musician, composer
Jean-Claude Van Damme, athlete (martial arts), actor
Tom Waits, musician, composer
Brian Wilson, musician, composer, arranger

Famous people (deceased) who had a confirmed diagnosis of bipolar disorder

Louis Althusser, 1918–1990, philosopher, writer
Clifford Beers, 1876–1943, humanitarian
Neal Cassady, 1926–1968, writer
Graham Greene, 1904–1991, writer
Frances Lear, 1923–1996, writer, editor, women's rights activist
Vivien Leigh, 1913–1967, actor
Robert Lowell, 1917–1977, poet
Burgess Meredith, 1908–1997, actor, director
Spike Milligan, 1919–2002, comic actor, writer
Theodore Roethke, 1908–1963, writer
Don Simpson, 1944–1996, movie producer
David Strickland, 1970–1999, actor
Joseph Vasquez, 1963–1996, writer, movie director
Mary Jane Ward, 1905–1981, writer
Virginia Woolf, 1882–1941, writer

Other famous people thought to have had bipolar disorder

William Blake, Napoleon Bonaparte, Agatha Christie, Winston Churchill, TS Eliot, F. Scott Fitzgerald, Cary Grant, Victor Hugo, Samuel Johnson, Robert E. Lee, Abraham Lincoln, Marilyn Monroe, Mozart, Isaac Newton, Plato (according to Aristotle), Edgar Allan Poe, St Francis, St John, St Theresa, Rod Steiger, Robert Louis Stevenson, Lord Tennyson, Mark Twain, Van Gogh, Walt Whitman, Tennessee Williams.

Historical perspective

Bipolar affective disorder has been known since ancient times. Hippocrates described patients as 'amic' and 'melancholic', and clear connections between melancholia and mania date back to the descriptions of the two syndromes by Aretaius of Cappadocia (c.150 BC) and Paul of Aegina (625–690). Thinking at that time reflected 'humoral' theories, with melancholia believed to be caused by excess of 'black bile' and mania by excess of 'yellow bile'.

Despite the view of some clinicians in the eighteenth century that melancholia and mania were interconnected (e.g. Robert James, 1705–1776), it was the middle of the nineteenth century before this was more widely accepted. In 1854 Jules Baillarger (1809–1890) published a paper in the *Bulletin of the Imperial Academy of Medicine* describing *la folie à double forme*, closely followed 2 wks later by a paper in the same journal by Jean-Pierre Falret (1794–1870), who claimed that he had been teaching students at the Salpêtrière about *la folie circulaire* for 10 years. Although the two men were to continue arguing about who originated the idea, they at least agreed that the illness was characterized by alternating periods of melancholia and mania, often separated by periods of normal mood. In 1899, Emil Kraepelin comprehensively described 'manic-depressive insanity' in the 6th edition of his textbook *Psychiatrie: Ein Lehrbuch für Studirende und Ärzte*. In the 5th edition he had already divided severe mental illnesses into those with a deteriorating course (i.e. schizophrenia and related psychoses) and those with a periodic course (i.e. the mood disorders). It was his view that the mood disorders 'represented manifestations of a single morbid process'.

At the turn of the twentieth century, hopes were high that understanding of the pathophysiology of mental illness might be within reach. In 1906, the German microbiologist August Wassermann discovered a method of detecting syphilitic infection in the CNS, and in the same year an effective treatment was developed by Paul Ehrlich using arsenic compounds. Syphilis was, at that time, one of the most common causes of severe (often mania-like) psychiatric symptoms—general paralysis of the insane. Reliably diagnosing and treating such a condition was a huge step forward. In cases of manic-depressive illness, however, neuropathologists failed to find any structural brain abnormalities. Although some still maintained it was a physical illness, caused by disruptions in biological functioning, the pervasive new psychodynamic theories regarded functional illnesses (i.e. schizophrenia and manic-depressive illness) as illnesses of the mind, not the brain. The idea that they could be understood and treated only if the traumatic childhood events, repressed sexual feelings, or interpersonal conflicts were uncovered, influenced psychiatric thinking for over half a century.

It was not until *specific* drug treatments for these functional illnesses were found that psychiatry came full circle again, and new life was breathed into the old search for *biological* mechanisms. In 1949 John Cade published a report on the use of lithium salts in manic patients, but it took nearly three decades, and the work of many psychiatrists, including Morgens Schou in Denmark and Ronald Fieve in the US, before lithium would become the mainstay of treatment for manic-depressive illness. Equally significant was the observation by Ronald Kuhn that when patients with 'manic-depressive psychosis' were treated with imipramine they could switch from depression to mania. That this did not occur in all patients with depression suggested that there was a different biological mechanism underlying depressive illness compared to manic-depressive illness. With different pharmacological agents treating different psychiatric disorders, the stage was set for classifying psychiatric disorders in line with their presumed differing aetiologies. The quest had begun to understand the biological mechanisms and, in doing so, to develop better treatments.

Mania/manic episode

Essence

A distinct period of abnormally and persistently elevated, expansive, or irritable mood, with 3 or more characteristic symptoms of mania (see Box 8.2. Both DSM-IV and ICD-10 specify the episode should last at least 1 wk, or less if admission to hospital is necessary. By definition, the disturbance is sufficiently severe to impair occupational and social functioning. Psychotic features may be present.

Clinical features

- Elevated mood (usually out of keeping with circumstances).
- Increased energy, which may manifest as:
  - over-activity;
  - pressured speech ('flight of ideas');
  - racing thoughts;
  - reduced need for sleep.
- Increased self-esteem, evident as:
  - over-optimistic ideation;
  - grandiosity;
  - reduced social inhibitions;
  - over-familiarity (which may be overly amorous);
  - facetiousness.
- Reduced attention/increased distractibility.
- Tendency to engage in behaviour that could have serious consequences:
  - preoccupation with extravagant, impracticable schemes;
  - spending recklessly;
  - inappropriate sexual encounters.
- Other behavioural manifestations:
  - excitement;
  - irritability;
  - aggressiveness;
  - suspiciousness.
- Marked disruption of work, usual social activities, and family life.

Psychotic symptoms

In its more severe form, mania may be associated with psychotic symptoms (usually mood-congruent, but may also be incongruent):

- Grandiose ideas may be delusional, related to identity or role (with special powers or religious content).
- Suspiciousness may develop into well-formed persecutory delusions.
- Pressured speech may become so great that clear associations are lost and speech becomes incomprehensible.
- Irritability and aggression may lead to violent behaviour.
- Preoccupation with thoughts and schemes may lead to self-neglect, to the point of not eating or drinking, and poor living conditions.
- Catatonic behaviour—also termed manic stupor.
- Total loss of insight.

Differential diagnosis
- Schizophrenia, schizoaffective disorder, delusional disorder, other psychotic disorders.
- Anxiety disorders/PTSD.
- Circadian rhythm disorders (see 📖 p. 436).
- ADHD/conduct disorder.
- Alcohol or drug misuse (e.g. stimulants, hallucinogens, opiates).
- Physical illness (e.g. hyper/hypothyroidism, Cushing's syndrome, SLE, MS, head injury, brain tumour, epilepsy, HIV and other encephalopathies, neurosyphilis, Fahr's disease).
- Other antidepressant treatment or drug-related causes (Box 8.2).

Management
- Exclusion of other causes and appropriate investigations (📖 p. 316).
- Address any specific psychosocial stressors.
- For specific management, see 📖 p. 326.

Box 8.2 Medications that may induce symptoms of hypomania/mania

- *Antidepressants:* drug-induced mania described with most antidepressants (or withdrawal, see 🕮 p. 964), less so with SSRIs and bupropion (also seen with ECT and light therapy).
- *Other psychotropic medication:*
  - *benzodiazepines*—may be confused with 'paradoxical' reactions (🕮 p. 929);
  - *antipsychotics*—olanzapine, risperidone;
  - *lithium*—toxicity, and when combined with TCAs;
  - *anticonvulsants* (rare)—carbamazepine (and withdrawal), valproate, gabapentin;
  - *psychostimulants*—fenfluramine, amfetamine, dexamfetamine, methylphenidate;
  - *other*—disulfiram.
- *Anti-Parkinsonian medication:* amantadine, bromocriptine, levodopa, procyclidine.
- *Cardiovascular drugs:* captopril, clonidine, digoxin, diltiazem, hydralazine, methyldopa withdrawal, procainamide, propranolol (and withdrawal), reserpine.
- *Respiratory drugs:* aminophylline, ephedrine, salbutamol, terfenadine, pseudoephedrine.
- *Anti-infection:* anti-TB medication, chloroquine, clarithromycin, dapsone, isoniazid, zidovudine.
- *Analgesics:* buprenorphine, codeine, indometacin, nefopam (IM), pentazocine, tramadol.
- *GI drugs:* cimetidine, metoclopramide, ranitidine.
- *Steroids:* ACTH, beclometasone, corticosteroids, cortisone, dexamethasone, DHEA, hydrocortisone, prednisolone, testosterone.
- *Other:* baclofen (and withdrawal), cyclizine, ciclosporin, interferon.

Hypomania/hypomanic episode

Essence
Three or more characteristic symptoms (see **Clinical features**) lasting at least 4 days (DSM-IV), and are clearly different from 'normal' mood (third-party corroboration). By definition, not severe enough to interfere with social or occupational functioning, require admission to hospital, or include psychotic features.

Clinical features
Hypomania shares symptoms with mania, but these are evident to a lesser degree and do not significantly disrupt work or lead to social rejection:
- Mildly elevated, expansive, or irritable mood.
- Increased energy and activity.
- Marked feelings of well-being, physical, and mental efficiency.
- Increased self-esteem.
- Sociability.
- Talkativeness.
- Over-familiarity.
- Increased sex drive.
- Reduced need for sleep.
- Difficulty in focusing on one task alone (tasks often started, but not finished).

Differential diagnosis
- Agitated depression.
- OCD/other anxiety disorders.
- Circadian rhythm disorders (see 📖 p. 436).
- Substance misuse/physical illness/medication-related (see 📖 p. 308, Box 8.2).

Management
- Exclusion of other possible causes with appropriate investigations (see 📖 p. 316).
- Address any specific psychosocial stressors.
- If sleep disturbance is a problem, consider use of an hypnotic.
- If episode is prolonged, discuss medication possibilities (see 📖 p. 326) and the possibility of prophylaxis (📖 p. 330).

Bipolar spectrum disorder

One view of the affective disorders is that they consist of a continuum (see Box 8.3) with bipolar spectrum sitting uneasily between cyclothymia and bipolar II. Whether or not such 'subsyndromal' disorders are of clinical relevance remains controversial and there are other unexpected diagnostic concerns (see 🕮 p. 318).

Proposed clinical features

Bipolar spectrum disorder is characterized by:[1]
- At least one major depressive episode.
- No spontaneous hypomanic or manic episodes.

The history will include some of the following:
- A family history of bipolar disorder in a first-degree relative.
- Antidepressant-induced mania or hypomania.
- Hyperthymic personality[2] (at baseline, non-depressed state).
- Recurrent major depressive episodes (>3).
- Brief major depressive episodes (on average, <3mths).
- Atypical depressive symptoms (DSM-IV criteria).
- Psychotic major depressive episodes.
- Early age of onset of major depressive episode (<age 25).
- Post-partum depression.
- Antidepressant 'wear-off' (acute but not prophylactic response).
- Lack of response to up to 3 antidepressant treatment trials.

Management

Patients with features of bipolar spectrum disorder may represent a subset of patients who do not respond well to antidepressants (often precipitating a switch to a hypomanic or manic episode) and for whom an anticonvulsant may be the drug of choice (e.g. valproate, see 🕮 p. 342).

Box 8.3 The 'affective continuum'

Dysthymia
Unipolar depression
Atypical depression
Psychotic depression $\Big\}$ Unipolar spectrum disorder
Recurrent depression
Cyclothymia
Bipolar spectrum disorder
Bipolar II
Bipolar I

---

1 Ghaemi SN, Ko JY, Goodwin FK (2002) 'Cade's disease' and beyond: misdiagnosis, antidepressant use, and a proposed definition for bipolar spectrum disorder. *Can J Psychiat* **47**: 125–34.
2 Characterized by cheerful, optimistic personality style, tendency to become easily irritated, extroverted and sociable, and requiring little sleep (less than 6hrs/night)—a lifelong disposition, unlike short-lived hypomania. Neither in ICD-10 nor DSM-IV, but significant overlap with narcissistic or antisocial personality.

Bipolar (affective) disorder 1: classification

Diagnostic classification (see Box 8.4 and Table 8.1)

ICD-10
Requires at least 2 episodes, one of which must be hypomanic, manic, or mixed, with recovery usually complete between episodes. Criteria for depressive episodes are the same as unipolar depression (see 📖 p. 236). Separate category (*manic episode*) for hypomania or mania (with or without psychotic symptoms) without history of depressive episodes. Cyclothymia included with dysthymia in *persistent mood disorders* section.

DSM-IV
Allows a single manic episode and cyclothymic disorder to be considered as part of bipolar disorder, and defines two subtypes (with additional specifiers):
- *Bipolar I disorder*: the occurrence of one or more manic episodes or mixed episodes, with or without a history of one or more depressive episodes.
- *Bipolar II disorder*: the occurrence of one or more depressive episodes accompanied by at least one hypomanic episode.
- *Severity specifiers*: mild, moderate, severe (with or without psychotic features); in partial or full remission.
- *Special syndrome specifiers:* with catatonic, melancholic, or atypical features; with post-partum onset.
- *Longitudinal course specifiers:* with or without full inter-episode recovery; with seasonal pattern; with rapid cycling.

Mixed episodes (DSM-IV and ICD-10)
- The occurrence of both manic/hypomanic and depressive symptoms in a single episode, present every day for at least 1wk (DSM-IV) or 2wks (ICD-10).
- Typical presentations include:
  - depression *plus* over-activity/pressure of speech;
  - mania *plus* agitation and reduced energy/libido;
  - dysphoria *plus* manic symptoms (with exception of elevated mood);
  - rapid cycling (fluctuating between mania and depression—4 or more episodes/yr)

Note: 'Ultra-rapid' cycling refers to the situation when fluctuations are over days or even hours.

'The clinical reality of manic-depressive illness is far more lethal and infinitely more complex than the current psychiatric nomenclature, bipolar disorder, would suggest. Cycles of fluctuating moods and energy levels serve as a background to constantly changing thoughts, behaviors, and feelings. The illness encompasses the extremes of human experience. Thinking can range from florid psychosis, or "madness", to patterns of unusually clear, fast and creative associations, to retardation so profound that no meaningful mental activity can occur. Behavior can be frenzied, expansive, bizarre, and seductive, or it can be seclusive, sluggish, and dangerously suicidal. Moods may swing erratically between euphoria and despair or irritability and desperation. The rapid oscillations and combinations of such extremes result in an intricately textured clinical picture. Manic patients, for example, are depressed and irritable as often as they are euphoric; the highs associated with mania are generally only pleasant and productive during the earlier, milder stages.'

Dr Kay Redfield Jamison (1993) Touched with fire: manic-depressive illness and the artistic temperament, pp. 47–8. New York: Free Press, Macmillan

Box 8.4 ICD-10 bipolar affective disorder

- Current episode, hypomanic.
- Current episode, manic without psychotic symptoms.
- Current episode, manic with psychotic symptoms.
- Current episode, mild or moderate depression.
- Current episode, severe depression without psychotic symptoms.
- Current episode, severe depression with psychotic symptoms.
- Current episode, mixed.
- Currently in remission.
- Other bipolar affective disorders: bipolar affective disorder, unspecified.

Table 8.1 DSM-IV bipolar disorder

Bipolar I disorder	Bipolar II disorder
Single manic episode	Most recent episode, hypomanic
Most recent episode, hypomanic	Most recent episode, depressed
Most recent episode, manic	
Most recent episode, mixed	**Cyclothymic disorder**
Most recent episode, depressed	
Most recent episode, unspecified	Bipolar disorder not otherwise specified

Bipolar (affective) disorder 2: clinical notes

Epidemiology

Lifetime prevalence 0.3–1.5% (0.8% bipolar I; 0.5% bipolar II); ♂ = ♀ (bipolar II and rapid cycling more common in ♀; 1st episodes: ♂ tend to be manic, ♀ depressive); no significant racial differences; age range 15–50+ yrs (peaks at 15–19yrs and 20–24yrs; mean 21yrs).

Course

Extremely variable. First episodes may be hypomanic, manic, mixed, or depressive. This may be followed by many years (5 or more) without a further episode, but the length of time between subsequent episodes may begin to narrow. There is often a 5–10-yr interval between age at onset of illness and age at first treatment or first admission to hospital. Often patients with recurrent depression have a first manic episode in later life (>50yrs). It is known that untreated patients may have more than 10 episodes in a lifetime, and that the duration and period of time between episodes stabilizes after the 4th or 5th episode. Although the prognosis is better for treated patients, there still remains a high degree of unpredictability.

Morbidity/mortality

Morbidity and mortality rates are high, in terms of lost work, lost productivity, effects on marriage (increased divorce rates) and the family, with attempted suicide in 25–50%, and completed suicide in 10% (♂ > ♀, usually during a depressive episode). Often significant comorbidity—esp. drug/alcohol misuse and anxiety disorders (both increase risk of suicide).

Differential diagnosis

Depends upon the nature of the presenting episode (See Mania/manic episode, 📖 p. 306, Hypomania/hypomanic episode, 📖 p. 310, and Depressive illness, 📖 p. 428).

Investigations

As for depression; full physical and routine blood tests to exclude any treatable cause, including FBC, ESR, glucose, U&Es, Ca^{2+}, TFTs, LFTs, drug screen. Less routine tests: urinary copper (to exclude Wilson's disease [rare]), ANF (SLE), infection screen (VDRL, HIV test). CT/MRI brain (to exclude tumour, infarction, haemorrhage, MS)—may show hyperintense subcortical structures (esp. temporal lobes), ventricular enlargement, and sulcal prominence; EEG (baseline and to rule out epilepsy). Other baseline tests prior to treatment should include ECG and creatinine clearance.

Management

See specific sections (□ p. 322) for management principles, other issues, treatment of acute manic episodes, depressive episodes, prophylaxis, and psychotherapeutic interventions.

Prognosis

Within the first 2 years of 1st episode, 40–50% of patients experience another manic episode. 50–60% of patients on lithium gain control of their symptoms (7% no recurrence; 45% some future episodes; 40% persistent recurrence). Often, the cycling between depression and mania accelerates with age. *Poor prognostic factors:* poor employment history; alcohol abuse; psychotic features; depressive features between periods of mania and depression; evidence of depression; male sex; treatment non-compliance. *Good prognostic factors:* manic episodes of short duration; later age of onset; few thoughts of suicide; few psychotic symptoms; few comorbid physical problems, good treatment response and compliance.

'I want to be bipolar ...'

A worrying trend in outpatient clinics is the 'expert' patient who has self-diagnosed bipolar disorder. One of the unexpected consequences of anti-stigma campaigns is the identification of individuals with celebrities who claim to have a psychiatric disorder (usually of a 'softer' variety—like bipolar II, rather than bipolar I). Whilst acceptance and more positive attitudes to psychiatric disorders are to be welcomed, it is still the provenance of the psychiatrist to legitimize such presumptive diagnoses. Good history taking is of paramount importance. It is essential that differentials and comorbidity are considered (e.g. personality traits, anxiety, alcohol and substance misuse). As far as possible, collateral information may help with possible recall bias and evidence of secondary gain prohibit the medicalization of difficult or imprudent behaviour. Clinicians must try and remain objective and not collude with the patient, professional colleagues, fashionable labelling (e.g. 'bipolar spectrum', see 📖 p. 312), or unsubstantiated claims of Big Pharma. Diagnosis carries not only far-reaching psychosocial consequences but also will often suggest a need for specific interventions which are not without risk.

The main differentials not to miss include:

- *Thyroid disorders:* may resemble depression or mania/hypomania; can be caused by lithium; may present subclinically as mixed states; and are treatable!

- *Substance abuse:* can mimic affective states; may unmask pre-existing illness/predisposition; may be a form of self-medication; should always be treated first.

- *ADHD: overlapping symptoms*—restlessness, hyperactivity, distractibility, impulsiveness, poor concentration/attention, temper dyscontrol; lifelong, pervasive not episodic; may respond to antidepressants and mood stabilizers.

- *Borderline PD:* stormy, unstable lifestyles; overly dramatic; intense unstable relationships; acutely sensitive to abandonment; unrealistically demanding of families and physicians; exhibiting self-defeating and self-destructive behaviours; heightened sense of personal rights (repeated vexatious complaints); frequently associated with substance abuse, self-harm (mutilation), and repeated suicidal acts.

- *Other PDs:* traits often seen in bipolar disorder: dependency, passive aggression, histrionics, paranoia, narcissism, hypochondriasis, manipulative antisocial traits. When these are secondary to bipolar disorder they tend to disappear between episodes, and with treatment, and the patient is more likely to be embarrassed and remorseful. Fixed PDs are often demanding, defiant, manipulative, self-defeating, actively undermine efforts to address needs, non-compliant with medication, abuse alcohol or substances, and end up in prison.

Bipolar affective disorder 3: aetiology

Despite significant research efforts the definitive pathophysiology of bipolar disorder remains elusive. There are many similarities with gene expression and neuroimaging studies of persons with schizophrenia and major depression, suggesting that mood disorders and schizophrenia may share a biological basis.

Genetic

Twin, family, and adoption studies point to a significant genetic contribution. First-degree relatives are 7× more likely to develop the condition than the general population (i.e. 10–15% risk). Children of a parent with bipolar disorder have a 50% chance of developing a psychiatric disorder (genetic liability appears shared for schizophrenia, schizoaffective, and bipolar affective disorder). MZ twins: 33–90% concordance; dizygotic (DZ) twins: ~23%.

Candidate genes

Results from 4 genome-wide association studies of large samples of subjects with bipolar disorder give combined support for 2 particular genes, ANK3 (ankyrin G) and CACNA1C (α1C subunit of the L-type voltage-gated calcium channel).[1] Other candidates are genes associated with biochemical pathways that lithium regulates, e.g. the phosphatidyl inositol pathway (diacylglycerol kinase eta [DGKH] gene); cell death/neuroprotection mechanisms (e.g. glycogen synthase kinase 3-beta [GSK3β]); or circadian periodicity (e.g CLOCK gene) (see Box 8.5). Postmortem studies found decreased levels of expression of oligodendrocyte-myelin-related genes implicating abnormal myelination in the illness.

Shared genetics with schizophrenia

As well as overlapping family susceptibility, there are emerging reports of shared genes, e.g. G72 on 13q34, which encodes d-amino acid oxidase activator (DAOA) and DISC1 (Disrupted in Schizophrenia 1) on 1q42. A large meta-analysis by the National Institutes of Health (NIH) on recent genome-wide association studies found evidence for a shared susceptibility locus around 6p22.1 known to harbour genes involved in immunity, and turning other genes on and off.[2]

Neuroimaging

A recent meta-analysis of structural and functional brain imaging found decreased activation and reduced grey matter in areas associated with emotional regulation, and increased activation in ventral limbic brain regions that mediate and generate emotional responses.[3]

Biochemical factors

There is increasing evidence of the importance of glutamate in bipolar disorder and major depression; the catecholamine hypothesis study suggests that an increase in epinephrine and norepinephrine causes mania, while a decrease causes depression; drugs that may cause mania (e.g. cocaine, L-dopa, amfetamines, antidepressants) suggest a role for DA and 5-HT; disruption of Ca^{2+} regulation may be caused by neurological insults, such as excessive glutaminergic transmission or ischaemia; hormonal imbalances and disruptions of the hypothalamic–pituitary–adrenal axis involved in homeostasis and stress response are also important.

Environmental factors

Stressful life events may lead to episodes. Pregnancy esp. carries a high risk of a mixed affective presentation or frank puerperal psychosis.

Box 8.5 Aetiological theories

Abnormal programmed cell death

Animal studies have recently shown that antidepressants, lithium, and valproate indirectly regulate a number of factors involved in cell survival pathways (e.g. CREB, BDNF, Bcl-2, and MAP kinases), perhaps explaining their delayed long-term beneficial effects (via under-appreciated neurotrophic effects, esp. in the frontal cortex and the hippocampus[1]). Neuroimaging studies also indicate cell loss in these same brain regions suggesting that bipolar affective disorder may result from abnormal programmed cell death (apoptosis) in critical neural networks involved in the regulation of emotion. Mood stabilizers and antidepressants may act to stimulate cell survival pathways and increase levels of neurotrophic factors that improve cellular resilience.

Kindling

An older hypothesis,[2] also drawing on animal models, it suggests a role for neuronal injury, through a mechanism involving electrophysiological kindling and behavioural sensitization. A genetically predisposed individual experiences an increasing number of minor neurological insults (e.g. due to drugs of abuse, excessive glucocorticoid stimulation, acute or chronic stress, or other factors), which eventually result in mania. After the 1st episode, neuronal damage may persist, allowing for recurrence with or without minor environmental or behavioural stressors (like epilepsy), which may result in further injury. This provides an explanation for later episodes becoming more frequent, why anticonvulsants may be useful in preventing recurrent episodes, and suggests that treatment should be as early as possible and long-term.

1 Manji HK, Duman RS (2001) Impairments of neuroplasticity and cellular resilience in severe mood disorders: implications for the development of novel therapeutics. *Psychopharmacol Bull* **35**: 5–49.

2 Post RM, Weiss SR (1989) Sensitization, kindling, and anticonvulsants in mania. *J Clin Psychiat* **50** (Suppl): 23–30.

1 Ferreira MA, O'Donovan MC, Meng YA, *et al.* (2008) Collaborative genome-wide association analysis supports a role for ANK3 and CACNA1C in bipolar disorder. *Nat Genet* **40**: 1056–8.

2 NIH News (2009) Schizophrenia and bipolar disorder share genetic roots. London: National Institutes of Health. ℘ http://www.nih.gov/news/health/jul2009/nimh-01.htm

3 Houenou J, Frommberger J, Carde S, *et al.* (2011) Neuroimaging-based markers of bipolar disorder: evidence from two meta-analyses. *J Affect Disord* **132**: 344–55.

Bipolar affective disorder 4: management principles

Acute episodes

This will depend upon the nature of the presenting episode (see 📖 p. 306, 📖 p. 310, and 📖 p. 312). Often the episode may require hospital admission (see **Hospital admission**, 📖 p. 323). Special consideration should also be given to certain specific issues related to the clinical presentation, the presence of concurrent medical problems, and particular patient groups, both in terms of setting and choice of treatment (see 📖 p. 324). Issues of prophylaxis (see 📖 p. 330) should be considered, and this may sometimes involve not only pharmacological, but also psychotherapeutic interventions (see 📖 p. 332).

Outpatient follow-up

Once the diagnosis has been clearly established, possible physical causes excluded, and the presenting episode effectively treated, follow-up has a number of key aims:

- Establishing and maintaining a therapeutic alliance.
- Monitoring the patient's psychiatric status.
- Providing education regarding bipolar disorder.
- Enhancing treatment compliance.
- Monitoring side-effects of medication and ensuring therapeutic levels of any mood stabilizer.
- Identifying and addressing any significant comorbid conditions (📖 p. 324).
- Promoting regular patterns of activity and wakefulness.
- Promoting understanding of and adaption to the psychosocial effects of bipolar disorder.
- Identifying new episodes early.
- Reducing the morbidity and sequelae of bipolar disorder.
- Maintaining a pragmatic view of how interventions will help—to reduce frequency and severity of episodes but perhaps not to eliminate them completely—bipolar disorder is a chronic condition.
- Providing an opportunity to discuss any new treatment developments in a balanced and evidence-informed manner.

Relapse prevention

A key part of psychiatric management is helping patients to identify precipitants or early manifestations of illness, so that treatment can be initiated early. This may be done as part of the usual psychiatric follow-up, or form part of a specific psychotherapeutic intervention (see 📖 p. 332), e.g. *insomnia* may often be either a precipitant, or an early indicator, of mania or depression—education about the importance of regular sleep habits and occasional use of an hypnotic (see 📖 p. 426) to promote normal sleep patterns may be useful in preventing the development of a manic episode. Other early or subtle signs of mania may be treated with the short-term use of benzodiazepines or antipsychotics. A good therapeutic alliance is critical, and the patient, who often has good insight, ought to feel that they can contact their clinician as soon as they are aware of these early warning signs. Use of a Mood Diary or Life Chart can help in this regard (see ☞ http://bipolarnews.org; select 'Life Charts' tab).

Hospital admission

Frequently acute episodes of bipolar disorder are severe enough to require hospital admission (often on a compulsory basis). Issues of safety and the provision of effective treatment will govern decisions about whether a patient can remain in the community.

Points to note

- Patients with symptoms of mania/hypomania or depression often have impaired judgement (sometimes related to psychotic symptoms), which may interfere with their ability to make reasoned decisions about the need for treatment.
- Risk assessment includes not only behaviours that may cause direct harm (e.g. suicide attempts or homicidal behaviour), but also those that may be indirectly harmful (e.g. overspending, sexual promiscuity, excessive use of drugs/alcohol, driving whilst unwell).
- Relapsing/remitting nature of the disorder makes it possible to work with the patient (when well) and their family/carers to anticipate future acute episodes—agree a treatment plan.

Clinical features and situations where admission may be necessary

- High risk of suicide or homicide.
- Illness behaviour endangering relationships, reputation, or assets.
- Lack of capacity to co-operate with treatment (e.g. directly due to illness, or 2° to availability of social supports/outpatient resources).
- Lack (or loss) of psychosocial supports.
- Severe psychotic symptoms.
- Severe depressive symptoms.
- Severe mixed states or rapid cycling (days/hours).
- Catatonic symptoms.
- Failure of outpatient treatment.
- Address comorbid conditions (e.g. physical problems, other psychiatric conditions, inpatient detoxification).

Suitable environment

During an acute manic episode, maintain a routine, calm environment (not always possible). A balance should be struck between avoiding over-stimulation (e.g. from outside events, TV, radio, lively conversation) and provision of space to walk or exercise to use up excess energy. Where possible, restrict access to alcohol and drugs. Regular observations by staff may be overly intrusive, and feel uncomfortable in a busy ward. Patients may make requests that may be reasonable, but not practical. Psychiatrist should adopt a pragmatic approach, listen to concerns, and balance risks. This may result in a difficult decision about whether to detain a patient to a hospital environment, which although far from ideal, is the 'least worst' option.

Other issues affecting management decisions

Specific clinical features

Certain clinical features will strongly influence the choice of treatment. For issues of substance misuse or other psychiatric morbidity these should be addressed directly (see specific sections).

- *Psychotic symptoms:* not uncommon for patients to experience delusions and/or hallucinations during episodes of mania or depression. *Management*—mood stabilizer with/without an antipsychotic; consider ECT; if severe consider admission to hospital.
- *Catatonic symptoms:* during a manic episode (manic stupor). *Management*—admit to hospital; exclude medical problem; clarify psychiatric diagnosis; if clear treat with ECT and/or benzodiazepine.
- *Risk of suicide:* assess nature of risk (see 📖 p. 51), note association with rapid cycling mood. If significant risk, or unacceptable uncertainty, admit to hospital (or if in hospital, increase level of observation), consider ECT.
- *Risk of violence:* assess nature of risk (see 📖 p. 692). Note increased risk with rapid mood cycling, paranoid delusions, agitation, and dysphoria. Admit to hospital, consider need for secure setting.
- *Substance-related disorders:* comorbidity is high, often confusing the clinical picture. Substance misuse may lead to relapse both directly and indirectly (by reducing compliance). Equally, alcohol consumption may increase when on lithium. *Management*—address issues of misuse; if detoxification considered, admit to hospital as risk of suicide may be increased.
- *Other comorbidities:* personality, anxiety or conduct disorder, ADHD.

Concurrent medical problems

The presence of other medical problems may affect the management either by exacerbating the course or severity of the disorder or by complicating drug treatment (i.e. issues of tolerability and drug interactions).

- *Cardiovascular/renal/hepatic disorders:* may restrict the choice of drug therapy or increase the need for closer monitoring (see 📖 pp. 972–7).
- *Endocrine disorders:* e.g. hypo/hyperthyoidism.
- *Infectious diseases:* e.g. HIV-infected patients may be more sensitive to CNS side-effects of mood stabilizers.
- *Use of steroids:* e.g. for treatment of asthma/IBS.

Special patient groups

- *Children and adolescents* (see 📖 p. 657). Lithium has been shown to be effective, but long-term effects on development have not been fully studied. Lithium may be excreted more quickly, allowing more rapid dose adjustments, but therapeutic levels are the same as for adults. Risks associated with other adjunctive agents (e.g. antipsychotics, antidepressants, benzodiazepines) should be considered separately. ECT is rarely used, but may be effective. Education, support, and other

specific psychosocial interventions should be considered (usually involving family, teachers, etc.).
- *The elderly* (see 📖 p. 521). When a first manic episode occurs in a patient after age 60, there is usually evidence of previous depressive episodes in their 40s and 50s. Full physical examination is necessary to exclude medical causes (esp. CNS disorders). Older patients may be more sensitive to the side-effects of lithium (particularly neurological) and may require lower therapeutic levels (i.e. below 0.7mmol/L).
- *Pregnancy and lactation* (see 📖 pp. 968–71). Consider ECT as first line for treatment of significant manic, depressed, or psychotically depressed episodes.

Published guidelines

There are now a number of guidelines that can help inform practice including the slightly ageing APA guideline (2002),[1] the Scottish SIGN guideline (2005),[2] the UK NICE guideline (2006),[3] and the BAP guideline (2009).[4] Many UK hospitals are also developing Integrated Care Pathways (IntCPs), which will include treatment guidelines based on these, as well as reflecting local custom and practice.

1 American Psychiatric Association (2002) Practice guideline for the treatment of patients with bipolar disorder. *Am J Psychiat* **159**(Suppl 4): 1–50. ℘ http://www.psychiatryonline.com/pracGuide/pracGuideTopic_8.aspx

2 Scottish Intercollegiate Guideline Network (2005) *Bipolar affective disorder: a national clinical guideline.* SIGN 82. ℘ http://www.sign.ac.uk/pdf/sign82.pdf

3 NICE (2006) Bipolar disorder. Transcranial magnetic stimulation for severe depression. Clinical Guideline CG38. ℘ http://www.nice.org.uk/nicemedia/live/11327/38391/38391.pdf

4 Goodwin GM, Consensus Group of the British Association for Psychopharmacology (2009) Evidence-based guidelines for treating bipolar disorder: revised second edition—recommendations from the British Association for Psychopharmacology. *J Psychopharmacol* **23**: 346–88. ℘ http://www.bap.org.uk/pdfs/Bipolar_guidelines.pdf

Treatment of acute manic episodes

For severe behavioural disorder

Follow local protocols for management (see 📖 p. 325). Pharmacological interventions should be regarded as separate from specific management of acute mania, although there is a degree of overlap. Evidence supports use of haloperidol and clonazepam, clinical practice the use of chlorpromazine and lorazepam or diazepam.

For severe/life-threatening manic episode (or previous good response/advance statement of preference)

ECT should be strongly considered as 1st line treatment and has been shown to be one of the best treatment options in acute mania.[1] Current practice reserves ECT for clinical situations where pharmacological treatments may not be possible, such as pregnancy or severe cardiac disease, or when the patient's illness is refractory to drug treatments.

If currently on antidepressant medication

Give consideration to reducing, stopping, or swapping to an alternative medication if manic episode related to commencement or recent dose change (or possible compliance issues).

Not currently on any treatment

The role of antipsychotic treatment

Most guidelines recommend use of one of the licensed second generation antipsychotics (SGAs) first line in view of ease of use, rapidity of action, and tolerability (see Table 8.2). There is a role for older antipsychotics too—a very recent meta-analysis found risperidone, olanzapine, and haloperidol among the best of the available options for the treatment of manic episodes.[2] Lithium or valproic acid would then be second line unless there is clear evidence of previous benefit.

Table 8.2 Licensed antipsychotics (UK). Starting doses and therapeutic ranges (see BNF for further details)

Drug	Starting dose	Therapeutic range
Olanzapine	15mg/day	5–20mg/day
Quetiapine	50mg bd	400–800mg/day
Risperidone	2mg/day	1–6mg/day
Aripiprazole	15mg/day	15–30mg/day
Asenapine	10mg bd	10–20mg/day

If already on valproic acid or lithium

- Ensure compliance and therapeutic dose.
- Consider adding antipsychotic treatment.

If already on antipsychotic medication
- Ensure compliance and therapeutic dose.
- Consider adding lithium or valproate.

Treatment notes
- *Lithium* (see 📖 p. 336): remains a first-line option for acute mania, with a response rate of around 80%. *Note:* Up to 2wks of treatment may be necessary to reach maximal effectiveness for manic patients. Due to this delayed effect, esp. for severe mania or psychotic symptoms, with associated acute behavioural disturbance, addition of an antipsychotic or a benzodiazepine usually required (see *Benzodiazepines*).
  - *Predictors of good response:* previous response to lithium, compliance with medication, >3 previous episodes, FHx of mood disorder, euphoria (not dysphoria), lack of psychotic symptoms or suicidal behaviour.
- *Valproate* (see 📖 p. 342): also effective in the treatment of acute mania. Well tolerated and has very few drug interactions, making it more suitable for combined treatment regimes. May also work faster than lithium, but not suitable for women of child-bearing age.
  - *Predictors of good response:* may be more effective in particular patients e.g. 'rapid cycling'—where some consider it first line, dysphoric mania, mixed episodes, stable or decreasing frequency of manic episodes, or less severe forms of bipolar spectrum disorders.
- *Benzodiazepines:* may reduce the need for using high antipsychotic doses just to achieve sufficient sedation. Clonazepam and lorazepam are most widely studied, alone or in combination with lithium,
- *Carbamazepine* (see 📖 p. 346): or its derivative, oxcarbazepine, may be effective, either alone or in combination with lithium or antipsychotics.[3] May be better tolerated in patients with comorbid drug or alcohol problems, obesity, or women of child-bearing age.
  - *Predictors of good response:* previous response to carbamazepine, poor compliance (due to wide therapeutic window), absence of psychotic symptoms, secondary mania (e.g. drug-induced, neurological disorder, brain injury), dysphoria, 'mixed' episode, rapid cycling, episode part of schizoaffective disorder.
- *Other anticonvulsants:* there is no current evidence to recommend use of any other anticonvulsant. The strongest evidence is for lamotrigine (see 📖 p. 331 and 📖 p. 348), but in depressive episodes, not mania or hypomania. Topiramate has shown some promise in both depressed and manic bipolar patients, with the added benefit of promoting weight loss. Overall, however, the evidence is still very limited.

1 Mukherjee S, Sackeim HA and Schnur DB (1994) Electroconvulsive therapy of acute manic episodes: a review of 50 years' experience. *Am J Psychol* **151**: 169–76.

2 Cipriani A, Barbui C, Salanti G, *et al.* (2011) Comparative efficacy and acceptability of antimanic drugs in acute mania: a multiple-treatments meta-analysis. *Lancet* **378**: 1306–15.

3 McElroy SL and Keck PE Jr (2000) Pharmacologic agents for the treatment of acute bipolar mania. *Biol Psychiat* **48**: 539–57.

Treatment of depressive episodes

Bipolar depression occurs more frequently, lasts longer, is more disruptive and is associated with greater risk of suicide than mania. Yet until recently research has focused more on treatment of mania and prophylaxis. The pharmacological treatment of depressive episodes in bipolar disorder represents a particular challenge.[1] Although almost all of the antidepressants used in the treatment of unipolar depression are effective in the treatment of bipolar depression, the response rates are lower and there is the risk of precipitating a manic episode or inducing/accelerating rapid cycling.[2] When symptoms are mild to moderate, consider combining pharmacological and psychological interventions (as for unipolar depression, 📖 p. 252).

If patient is already on prophylaxis

- Optimize (ensure compliance), check serum levels.
- Exclude/treat associated problems (e.g. hypothyroidism).
- Review need for other medications that may lower mood. Consider other conditions that may mimic or cause depression (📖 p. 248).
- Consider adding SSRI (in conjunction with prophylaxis).
- If not on antipsychotic then consider addition of quetiapine instead of SSRI (see **Treatment notes** 📖 p. 328).

If evidence of recent mood instability (manic/hypomanic episodes and depression)

- *1st line:* increase or (re)commence antimanic agent.
- *2nd line:* consider using lamotrigine.

If no response to SSRI

- Consider alternative antidepressant, e.g. mirtazapine, venlafaxine; or augmentation strategies (see **Treatment notes** 📖 p. 328).
- Consider addition of quetiapine or olanzapine if not currently on an antipsychotic (see **Treatment notes** 📖 p. 328).

For severe/life-threatening depressive episode (or previous good response/advance statement of preference)

- ECT should be strongly considered as 1st line treatment.
- Although well established for treatment of unipolar depressive disorder, ECT in bipolar disorder has not been fully researched, but should not be overlooked (esp. severe cases).
- Take care if the patient is on prophylaxis (see 📖 p. 287).

Following remission of depressive symptoms

- Taper antidepressants after 8wks of maintenance treatment.
- Continue mood stabilizer to prevent relapse.

Treatment notes

- *Choice of antidepressant:* although evidence is scarce, recent studies have suggested that the SSRIs may be better tolerated, work more quickly, and have a lower associated risk of inducing mania or rapid cycling compared to tricyclic antidepressants.[3] In general, choice will depend on issues of previous response, side-effects (both desired and undesired), and tolerability issues (see 📖 p. 266). As second-line treatment, an antidepressant may be better tolerated than a second mood stabilizer.

- *The role of antipsychotics:* quetiapine is licensed to treat depression in bipolar disorder (50mg nocte day 1, 100mg day 2, 200mg day 3, 300mg day 4; adjust according to response, usual dose 300mg nocte; max. 600mg daily). Efficacy has been demonstrated in 2 robust RCTs (BOLDER 1 & 2) and the EMBOLDEN I & II replication trials.[4] Olanzapine, as an olanzapine–fluoxetine combination (OFC), is licensed for bipolar depression in the USA as Symbyax® (6/25, 6/50 or 12/50mg/day). Not licensed for bipolar depression in the UK, but licensed for mania and propylaxis. Recommended as 2nd line after SSRIs in NICE (CG38, 2006) guidelines (see 📖 p. 325). Preliminary data suggest aripiprazole (15mg/day) may also be used.
- *Other anticonvulsants:* recent meta-analysis supports monotherapy with lamotrigine (licensed in USA, but not in UK; see 📖 p. 348), particularly for treatment-refractory bipolar depression.[5] Gabapentin appears much less effective. Controlled clinical trials comparing standard treatments for depression in patients with bipolar disorder are lacking. It is a widely accepted practice to add a second mood stabilizer to the treatment regimens of patients with bipolar disorder (e.g. carbamazepine or valproate). Be alert for evidence of lithium toxicity, even at 'normal' serum levels (see 📖 p. 339).
- *Alternative strategies/treatment resistance:* other suggested strategies include: the use of adjunctive tri-iodothyronine (T_3)—even if there is no evidence of clinical hypothyroidism;[6] and the novel use of inositol.[7] Evidence for omega-3 fatty acids is equivocal at best. For treatment-resistant depressive episodes, principles of management are as for unipolar depression (see 📖 p. 260).

1 Hirschfeld RM (2004) Bipolar depression: the real challenge. *Eur Neuropsychopharmacol* **14** (Suppl 2): S83–8.

2 Compton MT, Nemeroff CB (2000) The treatment of bipolar depression. *J Clin Psychiat* **61** (Suppl): 57–67.

3 Nemeroff CB, Evans DL, Gyulai L, *et al.* (2001) Double-blind, placebo-controlled comparison of imipramine and paroxetine in the treatment of bipolar depression. *Am J Psychol* **158**: 906–12.

4 For a review of the studies see: Bogart GT, Chavez B (2009) Safety and efficacy of quetiapine in bipolar depression. *Ann Pharmacother* **43**: 1848–56.

5 Geddes JR, Calabrese JR, Goodwin GM (2009) Lamotrigine for treatment of bipolar depression: independent meta-analysis and meta-regression of individual patient data from five randomised trials. *Br J Psychiat* **194**: 4–9.

6 Bauer M, Berghofer A, Bschor T, *et al.* (2002) Supraphysiological doses of L-thyroxine in the maintenance treatment of prophylaxis-resistant affective disorders. *Neuropsychopharmacol* **27**: 620–8.

7 Chengappa KN, Levine J, Gershon S, *et al.* (2000) Inositol as an add-on treatment for bipolar depression. *Bipolar Disord* **2**: 47–55.

Prophylaxis

Primary aim
Prevention of recurrent episodes (mania, hypomania, or depression).

Suicide prevention
Patients with bipolar disorder represent a group at high risk of suicide. Retrospective and prospective studies do suggest that long-term lithium therapy reduces the risk of suicide. There is still little data available on the anti-suicidal effects of other prophylactic treatments.

Indications
Following effective remission of acute symptoms of mania or bipolar depression; also recommended in bipolar II disorder.

Procedure following remission of acute symptoms of mania or depression
- Ensure therapeutic dose of mood stabilizer/optimal balance of risk–benefit for any antipsychotic medication.
- Withdraw gradually any additional antipsychotic or benzodiazepine used to manage acute symptoms.
- When euthymia achieved following depressive episode, consider tapering antidepressant after 8wks.
- Continue monitoring of side-effects, blood levels and physical checks as per protocols for individual agents (see 🔲 pp. 336–49).

Guiding principles
- Manage with lowest dose necessary of any maintenance medication.
- Aim for single agent if possible; most will require mood stabilizer + low-dose antipsychotic or mood stabilizer + antidepressant.
- Off-licence use of valproate or antipsychotic may be justified in the maintenance phase if there is good evidence of benefit in acute phase management (i.e. continuation is not unreasonable, perhaps at a lower dose, and few medications are licensed).
- 'Wait and see' policy for possible bipolar II disorder where use of mood stabilizer may prevent more serious later episodes should be discussed with the patient in light of detailed clinical interview (esp. high genetic risk), since treatments themselves are not without risks (evidence supports possible use of quetiapine or lamotrigine in this regard but these are off-licence indications).

Licensed treatments
- *Lithium* (🔲 p. 336): to date, remains the first-line choice for maintenance treatment in patients[1] especially with a 'classical' course of illness. Some subtypes of what has become known as the 'bipolar spectrum' may not respond as well to lithium. These include patients with mixed mania (i.e. depressive symptoms during manic episodes) and patients with rapid cycling mania. Emerging evidence would seem to suggest a role for anticonvulsants in these patients.

- *Carbamazepine* (see 📖 p. 342): appears to be effective in the long-term treatment of bipolar disorder, with an overall response rate of 63%. Although it does not have worldwide approval as yet, carbamazepine may be more effective in the treatment of bipolar spectrum than classical bipolar disorder.
- *Aripiprazole:* only licensed for continuation therapy when effective for management of acute mania (15–30mg/day).
- *Quetiapine:* only licensed for continuation therapy when effective for management of acute mania or bipolar depression (300–800mg/day).

Unlicensed treatments
- *Valproate/valproic acid* (see 📖 p. 346): has demonstrated efficacy in rapid cycling bipolar disorder and the added confidence of being the most widely prescribed therapy for bipolar depression, although unequivocal evidence of successful prophylaxis has not yet emerged. Indeed, the recent BALANCE study showed that both combination therapy (lithium plus valproate) and lithium monotherapy are more likely to prevent relapse than valproate monotherapy.[2]
- *Lamotrigine* (see 📖 p. 348): efficacy established in a pair of controlled studies for prevention of depression and, to a lesser extent, mania following discontinuation of other psychotropic medications.[3]
- *Other anticonvulsants:* there have been promising reports on the efficacy of oxcarbazepine, topiramate, gabapentin, and tiagabine, but the evidence is relatively weak.
- *Other antipsychotics:* olanzapine also appears to be effective either alone or in combination with lithium or valproate. Risperidone may also have an adjunctive or maintenance role. Older antipsychotics, including depots (usually low dose), are almost certainly effective but evidence is (unfortunately) lacking.
- *Alternative/augmentative agents:* a number of other compounds that may have some clinical utility include: Ca^{2+} channel antagonists such as verapamil, nifedipine, and nimodipine; thyroid hormones; tamoxifen; omega-3 fatty acids; and even vitamin/mineral supplements.

Risks of discontinuation
Substantial evidence exists that abrupt discontinuation of lithium is associated with an increased risk of relapse. The risk, particularly of mania, may be minimized by gradually reducing the lithium dose. Although comparable studies are not available for the anticonvulsants or SGAs, a similarly cautious approach would seem advisable.

1 Kessing LV, Hellmund G, Geddes JR, *et al.* (2011) Valproate v. lithium in the treatment of bipolar disorder in clinical practice: observational nationwide register-based cohort study. *Br J Psychiat* **199**: 57–63.

2 BALANCE investigators and collaborators (2010) Lithium plus valproate combination therapy versus monotherapy for relapse prevention in bipolar I disorder (BALANCE): a randomised open-label trial. *Lancet* **375**: 385–95.

3 Goodwin GM, Bowden CL, Calabrese JR, *et al.* (2004) A pooled analysis of 2 placebo-controlled 18-month trials of lamotrigine and lithium maintenance in bipolar I disorder. *J Clin Psychiat* **65**: 432–41.

Psychotherapeutic interventions

Most patients will struggle with some of the following issues:
- Emotional consequences of significant periods of illness and receiving the diagnosis of a chronic psychiatric disorder.
- Developmental deviations and delays caused by past episodes.
- Problems associated with stigmatization.
- Problems related to self-esteem.
- Fear of recurrence and the consequent inhibition of normal psychosocial functioning.
- Interpersonal difficulties.
- Issues related to marriage, family, child-bearing, and parenting.
- Academic and occupational problems.
- Other legal, social, and emotional problems that arise from illness-related behaviours.

For some patients, a specific psychotherapeutic intervention (in addition to usual psychiatric management and social support) will be needed to address these issues. Approaches include: psychodynamic, interpersonal, behavioural, and cognitive therapies. In addition, couple, family, and group therapy may be indicated for some patients. The selection of appropriate interventions is influenced by the local availability of such treatments, as well as the patient's needs and preferences.

Key elements of selected interventions[1]

- *Psychoeducation:*[2] key component to most therapies, psychoeducation goes further than simply delivering information, and does appear to reduce recurrence and relapse. Patients are given a theoretical and practical approach to understand their illness and the medication they are prescribed. Through understanding, patients can attain improved adherence to medication, recognize symptoms that might lead to decompensation, and recover occupational and social function.
- *CBT:*[3] time-limited, with specific aims: educate the patient about bipolar disorder and its treatment, teach cognitive behavioural skills for coping with psychosocial stressors and associated problems, facilitate compliance with treatment, and monitor the occurrence and severity of symptoms.
- *Interpersonal and social rhythm therapy (IPT/SRT):*[4] to reduce lability of mood by maintaining a regular pattern of daily activities, e.g. sleeping, eating, physical activity, and emotional stimulation. Evidence suggests IPT/SRT should be initiated immediately following an acute episode when individuals are most likely to make the lifestyle changes required to achieve social rhythm stability.
- *Family-focused therapy (FFT):*[5] usually brief, includes psychoeducation (of patient and family members) with specific aims: accepting the reality of the illness, identifying precipitating stresses and likely future stresses inside and outside the family, elucidating family interactions that produce stress on the patient, planning strategies for managing and/or minimizing future stresses, and bringing about the patient's family's acceptance of the need for continued treatment. Benefits

more pronounced in depressed patients and in those living in a high-expressed emotional environment.

- *Support groups:* May provide useful information about bipolar disorder and its treatment. Patients may benefit from hearing the experiences of others, struggling with similar issues. This may help them to see their problems as not being unique, understand the need for medication, and access advice and assistance with other practical issues. In the UK, groups such as the Manic Depression Fellowship, MIND, and SANE provide both support and educational material to patients and their families (see 📖 p. 1010).

'At this point in my existence, I cannot imagine leading a normal life without both taking lithium and having had the benefits of psychotherapy. Lithium prevents my seductive but disastrous highs, diminishes my depressions, clears out the wool and webbing from my disordered thinking, slows me down, gentles me out, keeps me out of a hospital, alive, and makes psychotherapy possible. But, ineffably, psychotherapy heals. It makes some sense of the confusion, reins in the terrifying thoughts and feelings, returns some control and hope and possibility of learning from it all. Pills cannot, do not, ease one back into reality; they only bring one back headlong, careening, and faster than can be endured at times. Psychotherapy is a sanctuary; it is a battleground; it is a place I have been psychotic, neurotic, elated, confused, and despairing beyond belief. But, always, it is where I have believed or have learned to believe – that I might someday be able to contend with all of this. No pill can help me deal with the problem of not wanting to take pills; likewise, no amount of psychotherapy alone can prevent my manias and depressions. I need both. It is an odd thing, owing life to pills, one's own quirks and tenacities, and this unique, strange, and ultimately profound relationship called psychotherapy.'

Dr Kay Redfield Jamison (1996) *An unquiet mind: a memoir of moods and madness*, pp. 88–9. London: Picador

1 Vieta E, Pacchiarotti I, Scott J, *et al.* (2005) Evidence-based research on the efficacy of psychologic interventions in bipolar disorders: a critical review. *Curr Psychiatry Rep* **7**: 449–55.

2 Colom F, Vieta E, Martinez-Aran A, *et al.* (2003) A randomized trial on the efficacy of group psychoeducation in the prophylaxis of recurrences in bipolar patients whose disease is in remission. *Arch Gen Psychiat* **60**: 402–7.

3 Lam DH, Watkins ER, Hayward P, *et al.* (2003) A randomized controlled study of cognitive therapy for relapse prevention for bipolar affective disorder: outcome of the first year. *Arch Gen Psychiatry* **60**:145–52.

4 Frank E, Kupfer DJ, Thase ME, *et al.* (2005) Two-year outcomes for interpersonal and social rhythm therapy in individuals with bipolar I disorder. *Arch Gen Psychiat* **62**: 996–1004.

5 Miklowitz DJ, George EL, Richards JA, *et al.* (2003) A randomized study of family-focused psychoeducation and pharmacotherapy in the outpatient management of bipolar disorder. *Arch Gen Psychiat* **60**: 904–12.

Cyclothymia

Previously regarded as a disorder of personality ('cyclothymic temperament'—see Box 8.6) mainly because of its early age of onset and relative stability throughout adult life, cyclothymia is now considered to be a mood disorder.[1]

Clinical features

- Persistent instability of mood, numerous periods of mild depression and mild elation, not sufficiently severe or prolonged to fulfil the criteria for bipolar affective disorder or recurrent depressive disorder.
- The mood swings are usually perceived by the individual as being unrelated to life events.

The diagnosis is difficult to establish without a prolonged period of observation or an unusually good account of the individual's past behaviour. In DSM-IV the symptoms must have been present for at least 2yrs, with no period lasting longer than 2mths in which they have been at a normal state. No mixed episodes may have occurred.

Epidemiology

- *Prevalence:* 3–6% of general population.
- *Age of onset:* usually early adulthood (i.e. teens or 20s), but sometimes may present later in life.
- Commoner in relatives of patients with bipolar affective disorder.

Differential diagnosis

Bipolar affective disorder, recurrent depressive disorder, drug or alcohol misuse, ADHD, conduct disorder, personality disorder (emotionally unstable), medical conditions (see 🛇 p. 307).

Course

Onset often gradual, making it difficult to pinpoint when symptoms began. Alternating ups and downs may fluctuate in hours, weeks, or months. Because mood swings are relatively mild and periods of mood elevation may be enjoyable (with increased activity and productivity, self-confidence, and sociability), cyclothymia frequently fails to come to medical attention. Person may often present either because of the impact of the depressive episodes on social and work situations, or because of problems related to comorbid drug or alcohol misuse. Usually runs a chronic course, persisting throughout adult life. In some cases symptoms may cease temporarily or permanently, or develop into more severe mood swings meeting the criteria for bipolar affective disorder or recurrent depressive disorder.

Management

- If pharmacological treatment is contemplated this usually consists of a trial of a mood stabilizer (e.g. lithium, low dose 600–900mg/day).

- Recently there has been a tendency to use anticonvulsants, such as valproate (500–750mg/day), carbamazepine, or lamotrigine, as these may be better tolerated. As yet there is no clear evidence to suggest any of these approaches is superior.
- At times of 'crisis' due to temperamental excesses a short course of a low-dose sedating antipsychotic (e.g. chlorpromazine 50mg nocte; risperidone 1mg nocte; olanzapine 2.5mg nocte; quetiapine 25–50mg nocte) may be helpful.
- Psychoeducation and insight-orientated psychotherapy may help the person to understand the condition, and allow them to develop better ways of coping.
- There is often a reluctance to continue to take medication as this not only treats the depressive episodes, but also may be perceived as 'blunting' creativity, productivity, or intellectual capacity.

Box 8.6 Kraepelin's 'cyclothymic temperament'

These are the people who constantly oscillate hither and thither between the two opposite poles of mood, sometimes 'rejoicing to the skies', sometimes 'sad as death'. Today lively, sparkling, beaming, full of the joy of life, the pleasure of enterprise, and the pressure of activity, after some time they meet us depressed, enervated, ill-humored, in need of rest, and again a few months later they display the old freshness and elasticity.

Kraepelin E (1896) Manic-depressive insanity and paranoia. (Extract from translation of the 8th edn of Kraepelin's textbook *Psychiatrie*)

Box 8.7 Schneider 1958

'(Kurt) Schneider (1958, in *Psychopathic Personalities*) admonished the kin of labile individuals (who might approximate what we might diagnose today as cyclothymia with borderline personality features) "on their bad days...to keep out of their way as far as possible" (p. 121). Cyclothymes, with some insight into their own temperament, would give the same advice to their loved ones. Cautious trial of anticonvulsants will often prove effective in those distressed enough by their behavior as to comply with such treatment.'

Extract from Akiskal HS (2001) Review article: dysthymia and cyclothymia in psychiatric practice a century after Kraepelin. *J Affect Disord* **62**: 17–31.

1 When Kahlbaum (1863) introduced the term 'cyclothymia' into modern psychiatry, he described it as the mildest form of manic–depressive disease. Kraepelin (1896) treated it the same way (see Box 8.6), but Schneider (1958) used the term cyclothymia synonymously with manic–depressive disease. He described and conceptualized the 'labile psychopath' as a personality disorder (see Box 8.7) as distinct from manic–depressive illness. Classification systems no longer reflect Schneider's view and both DSM-IV-TR and ICD-10 include cyclothymia within the affective (mood) disorders. Debate continues regarding the interface between such subthreshold affective conditions, personality, and temperament (see also 📖 p. 312 and 📖 p. 318).

Lithium

Despite problems with tolerability, lithium[1] still remains the gold standard in the treatment of bipolar affective disorder. The effectiveness of long-term treatment with lithium is supported by at least 9 controlled, double-blind studies,[2] far exceeding the available support for other alternatives to lithium treatment, although the last decade has seen an emerging literature supporting the use of anticonvulsant, antipsychotic, or sedative agents.

Mode of action

Uncertain numerous effects on biological systems (particularly at high concentrations). Lithium can substitute for Na^{2+}, K^+, Ca^{2+}, Mg^{2+} and may have effects on cell membrane electrophysiology. Within cells, lithium interacts with systems involving other cations, including the release of neurotransmitters and 2nd messenger systems, (e.g. adenylate cyclase, inositol 1,4,5,-triphosphate, arachidonate, protein kinase C, G proteins and calcium), effectively blocking the actions of transmitters and hormones. Also reduction in receptor up-regulation, perhaps explaining lithium's value as an adjunctive treatment.

Interactions

- *Increased plasma concentration (risk of toxicity even at therapeutic serum levels):* ACE inhibitors/angiotensin-II receptor antagonists, analgesics (esp. NSAIDs), antidepressants (esp. SSRIs), anti-epileptics, antihypertensives (e.g. methyldopa), antipsychotics (esp. haloperidol), calcium-channel blockers, diuretics, metronidazole.
- *Decreased plasma concentration (risk of decreased efficacy):* antacids, theophylline.
- *Other interactions:* anti-arrhythmics (e.g. amiodarone: increased risk of hypothyroidism), antidiabetics (may sometimes impair glucose tolerance), antipsychotics (increased risk of EPSEs), muscle relaxants (enhanced effect), parasympathomimetics (antagonizes neostigmine and pyridostigmine).

Guidelines on lithium therapy (Box 8.8)[3]

- *Prior to commencing lithium therapy:* physical examination, FBC, U&Es, TFTs, renal function (eGFR), baseline weight and height (BMI), if clinically indicated—ECG, pregnancy test.
- *Starting dose:* usually 400–600mg given at night, increased weekly depending on serum monitoring to max 2g (usual dose 800mg–1.2g)—actual dose depends upon preparation used (molar availability varies even when amounts (mg) are the same (see Table 8.3).
- *Monitoring:* check lithium level 7 days after starting and 7 days after each change of dose. Take blood samples 12hr post-dose.
- *Once a therapeutic serum level[4] has been established:* continue to check lithium level/eGFR every 3mths, TFTs every 6mths, monitor weight (BMI), and check for side-effects (see 📖 p. 338).

- *Stopping*: reduce gradually over 1–3mths, particularly if patient has history of manic relapse (even if started on other anti-manic agent).

Box 8.8 Safer lithium therapy

The UK National Patient Safety Agency (NPSA) issued a Patient Safety Alert (NPSA/2009/PSA005) on safer lithium therapy. This was in response to reports of harm caused to patients, including fatalities, by lithium therapy and was developed in collaboration with the Prescribing Observatory for Mental Health (POMH-UK) of the RCPsych, the National Pharmacy Association (NPA), other organizations, clinicians, and patients. It was designed to help NHS organizations, including community pharmacies, in England and Wales (and latterly Scotland) to take steps to minimize the risks associated with lithium therapy. The following recommendations were made:
- Patients should be monitored in accordance with NICE guidelines.
- There are reliable systems to ensure blood test results are communicated between laboratories and prescribers.
- Throughout their treatment patients receive appropriate ongoing verbal and written information and complete a record book.*
- Prescribers and pharmacists check that blood tests are monitored regularly and that it is safe to prescribe and/or dispense lithium.
- Systems are in place to identify and deal with medicines that might adversely interact with lithium therapy.

* The NPSA patient information booklet, lithium alert card and record book for blood tests can be downloaded from the RCPsych website: ℘ http://www.rcpsych.ac.uk/quality/quality,accreditationaudit/prescribingobservatorypomh/saferlithiumtherapy.aspx

Table 8.3 Lithium preparations (UK)

Preparation	Active component	Available strengths
Camcolit® (tablets)	Lithium carbonate	250/400mg (scored)
Li-liquid® (oral solution)	Lithium citrate	509mg/5mL
Liskonum® (tablets)	Lithium carbonate	450mg (scored)
Priadel® (tablets)	Lithium carbonate	200/400mg (scored)
Priadel® (liquid)	Lithium citrate	520mg/5mL

1 The use of lithium salts in the treatment of 'psychotic excitement' is usually credited to John Cade in 1949 (*Med J Aust* **2**: 349–52). However, this was a 'rediscovery' of the use of lithium to treat 'insanity' first described by Hammond WA, in 1871 (in *A treatise on diseases of the nervous system*. New York: Appleton, pp. 325–84).

2 Burgess S, Geddes J, Hawton K, *et al.* (2001) Lithium for maintenance treatment of mood disorders. *Cochrane Database System Rev* 3: Art. no.: CD003013.

3 NICE (2006) *Guideline on bipolar disorder*, CG38, including guidance on initiating, monitoring, stopping, and other risks associated with lithium therapy.

4 NICE suggests lithium levels between 0.6–0.8 mmol/L when prescribed for the first time. Those who have relapsed on lithium, or who still have subthreshold symptoms with functional impairment while on lithium, may warrant a trial of at least 6mths with levels between 0.8–1.0 mmol/L.

Lithium: adverse effects

As lithium is a highly toxic ion, safe and effective therapy requires monitoring of serum levels. Up to 75% of patients treated with lithium will experience some side-effects.[1]

Dose-related side-effects

Polyuria/polydipsia (reduced ability to concentrate urine due to antidiuretic hormone [ADH] antagonism), weight gain (effects on carbohydrate metabolism and/or oedema), cognitive problems (e.g., dulling, impaired memory, poor concentration, confusion, mental slowness), tremor, sedation or lethargy, impaired co-ordination, GI distress (e.g., nausea, vomiting, dyspepsia, diarrhoea), hair loss, benign leukocytosis, acne, and oedema.

Management

Usually dealt with by lowering the dose of lithium, or altering the dose schedule or formulation. If side-effects persist, additional medications may be necessary, e.g. β-blockers (tremor), thiazide or loop diuretics (polyuria, polydipsia or oedema), topical antibiotics or retinoic acid (acne). GI problems can be managed by administering lithium with meals or switching lithium preparations, such as lithium citrate.

Cardiac conduction problems

Usually benign ECG changes (e.g. T-wave changes, widening of QRS). Rarely, exacerbation of existing arrhythmias or new arrhythmias due to conduction deficits at the sinoatrial (SA) or atrioventricular (AV) nodes (contraindicated in heart failure, sick sinus syndrome).

Long-term effects

Renal function

10–20% of patients on long-term therapy demonstrate morphological kidney changes (interstitial fibrosis, tubular atrophy, and sometimes glomerular sclerosis). >1% may develop irreversible renal failure (rising serum creatinine) after 10yrs or more of treatment. If urea and creatinine levels become elevated, assess the rate of deterioration (see 🕮 p. 476); the decision whether to continue lithium depends on clinical efficacy and degree of renal impairment; seek advice from a renal specialist and a clinician with expertise in the management of bipolar disorder.

Subclinical/clinical hypothyroidism

5–35%, more frequent in women, tends to appear after 6–18mths of treatment, and may be associated with rapid cycling bipolar disorder. Although lithium-induced hypothyroidism is generally reversible on discontinuation, it does not constitute an absolute contraindication for continuing lithium treatment as the associated hypothyroidism is readily treated with levothyroxine.[2] It is worth noting that, in addition to the classic signs and symptoms of hypothyroidism, patients with bipolar disorder are also at risk of developing depression and/or rapid cycling as a consequence of suboptimal thyroid functioning. Should these symptoms occur and suboptimal thyroid functioning be confirmed, thyroid supplementation with or without lithium discontinuation is the treatment of choice.

Teratogenicity (see 📖 p. 968)

The much-quoted 400-fold increased risk of Ebstein's anomaly (a congenital malformation of the tricuspid valve) due to 1st trimester lithium exposure now appears to be substantially less than first reported—at most an eight-fold relative risk.[3] Other reported 2nd and 3rd trimester problems include polyhydramnios, premature delivery, thyroid abnormalities, nephrogenic diabetes insipidus, and floppy baby syndrome. The estimated risk of major congenital anomalies for lithium-exposed babies is 4–12% compared with 2–4% in untreated control groups.

Management

A balance needs to be struck between the risks of teratogenicity and the risks of relapse following discontinuation:[3]

- *Mild, stable forms of bipolar disorder:* lithium may be tapered down and stopped pre-pregnancy.
- *Moderate risk of relapse:* lithium should be tapered and discontinued during the first trimester (4–12wks after last menstrual period).
- *Severe forms of bipolar disorder, who are at high risk of relapse:* lithium should be maintained during pregnancy (with informed consent, appropriate counselling, prenatal diagnosis, and detailed ultrasound and echocardiography at 16–18wks gestation).

Toxicity

The usual upper therapeutic limit for 12-hr post-dose serum lithium level is 1.2mmol/L. With levels >1.5mmol/L most patients will experience some symptoms of toxicity; >2.0mmol/L definite, often life-threatening, toxic effects occur. There is often a narrow therapeutic window where the beneficial effects outweigh the toxic effects (esp. in older patients).

Early signs and symptoms Marked tremor, anorexia, nausea/vomiting, diarrhoea (sometimes bloody), with dehydration and lethargy.

As lithium levels rise Severe neurological complications—restlessness, muscle fasciculation/myoclonic jerks, choreoathetoid movements, marked hypertonicity. This may progress to ataxia, dysarthria, increased lethargy, drowsiness, and confusion/delirium. Hypotension and cardiac arrhythmias precede circulatory collapse, with emerging seizures, stupor, and eventual coma (high risk of permanent neurological impairment or death).

Management
- Education of patients (methods of avoiding toxicity, e.g. maintaining hydration and salt intake, and being alert to early signs and symptoms).
- Careful adjustment of dosage may be all that is required.
- In severe toxicity (e.g. following OD), rapid steps to reduce serum lithium level are urgently necessary. This may involve forced diuresis with intravenous isotonic saline, or in cases where toxicity is severe or accompanied by significant renal failure, haemodialysis.
- Review need for prophylaxis (see 📖 p. 330).

1 Goodwin FK, Jamison KR (1990) *Manic-depressive illness.* Oxford: Oxford University Press.

2 Bocchetta A, Bernardi F, Pedditzi M, *et al.* (1991) Thyroid abnormalities during lithium treatment. *Acta Psychiatr Scand* **83**: 193–8.

3 Cohen LS, Friedman JM, Jefferson JW, *et al.* (1994) A reevaluation of risk of *in utero* exposure to lithium. *J Am Med Ass* **271**: 146–50.

Valproate/valproic acid

In the UK, despite the widespread use of sodium valproate as a mood sta-bilizer, the only *licensed* preparation for bipolar affective disorder contains valproic acid as semisodium valproate (Depakote®). There are no pub-lished placebo-control trials of the efficacy of sodium valproate in bipolar affective disorder—despite data being published on tolerability (suggesting GI side-effects are less with Depakote®).

Psychiatric indications
- Acute mania (up to 56% effective); see 📖 p. 326.
- Acute depressive episode (in bipolar affective disorder) in combination with an antidepressant. Data limited; see 📖 p. 328.
- Prophylaxis of bipolar affective disorder—possibly more effective in rapid cycling; see 📖 p. 330.

Mode of action
Uncertain. Modulates voltage-sensitive Na channels, acts on second-messenger systems, and increases bioavailability of GABA (or mimics action at post-synaptic receptor sites) in the central nervous system.

Pharmacokinetics
Sodium valproate is available in tablet, liquid, solution, syrup, enteric-coated, and MR forms. Semisodium valproate (Depakote®) comes as enteric-coated tablets containing valproic acid and sodium valproate. They are both rapidly absorbed when taken orally (peak serum level for sodium valproate ~2hr; semisodium valproate 3–8hr) with a plasma half-life of 6–16hr (see Box 8.9 and Table 8.4).

Interactions
- Raised serum levels with phenobarbital, phenytoin, and antidepressants (TCAs, fluoxetine).
- Decreased serum levels with carbamazepine.
- Toxicity may be precipitated by other highly protein-bound drugs (e.g. aspirin), which can displace valproate from its protein-binding sites.

Side-effects and toxicity
- *Dose-related side-effects:* GI upset (anorexia, nausea, dyspepsia, vomiting, diarrhoea), raised LFTs, tremor, and sedation—if persistent, may require dose reduction, change in preparation, or treatment of specific symptoms (e.g. β-blocker for tremor; H_2-blocker for dyspepsia).
- *Unpredictable side-effects:* mild, asymptomatic leukopenia and thrombocytopenia (reversible upon drug reduction/discontinuation), hair loss (usually transient), increased appetite, and weight gain.
- *Rare, idiosyncratic side-effects:* irreversible hepatic failure, pancreatitis, agranulocytosis, polycystic ovaries/hyperandrogenism.
- *Toxicity/overdose:* wide therapeutic window; hence, unintentional overdose is uncommon. Signs of overdose include somnolence, heart block, eventually coma, and even death (haemodialysis may be needed).

Box 8.9 Treatment guidelines for sodium valproate

- Full medical history (particularly liver disease, haematological problems, and bleeding disorders)/full physical examination; check FBC, LFTs, baseline ECG, weight/height (BMI).
- *Sodium valproate:* start with a low, divided dose (e.g. 200mg bd or tds), increase every few days or every week by 200–400mg/day according to response and side-effects, up to a maximum of 2500mg/day, or until serum levels are 50–125mmol/L (see Table 8.4). Usual maintenance dose 1–2g/day.
- *Valproic acid as semisodium valproate:* start with 250mg tds (or up to 20mg/kg for acute manic episode) and increase every few days or every week by 250–500mg/day to a maximum of 2000mg/day, or until serum levels are 50–125mmol/L (see Table 8.4). Usual maintenance dose 1000–2000mg/day.
- Once the patient is stable, simplify regime.
- If GI upset is a problem with sodium valproate, consider changing to enteric-coated, slow-release (Epilim Chrono®), or Depakote®.
- If poor compliance is an issue, consider use of slow-release tablets.
- Once established, check FBC, LFTs, serum valproate level, and BMI every 6 months.

Points to note

- There is no well-established correlation between serum concentrations and mood-stabilizing effects. Best advice is to use similar doses and serum levels that are considered therapeutic for epilepsy.
- Closer clinical monitoring for side-effects may be necessary for patients who cannot reliably report early signs.

Table 8.4 Valproate/valproic acid preparations (UK)

Preparation	Active agent	Available strengths
Depakote®	Valproic acid	T 250/500mg
Convulex®	Valproic acid	C 150/300/500mg
Sodium valproate (generic)/ Orlept®	Sodium valproate	T 100/200/500mg L 200mg/5mL
Epilim®	Sodium valproate	T 100/200/500mg L 200mg/5mL
Epilim Chrono® (MR)	Sodium valproate	200/300/500mg
Epilim Chronosphere® (MR granules)	Sodium valproate	50/100/250/500 750/1000mg sachets
Episenta® (MR)	Sodium valproate	C 150/300mg Granules 500mg/1g
Epilim® intravenous	Sodium valproate	IV 400mg powder with 4mL water ampoule
Episenta®	Sodium valproate	IV 100mg/mL 3mL ampoule

Key
T: tablet; C: capsule; L: liquid

Carbamazepine

Psychiatric indications

- Acute mania (less effective than lithium/equivalent efficacy to antipsychotics)—alone or in combination with lithium—see ☐ p. 326.
- Acute depressive episode (in bipolar affective disorder)—alone or in combination with lithium—see ☐ p. 328.
- Prophylaxis of bipolar affective disorder—data limited—see ☐ p. 330.

Mode of action

Uncertain. Modulates sodium and calcium ion channels, receptor-mediation of GABA and glutamine, and various intracellular signalling pathways.

Pharmacokinetics

Carbamazepine is available in a variety of forms (solutions, suspensions, syrups, and chewable or slow-release formulations), all with similar bioavailability. Peak plasma concentrations between 4–8hrs (usually), may be as late as 26hrs. Plasma half-life 18–55hrs. With long-term use, carbamazepine induces its own metabolism, decreasing the half-life to 5–26hrs (Box 8.10 and Table 8.5).

Interactions

- Carbamazepine decreases the plasma levels of many drugs metabolized by the liver, e.g. antipsychotics, BDZs (except clonazepam), TCAs, other anticonvulsants, hormonal contraceptives, thyroid hormones.
- Carbamazepine serum concentrations can be increased by certain drugs, e.g. erythromycin, calcium channel blockers (diltiazem and verapamil, but not nifedipine or nimodipine), SSRIs.

Side-effects and toxicity

- *Unpredictable side-effects:* antidiuretic effects leading to hyponatraemia (6–31%), probably more common in the elderly, sometimes developing many months after starting treatment; decrease in total and free thyroxine levels/increase in free cortisol levels (rarely clinically significant).
- *Idiosyncratic side-effects:* agranulocytosis, aplastic anaemia, hepatic failure, exfoliative dermatitis (e.g. Stevens–Johnson syndrome), and pancreatitis (these side-effects usually occur within the first 3–6mths of treatment, rarely after longer periods). *Note:* routine blood monitoring does not reliably predict blood dyscrasias, hepatic failure, or exfoliative dermatitis—patient education about early symptoms and signs is essential.
- *Other rare side-effects:* systemic hypersensitivity reactions, cardiac conduction problems, psychiatric symptoms (including occasional cases of mania and psychosis), and, extremely rarely, renal problems (failure, oliguria, haematuria, and proteinuria).
- *Toxicity/overdose: early signs:* dizziness, ataxia, sedation, and diplopia. Acute intoxication may present as marked irritability, stupor, or even coma. May be fatal in overdose (if >6g ingested). *Symptoms of overdose*—nystagmus, ophthalmoplegia, cerebellar/extra-pyramidal

signs, impairment of consciousness, convulsions, respiratory depression, cardiac problems (tachycardia, hypotension, arrhythmias/ conduction disturbances), GI upset, and other anticholinergic symptoms. Significant overdose requires emergency medical management (i.e. close monitoring, symptomatic treatment, gastric lavage, and possible haemodialysis).

Box 8.10 Treatment guidelines for carbamazepine

* Full medical history (particularly liver disease, haematological problems, and bleeding disorders); physical examination; check FBC, LFTs, U&Es, baseline ECG and weight/height (BMI).
* Start with a low, divided dose (e.g. 200–600mg/day in 2–4 divided doses), increase every few days or every week by 200mg/day according to response and side-effects, up to 800–1200mg/day, with slower increases thereafter as indicated, to a maximum of 2000mg/ day, or until serum levels are 4–15g/mL (trough level—taken immediately prior to morning dose, and 5 days after dose change). See Table 8.5.
* Maintenance doses are usually around 1000mg/day (range 200–1600mg/day). *Doses higher than 1600mg/day are not recommended.*
* Check FBC, LFTs, and serum carbamazepine level every 2wks during first 2mths of treatment, then reduce monitoring to every 3mths, then every 6mths once well established (and monitor BMI).
* Once the patient is stable, simplify regimen and consider use of slow-release preparation, to enhance compliance.

Points to note
Closer clinical monitoring for side-effects may be necessary for patients who cannot reliably report early signs. If carbamazepine is combined with lithium, there may be increased risk of developing acute confusional state. Closer monitoring is advisable and minimization of the use or dose of other medications (e.g. antipsychotics, anticholinergics, BDZs) that may contribute to confusion.

Table 8.5 Carbamazepine preparations

Preparation	Formulation	Available strengths
Tegretol®	Tablet (also Chewtabs®)	100/200/400mg
	Liquid	100mg/5mL
	Suppositories	125/250mg
Tegretol® Prolonged Release	MR tablet	200/400mg
Carbagen® SR	MR capsule	200/400mg
Carbamazepine (generic)	Tablet	100/200/400mg

Lamotrigine

Psychiatric indications
- Maintenance treatment of bipolar disorder to delay relapse (depression, mania, hypomania, mixed episodes) – see 📖 p. 330.
- May be more effective than other mood stabilizers in preventing depressive episodes in bipolar disorder.

Mode of action
Unknown. Inhibits voltage-gated Na channels and glutamate release. Also has weak inhibitory effect on $5-HT_3$ receptors.

Pharmacokinetics
Rapidly and completely absorbed after oral administration with negligible first-pass metabolism (absolute bioavailability is 98%). Bioavailability is not affected by food/drug administration. Peak plasma concentrations occur anywhere from 1–5hrs following. Half-life 24hrs, and time to steady state is 5–8 days. Drug is 55% protein bound (Box 8.11).

Interactions
- *Certain medications have been shown to increase clearance of lamotrigine:* carbamazepine (40%), oxcarbazepine (30%), phenobarbital (40%), phenytoin (50%), ritonavir, methsuximide, rifampicin, primidone, and certain oestrogen-containing oral contraceptives.
- Valproate decreases the clearance of lamotrigine (i.e. more than doubles the elimination half-life of lamotrigine), so reduced doses (no greater than 50% usual dose) of lamotrigine should be given.

Side-effects and toxicity
- *Most common side-effects:* dizziness, headache, blurred/double vision, lack of co-ordination, sleepiness, nausea, vomiting, insomnia, and rash.
- *Rare side-effects:* rare incidence of multi-organ failure, various degrees of hepatic failure, aseptic meningitis, movement disorders.
- *Risk of rash:* 10–14% of patients receiving lamotrigine will develop a rash. Most are benign. A minority may be serious/life-threatening skin reactions requiring hospitalization, e.g. Stevens–Johnson syndrome, toxic epidermal necrolysis, angioedema, and a rash associated with a number of systemic manifestations (i.e. fever, lymphadenopathy, facial swelling, haematological, and hepatological abnormalities):
  - Most likely to occur within first 2–8wks of treatment. Risk of rash more likely when combined with valproate, exceeding recommended initial dose or recommended dose escalation.
  - Although most rashes resolve even with continuation of treatment, it is not possible to predict reliably which rashes will prove to be serious or life-threatening. Lamotrigine should ordinarily be discontinued at first sign of rash, unless the rash is clearly not drug-related.
  - Discontinuation of treatment may not prevent a rash from becoming life-threatening or permanently disabling/disfiguring.

- It is recommended that lamotrigine not be restarted in patients who discontinued due to rash associated with prior treatment (unless the potential benefits *clearly* outweigh the risks).
- *Other rare side-effects:* serious hypersensitivity reactions, blood dyscrasias (neutropenia, leukopenia, anaemia, thrombocytopenia, pancytopenia, and, rarely, aplastic anaemia and pure red cell aplasia), withdrawal seizures.

Box 8.11 Treatment guidelines for lamotrigine

- *Prior to starting:* pregnancy test (in women of child-bearing age).
- *As monotherapy:* start 25mg/day for weeks 1 and 2. Increase to 50mg/day for weeks 3 and 4. Increase by max 50–100mg/day every 1–2wks thereafter. Usual dose 100–200mg/day in 1–2 divided doses (max 500mg/day). See Table 8.6.
- *With valproate:* start 25mg every other day for weeks 1 and 2. Increase to 25mg/day for weeks 3 and 4. Increase by 25–50mg/day every 1–2wks. Usual dose 100–200mg/day in 1–2 divided doses.
- *With carbamazepine and NOT taking valproate:* start 50mg/day for weeks 1 and 2. Then 50mg bd for weeks 3 and 4. Increase by max 100mg/day every 1–2wks. Usual dose 200–400mg/day in 2 divided doses (up to 700mg/day sometimes needed).
- If a patient has discontinued lamotrigine for a period of more than 5 half-lives (i.e. 5 days) it is recommended that initial dosing recommendations and guidelines be followed.
- Although there is no well-established correlation between serum concentrations and mood-stabilizing effects, antiepileptic therapeutic serum levels are 8–10mg/mL.

Monitoring

- The value of monitoring plasma concentrations has not been established; however, due to drug interactions, monitoring of concomitant drugs may be indicated, particularly during dosage adjustments.
- Prior to treatment, the patient should be warned that a rash or other signs or symptoms of hypersensitivity (e.g. fever, lymphadenopathy, hives, painful sores in the mouth or around the eyes, or swelling of lips or tongue) warrant *urgent* medical assessment to determine if lamotrigine should be discontinued (see **side-effects and toxicity** 📖 p. 348).

Table 8.6 Lamotrigine preparations

Preparation	Formulation	Available strengths
Lamictal®	Tablet	25/50/100/200mg
	Dispersible tablet	2/5/25/100mg
Lamotrigine (generic)	Tablet	25/50/100/200mg
	Dispersible tablet	5/25/100mg

Anxiety and stress-related disorders

Introduction

If schizophrenia is 'the heartland of psychiatry', then the neurotic disorders surely make up much of the rest of the continent, in view of their prevalence in the general population (see Table 9.1) and the morbidity they cause.

As unpopular as the term 'neurosis' has become (for a historical perspective see 📖 p. 354), it is still retained in the ICD-10 in the rubric 'neurotic, stress-related, and somatoform disorders'. DSM-IV has effectively carved up the neuroses into anxiety disorders, somatoform disorders, dissociative disorders, and adjustment disorders. Here, we retain the use of 'neuroses' as shorthand for all these disorders, but will use the subdivisions when talking about the particular disorders.

We have all experienced anxiety symptoms, perhaps suffer from a particular 'phobia', or are a little bit obsessive about certain things, but to be clinically significant, these problems must be severe enough to cause marked distress and/or substantially interfere with our day-to-day lives. Because of the recognizable quality of some of the symptoms of neurotic disorders, it may be helpful to divide them into three categories:

The common neuroses

- *Anxiety/phobic disorders:* e.g. panic disorder, agoraphobia, generalized anxiety disorder (GAD), specific (understandable) phobias (e.g. snakes, spiders), hypochondriasis, social phobia.
- *Stress-related disorders:* e.g. acute stress reactions, adjustment disorder, post-traumatic stress disorder (PTSD).
- *Obsessive–compulsive disorder* (OCD).

The unusual neuroses (i.e. outwith 'normal' experience)

- *Anxiety/phobic disorders:* e.g. 'non-understandable' phobias (e.g. dirt, feathers), dysmorphophobia.
- 'Hysterical' conversion disorders.
- Dissociative/depersonalization–derealization disorder.
- Somatoform disorders.

'Culture-specific' disorders

Seen only in certain populations.
- Chronic fatigue syndrome (CFS)/eating disorders (see 📖 p. 398).
- Other 'culture-bound' disorders.

This chapter deals with the anxiety, phobic, and stress-related disorders. Other disorders are covered in Chapter 19, 📖 pp. 802–13 (conversion, somatization, CFS, hypochondriasis, dysmorphophobia), Chapter 10, 📖 p. 398, and Chapter 22, 📖 p. 914.

Points to note

- Anxiety symptoms are common in the general population.
- Comorbidity is frequent (other neuroses, depression, substance misuse, personality disorder).
- Anxiety disorders may often present with physical symptoms.

- Management will usually involve a combined approach (pharmacological and psychological).

Table 9.1 Prevalence of psychiatric disorders in the general population

Disorder	Rate (%)	
	Previous 6mths	Lifetime
Schizophrenia	0.9	1.5
Affective disorders	5.8	8.3
Substance abuse disorders	6.0	16.4
Anxiety disorders	8.9	14.6

Data derived from multiple community surveys.

Historical perspective

The term 'neurosis' was coined by William Cullen in 1777, replacing 'illness of the nerves' (coined by Robert Whytt in 1764 to replace the old 'vapours'), and meaning any disease of the nervous system without a known organic basis (which at the time also included epilepsy). Clinical descriptions of neurotic symptoms can be found in the works of Hippocrates. However, the 'illness' later vanished under the cloak of both pagan and Christian beliefs, with typical symptoms attributed to the work of spirits, possession, or divine punishment. It did not resurface properly until the Renaissance (the 1500s) thanks (in part) to the witchcraft trials, when doctors were called in to present diagnoses of known illnesses that could be mistaken for demonic possession (the first recorded 'medical defence'!). Although there was much debate, the brain became the final resting place as the organ most likely to be involved in the aetiology of the condition.

The history of the neuroses is tightly bound to the (re)discovery of hypnosis (formerly the remit of faith healing). The work of Franz-Anton Mesmer (1734–1815)—mesmerism—and James Braid (1795–1860)—braidism—was brought to France by Azam in 1859, coming to the attention of Charcot, whose experiments with hysterics would have a profound influence on one particular assistant—Sigmund Freud. Freud's first paper, published in 1886, shortly after his return to Vienna, was of a case of 'traumatic hysteria' in a male patient. It was his *Studies on hysteria*, written with Josef Breuer and published in 1895, that provided the starting point of his subsequent major concepts of psychoanalytical theory—including repression, psychic reality, and the subconscious.

The idea of repression of trauma (out of consciousness) and the appearance of 'defences' was highly influential, with the neuroses regarded as illnesses of the mind, needing psychotherapeutic treatment. Old arguments of emotional vs. physical factors resurfaced in the aftermath of the First World War, as some authorities found it difficult to attribute the illnesses seen in fit, healthy, young men (who had indisputably experienced traumatic events) to conversion hysteria or phobic neurosis. The encephalitis lethargicans epidemic in 1919, and the presence of numerous 'hysterical' symptoms (e.g. convulsions, mutism, feelings of passion, obsessions/compulsions, spasms) argued in favour of at least some of the neuroses having an organic basis.

In the 1920s, Walter Cannon proposed the concept of the 'emergency reaction', believing this 'fight-or-flight' response was mediated by the autonomic nervous system. He also noted that the physiological responses were too slow to account for feelings, and that some other 'neural mechanism' must be at work.

The dominance of the behaviourists in psychology relegated emotion to just another 'way of acting' in a particular situation (albeit internally perceived). Although an over-simplification, this led to the development of the 'conditioning theory' of anxiety. John Watson, the father of behaviourism, claimed to have produced an animal phobia in an 11-mth-old boy, 'little Albert', by making a loud clanging noise whilst the boy was playing with a rat. Watson proposed that neuroses arose out of traumatic learning situations and then persist to influence behaviour throughout life.

This was adapted by the 1930s to include the concept of 'instrumental conditioning' (association of an emotionally arousing stimulus and a neutral response), and, in the 1940s, Mowrer attempted to translate Freud's theory of anxiety neurosis into the language of learning theory: responses that reduce anxiety are learned—sometimes these reinforced behaviours may be aberrant, unhelpful, or simply bizarre, and present as neuroses. 'Avoidance' was postulated as the behaviour that was reinforced due to successfully removing a 'negative reinforcer' (e.g. fear). These ideas led to the rational treatment of phobias with desensitization techniques.

In the search for Cannon's neural mechanism, neurophysiologists used lesioning experiments to identify the thalamus as a critical gateway for stimuli, and the hypothalamus as mediating the physiological response (via the HPA axis)—the Cannon–Bard theory. Other theories emerged over the years (e.g. the Papez Circuit, 1937), and understanding the emotional life of the brain remains at the forefront of research (see *The emotional brain* by Joseph LeDoux, 1998).

Inviting as psychological explanations appeared, the late 1950s also heralded the arrival of the BDZs. 'Tranquillizers' (e.g. Miltown®, Librium®, Valium®) became the 'housewives' choice', effectively treating a multitude of neurotic symptoms. Unfortunately, the indiscriminate use of these drugs led to them being demonized as causing dependence problems (despite evidence for their effectiveness when properly used). The advent of the antidepressants artificially separated neurotic depression from the other neuroses, but nonetheless some utility was also seen in treating the anxiety disorders. A key study was the use of clomipramine in the treatment of OCD (see *The boy who couldn't stop washing* by Judith Rapoport, 1989). The fact that clomipramine was the most serotonergic of the TCAs paved the way for the second-generation antidepressants (the SSRIs) used in neuroses (previously thought only to be amenable to psychological approaches).

Brain imaging demonstrated underlying functional changes in OCD patients (in the frontal cortex [left orbital gyrus] and bilateral caudate nuclei), which 'normalized' after successful treatment with medication (and interestingly took longer with CBT techniques, although this took longer). For many patients with panic attacks, structural and functional changes were found in the temporal lobes. These findings resonated with the long-held observation that neurotic symptoms (e.g. anxiety, panic, somatic symptoms, depersonalization/derealization) were often reported in other 'organic' conditions (e.g. temporal lobe epilepsy).

Modern views are eclectic in their approach—e.g. the biopsychosocial model (see 📖 p. 245). For the neuroses, early environmental influences (including social factors like maternal deprivation) can alter the sensitivity of physiological stress responses in adulthood. Hence, the experience of stressors (psychological or physical) may lead (e.g. through the effects of stress hormones such as cortisol, and other neurophysiological mechanisms) to alterations in the structure and/or function of the brain, which in turn manifest as clinical symptoms (i.e. behavioural and/or emotional change).

Hyperventilation syndrome (HVS)[1]

Essence

Ventilation exceeds metabolic demands, leading to haemodynamic and chemical changes producing characteristic symptoms (dyspnoea, agitation, dizziness, atypical chest pain, tachypnoea, hyperpnoea, paraesthesias, and carpopedal spasm) usually in a young, otherwise healthy patient. HVS relatively common presentation; may be mistaken for panic disorder. Considerable overlap, hence inclusion here:

- 50–60% of patients with panic disorder or agoraphobia have symptoms of HVS.
- 25–35% of HVS patients have symptoms of panic disorder.

It may also be confused with other organic diseases, particularly of the cardiorespiratory system, due to the physical symptoms manifest.

Aetiology

Unknown, but certain stressors provoke an exaggerated respiratory response in some individuals (e.g. emotional distress, sodium lactate, caffeine, isoproterenol, cholecystokinin, and CO_2). HVS patients tend to use accessory muscles to breathe, rather than the diaphragm, resulting in hyperinflated lungs and perceived effort or dyspnoea when stressors induce the need to take a deep breath. This leads to anxiety, and triggers further deep breathing, setting up a vicious cycle.

Epidemiology ♀:♂=7:1, usually presents between 15 and 55yrs, but can occur at any age (except infancy).

Symptoms and signs

- *Cardiac*: chest pain/angina (atypical of cardiac origin: may last hours, not minutes; often relieved by exercise; GTN ineffective), ECG changes (prolonged QT, ST depression or elevation, and T-wave inversion).
- *Respiratory*: hyperpnoea, tachypnoea, dyspnoea, wheeze (bronchospasm secondary to low P_aCO_2). *Note*: in chronic forms hyperventilation may not be clinically apparent.
- *CNS* (due to reduced CBF 2° to hypocapnia): dizziness, weakness, confusion, agitation, depersonalization, visual hallucinations, syncope or seizure (rare), paraesthesias (usually upper limbs and bilateral), peri-oral numbness.
- *GI*: bloating, belching, flatus, epigastric pressure (due to aerophagia), dry mouth (due to mouth breathing and anxiety).
- *Metabolic* (due to electrolyte disturbance 2° to respiratory alkalosis): acute hypocalcaemia (signs: carpopedal spasm, muscle twitching, +ve Chvostek and Trousseau signs, and prolonged QT interval), hypokalaemia (with generalized weakness), acute hypophosphataemia (may contribute to paraesthesias and generalized weakness).

Differential diagnosis

Extensive. Diagnosis of exclusion—acute respiratory distress syndrome (ARDS), (venous) air embolism, asthma, atrial fibrillation (AF), atrial flutter, cardiomyopathy, chronic obstructive pulmonary disease (COPD), costochondritis, diabetic ketoacidosis (DKA), hyperthyroidism, metabolic acidosis, methaemoglobinaemia, MI, nasopharyngeal stenosis, panic (and other anxiety) disorder, pleural effusion, pneumonia, pneumothorax, pulmonary embolism (PE), smoke inhalation, CO poisoning, withdrawal syndromes.

Investigations

- Unless there is a clear history of HVS, any first presentations of hyperventilation should be referred for exclusion of serious underlying medical problems (see **Differential diagnosis**).
- These investigations may include full physical, FBC, U&Es, TFTs, glucose, Ca^{2+}, PO_4, pulse oximetry, arterial blood gas (ABG) (in HVS: pH normal, P_aCO_2 and HCO_3 low), toxicology, ELISA d-dimer (PE), ECG, CXR, and possibly V/Q scan.
- Repeating these investigations at later presentations should only be done if there are new clinical findings.

Management

Acute management

If serious underlying pathology excluded, management includes:

- Reassuring the patient.
- Alleviating severe anxiety (e.g. use of BDZs).
- Establishment of normal breathing pattern (instructing the patient to breathe more abdominally using the diaphragm; physically compressing the upper chest and instructing the patient to exhale maximally to reduce hyperinflation).

Note: use of rebreathing techniques (e.g. into a paper bag) is no longer recommended due to reports of significant hypoxia and death. This form of rebreathing may be unsuccessful anyway because very distressed patients have difficulty complying with the technique and because CO_2 itself may be a chemical trigger for anxiety.

Further management

- Education: e.g. hyperventilation, relaxation, and breathing techniques ('provocation' should only be performed in this setting).
- Formal breathing retraining (usually provided by physiotherapists) is available in some centres.
- Beta-blockers and BDZs may be of some use. Some success reported for use of antidepressants in preventing further episodes.
- If there is clear psychiatric morbidity (e.g. anxiety or depression), this should also be specifically addressed.

1 Formerly known as Da Costa syndrome. Other archaic terms include: cardiac neurasthenia, cardiac neurosis, circulatory neurasthenia, disordered action of the heart (DAH), effort syndrome, hyperdynamic–adrenergic circulatory state, hyperkinetic heart syndrome, irritable heart, neurocirculatory asthenia, soldier's heart, vasoregulatory asthenia.

Panic¹ disorder 1: clinical features

Essence
- *Panic attack:* period of intense fear characterized by a constellation of symptoms (see Box 9.1) that develop rapidly, reach a peak of intensity in about 10min, and generally do not last longer than 20–30min (rarely over 1hr). Attacks may be either *spontaneous* ('out of the blue') or *situational* (usually where attacks have occurred previously). Sometimes attacks may occur during sleep (*nocturnal panic attacks*), and rarely, physiological symptoms of anxiety may occur without the psychological component (*non-fearful panic attacks*).
- *Panic disorder:²* Recurrent panic attacks, which are not 2° to substance misuse, medical conditions, or another psychiatric disorder. Frequency of occurrence may vary from many attacks a day to only a few a year. Usually a persistent worry about having another attack or consequences of the attack (which may lead to phobic avoidance of places or situations—see 📖 p. 364), and significant behavioural changes related to attack.

Symptoms/signs (see Box 9.1)
- Physical symptoms/signs related to autonomic arousal (e.g. tremor, tachycardia, tachypnoea, hypertension, sweating, GI upset), often compounded by HVS (in 50–60% of cases, see 📖 p. 356).
- Concerns of death from cardiac or respiratory problems may be a major focus, leading to patients presenting (often repeatedly) to emergency medical services.
- Panic disorder may be undiagnosed in patients with 'unexplained' medical symptoms (chest pain, back pain, GI symptoms including IBS, fatigue, headache, dizziness, or multiple symptoms).
- Thoughts of suicide (or homicide) should be elicited; acute anxiety (particularly when recurrent) can lead to impulsive acts (usually directed towards self). *Note:* risk of attempted suicide substantially raised where comorbid depression, or alcohol or substance misuse.

Epidemiology³
Lifetime prevalence (NCS-R): 1.5–3.7% for panic disorder, 7–9% for panic attacks. Rates much higher in medical clinic samples, e.g. dizziness clinics (15%), cardiac clinics (16–65%), HVS clinics (25–35%). Women are 2–3 times more likely to be affected than men. *Age of onset* has a bimodal distribution with highest peak incidence at 15–24yrs and a second peak at 45–54yrs. Rare after age 65 (0.1%). *Other risk factors* include: being widowed, divorced, or separated; living in a city; limited education; early parental loss; physical or sexual abuse.

Comorbidity
Agoraphobia (community surveys: 30–50%; psychiatric clinics: 75%), depressive disorder (up to 68%), other anxiety and related disorders (up to 50%—e.g. social phobia, OCD), alcohol (up to 30%) and substance misuse, bipolar affective disorder (20%), medical conditions (e.g. mitral valve prolapse, hypertension, cardiomyopathy, COPD, HVS, IBS, migraine).

Differential diagnosis

Other anxiety or related disorder (panic attacks may be part of the disorder), substance or alcohol misuse/withdrawal (e.g. amfetamines, caffeine, cannabis, cocaine, theophylline, sedative-hypnotics, steroids), mood disorders, psychiatric disorders secondary to medical conditions, medical conditions presenting with similar symptoms (e.g. endocrine: carcinoid syndrome, Cushing's disease/syndrome, hyperthyroidism, hypoglycaemia, hypoparathyroidism, phaeochromocytoma; haematological: anaemia; cardiac: arrhythmias (supraventricular), atypical chest pain, mitral valve prolapse, MI; respiratory: COPD, asthma, HVS; neurological: epilepsy—esp. TLE, vestibular dysfunction).

Investigations

No specific tests for panic disorder; basic investigations should be performed to exclude physical causes (e.g. FBC, U&Es, glucose, TFTs, ECG; if supported by history/physical examination: toxicology, Ca^{2+}, urinary vanillyl mandelic acid [VMA]/plasma homovanillic acid [pHVA], echo, and EEG).

Box 9.1 Symptoms associated with panic attacks

In order of frequency of occurrence:
- Palpitations, pounding heart, or accelerated heart rate.
- Sweating.
- Trembling or shaking.
- Sense of shortness of breath or smothering.
- Feeling of choking or difficulties swallowing (globus hystericus).
- Chest pain or discomfort.
- Nausea or abdominal distress.
- Feeling dizzy, unsteady, light-headed, or faint.
- Derealization or depersonalization (feeling detached from oneself or one's surroundings).
- Fear of losing control or going crazy.
- Fear of dying (angor animus).
- Numbness or tingling sensations (paraesthesia).
- Chills or hot flashes.

---

1 'Panic' derives from the Greek god Pan, who was in the habit of frightening humans and animals 'out of the blue'.

2 ICD-10 and DSM-IV disagree on nature of panic disorder. ICD-10 regards true panic attacks as not being *situational*, and DSM-IV allows for both *spontaneous* and *situational*. Hence, DSM-IV includes agoraphobia within panic disorder (as a special case of *situational panic disorder* (panic disorder with agoraphobia), whereas ICD-10 separates agoraphobia (under the rubric 'phobic anxiety disorders') from panic disorder (under the rubric 'other anxiety disorders'). 'Agoraphobia with panic disorder' allowed in ICD-10 when there is avoidance of places or situations where to have a spontaneous panic attack would be difficult or embarrassing.

3 Kessler RC, Chiu WT, Jim R, et al. (2006) The epidemiology of panic attacks, panic disorder, and agoraphobia in the national comorbidity survey replication. *Arch Gen Psychiat* **63**: 415–24.

Panic disorder 2: aetiological models

A number of theories, based primarily on successful pharmacological treatment, explain the biological basis of panic disorder.

- *The serotonergic model:* exaggerated post-synaptic receptor response to synaptic serotonin, possibly 2° to subsensitivity (reduced binding) at 5-HT_{1A} receptors and 5-HT transporters.
- *The noradrenergic model:* increased adrenergic activity, with hypersensitivity of presynaptic α_2 receptors. (Locus coeruleus activity affects the hypothalamic–pituitary–adrenal axis and the firing rate is increased in panic.)
- *The GABA model:* decreased inhibitory receptor sensitivity (impaired GABA neuronal response to BDZs), with resultant excitatory effect.
- *Cholecystokinin–pentagastrin model:* pentagastrin induces panic in a dose-dependent fashion in patients with panic disorder. Gene studies also implicate CCK gene polymorphisms in panic disorder (see **The genetic hypothesis**).
- *The lactate model:* postulated aberrant metabolic activity induced by lactate, from studies involving exercise-induced panic attacks (replicated by IV lactate infusion).
- *The false suffocation carbon dioxide hypothesis:* explains panic phenomena by hypersensitive brainstem receptors.
- *The neuroanatomical model:* suggests that panic attacks are mediated by an overactive 'fear network' in the brain that involves the amygdala, hippocampus, periaqueductal grey, locus coeruleus, thalamus, cingulate, and orbitofrontal areas.

The genetic hypothesis

Panic disorder has moderate heritability of around 25–50% (from family and twin studies). Most studies to date suggest that *vulnerability* is genetically determined, but critical stressors are required to develop clinical symptoms (e.g. separation/loss event, adjusting to a new role, relationship problems, physiological stress: childbirth, surgery, hyperthyroidism). Replicated linkages have been found with chromosomes 13q, 22q, 7p, and 9q31. Candidate genes include ADOR2A, 10832/T, CCK and those coding for 5-HT1A, 5-HT2A, COMT, and linked to the CRH gene.[1]

1 Arnold PD, Zai G, Richter MA (2004) Genetics of anxiety disorders. *Curr Psychiat Rep* **6**: 243–54.

Panic disorder 3: management guidelines

Combination of pharmacological and psychological treatments may be superior to single approach. Choice of initial approach will depend upon patient preference, past history of previous treatment, costs, and availability (as well as local guidelines, e.g. NICE guidance CG113).[1] For emergency treatment of a panic attack, see Box 9.2.

Pharmacological

Current evidence does not suggest any superior efficacy between SSRIs, SNRIs, BDZs, TCAs, and MAOIs. Other factors will determine the choice of medication (see 🔲 p. 266).

- *SSRIs:* in the UK citalopram (20–30mg), escitalopram (5–10mg), paroxetine (10–40mg), and sertraline (50–200mg) are all licensed for panic disorder (and recommended as 1st line by NICE). In view of the possibility of initially increasing panic symptoms, start with lowest possible dose and gradually increase. Evidence of beneficial effect may take up to 12wks and high doses may be necessary.
- *Alternative antidepressants (unlicensed in the UK):* SNRIs (e.g. venlafaxine), TCAs (e.g. imipramine, clomipramine), MAOIs (e.g. phenelzine)—thought by some clinicians to be superior to TCAs (for severe, chronic symptoms), RIMAs (e.g. moclobemide).
- *BDZs* (e.g. alprazolam or clonazepam): not recommended by NICE. Should be used with caution (due to potential for abuse or dependence and cognitive impairment), but may be effective for severe, frequent, incapacitating symptoms. Use for 1–2wks in combination with an antidepressant may 'cover' symptomatic relief until the antidepressant becomes effective. *Note:* 'anti-panic' effects do not show tolerance, although sedative effects do.
- *Limited benefit:* little evidence to support use of bupropion, mirtazapine, inositol, reboxetine, atypical antipsychotics, anticonvulsants, and, perhaps surprisingly, propranolol.
- *Second-line treatment:* consider change to a different class agent (i.e. TCA, SNRI, SSRI, MAOI), addition of BDZ (or a different BDZ), trial of bupropion, or for severe symptoms an atypical antipsychotic (e.g. olanzapine or risperidone).
- *If successful:* continue treatment for 12–18mths before trial discontinuation (gradually tapering of dose over 2–4mths). Do not confuse 'withdrawal' effects (10–20% of patients) with re-emergence of symptoms (50–70% of patients). If symptoms recur, continue for ~1yr before considering second trial discontinuation. (*Note:* patient may wish to continue treatment, rather than risk return of symptoms).

Psychological

- *CBT—behavioural methods*: to treat phobic avoidance by exposure, use of relaxation, and control of hyperventilation (have been shown to be 58–83% effective).[2] *Cognitive methods:* teaching about bodily responses associated with anxiety/education about panic attacks, modification of thinking errors.[3]

- *Psychodynamic psychotherapy:* there is some evidence for brief dynamic psychotherapy, particularly 'emotion-focused' treatment (e.g. 'panic-focused psychodynamic psychotherapy'),[4] where typical fears of being abandoned or trapped are explored.

Issues of comorbidity

- In view of high levels of comorbidity, treatment of these conditions should not be neglected.
- For the other anxiety disorders and depression, this issue is somewhat simplified by the fact that SSRIs and other antidepressants have been shown to be effective for these conditions, too. However, behavioural interventions (e.g. for OCD, social phobia) should also be considered.
- Alcohol/substance abuse may need to be addressed first, but specific treatment for persistent symptoms of panic ought not to be overlooked.

Course

- Most patients seeking treatment have already experienced chronic symptoms for 10–15yrs.
- Untreated, the disorder runs a chronic course.
- With treatment, functional recovery is seen in 25–75% after the first 1–2yrs, falling to 10–30% after 5yrs. Long-term, around 50% will experience only mild symptoms.
- Poor responses associated with: very severe initial symptoms, marked agoraphobia, low socio-economic status, less education, long duration of untreated symptoms, restricted social networks (including loss of a parent, divorce, remaining unmarried), and presence of personality disorder.

Box 9.2 Emergency treatment of an acute panic attack

- Maintain a reassuring and calm attitude (most panic attacks resolve spontaneously within 30min).
- If symptoms are severe and distressing consider prompt use of BDZs (immediate relief of anxiety may help reassure the patient, provide confidence that treatment is possible, and reduce subsequent 'emergency' presentations).
- If first presentation, exclude medical causes (may require admission to hospital for specific tests).
- If panic attacks are recurrent, consider differential diagnosis for panic disorder and address underlying disorder (may require psychiatric referral).

1 For full NICE guidance see: http://www.nice.org.uk/nicemedia/live/13314/52599/52599.pdf (issued Jan. 2011)

2 Ballenger JC et al. (1997) Panic disorder and agoraphobia. In *Treatments of psychiatric disorders,* vol. 2, 2nd edn, pp. 1421–52. Washington, DC: American Psychiatric Press.

3 Barlow DH and Craske MG (1988) *Mastery of your anxiety and panic.* State University for New York at Albany, Center for Stress and Anxiety Disorders.

4 Milrod B, Leon AC, Busch E, et al. (2007) A randomized controlled clinical trial of psychoanalytical psychotherapy for panic disorder. *American Journal of Psychiatry* **164**: 265–72.

Agoraphobia[1]

Essence
Anxiety and panic symptoms associated with places or situations where escape may be difficult or embarrassing (e.g. of crowds, public places, travelling alone or away from home), leading to avoidance.

Epidemiology[2]
Prevalence (6mths) 2.8–5.8% (ECA); ♂:♀ = 1:3; as for panic disorder, there is bimodal distribution, with the first being somewhat broader (15–35yrs). In later life agoraphobic symptoms may develop 2° to physical frailty, with associated fear of exacerbating medical problems or having an accident.

Aetiology
- *Genetic:* both genetic and environmental factors appear to play a role. The predisposition towards overly interpreting situations as dangerous may be genetic, and some commentators suggest an ethological factor involving an evolutionarily determined vulnerability to unfamiliar territory. First-degree relatives also have an increased prevalence of other anxiety and related disorders (e.g. panic disorder, social phobia), alcohol misuse, and depressive disorders.
- *Psychoanalytical:* unconscious conflicts are repressed and may be transformed by displacement into phobic symptoms.
- *Learning theory:* conditioned fear responses lead to learned avoidance.

Comorbidity
Panic disorder, depressive disorder, other anxiety and related disorders (e.g. 55% also have social phobia), alcohol and substance misuse.

Differential diagnosis
Other anxiety and related disorders (esp. generalized anxiety disorder, social phobia, OCD), depressive disorders, secondary avoidance due to delusional ideas in psychotic disorders.

Management
- **Pharmacological** *Antidepressants:* as for panic disorder. BDZs short-term use only (may reinforce avoidance)—most evidence for alprazolam/clonazepam.
- **Psychological** *Behavioural methods:* exposure techniques (focused on particular situations or places), relaxation training, and anxiety management. *Cognitive methods:* teaching about bodily responses associated with anxiety/education about panic attacks, modification of thinking errors.

1 Literally 'fear of the market place' (Greek).
2 Whether or not agoraphobia differs from panic disorder in neurobiology or simply represents a more severe form of panic disorder remains controversial. The similarities of epidemiology, genetics, environmental precipitants, and effective treatments are hard to ignore. NCS-R data (2006) suggest that pure agoraphobia does occur, but it is rarer than earlier epidemiological studies would suggest (e.g. the ECS) with a lifetime prevalence of 1.3% and ♂:♀ = 2:3.

Simple or specific phobias

Essence
Recurring excessive and unreasonable psychological or autonomic symptoms of anxiety, in the (anticipated) presence of a specific feared object or situation (see Box 9.3 for glossary) leading, whenever possible, to avoidance. DSM-IV distinguishes 5 subtypes: animals, aspects of the natural environment, blood/injection/injury, situational, and 'other'.

Epidemiology
Prevalence: (NCS-R) lifetime 12.5%, 12mths 8.7%, 6mths (ECA) 4.5–11.9%; ♂:♀ (all) = 1:3; animal/situational phobias may be more common in ♀; mean age of occurrence is 15yrs: onset for animal phobias ~7yrs, blood/injection/injury ~8yrs, situational phobias ~20yrs.

Aetiology
- *Genetic:* both genetic and environmental factors play a role. MZ:DZ = 25.9%:11.0%[1] for animal phobia, situational phobia roughly equal suggesting stronger role for the environment.
- *Psychoanalytical:* manifest fear is the symbolic representation of an unconscious conflict, which has been repressed and displaced into phobic symptoms.
- *Learning theory:* conditioned fear response related to a traumatic situation, with learned avoidance (trigger to the conditioned response may be a reminder of the original situation). Observational and informational learning also appear to be important, and 'preparedness' theory (Marks)[2] suggests that fear of certain objects may be evolutionarily adaptive (related to survival of the individual or species), selectively acquired, and difficult to extinguish.

Comorbidity
The lifetime risk for patients with specific phobias experiencing at least one other lifetime psychiatric disorder is reportedly over 80% (NCS), particularly other anxiety disorders (panic, social phobia) and mood disorders (mania, depression, dysthymia). However, rates of substance misuse are considerably less than in other anxiety disorders.

Differential diagnosis
Panic disorder (fear of having further panic attack), agoraphobia, social phobia, hypochondriasis (fear of having a specific serious illness), OCD (avoidance/fear of an object or situation due to obsessional thoughts, ideas, or ruminations), psychosis (avoidance due to delusional idea of threat—fears tend to be overly excessive).

Management
Psychological
- *Behavioural therapy:* exposure is the treatment of choice: methods aim to reduce the fear response, e.g. Wolpe's systematic desensitization[3] with relaxation and graded exposure (either imaginary or *in vivo*).

Recent studies have utilized virtual environments (virtual reality exposure: VRE).
- *Other techniques:* reciprocal inhibition, flooding (not better than graded exposure), and modelling.
- *Cognitive methods:* education/anxiety management, coping skills/ strategies, and cognitive restructuring—may enhance long-term outcomes.
- *Pharmacological:* generally not used, except in severe cases to reduce fear/avoidance (with BDZs, e.g. diazepam) and allow the patient to engage in exposure. May reduce the efficacy of behaviour therapy by inhibiting anxiety during exposure. β-blockers may be helpful, but reduce sympathetic arousal not subjective fear. Clear secondary depression may require an antidepressant.

Course

Without treatment, tends to run a chronic, recurrent course. However, individuals may not present unless life changes force them to confront the feared object or situation.

Box 9.3 Specific phobias—selected glossary

Accidents	Dystychiphobia
Animals	Zoophobia
Ants	Myrmecophobia
Automobiles	Amaxophobia, motorphobia
Bees	Apiphobia, melissophobia
Birds	Ornithophobia
Blood	Haemophobia
Bridges	Gephyrophobia
Cats	Felinophobia
Choking/being smothered	Anginaphobia, pnigophobia, pnigerophobia
Contamination, dirt, or infection	Molysomophobia, mysophobia
Creepy, crawly things	Herpetophobia
Crossing streets	Agyrophobia
Darkness	Nyctophobia, scotophobia
Dentists	Dentophobia, odontophobia
Depth	Bathophobia
Doctors	Iatrophobia
Dogs or rabies	Cynophobia
Everything	Panophobia, panphobia, pamphobia
Feathers	Pteronophobia
Flying	Aviophobia
Forests, at night	Nyctohylophobia
Frogs	Batrachophobia
Hair, fur, or animal skins	Chaetophobia, trichophobia, doraphobia
Horses	Equinophobia, hippophobia
Hospitals	Nosocomephobia
Injections	Trypanophobia
Jumping	Catapedaphobia
Lightning and thunder	Brontophobia, karaunophobia
Moths	Mottephobia
Needles	Aichmophobia, belonephobia
Open high places	Aeroacrophobia
Operations: surgical	Tomophobia
Places: enclosed	Claustrophobia
Railways/trains	Siderodromophobia
Rain	Ombrophobia, pluviophobia
Rats	Zemmiphobia
Reptiles	Herpetophobia
Snakes	Ophidiophobia
Spiders	Arachnophobia
Vomiting	Emetophobia
X-rays	Radiophobia

1 Kendler KS, Neale MC, Kessler RC, *et al.* (1992) The genetic epidemiology of phobias in women. The interrelationship of agoraphobia, social phobia, situational phobia, and simple phobia. *Arch Gen Psychiat* **49**: 273–81.
2 Marks IM (1969) *Fears and phobias.* New York: Academic Press.
3 Wolpe J (1973) *The practice of behaviour therapy,* 2nd edn. New York: Pergamon.

Social phobia

Essence
Symptoms of incapacitating anxiety (psychological and/or autonomic) are not 2° to delusional or obsessive thoughts and are restricted to particular social situations, leading to a desire for escape or avoidance (which may reinforce the strongly held belief of social inadequacy).

Epidemiology
Lifetime rates vary from 2.4% (ECA) to 12.1% (NCS-R), 12-mth prevalence 6.8% (NCS-R); ♂ = ♀ for those seeking treatment (however, community surveys suggest ♂ > ♀); bimodal distribution with peaks at 5yrs and between 11–15yrs (ECA)—often patients do not present until they are in their 30s.

Aetiology
Both genetic and environmental factors play a role. MZ:DZ = 24.4%:15.3%.[1] The predisposition towards overly interpreting situations as dangerous may be genetic, whereas individual interpretations of social cues may be environmentally determined[2] (i.e. the particular trigger for the conditioned fear response depends on the social situation in which first episode of anxiety experienced). Responses may be learned from observing parents. Imaging studies show increased activity in individuals with social anxiety in fear networks (prefrontal cortex, amygdala, hippocampus) during anxiety-provoking tasks.[3] Response to antidepressants suggests there may be dysregulation of 5-HT, NE, or DA systems.

Symptoms/signs
Somatic symptoms include blushing, trembling, dry mouth, perspiration when exposed to the feared situation, with excessive fear (which is recognized as such by the patient) of humiliation, embarrassment, or others noticing how anxious they are. Individuals are often characteristically self-critical and perfectionistic. Avoidance of situations may lead to difficulty in maintaining social/sexual relationships, educational problems (difficulties in interactions with other students/oral presentations), or vocational problems (work in less demanding jobs, well below their abilities). Thoughts of suicide are relatively common.

Comorbidity[4]
There is a high level of psychiatric comorbidity with the most common disorders including simple phobia, agoraphobia, panic disorder, generalized anxiety disorder, PTSD, depression/dysthymia, and substance misuse.

Differential diagnosis
Other anxiety and related disorders (esp. generalized anxiety disorder, agoraphobia, OCD), poor social skills, anxious/avoidant personality traits, depressive disorders, secondary avoidance due to delusional ideas in psychotic disorders, and substance misuse

Management

- *Psychological:* CBT, in either an individual or group setting (CBGT),[5] should be considered as a first-line therapy (with SSRIs/MAOIs) and may be better at preventing relapse. Components of this approach include relaxation training/anxiety management (for autonomic arousal), social skills training, integrated exposure methods (modelling and graded exposure), and cognitive restructuring.
- *Pharmacological:* β-blockers (e.g. atenolol) may reduce autonomic arousal, particularly for 'specific social phobia' (e.g. performance anxiety). For more generalized social anxiety, both SSRIs (e.g. escitalopram [licensed: 10mg/day initially; range 5–20mg/day], fluoxetine [unlicensed], fluvoxamine [unlicensed], paroxetine [unlicensed], sertraline [licensed: 25mg/day increased to 50mg/day after 1wk; max 200mg/day]), SNRIs (e.g. venlafaxine [licensed: 75mg/day]), and MAOIs (e.g. phenelzine [unlicensed]) are significantly more effective. Other treatment possibilities include RIMAs (e.g. moclobemide [licensed: 300mg/day for 3 days, then 600mg/day in 2 divided doses]) or the addition of a BDZ (e.g. clonazepam, alprazolam) or buspirone (to augment SSRI). Limited evidence for anticonvulsants (e.g. gabapentin, pregabalin, levetiracetam, valproate [all unlicensed]).

Course

- Without treatment, social phobia may be chronic lifelong condition.
- Course does not appear to be related to gender, age of onset, duration of illness, level of premorbid functioning, lifetime history of anxiety or depressive disorders.
- Extreme childhood shyness and behavioural inhibition may be early manifestations of social phobia.
- With treatment, response rates may be up to 90%, especially with combined approaches.
- Medication best regarded as long-term, as relapse rates are high on discontinuation.

1 Kendler KS, Neale MC, Kessler RC, *et al.* (1992) The genetic epidemiology of phobias in women. The interrelationship of agoraphobia, social phobia, situational phobia, and simple phobia. *Arch Gen Psychiat* **49**: 273–81.
2 Rapee RM, Heimberg RG (1997) A cognitive-behavioral model of anxiety in social phobia. *Behav Res Ther* **35**: 741–56.
3 Stein MB, Goldin PR, Sareen J, *et al.* (2002) Increased amygdala activation to angry and contemptuous faces in generalized social phobia. *Arch Gen Psychiat* **59**: 1027–34.
4 Schneier FR, Johnson J, Hornig CD, *et al.* (1992) Social phobia. Comorbidity and morbidity in an epidemiologic sample. *Arch Gen Psychiat* **49**: 282–8.
5 Heimberg RG, Becker RE (2002) *Cognitive-behaviour group therapy [CBGT] for social phobia: basic mechanisms and clinical strategies.* New York: Guildford Press.

Generalized anxiety disorder (GAD)

Essence
'Excessive worry' (generalized free-floating persistent anxiety) and feelings of apprehension about everyday events/problems, with symptoms of muscle and psychic tension, causing significant distress/functional impairment.

Symptoms/signs
See Box 9.4.

Epidemiology
Prevalence: 6mths (ECA) 2.5–6.4%, 12mths (NCS-R) 3.1%, lifetime (NCS-R) 5.7%; lowest in 18–29yrs (4.1%) and 60+yrs (3.7%); highest 45–59yrs (7.7%); ♀>♂ esp. early onset (associated with childhood fears and marital/sexual disturbance); later onset often after a stressful event; single (~30% never marry); unemployed.

Aetiology (triple vulnerability model)[1]
- *Generalized biological vulnerability:*
  - *Genetic*—modest role, shared heritability with depression.
  - *Neurobiological*—human studies limited. Animal work implicates norepinephrine system: diminished autonomic nervous system responsiveness (? down-regulation of α_2 receptors); HPA axis: loss of regulatory control of cortisol (~1/3 of GAD patients show reduced cortisol suppression using the dexamethasone suppression test [DMST]); amygdala and stria terminalis—possible sustained or repeated activation by CRF due to stress; septohippocampal ('behavioural inhibition') system: sustained activation moderated by ascending 5-HT and NE systems; BDZ-GABA system: reduced expression of peripheral BDZ receptors due to high cortisol levels; other neurotransmitter systems: dysregulation of 5-HT systems, cholecystokinin (CCK-4 and CCK-8S).
- *Generalized psychological vulnerability:*
  - *Diminished sense of control*—trauma or insecure attachment to primary caregivers, leading to intolerance of uncertainty.
  - *Parenting*—overprotective or lacking warmth, leading to low perceived control over events.
- *Specific psychological vulnerability: stressful life events*—trauma (e.g. early parental death, rape, war) and dysfunctional marital/family relationships.

Comorbidity
Other anxiety disorders (simple phobias, social phobia, panic disorder), depression/dysthymia, alcohol and drug problems, other 'physical' conditions (e.g. IBS, HVS, atypical chest pain).

Box 9.4 Symptoms of GAD (present most days for at least 6mths)

- *DSM-IV:* at least 3 (or 1 in children) out of:
  - restlessness or feeling keyed up or on edge;
  - easy fatiguability;
  - concentration difficulties or 'mind going blank';
  - irritability;
  - muscle tension;
  - sleep disturbance.
- *ICD-10:* at least 4 (with at least 1 from 'autonomic arousal') out of:
  - *Symptoms of autonomic arousal*—palpitations/tachycardia; sweating; trembling/shaking; dry mouth.
  - *'Physical' symptoms*—breathing difficulties; choking sensation; chest pain/discomfort; nausea/abdominal distress.
  - *Mental state symptoms*—feeling dizzy, unsteady, faint or light-headed; derealization/depersonalization; fear of losing control, 'going crazy', passing out, dying.
  - *General symptoms*—hot flushes/cold chills; numbness or tingling.
  - *Symptoms of tension*—muscle tension/aches and pains; restlessness/ inability to relax; feeling keyed up, on edge, or mentally tense; a sensation of a lump in the throat or difficulty swallowing.
  - *Other*—exaggerated responses to minor surprises/being startled.
  - *Concentration difficulties/'mind going blank'*—due to worry or anxiety; persistent irritability; difficulty getting to sleep due to worrying.

Differential diagnosis
'Normal worries', depression, mixed anxiety/depression, other anxiety disorders (the anxiety is more focused), drug and alcohol problems, medical conditions (see Box 9.5), side-effects of prescribed medications (see Box 9.6).

Management
- *Psychological:* generally less effective than in the other anxiety disorders (lack of situational triggers); some evidence for CBT[2] combining behavioural methods (treat avoidance by exposure, use of relaxation and control of hyperventilation) and cognitive methods (teaching about bodily responses related to anxiety/education about panic attacks, modification of thinking errors).
- *Pharmacological:* directed towards predominant anxiety symptoms:
  - *psychic symptoms*—buspirone[3] (beneficial effects may take 2–4wks);
  - *somatic symptoms*—BDZs[2] (e.g. lorazepam, diazepam);
  - *depressive symptoms*—TCAs (unlicensed—imipramine, clomipramine), trazodone (licensed 75–300mg/day), SNRIs (licensed—duloxetine 30–60mg/day, venlafaxine 75–225mg/day), SSRIs[2] (licensed—escitalopram 10–20mg/day, paroxetine 20–50mg/ day);

- *cardiovascular symptoms* or *autonomic symptoms*—β-blockers (e.g. atenolol); *other licensed treatments* pregabalin (start 150mg/day; max 600mg/day; in divided doses).
- *Physical:* psychosurgery (very rare)—for severe/intractable anxiety.

Course

Chronic and disabling, prognosis generally poor, remission rates low (~30% after 3yrs, with treatment); 6-yr outcome—68% mild residual symptoms, 9% severe persistent impairment. Often comorbidity becomes more significant (esp. alcohol misuse) and this worsens the prognosis.

Box 9.5 **Medical conditions associated with anxiety-like symptoms**

- *CVS:* arrhythmias, IHD, mitral valve disease, cardiac failure.
- *Respiratory:* asthma, COPD, HVS, PE, hypoxia.
- *Neurological:* TLE, vestibular nerve disease.
- *Endocrine:* hyperthyroidism, hypoparathyroidism, hypoglycaemia, phaeochromocytoma.
- *Miscellaneous:* anaemia, porphyria, SLE, carcinoid tumour, pellagra.

Box 9.6 **Prescribed medications causing anxiety-like symptoms**

- *CVS:* antihypertensives, anti-arrhythmics.
- *Respiratory:* bronchodilators, α_1/β-adrenergic agonists.
- *CNS:* anaesthetics, anticholinergics, anticonvulsants, anti-Parkinsonian agents, antidepressants, antipsychotics, disulfiram reactions, withdrawal from BDZs and other sedatives.
- *Miscellaneous:* levothyroxine, NSAIDs, antibiotics, chemotherapy.

1 Suarez L, Bennett SM, Goldstein CM, *et al.* (2008) Understanding anxiety disorders from a 'triple vulnerability' framework. In: Antony MM and Stein MB, eds, *Handbook of anxiety and anxiety disorders*. New York: Oxford University Press.
2 NICE recommends SSRIs as first-line treatment (+CBT) and does not recommend BDZs for more than 2–4wks. See: ℛ http://www.nice.org.uk/nicemedia/live/13314/52599/52599.pdf
3 Buspirone should be considered as an alternative to BDZs when sedative effects are unwanted (e.g. drivers of vehicles, pilots, machine operators), in patients with a personal/family history of drug misuse, or for those already taking other CNS depressants.

Obsessive–compulsive disorder (OCD)

Essence

A common, chronic condition, often associated with marked anxiety and depression, characterized by 'obsessions' (see 🕮 p. 101) and 'compulsions' (see 🕮 p. 89). Obsessions/compulsions must cause distress or interfere with the person's social or individual functioning (usually by wasting time), and should not be the result of another psychiatric disorder. At some point in the disorder, the person recognizes the symptoms to be excessive or unreasonable.

Content of obsessions/compulsions Checking (63%), washing (50%), contamination (45%), doubting (42%), bodily fears (36%), counting (36%), insistence on symmetry (31%), aggressive thoughts (28%).

Epidemiology Mean age: 20yrs, 70% onset before age 25yrs, 15% after age 35yrs, ♀=♂, prevalence: 0.5–3% of general population.

Aetiology of OCD

- *Neurochemical:* dysregulation of the 5-HT system (possibly involving 5-HT$_{1B}$, or 5-HT/DA interaction).
- *Immunological:* cell-mediated autoimmune factors may be associated e.g. against basal ganglia peptides—as in Sydenham's chorea.
- *Imaging: CT and MRI:* bilateral reduction in caudate size. *PET/SPECT:* hypermetabolism in orbitofrontal gyrus, basal ganglia (caudate nuclei), and cingulum that 'normalizes' following successful treatment (either pharmacological or psychological).
- *Genetic:* suggested by family and twin studies (3–7% of first-degree relatives affected, MZ: 50–80% DZ: 25%), no candidate genes as yet identified, but polymorphisms of 5-HT$_{1B\beta}$ have been replicated.
- *Psychological:* defective arousal system and/or inability to control unpleasant internal states. Obsessions are conditioned (neutral) stimuli, associated with an anxiety-provoking event. Compulsions are learned (and reinforced) as they are a form of anxiety-reducing avoidance.
- *Psychoanalytical:* Freud coined the term 'obsessional neurosis', thought to be the result of regression from oedipal stage to pre-genital anal–erotic stage of development as a defence against aggressive or sexual (unconscious) impulses. *Associated defences:* isolation, undoing, and reaction formation. Symptoms occur when these defences fail to contain the anxiety.

Associations

Avoidant, dependent, histrionic traits (~40% of cases), anankastic/obsessive–compulsive traits (5–15%) prior to disorder. In schizophrenia, 5–45% of patients may present with symptoms of OCD (schizo-obsessives—poorer prognosis). Sydenham's chorea (up to 70% of cases) and other basal ganglia disorders (e.g. Tourette's syndrome, post-encephalitic Parkinsonism).

Comorbidity

Depressive disorder (50–70%), alcohol- and drug-related disorders, social phobia, specific phobia, panic disorder, eating disorder, PTSD, tic disorder (~40% in juvenile OCD) or Tourette's syndrome.

Differential diagnosis

'Normal' (but recurrent) thoughts, worries, or habits (do not cause distress or functional impairment); anankastic PD/OCD; schizophrenia; phobias; depressive disorder; hypochondriasis; body dysmorphic disorder; trichotillomania.

Management[1]

- Psychological
  - CBT—recommended by NICE, but essentially takes a behavioural approach, including exposure and response prevention (ERP).
  - Behavioural therapy—response prevention useful in ritualistic behaviour; thought stopping may help in ruminations; exposure techniques for obsessions.
  - Cognitive therapy—so far not proven effective.
  - Psychotherapy—supportive: valuable (including family members, use of groups); psychoanalytical: no unequivocal evidence of effectiveness (insight-orientated psychotherapy may be useful in some patients).
- Pharmacological:
  - Antidepressants SSRIs (licensed): escitalopram (10–20mg/day), fluoxetine (20–60mg/day), fluvoxamine (100–300mg/day), sertraline (150mg/day), or paroxetine (40–60mg/day) should be considered first-line (no clear superiority of any one agent, high doses usually needed, at least 12wks for treatment response, long-term therapy). Clomipramine (e.g. 250–300mg) has specific anti-obsessional action (NICE second-line choice). Other (unlicensed) agents include citalopram (20–60mg/day; NICE recommended alone or in combination with clomipramine), venlafaxine (225–300mg).
  - Augmentative strategies: antipsychotic (risperidone, haloperidol, pimozide)—esp. if psychotic features, tics, or schizotypal traits (less evidence for olanzapine, quetiapine, aripiprazole); buspirone/short-term clonazepam (not NICE recommended)—if marked anxiety.
- Physical:
  - ECT—consider if patient suicidal or severely incapacitated.
  - Psychosurgery may be considered for severe, incapacitating, intractable cases (i.e. treatment-resistant: 2 antidepressants, 3 combination treatments, ECT, and behavioural therapy), where the patient can give informed consent—e.g. stereotactic cingulotomy (reported up to 65% success). In theory, disrupts the neuronal loop between the orbitofrontal cortex and the basal ganglia.
  - Deep brain stimulation (DBS) efficacy remains to be established (severe refractory cases).

Course

Often sudden onset (after stressful event, e.g. loss, pregnancy, sexual problem), presentation may be delayed by 5–10yrs due to secrecy, symptom intensity may fluctuate (contact-related/phasic) or be chronic.

Outcome

20–30% significantly improve, 40–50% show moderate improvement, but 20–40% have chronic or worsening symptoms. Relapse rates are high after stopping medication. Suicide rates increased esp. if there is secondary depression.

Prognostic factors

• *Poor prognosis:* giving in to compulsions, longer duration, early onset, male, presence of tics, bizarre compulsions, hoarding, symmetry, comorbid depression, delusional beliefs or over-valued ideas, personality disorder (esp. schizotypal PD).
• *Better prognosis:* good premorbid social and occupational adjustment, a precipitating event, episodic symptoms, less avoidance.

Exceptional stressors and traumatic events

ICD-10 definition
'Common-sense' approach: 'a stressful event or situation...of an exceptionally threatening or catastrophic nature, which is likely to cause pervasive distress in almost anyone'. Includes traumatic events (e.g. rape, bombing, criminal assault, natural catastrophe), and unusual sudden changes in the social position and/or network of the individual (e.g. domestic fire, multiple bereavement).

DSM-IV definition
Narrower criteria. Traumatic event must have involved actual or threatened death or serious injury, or threat to the physical integrity of self or others. The person's response to the traumatic event must have involved intense fear, helplessness, or horror (disorganized/agitated behaviour in children).

Type I and Type II trauma (see Box 9.7)
The ICD-10 and DSM-IV definitions describe what has been termed:
- *Type I trauma*: single, dangerous and overwhelming events comprising isolated (often rare) traumatic experiences of sudden, surprising, devastating nature, with limited duration.
- *Type II trauma*: due to sustained and repeated ordeal stressors (series of traumatic events or exposure to prolonged trauma); may be variable, multiple, chronic, repeated, and anticipated, usually of intentional human design (e.g. ongoing physical or sexual abuse, combat). May lead to 'complex PTSD'. Symptoms include: somatization, dissociation, detachment from others, restricted range or dysregulation of affect, emotional lability (poor impulse control, self-destructive behaviour, pathological patterns of relationships), and emotional numbing. ICD-10 acknowledges this type of reaction with the diagnosis '*enduring personality changes after catastrophic experience*', whereas DSM-IV does not currently include the much debated diagnosis 'DESNOS' (disorders of extreme stress not otherwise specified).

How common are these events?
Using DSM-IV criteria, up to 80% of men and 75% of women[1] experience at least one traumatic event in their lifetime (but see cautionary notes in Box 9.8). Common events include sudden death of a loved one, accidents, fire, flood, natural disasters, or being a witness to severe injury (or murder).

Box 9.7 Continued debate

- Both of the ICD-10 and DSM-IV definitions fail to address 'low-magnitude stressors' (e.g. divorce, job loss, failing exams) even though 0.4% of the population may develop 'PTSD-like' symptoms.[1]
- Equally, 'common' events (e.g. RTAs, sexual assault) quite often lead to PTSD-like symptoms.
- Even perpetrators (albeit 'unwilling') of traumatic events (e.g. war-related crimes, torture) may experience PTSD-like symptoms (associated with feelings of shame or guilt).
- Emphasis on life-threatening events/threats to physical integrity may also be too restrictive. The perception of threat to, or loss of, autonomy and mental defeat may actually be more significant than physical assault—seen in studies of victims of sexual/physical assault and political prisoners.
- Whether diagnosis should be made on the basis of symptom clusters, rather that any definition of what constitutes a 'valid' traumatic event becomes academic when a patient presents with clinically significant problems (although it may generate much heat when issues of compensation are involved).

1 McNally RJ (2000) Post traumatic stress disorder. In: Millon T, Blaney PH, David RD, eds, *Oxford textbook of psychopathology.* Oxford: Oxford University Press.

Box 9.8 Recovered and false memories

- Survivors of traumatic events, esp. child abuse, sometimes claim to have recovered memories after a long period of time.
- Organizations such as the False Memory Syndrome Foundation (USA) and the False Memory Society (UK) suggest that many, if not all, of these recovered memories are the product of inappropriate therapeutic suggestion.
- The possibility of false accusations of supposed perpetrators, disruption of families, and accusations of malpractice against therapists have meant that debate is polarized and subsequently the literature is very difficult to interpret.
- Few would disagree with Lindsay & Read's summary (1995):[1] 'In our reading, the scientific evidence has clear implications...memories recovered via suggestive memory work by people who initially denied any such history should be viewed with skepticism, but there are few grounds to doubt spontaneously recovered memories of common forms of child sexual abuse or recovered memories of details of never-forgotten abuse. Between these extremes lies a grey area within which the implications of existing scientific evidence are less clear and experts are likely to disagree.'

1 Lindsay DS and Read JD (1995) 'Memory work' and recovered memories of childhood sexual abuse: scientific evidence and public, professional and personal issues. *Psychol Publ Policy Law* **1**: 846–908.

1 Stein MB, Walker JR, Hazen AL, *et al.* (1997) Full and partial posttraumatic stress disorder: findings from a community survey. *Am J Psychol* **154**: 1114–19.

Acute stress reaction (ICD-10)

Essence
A transient disorder (lasting hours or days) that may occur in an individual as an immediate (within 1hr) response to exceptional stress (e.g. natural catastrophe, major accident, serious assault, warfare, rape, multiple bereavement, fire). The stressor usually involves severe threat to the security or physical integrity of the individual or of a loved person(s).

Symptoms/signs
Symptoms tend to be mixed/changeable with an initial state of daze, followed by depression, anxiety (as for GAD, see 📖 p. 372), anger, or despair. Presence of social withdrawal, narrowed attention, disorientation, aggression, hopelessness, over-activity, or excessive grief defines mild (none of these symptoms present), moderate (2 present), or severe (4 present, or dissociative stupor) forms.

Epidemiology
Incidence variable across studies, but estimated around 15–20% of individuals following exceptional stress.

Aetiology
No specific theories, as it is a transient disorder.

Risk factors
Physical exhaustion, presence of other organic factors, elderly.

Differential diagnosis
PTSD ('exceptional trauma', delayed or persistent symptoms, re-experiencing of the traumatic event), adjustment disorder (not necessarily exceptional stressor, wider range of symptoms), concussion/mild brain injury (neuropsychological testing cannot always distinguish), brief psychotic disorder, dissociative disorders (no clear stressor), substance misuse.

Management
By definition, no specific treatment needed. Ensure other needs are addressed, i.e. safety, security, practical assistance, social supports.

Outcome
- Once the stressor is removed, symptoms resolve (usually) within a few hours.
- If the stress continues, the symptoms tend to diminish after 24–48hrs and are minimal within about 3 days.

Acute stress disorder (DSM-IV)

Essence
Clear overlap with 'acute stress reaction' (symptoms of dissociation, anxiety, hyperarousal), but greater emphasis on dissociative symptoms, onset within 4wks, lasting 2 days to 4wks (after which diagnosis changes to PTSD).

Symptoms/signs
As for PTSD—re-experiencing of events, avoidance, and hyperarousal (but lasting no more than 4wks).

Epidemiology
Incidence depends on trauma: e.g. 13–14% in RTA survivors, 19% in victims of assault, 33% in victims of mass shooting.

Aetiology
Similar to PTSD.
- *Psychological:* 're-experiencing symptoms'. Fear response to harmless situations associated with original trauma, perhaps due to emotional memories (i.e. having personal significance). Remodelling underlying schemas requires holding trauma experiences in 'active' memory until the process is complete (working through). *Dissociation*—a mechanism of avoiding overwhelming emotion (i.e. 'thinking without feeling'), which, if persistent, delays the process of integration.
- *Biological:* neurophysiological changes leading to permanent neuronal changes as a result of the effects of chronic stress or persistent re-experiencing of the stressful event. *Neurotransmitters implicated*— cathecholamines, 5-HT, GABA, opioids, and glucocorticoids.

Risk factors
Previous history of psychiatric disorder, previous traumatic event(s), pre-morbid depression, or dissociative symptoms.

Comorbidity
Similar to PTSD (i.e. depression, substance misuse).

Differential diagnosis
PTSD (timeframe >4wks duration), adjustment disorder (doesn't meet criteria for 'traumatic' event—see [book icon] p. 380; wider range of symptoms), concussion/mild brain injury (neuropsychological testing cannot always distinguish), brief psychotic disorder, dissociative disorders (no clear stressor), substance misuse.

Management
- *Simple practical measures:* e.g. support, advice regarding police procedures, insurance claims, dealing with the media, course and prognosis, may be all that is required.
- *Psychological:*
  - *Debriefing*—may be useful for certain individuals (needing supportive therapy), but reviews suggest there is little positive benefit of single session debriefing and may worsen outcome![1]

- *CBT*—brief interventions (education, relaxation, graded *in vivo* exposure, and cognitive restructuring) may reduce development of chronic problems/PTSD (not immediate, but ~2wks after the event appears best).
- *Pharmacological:* TCAs, SSRIs, and BDZs may be useful for clinically significant symptoms (evidence lacking).

Outcome

By definition, either self-limiting or continues into PTSD.

1 Rose SC, Bisson J, Churchill R and Wessely S (2002) *Psychological debriefing for preventing post traumatic stress disorder (PTSD).* Cochrane Database of Systematic Reviews: CD000560.

Adjustment disorders

Adjustment disorders sit uneasily between what are regarded as normal or just 'problematic' difficulties and the major psychiatric diagnoses. They must occur within 1 (ICD-10) or 3mths (DSM-IV) of a particular psychosocial stressor, and should not persist for longer than 6mths after the stressor (or its consequences) is removed (except in the case of 'prolonged depressive reaction' in ICD-10). Symptoms are 'clinically significant' due to marked distress, or impairment of normal functioning, and may be 'subthreshold' (due to symptom or duration criteria) manifestations of mood disorders, anxiety disorders, stress-related disorders, somatoform disorders, or conduct disorders.

Subclassification

- *ICD-10:* brief depressive reaction (>1mth), prolonged depressive reaction (>6mths, but <2yrs), mixed anxiety and depressive reaction, predominant disturbance of other emotions, predominant disturbance of conduct, mixed disturbance of emotion and conduct, and other specified predominant symptoms. Allows inclusion of bereavement/ grief reactions.
- *DSM-IV:* depressed mood, anxious mood, mixed anxious and depressed mood, disturbance of conduct, mixed disturbance of emotions and conduct, and unspecified. Specifically excludes bereavement reactions (see 🕮 p. 388). 'Acute' disorders <6mths; 'chronic' disorders >6mths.

Epidemiology

Prevalence in inpatient/outpatient psychiatric populations is conservatively estimated at around 5%. In general hospital settings it may be as high as 20% (physical illness being the primary stressor for up to 70% of these cases).

Aetiology

By definition the problems are caused by an identifiable stressor. Individual predisposition plays a greater role than in other conditions, but symptoms would not have arisen without the stressor.

Comorbidity

Possibly higher incidence of alcohol-related problems than the general population, but no different from other psychiatric disorders.

Differential diagnosis

Diagnostic uncertainty may arise if debate surrounds whether the stressor is sufficiently severe to be labelled 'exceptional' or 'traumatic' (acute stress reaction/disorder or PTSD may be considered). Equally, it may be difficult to determine whether symptoms (e.g. low mood, anxiety, sleep disturbance, anorexia, lack of energy) are attributable to a medical disorder or are primarily psychiatric in nature. Use of alcohol and drugs (illicit and prescribed) may complicate the picture.

Management

- *Psychological:* the mainstay of management is essentially supportive psychotherapy to enhance the capacity to cope with a stressor that cannot be reduced or removed, and to establish sufficient support (esp. practical help, e.g. provision of carers/childcare, financial support and benefits, occupational therapy [OT] assessment, contact with specific support groups) to maximize adaption. Ventilation/verbalization of feelings may be useful in preventing maladaptive behaviours (e.g. social isolation, destructive behaviours, suicidal acts) and understanding the 'meaning' of the stressor to the individual may help correct cognitive distortions.
- *Pharmacological:* the use of antidepressants or anxiolytics/hypnotics may be appropriate where symptoms are persistent and distressing (e.g. prolonged depression/dysphoria), or where psychological interventions have proved unsuccessful.

Outcome

- 5-yr follow-up suggests recovery in ~70% (adolescents: ~40%), intervening problems in ~10% (adolescents: ~15%), and development of major psychiatric problems in ~20% (adolescents: ~45%).
- In adults, further psychiatric problems are usually depression/anxiety or alcohol-related problems.

⚠ There is a very real risk of suicide and self-harm (esp. in younger populations). Additional risk factors include poor psychosocial functioning, previous psychiatric problems, personality disorder, substance misuse, and mixed mood/behavioural symptoms. *Do not ignore.*

Normal and abnormal grief reactions

Controversy surrounds how we should regard normal/abnormal grief, and whether they are distinct from depression or other stress-related disorders.[1] It is very common for those suffering bereavement to have depressive symptoms. However, it is less common for people to experience a clear depressive episode that requires treatment.[2] Normal grief is variable in its intensity and duration. Some commentators regard bereavement as just another stressor and argue that, depending on the phenomenology, grief may be regarded as an acute stress reaction/disorder, an adjustment disorder, or even a form of PTSD ('traumatic grief'). Just as the former reactive/endogenous debate surrounding depression has led to recommendations that 'clinical' symptoms should be treated, a bereaved person should not be denied effective treatment on the basis of 'understandability', nor should arbitrary timeframes (e.g. less than 4wks [ICD-10], less than 2mths [DSM-IV]) become more important than assessment of clinical need.

Definitions
- Bereavement: any loss event, usually the death of someone.
- Grief: feelings, thoughts, and behaviour associated with bereavement.
  - 'Normal' —typical symptoms experienced after bereavement include: disbelief, shock, numbness, and feelings of unreality; anger; feelings of guilt; sadness and tearfulness; preoccupation with the deceased; disturbed sleep and appetite and, occasionally, weight loss; seeing or hearing the voice of the deceased. Usually these symptoms gradually reduce in intensity, with acceptance of the loss and readjustment. A typical 'grief reaction' lasts up to 12mths (mean 6mths), but cultural differences exist. Intensity of grief is usually greatest for the loss of a child, then spouse or partner, then parent.
  - 'Abnormal (pathological/morbid/complicated)'—grief reaction that is very intense, prolonged, delayed (or absent), or where symptoms outside normal range are seen, e.g. preoccupation with feelings of worthlessness, thoughts of death, excessive guilt, marked slowing of thoughts and movements, a prolonged period of not being able to function normally, hallucinatory experiences (other than the image or voice of the deceased)[3] (see Box 9.9).

Risk factors for depression following a bereavement
Previous history of depression, intense grief or depressive symptoms early in the grief reaction, few social supports, little experience of death, 'traumatic' or unexpected death.

Management
Generally 'normal' grief does not require specific treatment, although BDZs may be used to reduce severe autonomic arousal or treat problematic sleep disturbance in the short-term. Where there are features of 'abnormal' grief, or where there are clinical symptoms of depression/anxiety, treatment with antidepressants ought to be considered, along with culturally appropriate supportive counselling[1] (e.g. through organizations such as CRUSE).

Box 9.9 Prolonged Grief Disorder (PGD) (aka Complicated Grief Disorder, Traumatic Grief)

Prigerson et al.[1], a group of international researchers, have attempted to refine this syndrome for inclusion in DSM-V and ICD-11 with criteria to identify bereaved persons at heightened risk for enduring distress and dysfunction. Criteria require reactions to a significant loss that involve the experience of yearning (e.g., physical or emotional suffering as a result of the desired, but unfulfilled, reunion with the deceased) and at least 5 of the following 9 symptoms experienced at least daily or to a disabling degree:
- feeling emotionally numb, stunned, or that life is meaningless;
- experiencing mistrust;
- bitterness over the loss;
- difficulty accepting the loss;
- identity confusion;
- avoidance of the reality of the loss;
- difficulty moving on with life.

Symptoms must be present at sufficiently high levels at least 6mths from the death and be associated with functional impairment.

[1] Prigerson HG, Horowitz MJ, Jacobs SC, et al. (2009) Prolonged grief disorder: Psychometric validation of criteria proposed for DSM-V and ICD-11. *PLoS Med* **6**:e1000121. Epub.

Near the end of his life Sigmund Freud was consulted by a woman who had become depressed following the death of her husband. After listening to her, Freud quietly stated, 'Madam, you do not have a neurosis, you have a misfortune'.

Wahl CW (1970) *Arch Found Thanatol* **1**: 137.

'I know of only one functional psychiatric disorder, whose cause is known, whose features are distinctive, and whose course is usually predictable, and this is grief, the reaction to loss. Yet this condition has been so neglected by psychiatrists that until recently it was not even mentioned in the indexes of most of the best-known general textbooks of psychiatry.'

Parkes CM (1986) *Bereavement studies of grief in adult life*. 2nd edn. Tavistock Publications, London and New York.

1 Stroebe MS, Hanson RO, Stroebe W, et al. (eds) (2007) *Handbook of bereavement research and practice: 21st century perspectives*. Washington, DC: American Psychological Association Press.
2 Results vary, e.g. in one study 16% of late-life widows had depression 13mths after bereavement. Zisook S, Paulus M, Shuchter SR, and Judd LL (1997) The many faces of depression following spousal bereavement. *J Affect Disord* **45**: 85–95.
3 Parkes CM (1986) *Bereavement: studies of grief in adult life*, 2nd edn. International Universities Press.

Post-traumatic stress disorder 1: diagnosis

Essence

Severe psychological disturbance following a traumatic event (see 📖 p. 380) characterized by involuntary re-experiencing of elements of the event, with symptoms of hyperarousal, avoidance, emotional numbing.

Symptoms/signs

Symptoms arise within 6mths (ICD-10) of the traumatic event (delayed onset in ~10% of cases) or are present for at least 1mth, with clinically significant distress or impairment in social, occupational, or other important areas of functioning (DSM-IV). Both ICD-10 and DSM-IV include:

- 2 or more 'persistent symptoms of increased psychological sensitivity and arousal' (not present before exposure to the stressor): difficulty falling or staying asleep; irritability or outbursts of anger; difficulty in concentrating; hypervigilance; exaggerated startle response.

Other ICD-10 criteria

- Persistent remembering or 'reliving' of the stressor in intrusive flashbacks, vivid memories, or recurring dreams; and in experiencing distress when exposed to circumstances resembling or associated with the stressor.
- Actual or preferred avoidance of circumstances resembling or associated with the stressor which was not present before exposure to the stressor.
- Inability to recall, either partially or completely, some important aspects or the period of exposure to the stressor.

Other DSM-IV criteria (see Box 9.10)

Epidemiology

Risk of developing PTSD after a traumatic event 8–13% for men, 20–30% for women. Lifetime prevalence estimated as 7.8% (♂:♀ = 1:2).[1] Cultural differences exist. Some types of stressor are associated with higher rates of PTSD (e.g. rape, torture, being a prisoner of war).

Aetiology

- *Psychological/biological:* see 📖 p. 384.
- *Neuroimaging:* reduced hippocampal volume (may relate to appreciation of safe contexts and explicit memory deficits). Dysfunction of the amygdala, hippocampus, septum, and prefrontal cortex may lead to enhanced fear response. High arousal appears to be mediated by anterior cingulate, medial prefrontal cortex, and thalamus; dissociation by parietal, occipital, and temporal cortex.
- *Genetic:* higher concordance rates seen in MZ than DZ twins.

Risk factors

- *Vulnerability factors:* low education, lower social class, Afro-Carribbean/ Hispanic, female gender, low self-esteem/neurotic traits, previous (or

family) history of psychiatric problems (esp. mood/anxiety disorders), previous traumatic events (including adverse childhood experiences and abuse).
- *Peri-traumatic factors:* trauma severity, perceived life threat, peri-traumatic emotions, peri-traumatic dissociation.
- *Protective factors:* high IQ, higher social class, Caucasian, male gender, psychopathic traits, chance to view body of dead person.

Comorbidity (may be primary or secondary)
Depressive/mood disorders, other anxiety disorders, alcohol and drug misuse disorders, somatization disorders.

Differential diagnosis
Acute stress reaction/disorder, enduring personality change after a cata-strophic event (duration at least 2yrs, see 📖 p. 380), adjustment disorder (less severe stressor/different symptom pattern), other anxiety disorder, depressive/mood disorder, OCD, schizophrenia (or associated psychosis), substance-induced disorders.

Box 9.10 Other DSM-IV criteria
Traumatic event is persistently re-experienced in 1 (or more) of the following ways:
- Recurrent and intrusive distressing recollections of the event, including images, thoughts, or perceptions (or repetitive play in which themes or aspects of the trauma are expressed in children).
- Recurrent distressing dreams of the event (or frightening dreams without recognizable content in children).
- Acting or feeling as if the traumatic event were recurring (or trauma-specific re-enactment in children).
- Intense psychological distress at exposure to internal or external cues that symbolize or resemble an aspect of the traumatic event.
- Physiological reactivity at exposure to internal or external cues that symbolize or resemble an aspect of the traumatic event.

Persistent avoidance of stimuli associated with the trauma and numbing of general responsiveness (not present before the trauma), as indicated by 3 (or more) of:
- Efforts to avoid thoughts, feelings, or conversations associated with the trauma.
- Efforts to avoid activities, places, or people that arouse recollections of the trauma.
- Inability to recall an important aspect of the trauma.
- Markedly diminished interest or participation in significant activities.
- Feeling of detachment or estrangement from others.
- Restricted range of affect.
- Sense of foreshortened future.

1 Kessler RC, Sonnega A, Bromet E, et al. (1995) Posttraumatic stress disorder in the National Comorbidity Survey. *Archives of General Psychiatry* **52**: 1048–60.

Post-traumatic stress disorder 2: management[1]

Psychological

Meta-analyses support the superior efficacy of trauma-focused treatments,[2] specifically trauma-focused CBT and EMDR. These are recommended as first-line treatments in all recent guidelines.

- *CBT:* includes elements of: education about the nature of PTSD, self-monitoring of symptoms, anxiety management, breathing techniques, imaginal reliving, exposure to anxiety-producing stimuli in a supportive environment, cognitive restructuring (esp. for complicated trauma), anger management.
- *Eye movement desensitization and reprocessing (EMDR):*[3] novel treatment using voluntary multi-saccadic eye movements to reduce anxiety associated with disturbing thoughts and help process the emotions associated with traumatic experiences (see Box 9.11).
- *Other psychological treatments:*
  - *Psychodynamic therapy*—focus on resolving unconscious conflicts provoked by the stressful events, the goal being to understand the meaning of the event in the context of the individual.
  - *Stress management (stress inoculation)*—teaching skills to help cope with stress, such as relaxation, breathing, thought stopping, assertiveness, positive thinking.
  - *Hypnotherapy*—use of focused attention to enhance control over hyperarousal and distress, enabling recollection of traumatic event. Concern over possible induction of dissociative states.
  - *Supportive therapy*—non-directive, non-advisory method of exploring thoughts, feelings, and behaviours to reach clearer self-understanding.

Pharmacological

Medication may be considered when there is severe ongoing threat, if the patient is too distressed or unstable to engage in psychological therapy, or fails to respond to an initial psychological approach.

- *SSRIs* (e.g. paroxetine 20–40mg/day; sertraline 50–200mg/day) are licensed for PTSD, and their use supported by systematic review.[4] Other unlicensed possibilities include: fluoxetine, citalopram, escitalopram, and fluvoxamine.
- *Other antidepressants:* although unlicensed there is some evidence for TCAs (e.g. amitriptyline, imipramine); MAOIs (e.g. phenelzine) may also reduce anxiety (over-arousal), intrusiveness, and improve sleep; venlafaxine; mirtazapine.

It may be helpful to target specific symptoms:

- *Sleep disturbance* (including nightmares): may be improved by mirtazapine (45mg/day), levomepromazine, prazosin (mean dose 9.5mg/day), or specific hypnotics (e.g. zopiclone, zolpidem).
- *Anxiety symptoms/hyperarousal:* consider use of BDZs (e.g. clonazepam 4–5mg/day), buspirone, antidepressants, propranolol.

- *Intrusive thoughts/hostility/impulsiveness:* some evidence for use of carbamazepine, valproate, topiramate, or lithium.
- *Psychotic symptoms/severe aggression or agitation:* may warrant use of an antipsychotic (some evidence for olanzapine, risperidone, quetiapine, clozapine, aripiprazole).

Outcome

- ~50% will recover within 1st year, ~30% will run a chronic course.
- Outcome depends on initial symptom severity.
- Recovery will be helped by: good social support; lack of −ve responses from others; absence of 'maladaptive' coping mechanisms (e.g. avoidance, denial, 'safety behaviours', not talking about the experience, thought suppression, rumination); no further traumatic life events (2° problems such as physical health, acquired disability, disfigurement, disrupted relationships, financial worries, litigation).

◆ Box 9.11 EMDR controversy

In 1987 Francine Shapiro, a California psychologist in private practice, whilst walking in the woods, preoccupied with disturbing thoughts, discovered her anxiety improved during the walk. She realized that she had been moving her eyes back and forth, from one side of the path to the other, while walking. Shapiro tried out variants of this procedure with her clients and found that they felt better, too. Her findings were published in 1989 and EMDR was born.

Initially developed to help clients with PTSD and other anxiety disorders, therapists have since extended EMDR to other conditions, including depression, sexual dysfunction, schizophrenia, eating disorders, and stress associated with illnesses such as cancer. Like other serendipitous discoveries the claims for EMDR were treated with a healthy dose of scepticism, esp. when its proponents tried to explain 'how' it worked, using erroneous theories of memory, right–left brain imbalance, and REM-sleep-like processing. It became associated with alternative therapies, such as Roger Callahan's Thought Field Therapy and Gary Craig's Emotional Freedom Therapy. These therapies have all the hallmarks of pseudoscience (see 📖 p. 20).

Although the mechanism of action of EMDR is not fully understood, it has been shown that the eye movements are *not* a necessary component of the therapy. In fact, well-established psychological principles of attention, imaginal exposure, and methods of relaxation are probably sufficient to explain the efficacy of the EMDR procedure.

1 NICE (2005) *PTSD: the management of PTSD in adults and children in primary and secondary care*. Clinical guideline CG26. Available at: 🔗 http://www.nice.org.uk/CG26
2 Bisson J, Ehlers A, Matthews R, *et al.* (2007) Systematic review and meta-analysis of psychological treatments for post-traumatic stress disorder. *Br J Psychiat* **190**: 97–104.
3 Shapiro F (1995) *Eye movement desensitization and reprocessing: basic principles, protocols, and procedures.* New York: Guildford Press.
4 Stein DJ, Ipser JC, and Seedat S (2006) Pharmacotherapy for posttraumatic stress disorder (PTSD). *Cochrane Database System Rev* Issue 1.

Depersonalization (derealization) syndrome

Essence

A rare disorder, characterized by persistent or recurrent episodes of a distressing feeling of unreality or detachment. This may be in relation to the outside world (derealization) or the person's own body, thoughts, feelings, or behaviour (depersonalization). It is viewed as a dissociative disorder (DSM-IV) or an anxiety/stress-related disorder (ICD-10).

Clinical features

- Patients may find it difficult to describe their experiences, often reporting feeling 'as if' they are a passive observer of what is going on around them or their own actions. This may be accompanied by an emotional numbness (inability to experience feelings) and the impression of being in a dream- or trance-like state.
- There may also be the experience of alterations in the perception of objects or people, appearing unfamiliar or different in respect to usual colour, shape, distance, or size. Insight tends to be preserved (unlike 'passivity phenomena' in psychoses): the patient recognizes the experiences as abnormal, and often finds them unpleasant, distressing, and anxiety-provoking.

Epidemiology[1]

Up to 50% of 'normal' individuals may experience depersonalization in their lifetime (usually in the context of psychological distress) with 1–2% having more chronic symptoms. In psychiatric populations it is a very common experience (lifetime prevalence ~80%), with persistent symptoms (and associated functional impairment) in ~12%. In clinical populations ♂:♀ = 1:2 whereas in the general population ♂ = ♀. Age of onset usually adolescence/early adulthood (may go undetected in children).

Aetiology

- *Psychoanalytical:* ego defence against painful and conflicting memories, impulses, or affects; usually rooted in childhood trauma.[2]
- *Psychological:* adaptive response to overwhelming stress, allowing continued function by protecting against potentially overwhelming anxiety. Specific precipitant(s) may not be readily identifiable.
- *Biological:* altered function in systems central to integrated processing of information in the brain (with functional localization in the parietotemporal and limbic areas), where serotonergic mechanisms play a key role.[3] Appears to be a role for the effects of illicit drugs with 10–20% of patients describing symptoms first occurring in the context of drug use (especially cannabis).

Comorbidity

Anxiety disorders (particularly phobias, panic disorder, OCD), depressive disorders, personality disorders (anankastic/obsessional, BPD).

Differential diagnosis

Depersonalization may be experienced in the context of sleep or sensory deprivation, being in unfamiliar surroundings, or an acutely stressful/

traumatic situation. May also be a symptom in schizophrenia/psychosis (usually accompanied by a delusional explanation, e.g. Cotard delusion), mood or anxiety disorders, acute intoxication/withdrawal from alcohol, illicit substances (particularly cannabis or hallucinogens), or medication, and in organic disorders (hyperventilation, hypoglycaemia, migraine and epilepsy, usually brief stereotyped episodes, or other neurological conditions).

Management[4]

- Use of rating scales (e.g. The Cambridge Depersonalization Scale)[5] may assist assessment of treatment response.
- Exclude organic causes with appropriate investigations, which may sometimes include brain imaging (CT/MRI) and EEG.
- Comorbid psychiatric conditions should be identified and treated. Despite successful treatment, depersonalization may persist.
- Evidence for successful management of depersonalization syndrome is poor. No drugs are licensed for use in the UK.
- Some evidence supports a role for SSRIs (usually citalopram or escitalopram) alone or in combination with lamotrigine (up to 500mg/day).
- Where there is marked anxiety, clonazepam (0.5–4mg/day) may be useful; anecdotal evidence supports clomipramine (if obsessional symptoms are marked), naltrexone, and bupropion.
- CBT is the only psychological treatment shown to be beneficial in an open trial, particularly in tackling anxieties, ruminations, and avoidance behaviours relating to identifiable stressors.
- Other psychotherapeutic approaches: acceptance and understanding of symptoms; identification of 'putative' defence functions; identifying underlying psychopathology; integration of traumatic experiences and memories.

Course

- Onset is usually sudden, with symptoms persisting only for a brief period. Gradual onset does occur and course is very variable—both episodic and continuous. Occasionally symptoms may persist for hours, days, weeks, months, or even years (rare).
- Resolution tends to be gradual. Recurrent episodes generally occur in the context of recurring (perceived) stressful situations or fatigue.
- Chronic symptoms run a fluctuating course, and may be treatment-resistant.

1 Hunter ECM, Sierra M, and David AS (2004) The epidemiology of depersonalization and derealisation: a systematic review. *Soc Psychiat Psychiat Epidemiol* **39**: 9–18.

2 Dangers of attributing present psychopathology to childhood events cannot be overstated. Recently illustrated by high-profile cases of alleged 'recovered memories' (see Box 9.8). Regard unsubstantiated claims of childhood (or other) abuse with extreme caution. Psychodynamic notion of 'repression' is intellectually dubious, and significance of childhood trauma, even in empirical studies, finds little support. See Pope HG (1997) *Psychology astray: fallacies in studies of 'repressed memory' and childhood trauma.* Boca Raton: Upton.

3 As early as 1935, Mayer-Gross thought psychological explanations to be of 'limited value', seeing depersonalization as 'an unspecific preformed functional response of the brain'. Mayer-Gross W (1935) On depersonalization. *Br J Med Psychol* **XV**(2): 103–26.

4 Medford N, Sierra M, Baker D, *et al.* (2005) Understanding and treating depersonalization disorder. *Adv Psychiat Treat* **11**: 92–100.

5 ℘ http://www.iop.kcl.ac.uk/iopweb/blob/downloads/locator/l_911_Scale3.pdf

Eating and impulse-control disorders

Anorexia nervosa 1: overview

Essence
Condition most commonly seen in young women in which there is marked distortion of body image, pathological desire for thinness, and self-induced weight loss by a variety of methods. Significant mortality: 10–15% (2/3 physical complications, 1/3 suicide).

Epidemiology
$\male$:$\female$ = 1:10; mean age of onset: $\female$ 16–17yrs (rarely >30yrs); $\male$ ~ 12yrs. Incidence ~0.5% of adolescent and young women. Community samples suggest equal distribution across the social classes, but clinic samples show excess of upper/middle classes.

Diagnostic criteria
- **Low body weight**—15%+ below expected, BMI 17.5 or less (see Box 10.1 for calculation).
- **Self-induced weight loss**—avoidance of 'fattening' foods, vomiting, purging, excessive exercise, use of appetite suppressants.
- **Body image distortion**—'dread of fatness': over-valued idea, imposed low weight threshold.
- **Endocrine disorders**—HPA axis: e.g. amenorrhoea, reduced sexual interest/impotence, raised GH levels, raised cortisol, altered TFTs, abnormal insulin secretion.
- **Delayed/arrested puberty**—if onset pre-pubertal.

Note: in 'atypical' cases one or more of these key features may be absent, or all are present but to a lesser degree.

Aetiology
- **Genetic** Concordance rates MZ:DZ = 65%:32%, female siblings: 6–10%.
- **Adverse Life events** No excess of childhood physical or sexual abuse (compared to psychiatric controls).
- **Psychodynamic models**
  - Family pathology—enmeshment, rigidity, over-protectiveness, lack of conflict resolution, weak generational boundaries.
  - Individual pathology—disturbed body image (due to dietary problems in early life, parents' preoccupation with food, lack of a sense of identity).
  - Analytical model—regression to childhood, fixation on the oral stage, escape from the emotional problems of adolescence.
- **Biological**
  - Hypothalamic dysfunction—? cause or consequence.
  - Neuropsychological deficits—reduced vigilance, attention, visuospatial abilities, and associative memory (correct with weight gain).
  - Brain imaging CT: 'pseudoatrophy'/sulcal widening and ventricular enlargement (corrects with weight gain). Functional imaging: unilateral temporal lobe hypoperfusion perhaps related to visuospatial problems/body image distortion.

Differential diagnosis
- Chronic debilitating physical disease.
- Brain tumours.
- GI disorders (e.g. Crohn's disease, malabsorption syndromes).
- Loss of appetite (may be secondary to drugs, e.g. SSRIs, amfetamines).
- Depression/OCD (features of which may be associated).

Box 10.1 BMI (body mass index)*

BMI is a ratio between weight and height, which correlates with body fat, and is used to evaluate if a person is at an unhealthy weight (given a certain height). BMI value is more useful for predicting health risks than the weight alone (for adults aged 18+ yrs).

To calculate BMI the following formulae are used:

$$BMI = \frac{Weight\ (in\ kilos)}{Height\ (in\ metres)^2}$$

or

$$BMI = \frac{Weight\ (in\ pounds) \times 704.5}{Height\ (in\ inches)^2}$$

Range			
Women	**Men**	**Interpretation**	**Risk to health**
<19.1	<20.7	Underweight	The lower the BMI, the greater the risk
19.1–25.8	20.7–26.4	Ideal weight	Normal, very low risk
25.8–27.3	26.4–27.8	Marginally overweight	Some risk
27.3–32.2	27.8–31.1	Overweight	Moderate risk
32.3–44.8	31.1–45.4	Very overweight or obese	High risk
>44.8	>45.4	Morbid obesity	Very high risk

Note: BMI is less reliable for: children and teenagers (ranges are based on adult heights), competitive athletes and bodybuilders (muscle weight may skew the results), pregnant or nursing women, and people over 65.

* The formula for BMI was developed by the Belgian statistician Adolphe Quetelet in the nineteenth century and is sometimes referred to as 'Quetelet's formula'.

Anorexia nervosa 2: physical consequences

Common problems
Mainly due to the effects of starvation or vomiting:
- **Oral** Dental caries.
- **Cardiovascular** Hypotension; prolonged QT; arrhythmias; cardiomyopathy.
- **Gastrointestinal** Prolonged GI transit (delayed gastric emptying, altered antral motility, gastric atrophy, decreased intestinal mobility); constipation. *Note:* prokinetic agents may accelerate gastric emptying and relieve gastric bloating, which can accelerate resumption of normal eating habits.
- **Endocrine and metabolic** Hypokalaemia; hyponatraemia; hypoglycaemia; hypothermia; altered thyroid function; hypercortisolaemia; amenorrhoea; delay in puberty; arrested growth; osteoporosis.
- **Renal** Renal calculi.
- **Reproductive** Infertility; low birth-weight infant.
- **Dermatological** Dry scaly skin and brittle hair (hair loss); lanugo (fine downy) body hair.
- **Neurological** Peripheral neuropathy; loss of brain volume: ventricular enlargement, sulcal widening, cerebral atrophy (pseudoatrophy—corrects with weight gain).
- **Haematologic** Anaemia; leukopenia; thrombocytopenia.

Cardiac complications
- The most common cause of death (mortality rate 7–10%).
- Findings may include:
  - Significant bradycardia (30–40bpm).
  - Hypotension (systolic <70mmHg).
  - ECG changes (sinus bradycardia, ST-segment elevation, T-wave flattening, low voltage, and right axis deviation) may not be clinically significant unless there are frequent arrhythmias (QT prolongation may indicate increased risk for arrhythmias and sudden death).
  - Echocardiogram may reveal decreased heart size, decreased left ventricular mass (with associated abnormal systolic function), and mitral valve prolapse (without significant mitral regurgitation). These changes reflect physiological response to malnutrition and will recover on refeeding.

Amenorrhoea
- Included in the diagnostic criteria, due to hypothalamic dysfunction (hypothalamic–pituitary–ovarian axis) with low levels of follicle-stimulating hormone (FSH) and luetinizing hormone (LH), despite low levels of oestrogen (reversion to the pre-pubertal state occurs with LH response to GnRH blunted leading to amenorrhoea).
- Consequences include reduced fertility, multiple small follicles in the ovaries, decreased uterine volume, and atrophy.

Note: weight loss, excessive exercise, and stress are also important. However, amenorrhoea can persist (in 5–44% of cases) even after recovery and return to normal weight.

Osteopenia

Both cortical and trabecular bone are affected, and osteopenia persists despite oestrogen therapy. Contributing to bone loss are low levels of progesterone and decreased IGF-1 levels.

Treatment

- No specific treatment exists; however, 1000–1500mg/d of dietary calcium and 400IU of vitamin D is recommended to prevent further bone loss and maximize peak bone mass.
- Exercise and HRT, although of benefit in adult women, may be harmful for adolescents with anorexia nervosa (causing premature closure of bone epiphysis).

Box 10.2 Physical signs

- loss of muscle mass
- dry skin
- brittle hair and nails
- callused skin over interphalangeal joints (Russell sign)
- anaemia
- hypercarotinaemia (yellow skin and sclera)
- fine, downy, lanugo body hair
- eroded tooth enamel
- peripheral cyanosis
- hypotension
- bradycardia
- hypothermia
- atrophy of the breasts
- swelling of the parotid and submandibular glands
- swollen tender abdomen (intestinal dilatation due to reduced motility and constipation)
- peripheral neuropathy

Anorexia nervosa 3: assessment

Full psychiatric history (Box 10.3)
- Establish the context in which the problems have arisen (to inform development of a treatment plan).
- Confirm the diagnosis of an eating disorder.
- Assess risk of self-harm/suicide.

Box 10.3 Commonly reported psychiatric symptoms

- Concentration/memory/decision-making problems
- Irritability
- Depression
- Low self-esteem
- Loss of appetite
- Reduced energy
- Insomnia
- Loss of libido
- Social withdrawal
- Obsessiveness regarding food

Full medical history (Box 10.4)
- Focus on the medical complications of altered nutrition (📖 p. 400).
- Detail weight changes, dietary patterns, and excessive exercise.

Box 10.4 Symptoms commonly elicited on systemic enquiry

- General physical health concerns
- Amenorrhoea
- Cold hands and feet
- Weight loss
- Constipation
- Dry skin
- Hair loss
- Headaches
- Fainting or dizziness
- Lethargy

Physical examination
- Determine weight and height (calculate BMI—see 📖 p. 399).
- Assess physical signs of starvation and vomiting (📖 p. 400).
- Routine and focused blood tests (see Box 10.5).
- ECG (and echocardiogram if indicated).

Box 10.5 Blood tests

FBC Haemoglobin (Hb) usually normal or elevated (dehydration); if anaemic, investigate further. Leukopenia and thrombocytopenia seen.

ESR Usually normal or reduced; if elevated, look for other organic cause of weight loss.

U&Es Raised urea and creatinine (dehydration), hyponatraemia (excessive water intake or syndrome of inappropriate antidiuretic hormone secretion [SIADH]—neurogenic diabetes insipidus, affecting 40%, may be treated with vasopressin, but is reversible following weight gain), hypokalaemic/hypochloraemic metabolic alkalosis (from vomiting), metabolic acidosis (laxative abuse). Other abnormalities may include hypocalcaemia, hypophosphataemia, hypomagnesaemia.

Glucose Hypoglycaemia (prolonged starvation and low glycogen stores).

LFTs Minimal elevation.

TFTs Low T_3/T_4, increased rT_3 (euthyroid sick syndrome—an adaptive mechanism; hormonal replacement not necessary; reverts to normal on refeeding).

Albumin/total protein Usually normal.

Cholesterol May be dramatically elevated (starvation)—secondary to decreased T_3 levels, low cholesterol binding globulin, and leakage of intrahepatic cholesterol.

Endocrine Hypercortisolaemia, ↑GH levels, ↓ luetinizing hormone releasing hormone (LHRH), ↓LH, ↓FSH, ↓oestrogens, and ↓progestogens.

Anorexia nervosa 4: management

General principles
- Most patients will be treated as outpatients.
- A combined approach is better:
  - **Pharmacological** Fluoxetine (especially if there are clear obsessional ideas regarding food); previously TCAs or chlorpromazine used for weight gain.
  - **Psychological** Family therapy (more effective in early onset), individual therapy (behavioural therapy = CBT; may improve long-term outcome).
  - **Education** Nutritional education (to challenge over-valued ideas), self-help manuals ('bibliotherapy').
- Hospital admission should only be considered if there are serious medical problems (see Box 10.6).
  - Compulsory admission may be required: feeding is regarded as 'treatment' (*Note:* ethical issue regarding patient's 'right to die' vs. their 'right to treatment').

Box 10.6 Criteria for admission to hospital

Inpatient management may be necessary for patients with significant medical or psychiatric problems:
- Extremely rapid or excessive weight loss that has not responded to outpatient treatment.
- Severe electrolyte imbalance (life-threatening risks due to hypokalaemia or hyponatraemia).
- Serious physiological complications, e.g. temperature < 36°C; fainting due to bradycardia (PR <45bpm) and/or marked postural drop in BP.
- Cardiac complications or other acute medical disorders.
- Marked change in mental status due to severe malnutrition.
- Psychosis or significant risk of suicide.
- Failure of outpatient treatment (e.g. inability to break the cycle of disordered eating or engage in effective outpatient psychotherapy).
Admission should not be viewed as punishment by the patient and the goals of inpatient therapy should be fully discussed with the patient (and their family):
- Addressing physical and/or psychiatric complications.
- Development of a healthy meal plan.
- Addressing underlying conflicts (e.g. low self-esteem, planning new coping strategies).
- Enhancing communication skills.

Risks of re-feeding

With re-feeding, cardiac decompensation may occur, especially during the first 2wks (when the myocardium cannot withstand the stress of an increased metabolic demand). Symptoms include excessive bloating, oedema, and, rarely, congestive cardiac failure (CCF).

To limit these problems:

- Measure U&Es and correct abnormalities before re-feeding.
- Recheck U&Es every 3 days for the first 7 days and then weekly during re-feeding period.
- Attempt to increase daily caloric intake slowly by 200–300kcal every 3–5 days until sustained weight gain of 1–2 pounds/wk is achieved.
- Monitor patient regularly for development of tachycardia or oedema.

Prognosis

- If untreated, this condition carries one of the highest mortality figures for any psychiatric disorder (10–15%).
- If treated, 'rule of thirds' (1/3 full recovery, 1/3 partial recovery, 1/3 chronic problems).
- Poor prognostic factors include:
  - chronic illness
  - late age of onset
  - bulimic features (vomiting/purging)
  - anxiety when eating with others
  - excessive weight loss
  - poor childhood social adjustment
  - poor parental relationships
  - male sex.

Bulimia nervosa

Essence
Characterized by recurrent episodes of binge eating, with compensatory behaviours and overvalued ideas about 'ideal' body shape and weight. Often there is a past history of anorexia nervosa (30–50%) and body weight may be normal.

Epidemiology
Incidence 1–1.5% of women, with mid-adolescent onset, and presentation in early 20s.

Aetiology
Similar to anorexia nervosa, but also evidence for associated personal/family history of obesity, and family history of affective disorder and/or substance misuse. Possible 'dysregulation of eating', related to serotonergic mechanisms (?supersensitivity of 5-HT$_{2C}$ secondary to ↓5-HT).

Diagnostic criteria (see Box 10.7)
- Persistent preoccupation with eating
- Irresistible craving for food
- 'Binges'—episodes of overeating
- Attempts to counter the 'fattening' effects of food (self-induced vomiting, abuse of purgatives, periods of starvation, use of drugs, e.g. appetite suppressants, thyroxine, diuretics)
- Morbid dread of fatness, with imposed 'low weight threshold'
Note: in 'atypical' cases, one or more of these features may be absent.

Physical signs
- May be similar to anorexia nervosa (🕮 p. 400), but less severe.
- Specific problems related to 'purging' include:
  - Arrhythmias
  - Cardiac failure (sudden death)
  - Electrolyte disturbances (↓K$^+$, ↓Na$^+$, ↓Cl$^-$, metabolic acidosis [laxatives] or alkalosis [vomiting])
  - Oesophageal erosions
  - Oesophageal/gastric perforation
  - Gastric/duodenal ulcers
  - Pancreatitis
  - Constipation/steatorrhoea
  - Dental erosion
  - Leukopenia/lymphocytosis

Investigations
As for Anorexia nervosa (🕮 p. 402).

Differential diagnosis
- Upper GI disorders (with associated vomiting)
- Brain tumours
- Personality disorder
- Depressive disorder
- OCD

- Drug-related increased appetite (see 🕮 p. 930)
- Other causes of recurrent overeating (e.g. menstrual-related syndromes— 🕮 p. 464, Kleine–Levin syndrome— 🕮 p. 434)

Comorbidity
- Anxiety/mood disorder
- 'Multiple dyscontrol behaviours' e.g.:
  - Cutting/burning
  - Overdose
  - Alcohol/drug misuse
  - Promiscuity
  - Other impulse disorders (🕮 pp. 408–11)

Treatment
- **General principles**
  - Full assessment (is for anorexia nervosa—see 🕮 p. 402).
  - Usually managed as an outpatient.
  - Admission only for suicidality, physical problems, extreme refractory cases, or if pregnant (due to increased risk of spontaneous abortion).
  - Combined approaches improve outcome.
- **Pharmacological**
  - Most evidence for high-dose SSRIs (fluoxetine 60mg)—long-term treatment necessary (>1yr).
- **Psychotherapy**
  - Best evidence for CBT.
  - IPT may be as effective long-term, but acts less quickly.
  - Guided self-help is a useful first step (e.g. bibliotherapy), with education and support often in a group setting.

Prognosis
Generally good, unless there are significant issues of **low self-esteem** or evidence of **severe personality disorder**.

Box 10.7 The SCOFF[1] questions

These questions are useful as a screening tool for eating disorders (both anorexia and bulimia nervosa) in primary care. They have low sensitivity, and a score of 2+ 'yes' answers indicates that a further more detailed history is indicated, before considering treatment or referral.
- Do you make yourself Sick because you feel uncomfortably full?
- Do you worry you have lost Control over how much you eat?
- Have you recently lost more than One stone in a 3-month period?
- Do you believe yourself to be Fat when others say you are too thin?
- Would you say that Food dominates your life?

1 Morgan JF, Reid F, and Lacey JH (1999) The SCOFF questionnaire: assessment of a new screening tool for eating disorders. *Br Med J* **319**: 1467–8.

Impulse-control disorders 1[1]

Impulse-control disorders (ICDs) are disorders in which a person acts on a certain impulse, that is potentially harmful, but they cannot resist. There is usually an increasing sense of arousal or tension prior to committing or engaging in the act and an experience of pleasure, gratification, or release of tension at the time of committing the act (*Note:* this distinguishes these disorders from OCD where acts are not in themselves pleasurable).

Intermittent explosive disorder (IED)[1]

Although not specifically recognized in ICD-10 and often subsumed under Emotionally Unstable PD, DSM-IV distinguishes IED for individuals who have extreme explosive behaviours out of proportion to the actual trigger (e.g. a person who feels insulted by a coworker may go into the lunch area and rip down the cabinets and throw the chairs, only to later feel very guilty and embarrassed). IED may have a lifetime prevalence up to 2–11%, and occurs most often in young men. Episodes are typically infrequent (not a personality trait per se) in occurrence, and last only 20mins or less. Other symptoms may include tingling, tremor, palpitations, chest tightness, head pressure, hearing an echo.

Clinical features
- Several discrete episodes of failure to resist aggressive impulses that result in serious assaultive acts or destruction of property.
- The degree of aggressiveness expressed during the episodes is grossly out of proportion to any precipitating psychosocial stressors.
- Not due to another disorder or substance use.

Differential diagnosis ADHD, bipolar disorder, conduct disorder, personality disorder.

Treatment Evaluate and treat comorbid disorders. IED is challenging to treat, and most efforts are focused on minimizing aggression. There is some evidence for the use of mood stabilizers (lithium, semisodium valproate, maybe carbamazepine), phenytoin, SSRIs, β-blockers (best evidence if brain damage is present), α2-agonists (clonidine), and antipsychotics.

Kleptomania[1,2]

Failure to resist impulses to steal items that are not needed for their personal use or monetary value. Usually women, mean age 36, mean duration of illness 16yrs (often childhood onset). Accounts for about 5% of stealing in USA.

Clinical features
- Recurrent failure to resist impulses to steal objects that are not needed for personal use or for their monetary value.
- Increasing sense of tension immediately before committing the theft.
- Pleasure, gratification, or relief at the time of committing the theft.
- The stealing is not committed to express anger or vengeance and is not in response to a delusion or a hallucination.

- The stealing is not better accounted for by conduct disorder, a manic episode, or antisocial personality disorder.

Differential diagnosis Shoplifting (actions are usually well-planned and motivated by need or monetary gain), antisocial personality disorder, OCD, depression.

Comorbidity Eating disorders, substance abuse, depression. May be precipitated by major stressors (e.g. loss events).

Treatment SSRIs (e.g., fluoxetine); psychotherapy (e.g. CBT, family therapy).

Pyromania[3]

The presence of multiple episodes of deliberate and purposeful fire-setting, leading to property damage, legal consequences, and injury or loss of life. It is rare in children; more common in male adolescents, particularly those with poor social skills and learning difficulties.

Clinical features

- Tension or affective arousal before the act.
- Fascination with, interest in, or attraction to fire and its situational contexts.
- Pleasure, gratification, or relief when setting fires, or when witnessing or participating in the aftermath.
- Evidence of advance preparation.
- Indifference to consequences on property or life.
- Not for financial gain, to express sociopolitical ideology, to conceal criminal activity, as an expression of anger or vengeance, to improve one's living circumstances, due to delusions or hallucinations, or as a result of impaired judgement.

Differential diagnosis Conduct disorder, ADHD, adjustment disorder, other major affective or psychotic disorder.

Comorbidity Substance misuse, past history of sexual or physical abuse, antisocial personality disorder.

Treatment Should address any underlying or comorbid psychiatric disorder. Psychotherapeutic intervention may be helpful (e.g. CBT).

1 Dell'Osso B, Altamura AC, Allen A, *et al.* (2006) Epidemiologic and clinical updates on impulse control disorders: a critical review. *Eur Arch Psychiat Clin Neurosci* **256**: 464–75.
2 McElroy SL, Pope HG Jr, Hudson JI, *et al.* (1991) Kleptomania: a report of 20 cases. *Am J Psychol* **148**: 652–7.
3 Puri BK, Baxter R, Cordess CC (1995) Characteristics of fire-setters. A study and proposed multiaxial psychiatric classification. *Br J Psychiat* **166**: 393–6.

Impulse-control disorders 2

Pathological gambling disorder[1]

Persistent and recurrent maladaptive patterns of gambling behaviour that may lead to significant personal, family, and occupational difficulties. The disorder is felt to start in adolescents, where the prevalence is 4–7%. Prevalence in adults is reported around 1–3%, whereas around 80% of the general population consider themselves 'recreational gamblers'.

Diagnostic criteria

- Preoccupation with gambling (thinking of past gambling experiences, planning the next experience, or thinking of ways to get money to gamble).
- Needing to gamble with larger amounts of money to get the same feeling of excitement.
- Unsuccessful attempts to stop gambling or to cut down.
- Restlessness or irritability when trying to cut down or stop gambling.
- Gambling to escape from problems or to relieve feelings of anxiety, depression, or guilt.
- Chasing losses (return after losing to get even).
- Lying to family or friends about gambling.
- Committing illegal acts to finance gambling.
- Has lost or jeopardized a significant relationship, job, career, or educational opportunities because of gambling.
- Relies on family or friends for money to relieve financial problems caused by gambling.
- The gambling behaviour is not better accounted for by a manic episode.

Comorbidity Highly comorbid with mood disorders (both depression and bipolar), substance abuse or dependence. Other associations seen with ADHD, other impulse control disorders, personality disorders (esp. cluster B DSM-IV).

Treatment Exclusion and treatment of any comorbid psychiatric disorder. Proposed specific treatments to control addictive behaviour include SSRIs (e.g., fluoxetine, fluvoxamine, paroxetine, citalopram), lithium, clomipramine, and naltrexone. CBT may also help reduce preoccupation with gambling.

Trichotillomania[2]

Recurrent pulling of one's own hair, exacerbated by stress or relaxation (e.g. reading, watching TV). Feelings of tension are relieved by pulling hair. Usually involves the scalp, but may include eyelashes, eyebrows, axillae, pubic, and any other body regions. In children, ♀ = ♂, often with a limited course. In adults, ♀ 3.4% > ♂ 1.5%, with a chronic or episodic course. Lifetime prevalence rate of 1–2%.

Clinical features

- Recurrent pulling out of one's hair resulting in noticeable hair loss.
- An increasing sense of tension immediately before pulling out the hair or when attempting to resist the behaviour.

- Pleasure, gratification, or relief when pulling out the hair.
- The disturbance is not better accounted for by another mental disorder and is not due to a general medical condition (e.g., a dermatological condition).
- The behaviour causes clinically significant distress or impairment in social or occupational functioning.

Associated features Examining hair root, pulling strands between teeth, trichophagia (eating hairs), nail biting, scratching, gnawing, excoriation.

Differential diagnosis OCD, Tourette's syndrome, pervasive developmental disorder (e.g. autism), stereotyped behaviour, factitious disorder.

Comorbidity Depressive disorder, generalized anxiety disorder, OCD, personality disorder.

Treatment Address any comorbid disorder. CBT/behavioural modification (substitution, positive/negative reinforcement) is key to treatment. There is some evidence for use of SSRIs, clomipramine, pimozide, risperidone, and lithium.

1 Grant J, Potenza E, Marc N (2004) Impulse control disorders: clinical characteristics and pharmacological management. *Ann Clin Psychiat* **16**(1): 27–34.
2 Walsh KH and McDougle CJ (2001) Trichotillomania. Presentation, etiology, diagnosis and therapy. *Am J Clin Dermatol* **2**: 327–33.

Sleep disorders

Introduction

Disorders of sleep and wakefulness are a somewhat marginalized concern to most psychiatrists. Even taking a look at ICD-10 or DSM-IV reveals a disappointing paucity of clinical interest, which belies the advances which have taken place in sleep research in recent decades and their relevance to psychiatric training and practice. This is partly due to the fact that sleep research had focused on the physical causes of insomnia, such as obstructive sleep apnoea (see 📖 p. 428)—which is more the remit of respiratory physicians—or the neurological presentations, such as narcolepsy—which have yielded interesting genetic and neurobiological findings (see 📖 p. 432). Having ventured down the cul-de-sac of dream/psychosis research in the 1960s and '70s, few psychiatric units in the UK or Ireland still have facilities to conduct inpatient sleep monitoring. As a result we have to rely on good relations with our physician colleagues in order to appropriately investigate possible sleep disorders (see Box 11.1 for a brief history).

Relevance to psychiatric practice

Aside from the common-sense notion that 'getting a good night's sleep' is good for mental health, it is vital that mental health professionals understand the effects that mental disorder and treatment may have on the normal sleep–wake cycle (see 📖 pp. 454–9). Perhaps even more important is the need to recognize that disorders of sleep and wakefulness may themselves manifest bizarre and difficult to explain psychiatric symptoms, such as hypnic hallucinations and REM-sleep behaviour, which ought not to be labelled as 'psychotic' in nature (see 📖 p. 440 for cautionary notes). Psychiatrists also should be aware of principles of good sleep hygiene (see 📖 p. 426) and not always be reaching for the prescription pad to sort out sleeping difficulties!

The International Classification of Sleep Disorders

In 2005 the American Academy of Sleep Medicine (AASM) published a revised form of its International Classification of Sleep Disorders (ICSD-2). Its stated goals were:

- To describe all currently recognized sleep and arousal disorders, and to base the descriptions on scientific and clinical evidence.
- To present the sleep and arousal disorders in an overall structure that is rational and scientifically valid.
- To render the sleep and arousal disorders as compatible with ICD-9 and ICD-10 as possible.

In this chapter, we have adhered to the structure laid out in ICSD-2 for the clinical syndromes, rather than the much broader categories of ICD-10 or DSM-IV (see 📖 p. 1034) as not only does this provide a more valid way of conceiving the disorders but also it is likely that future classifications in ICD and DSM will follow the lead of the AASM. Key ICSD-2 groupings include:

- Insomnias.
- Sleep-related breathing disorders.
- Hypersomnias of central origin not due other causes.
- Circadian rhythm disorders.

- Parasomnias.
- Sleep-related movement disorders.
- Isolated symptoms, apparently normal variants, and unresolved issues.
- Other sleep disorders.

Box 11.1 A brief history of sleep research

Interest in disorders of sleep and wakefulness truly began when, in 1880, Gélineau described 14 cases of hypersomnia, distinguished 1° from 2° hypersomnia and coined the term 'narcolepsy' (Gk. 'seized by somnolence'). In 1902, Loewenfeld noticed the common association between the sleep attacks and paralysis during bouts of laughter, anger, or other strong emotions. This was referred to as 'cataplectic inhibition' by Henneberg in 1916 and later as 'cataplexy' (Gk. 'stupefaction' or literally 'strike down') by Adie in 1926. The term 'sleep paralysis'—a brief episodic loss of voluntary movement that occurs on falling asleep or awakening—was introduced by Wilson in 1928, although Mitchell had previously described the phenomenon as 'night palsy' as early as 1876.

In 1903, the work of Cajal and Tello on the morphological changes in reptilian brains during hibernation led to a number of neuronal theories of sleep. These culminated in von Economo's work in patients dying from encephalitis lethargicans, following the 1917 epidemic. The idea that there were centres in the brain that controlled sleep caught the imagination of neuroscientists, focused attention on the hypothalamus, and laid the foundations for further neurophysiological and neuropathological research.

In 1924, Berger succeeded in recording the first human EEG. Filled with doubt, it took him 5 years to publish his first paper in 1929, but he was the first to show that cerebral electrical activity was different during sleep than arousal. It took some time for EEG to be accepted, but, in 1937, Loomis documented the slow wave EEG patterns of non-REM (NREM) sleep (SWS). The major breakthrough came in 1949 when Moruzzi and Magoun first investigated the neural components regulating the brain's sleep-wake mechanisms, discovering the relationship between the reticular formation (RAS) and EEG activation during transitions between sleep and wakefulness.

This was followed in 1953 by Kleitman and Aserinsky publishing a paper in *Science* that described the rapid eye movement (REM) stage of sleep and proposed a correlation with dreaming. With his student, Dement, Kleitman also described the 'typical' architecture of sleep in 1957. Dement went on to show that REM sleep was characterized by a characteristic desynchronized, 'active' pattern, a finding confirmed by Jouvet in 1959. Jouvet described the controlling centres in the brainstem, clarified the role of the pontine centres, and in 1962, presented a clear neurophysiological framework for the generation of REM sleep with associated muscle atonia.

The first specific treatment for a sleep disorder came in 1959 when Yoss and Daly used methylphenidate (Ritalin) to treat narcolepsy and in 1965 Oswald and Priest began using the sleep laboratory to evaluate sleeping pills. Also in 1965 Gastaut and colleagues in Marseilles and Jung and Lugaresi in Bologna independently described obstructive sleep apnoea (OSA) and a variety of surgical treatments was proposed.

The publication of Rechtschaffen and Kale's *Manual of standardized terminology, techniques and scoring system for sleep stages of human subjects* in 1968, the identification of the suprachiasmatic nuclei (SCN) as the site of the biological clock in 1971, the first formal classification of sleep disorders in 1979, and the introduction of CPAP to treat OSA by Sullivan and colleagues in 1981, were all significant advances in the diagnosis, treatment, and neurobiology of specific sleep disorders and set the stage for the next generation of sleep researchers.

Normal sleep: stages and cycles

Sleep normally follows a typical pattern of stages and cycles that can be objectively measured using electroencephalography (EEG; see Fig. 11.1).[1,2]

Non-REM (NREM) sleep stages[3]

N1 (light sleep) As wakefulness declines, posterior α activity (8–13Hz) disappears, with slow θ (4–7Hz) and δ (0.5–2Hz) activity emerging, plus occasional vertex waves. This stage lasts only a few minutes, but may recur briefly during the night during sleep stage transitions or following body movements. Sudden twitches and hypnic jerks may be associated with the onset of sleep during N1. Hypnagogic hallucinations may also be experienced during this stage. During N1, there is loss of some muscle tone and most conscious awareness of the external environment.

N2 Characterized by sleep spindles (0.5s phases fast activity, maximal at the vertex) ranging from 11 to 16Hz (most commonly 12–14Hz) and K-complexes (symmetrical high-voltage vertex waves) that arise both spontaneously and in response to sudden stimuli. During this stage, muscular activity as measured by EMG decreases, and conscious awareness of the external environment disappears. This stage occupies 45–55% of total sleep in adults. This lasts 15–30min, followed by the gradual appearance of high-voltage waves (>75μV) in the delta range in a semi-symmetrical distribution over both hemispheres occupying less than 20% of the EEG recording.

N3 (deep or slow wave sleep [SWS]) Defined by the presence of a minimum of 20% δ waves (0.5–2 Hz; peak-to-peak amplitude >75μV). This is the stage in which parasomnias such as night terrors, nocturnal enuresis, sleepwalking, and somniloquy occur. Other texts may still describe stage 3 sleep (S3) with 20–50% δ waves and stage 4 sleep (S4) with greater than 50% δ waves; these have officially been combined as stage N3[3]. N3 lasts 30–45min, before reversion to N2.

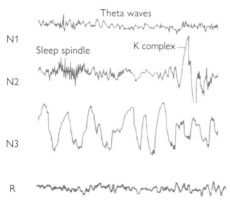

Fig. 11.1 Sleep stages: characteristic EEG traces.

REM sleep (stage R)

The end of the first sleep cycle is marked by a brief period of arousal before the onset of REM sleep. This has characteristic low-voltage, desynchronized EEG activity with associated muscle atonia (paralysis may be necessary to protect organisms from self-damage through physically acting out scenes from the often-vivid dreams that occur during this stage) and episodic *rapid eye movements* (REM). Occasional bursts of EMG activity (myoclonia) may be seen in association with the phasic eye movements. There are no sleep spindles or K complexes and α activity is rarely seen.

Sleep cycles

A typical night's sleep has 4 or 5 cycles of these sequential stages, each lasting 90–110min (see Fig. 11.2). As the night progresses, the amount of time spent in δ sleep decreases, with consequent increase in REM sleep. Hence, the first REM period may last 5–10min, while the last, just before waking, may last up to 40min. Although the total amount of sleep needed varies between individuals and with age, total sleep time in adults is usually between 5 and 9hrs. Remarkably, REM sleep occupies 20–25% of the total sleep time in all ages.

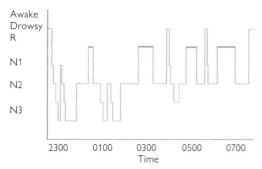

Fig. 11.2 Typical hypnogram.

1 Rechtschaffen A and Kales A (1968) *A manual of standardized terminology, techniques and scoring system for sleep stages of human subjects.* Washington, DC: US Government Printing Office, Public Health Service.

2 Iber C, Ancoli-Israel S, Chesson A, *et al.* (eds) (2007) *The AASM manual for the scoring of sleep and associated events: rules, terminology, and technical specification.* Westchester: American Academy of Sleep Medicine.

3 In 2007, the American Academy of Sleep Medicine (AASM) modified the Rechtschaffen and Kales (R&K) standard guidelines for sleep classification (1968). One of the major changes was a change in terminology: in the AASM classification, NREM sleep stages formerly called stage 1, 2, 3, and 4 (S1,S2,S3, S4) are referred to as N1, N2, and N3, with N3 reflecting slow wave sleep (SWS, R&K stages S3 + S4); REM sleep is referred to as stage R. The new manual also clarifies the definition of the sleep–wake transition, sleep spindles, K-complexes, slow wave sleep, and REM sleep, as well as arousals and major body movements.

Assessment of sleep disorders

Sleep history

Always try to obtain a third-party account from the patient's bed partner, or from an informant such as a parent or carer. The main areas covered should include:

- *The presenting complaint(s):*
  - Onset, duration, course, frequency, severity, effects on everyday life.
  - Pattern of symptoms, timing, fluctuations, exacerbating/relieving factors, environmental factors, relevant current stressors.
- *The usual daily routine:*
  - Waking (time, method, e.g. alarm, natural), usual morning routine.
  - Daily activities (start/finish times), any daily naps (when, duration).
  - Bedtime (preparations for bed, time of going to bed, time of falling asleep, activities in bed, e.g. TV, reading, sex).
- *Description of sleep:*
  - Behaviour whilst asleep.
  - Dreams/nightmares.
  - Episodes of wakening (and how they are dealt with).
  - Quality and satisfaction with sleep.
- *Daytime somnolence:*
  - General level of alertness during the day.
  - When/if sleep occurs (e.g. when active, mealtimes, walking, driving, operating machinery).
  - Effects on work/social activities.
  - Any periods of confusion.
  - Any episodes of collapse.

Family history

Past and current history of medical or psychiatric problems

Drug and alcohol history

- General review of regular medications (alerting/sedating effects), including timing of administration.
- Specific questions regarding: caffeine-containing drinks (tea, coffee, soft drinks), smoking, alcohol, other recreational drugs.

Previous treatments

- Types of treatment tried.
- Benefits/problems/side-effects.

Third-party/other information

- Breathing problems (snoring, gasping, choking, stopping breathing).
- Motor activity (muscle twitches, limb movements, unusual or complex behaviours, e.g. sleep-talking/sleepwalking/dream enactment).
- Frequency of occurrence and any clear pattern.
- Any recent mood changes.
- Any recent change in use of drugs or alcohol.

Methods of further assessment

Sleep diary

To create a record of the sleep–wake pattern over a 2-wk period in order to clarify any pattern or particular factors that may be present. Important information includes: daily activities, pattern of sleeping, mealtimes, consumption of alcohol/caffeine/other drugs, exercise, and daytime sleepiness/napping.

Video recording

A useful component of assessment, particularly for the parasomnias. Routinely used in sleep laboratory studies; however, home videos of sleep-related behaviour may be just as informative.

Actigraphy

A method of both quantifying circadian sleep–wake patterns and identifying movement disorders occurring during sleep. Actigraphs incorporate a piezoelectric motion sensor, often in a wristwatch-like unit, that collects data on movement over several days, for later computer analysis.

Indications

Circadian rhythm sleep disorders, jet lag, paediatric sleep disorders, monitoring leg movements (e.g. in 'restless leg syndrome' or periodic movements of sleep) or other movement disorders (e.g. Parkinsonian tremor).

Polysomnography

Detailed recording of a variety of physiological measures including EEG, electro-oculogram (EOG), and EMG. Other parameters may be added as required: ECG, respiratory monitoring (nasal/oral airflow, diaphragm EMG), pulse oximetry, actigraphy, penile tumescence, and oesophageal pH (for oesophageal reflux). Audio and video recording help to assess nocturnal behaviours, vocalizations, and snoring. Time coding of all these measures allows temporal correlations to be made of the various parameters. In general, one night of testing, followed by a daytime multiple sleep latency test (MSLT), is sufficient to diagnose most conditions.

Indications

Hypersomnia (where common extrinsic causes, e.g. medication, shift work, have been excluded; to diagnose suspected periodic limb movements of sleep, sleep apnoea, or narcolepsy), insomnia (where periodic limb movements of sleep or sleep apnoea are suspected and initial treatment has been ineffective), parasomnias (where the clinical history is unclear, initial treatment has been unsuccessful, and polysomnography is likely to aid the diagnosis, e.g. REM sleep behaviour disorder or multiple parasomnias), to validate the accuracy of a sleep complaint (where a more objective measure is needed), to assess the benefits of treatment (e.g. continuous positive airway pressure [CPAP]), suspected nocturnal epilepsy, serious cases of sleep-related violence.

Multiple sleep latency test (MSLT)

Devised to assess daytime somnolence, but also helps in identifying daytime REM sleep, for example in narcolepsy. The patient is put to bed at 2-h intervals starting at 8a.m. with the objective of measuring time to sleep onset (*sleep latency*). In adults a mean sleep latency of 5min or less indicates a pathological level of daytime somnolence; 5–10min is 'indeterminate' but may reflect a primary psychiatric disorder; over 10min is regarded as normal. The ICSD-2 suggests specific MSLT criteria for a diagnosis of narcolepsy (see p. 433).

Insomnia 1: overview

Essence

Persistent problems (at least 3 days/wk for 1mth) falling asleep, maintaining sleep, or poor quality of sleep. Individuals are preoccupied and excessively concerned with their sleep problems, distressed by them, and social or occupational functioning is affected. Insomnia may be primary—caused by both extrinsic and intrinsic factors—or secondary to medical or psychiatric illness, other sleep disorders, or substance misuse. When it is difficult to determine the direction of the association the term comorbid insomnia is preferred.

Prevalence

Common complaint (~30% general population), ♀ > ♂, greater in the elderly. 'Clinically significant insomnia' (causing marked personal distress or interference with social and occupational functioning) 9–12%.

Primary causes (see Table 11.1)

- *Psychophysiological insomnia:* difficulty initiating and maintaining sleep, with associated somatized tension anxiety: over-concern with inability to sleep, and learned sleep prevention.
- *Paradoxical insomnia:* also called 'sleep state misperception': patient complains of little or no sleep without objective evidence of sleep disturbance.
- *Adjustment sleep disorder:* sleep disturbance temporally related to stress, conflict, or environmental change, causing emotional arousal. Disorder usually resolves once the stressor is no longer present.
- *Inadequate sleep hygiene:* clinically significant disruption of the normal sleep–wake schedule due to a wide range of daily living activities (e.g. level of coffee consumption, frequent late nights) is inconsistent with the maintenance of good-quality sleep and full daytime alertness. Understanding the contribution of each factor and taking steps to eliminate or minimize their effects usually sorts out the problem.
- *Idiopathic insomnia:* Rare, lifelong inability to sleep adequately.
- *Behavioural insomnia of childhood:* includes two common subtypes:
  - *Limit-setting sleep disorder*—estimated prevalence 5–10% in children, characterized by inadequate enforcement of bedtimes by a caregiver, with resultant stalling or refusal to go to bed at an appropriate time.
  - *Sleep-onset association disorder*—occurring mainly in children aged 6mths to 3yrs, sleep onset is impaired by the absence of a certain object (e.g. favourite toy) or set of circumstances (specific routine, TV, night-light).
  - Less commonly: *nocturnal eating (drinking) syndrome*—primarily a childhood problem (prevalence 5% in children aged 6mths to 3yrs), with marked decrease after weaning, characterized by recurrent awakenings and inability to return to sleep without eating or drinking.
- *Other sleep disorders:*
  - *Environmental sleep disorder*—common transient sleep disturbance due to disturbing environmental factor(s) (e.g. heat, cold, noise,

light, excessive movement of bed partner, danger, allergens, hospitalization, unfamiliar surroundings) leading to insomnia or excessive sleepiness.
- *Altitude insomnia*—unusual form of acute insomnia, accompanied by headaches, loss of appetite, and fatigue, occuring at high altitudes in the absence of administered oxygen. Seen in 25% of individuals who ascend above 2000m above sea level, and in most individuals above 4000m.
- *Food allergy insomnia*—a rare disorder of initiating and maintaining sleep due to an allergic response to food allergens.

Secondary or comorbid causes

- *Sleep disorders classified elsewhere:* sleep-related breathing disorders (□ p. 428); circadian rhythm disorders (□ p. 436); sleep-related movement disorders (□ p. 450).
- *Insomnia due to medical condition:* pain (arthritis, peptic ulcer, headache), respiratory disorders (COPD, cystic fibrosis, asthma), diabetes, Parkinson's disease, endocrine disorders (Addison's disease, Cushing's syndrome).
- *Insomnia due to mental disorder* (see □ pp. 454–7).
- *Drugs and alcohol* (see also □ p. 458). Antidepressants (e.g. MAOIs, SSRIs, venlafaxine, reboxetine); anti-Parkinsonian medication; bronchodilators (e.g. aminophylline, theophylline, pseudoephedrine); cardiovascular medication (e.g. β-blockers, clonidine, high-dose digoxin, verapamil); chemotherapy agents; corticosteroids/anabolic steroids; NSAIDs (high-dose); stimulants (e.g. dexamfetamine methylphenidate, amfetamine cocaine, caffeine, nicotine); levothyroxine withdrawal/dependency (e.g. hypnotics, opiates, alcohol, or cannabis).

Table 11.1 Classification of insomnia with diagnostic codes

ICSD-2	ICD-10	DSM-IV-TR
Psychophysiological insomnia	F51.04	307.42
Paradoxical insomnia	F51.03	307.42
Adjustment insomnia	F51.02	307.42
Inadequate sleep hygiene	Z72.821	307.42
Idiopathic	F51.01	307.42
Insomnia due to mental disorder	F51.05	327.02
Behavioural insomnia of childhood	Z73.81	307.42
Insomnia due to a medical condition	G47.09	327.01
Insomnia due to a drug or substance	F11–19.x	291.85
Insomnia due to alcohol	F10.x	291.82
Physiological (organic) insomnia, unspecified	G47.00	
Insomnia not due to a substance or known physiological condition, unspecified	F51.09	

Insomnia 2: general management strategies

Education about sleep Many myths surround sleep and the clinician should be able to educate the patient about the stages of sleep, sleep cycles, changes in sleep patterns with age, and the nature of the particular sleep problem or disorder the patient presents with.

Sleep hygiene

Establishing good sleep habits

Control environmental factors (noise, light, temperature); 'wind down' time (~1hr) before going to bed: distract from the day's stresses (reading, watching television, listening to music, having a warm bath); avoidance of caffeine-containing drinks after about 16.00hr; not smoking for at least 1 hr before bed; regular exercise (not late at night); late 'tryptophan' snack (warm milk or other milky drink); avoid naps during the day (or confine naps to the early afternoon, not longer than ~40min); set aside time during the day to reflect on problems and stresses.

Stimulus control

Go to bed only when sleepy; avoid other activities (with the exception of sex) whilst in bed; if sleep does not occur, do not remain in bed for more than 10–20min, get up and go to another room (without turning on all the lights), returning to bed only when sleepy; establish a regular time to get up, with no more than 1hr variation (even at weekends and during holidays).

Relaxation training The regular practice of relaxation techniques during the day (particularly progressive relaxation) may help to provide patients with the means to reduce general arousal, which can be used if necessary whilst in bed.

Sleep restriction When sleep is fragmented, a sleep restriction strategy may help to reduce total time spent in bed and improve quality of sleep by 'consolidation'. There are a number of steps to sleep restriction, and to complete the programme does require motivation and encouragement (see Box 11.2).

Medication

Despite prevailing public perception that insomnia is best treated by use of a sleeping tablet—prescribing should be last option, rather than first. Before a hypnotic is prescribed, cause of insomnia should be established, possible underlying factors addressed, and any primary medical or psychiatric disorder effectively treated. Should only be used to treat insomnia when it is severe, disabling, or subjects individual to extreme distress. Ideally, hypnotics should be short-term adjuncts to other forms of therapy and avoid prolonged administration. Interrupted courses (i.e. 5 nights with medication, 2 without) for no more than 4wks may help avoid tolerance and reduce 'rebound insomnia' often accompanying cessation. Choices (see Table 11.2) include: benzodiazepines, the 'Z-drugs' (zopiclone, zolpidem, zapeplon—usually first line), chloral hydrate, sedating antidepressants (e.g. trazodone, mirtazapine), sedating antipsychotic, and possibly melatonin agonists.

Box 11.2 Sleep restriction

- Keep a sleep diary for 5–14 days to allow the calculation of total sleep time (TST) and sleep efficiency (SE).
- TST = (total time spent in bed) – (time spent awake during night).
- SE = (TST × 100)/total time spent in bed.
- For first few nights of a sleep restriction programme spend only the same number of hours in bed as the average TST for the past week. No naps allowed during the day (despite initial tiredness).
- Continue to keep sleep diary. When the calculated mean SE for 5 nights reaches 85% or better, go to bed 15min earlier.
- Repeat procedure with increases of 15min if mean SE remains 85% or better, or decreases of 15min if the mean SE falls below 85%, until a satisfactory amount of night-time sleep is achieved.

Table 11.2 Pharmacokinetic data for drugs used as hypnotics (in order of decreasing T_{half})[1]

Drug	Availability (%)	Plasma bound (%)	Time to T_{max} (hr)	T_{half} (hr)
Mirtazapine	50	85	0.25–2	16.3–40
Nitrazepam	78	85–87	0.5–5	15–40
Olanzapine	60	93	5–6	24–30
Temazepam	91	96–98	0.75–3	2–25
Promethazine	12.3–25	—	4.39	18.6
Trazodone	60–80	89–95	1–2	6–15
Lormetazepam	70–80	92	2	7.9–12
Chloral hydrate[2]	—	35	0.76–8.2	9.3–10.9
Quetiapine	—	83	1–2	5.3–7
Zopiclone	70–80	45–80	0.25–1.5	3.5–6.5
Zolpidem	70	90–92	0.5–2.6	1.5–4.5
Agomelatine[3]	<5	95	1–2	1–2
Zaleplon	30	60	0.25–1.5	0.9–1.1

1 BAP Consensus Guidelines (2010) http://www.bap.org.uk/pdfs/BAP_Sleep_Guidelines.pdf
2 T_{half} is so short, values are for the primary active metabolite trichloroethanol
3 Source: http://www.servier.co.uk/products/valdoxan/

Sleep-related breathing disorders

Essence

Sleep-related breathing disorders (see Table 11.3) commonly lead to chronic insomnia and daytime tiredness. Caused by CNS dysfunction, pathological processes affecting normal lung function, and environmental factors. Obstructive sleep apnoea often missed in psychiatric patients despite obvious risk factors (see **Central sleep apnoea syndromes**. Associated with significant comorbidity including: hypertension, arrhythmias and conduction disturbances, cardiac or cerebral ischaemia, functional cognitive impairment, and depression.

Central sleep apnoea syndromes

- *Primary central sleep apnoea:* disorder of unknown aetiology characterized by recurrent episodes of breathing cessation during sleep without associated respiratory effort. Usually leads to EDS, insomnia, or breathing difficulties during sleep. PSG shows no evidence of hypercapnia and 5+ episodes of apnoea per hour of sleep.
- *Central sleep apnoea including Cheyne–Stokes breathing pattern:* recurrent apnoeas and/or hypopnoeas alternating with prolonged hyperpnoea in a crescendo–decrescendo pattern. Seen in NREM sleep; associated with heart or renal failure, and cerebrovascular disorders.
- *Central sleep apnoea due to a drug or substance:* most commonly associated with long-term opioid use, due to suppression of respiration through μ-receptors in the ventral medulla.
- *Other causes of central sleep apnoea:*
  - *high-altitude breathing pattern*—seen in most people at elevations of >2600m; characterized by 12–34s cycles of apnoea or hyperpnoea;
  - *other medical conditions*—vascular, neoplastic, degenerative, demyelinating or traumatic condition involving the brain stem;
  - *primary sleep apnoea of infancy*—developmental or secondary to other medical problems—includes 'apnoea of prematurity' and 'apnoea of infancy').

Obstructive sleep apnoea[1,2] (Pickwickian syndrome)

Repeated episodes of upper airway obstruction (hypopnoeas) or cessation of breathing (apnoeas) during sleep, usually associated with reduced blood O_2 saturation, daytime somnolence, loud snoring, and dry mouth. Usually middle-aged, overweight males. Prevalence 1–2%. PSG showing 5+ respiratory events: apnoeas, hyponoeas, or respiratory effort-related arousals, makes the diagnosis. In children, cortical arousals less likely possibly due to a higher arousal threshold.

Management

- *General:* weight loss, avoidance of sedative drugs, reduction of alcohol consumption/smoking, alternative sleeping position (not lying on back).
- *Specific:* oral appliances (for mild cases, e.g. sleep and nocturnal obstructive apnoea redactor [SNOAR]); continuous positive airway pressure (CPAP);[3] bi-level positive airways pressure (BiPAP).
- *Surgical* (for severe cases): nasal reconstruction, tonsillectomy, uvulopalatopharyngoplasty (UPPP), bimalleolar advancement, and rarely tracheostomy.

Other causes

Sleep-related hypoventilation/hypoxaemic syndromes are caused by a variety of disorders including: *idiopathic, congenital central alveolar hypoventilation* ('Ondine's curse': the extremely rare failure of automatic central control of breathing in infants who do not breathe spontaneously, or only shallowly and erratically). *Medical conditions* (specific pulmonary disease: COPD, cystic fibrosis, and interstitial lung disease; other causes of abnormality in lung or vascular pathology, lower airways obstruction, neuromuscular or chest wall disorders.)

Table 11.3 Classification of sleep-related breathing disorders with diagnostic codes

ICSD-2	ICD-10	DSM-IV-TR
Primary central sleep apnoea	G47.31	780.57
Central sleep apnoea including Cheyne–Stokes breathing pattern	G47.39	780.57 or 327.xx
Central sleep apnoea including high-altitude periodic breathing	G47.37	780.57 or 327.xx
Central sleep apnoea due to a medical condition not Cheyne–Stokes breathing pattern		327.xx
Central sleep apnoea due to a drug or substance	F10–19.x	
Primary sleep apnoea of infancy	P28.3	
Obstructive sleep apnoea, adult	G47.33	780.57
Obstructive sleep apnoea, paediatric	G47.33	780.57
Sleep-related non-obstructive alveolar hypoventilation, idiopathic	G47.34	780.57
Sleep-related hypoventilation/hypoxaemia due to lower airways obstruction	G47.36	
Sleep-related hypoventilation/hypoxaemia due to neuromuscular and chest wall disorders	G47.36	
Sleep-related hypoventilation/hypoxaemia due to pulmonary parenchymal or vascular pathology	G47.36	
Congenital central alveolar hypoventilation syndrome	G47.35	
Sleep apnoea/sleep-related breathing disorder, unspecified	G47.30	780.57

1 SIGN Guideline 73 (Jun 2003). ℘ http://www.sign.ac.uk/pdf/sign73.pdf
2 Morgenthaler TI, Kapen S, Lee-Chiong T, et al. (2006) Standards of Practice Committee, American Academy of Sleep Medicine. Practice parameters for the medical therapy of obstructive sleep apnea. *Sleep* **29:** 1031–5.
3 NICE (Mar 2008) *Technology appraisal 139 for CPAP treatment of OSA/hypopnoea syndrome.* ℘ http://www.nice.org.uk/nicemedia/pdf/TA139Guidance.pdf

Hypersomnia 1: overview

⚠ *Excessive sleepiness is a leading cause of road traffic accidents.*

Essence

'Hypersomnia' covers a number of different forms of excessive daytime sleepiness (EDS). Patient may complain of 'sleep attacks' (recurrent daytime sleep episodes that may be refreshing or unrefreshing), 'sleep drunkenness' (prolonged transition to a fully aroused state on waking), lengthening of night-time sleep, almost constant EDS, even recurrent periods of more or less permanent sleep lasting several days over several months. Diagnosis and treatment particularly relevant when the individual works in an industry or profession where vigilance and concentration are essential (e.g. hospital workers, pilots, train drivers, the military). The most commonly used rating scale is the Epworth Sleepiness Scale (see Table 11.4).

Prevalence Common: moderate (occasional) EDS reported in up to 15% in the general population (severe EDS ~5%).

Differential diagnosis (see Table 11.5)

- *Narcolepsy:* with or without cataplexy (📖 p. 432).
- *Recurrent hypersomnia:* Kleine–Levin syndrome, menstrual-related hypersomnia, see 📖 p. 434.
- *Idiopathic hypersomnia:* with or without long sleep time (📖 p. 434).
- *Behaviourally-induced insufficient sleep syndrome* (📖 p. 435).
- *Hypersomnia due to a medical condition:* neurological (altered ICP, diencephalic tumours, thalamic infarcts, Parkinson's disease, multiple system atrophy, NPH, Arnold–Chiari malformation, myotonic dystrophy, head injury—'post-traumatic hypersomnia': lesions (when they can be demonstrated) generally involve the brain stem (the tegmentum of the pons or thalamic projections) or the posterior hypothalamus), infectious (EBV, atypical viral pneumonia, hep B, Guillain–Barré syndrome, viral encephalitis, sleeping sickness [trypanosomiasis—sleepiness, headache, trembling, dyskinesias, choreoathetosis, mood changes]), metabolic, and endocrine disorders (hypothyroidism, acromegaly, cause OSA).
- *Hypersomnia due to a drug, substance or alcohol* (see 📖 p. 458): includes dependency-related sleep disorders (alcohol, hypnotics, opiates), toxins (arsenic, bismuth, mercury, copper, other heavy metals, carbon monoxide, vitamin A), medication-related (e.g. anticonvulsants, antidepressants, anti-emetics, antihistamines, anti-Parkinsonian drugs, antipsychotics, anxiolytics/hypnotics, clonidine, methyldopa, prazosin, reserpine, hyoscine, progestogens).
- *Hypersomnia not due to a substance or known physiological condition* (see 📖 p. 454): essentially psychiatric causes.
- *Hypersomnia associated with other sleep disorders:* e.g. sleep apnoea syndromes (📖 p. 428), PLMS (📖 p. 450), circadian rhythm disorders, e.g. DSPS (📖 p. 436).

Table 11.4 Epworth Sleepiness Scale (ESS)[1]

Chance of dosing situation	Score[2]
Sitting and reading	0 1 2 3
Watching television	0 1 2 3
Sitting inactive in a public place (e.g. in a theatre or a meeting)	0 1 2 3
As a passenger in a car for an hour without a break	0 1 2 3
Lying down to rest in the afternoon when circumstances permit	0 1 2 3
Sitting and talking to someone	0 1 2 3
Sitting quietly after a lunch without alcohol	0 1 2 3
In a car, while stopped for a few minutes in traffic	0 1 2 3

1 Johns MW (1991) A new method for measuring daytime sleepiness: the Epworth Sleepiness Scale. *Sleep* **14**: 540–5.
2 Patient is instructed to use scale to choose most appropriate number for each situation: 0 = no chance of dozing, 1 = slight chance, 2 = moderate chance, 3 = high chance. Maximum score on this scale is 24; however, scores >10 often considered to be consistent with some degree of daytime sleepiness, while scores >15 considered to be consistent with EDS.

Table 11.5 Classification of hypersomnia not due to sleep-related breathing disorders with diagnostic codes

ICSD-2	ICD-10	DSM-IV-TR
Narcolepsy with cataplexy	G47.41	
Narcolepsy without cataplexy	G47.419	
Narcolepsy due to medical condition with cataplexy	G47.42	
Narcolepsy due to medical condition without cataplexy	G47.42	
Narcolepsy, unspecified		347.00
Recurrent hypersomnia	G47.13	307.44
Idiopathic hypersomnia with long sleep time	G47.11	307.44
Idiopathic hypersomnia without long sleep time	G47.12	307.44
Behaviourally induced insufficient sleep syndrome	F51.12	
Hypersomnia due to a medical condition	G47.14	327.14
Hypersomnia due to a drug or substance	F10–19	292.85
Hypersomnia due to alcohol	F10–19	292.82
Hypersomnia not due to a substance or known physiological condition	F51.19	327.15
Physiological (organic) hypersomnia, unspecified	G47.10	

Hypersomnia 2: narcolepsy

First described by Westphal in 1877[1] and given it name by Gélineau in 1880,[2] narcolepsy is now divided into three separate entities: narcolepsy with cataplexy, without cataplexy, and due to medical disorder (see Table 11.5). Narcolepsy seriously impacts on education, work, relationships, ability to drive, recreational activities, and can have negative effects on self-esteem and mood.

Narcolepsy with cataplexy

Prevalence The most common neurological cause of hypersomnia, estimated prevalence 0.20–0.40 per 1000 in the general population. Sex ratio is equal. Age range: 10–50+yrs (70–80% before 25yrs).

Aetiology May be due to hypocretin deficiency.

Clinical features

- *The classical 'tetrad' of symptoms:[3] excessive sleepiness, cataplexy, sleep paralysis, and hypnagogic hallucinations* are suffered by only a minority of patients with narcolepsy.
- Excessive daytime sleepiness and associated cataplexy (sudden bilateral loss of muscle tone, with preserved consciousness, triggered by a strong emotional reaction such as laughter or anger) are by far the most common complaints. More often a cataplectic attack will be partial, e.g. involving jaw muscles (difficulty with articulation), facial muscles (grimacing), or thigh muscles (brief unlocking of the knees). Attacks vary from seconds to minutes, with a frequency of a few a year to several a day, and very rarely repeated 'status cataplecticus'.
- Other REM sleep phenomena also occur, but are not necessary for the diagnosis to be made. These include sleep paralysis (sometimes up to 10min long) and vivid hallucinations on falling asleep (hypnagogic) or, less commonly, waking up (hypnopompic).
- Sleep may also be disturbed due to frequent awakenings, disturbing dreams, sleep-talking, and REM-related sleep behaviours (from phasic muscle twitching to more dramatic dream enactment).

Course Usually chronic, although some of the symptoms may improve or remit. Hallucinations and sleep paralysis present variably, and sometimes cataplexy may disappear over time. Poor sleep quality tends to persist. Treatments are directed at the most troublesome symptoms.

Differential diagnosis

- Sleep attacks in narcolepsy are usually irresistible and refreshing, whereas in other forms of hypersomnia they tend to be more frequent, of longer duration, easier to resist, and unrefreshing.
- The attacks also tend to occur in unusual and often dangerous situations in narcolepsy (e.g. talking, eating, standing, walking, or driving).
- Disturbances and shortening of nocturnal sleep are more common in narcolepsy—in other causes of hypersomnia nocturnal sleep is usually prolonged and there is difficulty in waking in the morning.

Investigations

- *Polysomnography* (sleep EEG and MSLT): sleep onset REM period (SOREMP) is highly specific (25–50% of cases); increased N1 sleep and repeated awakenings. ICSD-2 criteria: sleep latency of 10min or less, REM sleep latency of 20min or less, MSLT: mean sleep latency of 8min or less, and two or more SOREMPs.
- *CSF hypocretin-1 levels:* levels below 110pg/mL are highly specific and sensitive for narcolepsy with cataplexy (in 10% levels may be normal).
- *HLA (human leukocyte antigen) typing:* there is a strong association between HLA-DR2 haplotypes coded on chromosome 6 and narcolepsy: HLA DQB1*0602 and DQA1*0102 are found in up to 85–95% of individuals, compared with 12–38% in the general population.

Management

- *Daytime somnolence* Regular naps, stimulants (modafinil, methylphenidate, dexamfetamine). Possibly sodium oxybate (GHB).
- *Cataplexy* TCAs (clomipramine 10–75mg/day is licensed) or SSRIs (and possibly other antidepressants: venlafaxine, nefazodone, mirtazapine, atomoxetine). These drugs may also improve REM-related symptoms, hypnagogic/hypnopompic hallucinations, and sleep paralysis. *Note:* abrupt withdrawal of antidepressants may potentially cause cataplectic episodes or even 'status cataplecticus'. Sodium oxybate is newly licensed for cataplexy,[4] is not associated with a rebound cataplexy on withdrawal, but can cause significant side-effects (nausea, nocturnal enuresis, confusional arousals, headache) and there is a danger of abuse.
- *Other treatments for poor sleep and REM-related symptoms:* benzodiazepines (e.g. clonazepam) and possibly sodium oxybate.

Narcolepsy without cataplexy

The occurrence of EDS and irresistible episodes of sleep without associated cataplexy. Other features may also be present, e.g. automatic behaviour, hypnic hallucinations or sleep paralysis. Nocturnal sleep is usually less disturbed than in narcolepsy with cataplexy. PSG with MSLT showing mean sleep latency of <8min and >2 SOREMPs is required for diagnosis. Cataplexy may develop later in the course of the disorder.

Narcolepsy due to medical condition

An extremely rare form of narcolepsy, ICSD-2 requires the following criteria:

- The co-occurrence of EDS with cataplexy.
- PSG with MSLT showing mean sleep latency of <8min and >2 SOREMPs.
- CSF hypocretin-1 levels less than 110pg/mL (provided the patient is not comatose).
- A consistent chronological link with the presumed underlying causative medical condition.

---

1 Westphal C (1877) Eigentümliche mit Einschlafen verbundene Anfälle. *Arch Psychiat Nervenkrankeheiten* **7**: 631–5.

2 Gélineau J (1880) De la narcolepsie. *Gaz Hôp (Paris)* **53**: 626–8; 635–7.

3 Yoss RE, Daly DD (1957) Criteria for the diagnosis of the narcoleptic syndrome *Mayo Clin Proc* **32**: 320–8.

4 http://www.ukmi.nhs.uk/NewMaterial/html/docs/SodiumOxybateNMP0603.pdf

Hypersomnia 3: other causes

Recurrent hypersomnia

Kleine–Levin syndrome[1]

A rare syndrome of 'periodic somnolence and morbid hunger', occurring almost exclusively in male adolescents, usually following a course of decreasing frequency of attacks, which may persist for many years before complete cessation.

Clinical features

Periods lasting from days to weeks of attacks of hypersomnia accompanied by excessive food intake (megaphagia). Other behavioural symptoms may occur including sexual disinhibition (which may appear compulsive in nature), along with a variety of other psychiatric symptoms such as confusion, irritability, restlessness, euphoria, hallucinations, delusions, and schizophreniform states. Attacks may occur every 1–6mths, and last from 1 day to a few weeks. Between attacks the patients recover completely, and the syndrome may easily be confused for other neurological, metabolic, or psychiatric disease.

Management

- *Hypersomnia*: stimulants (only effective for short periods of time).
- *Preventative measures*: for sufficiently frequent episodes causing major disruption of social or occupational functioning—lithium, carbamazepine, or valproate.

Menstrual-related hypersomnia

Characterized by excessive daytime sleepiness preceding menstruation, with detectable alterations in polysomnography when symptomatic.

Aetiology Unknown; no clear hormonal differences have been found.

Management Stimulants—reserved only for symptomatic periods.

Idiopathic hypersomnia[2]

Clinical features

- *With long sleep time (polysymptomatic form):* nocturnal sleep is prolonged (10hrs or more), with sleep drunkenness on waking, and constant or recurrent EDS with frequent, unrefreshing naps.
- *Without long sleep time (monosymptomatic form):* EDS alone.

Course A chronic condition with marked impact on social and occupational functioning.

Diagnosis Detailed history (to exclude other causes of hypersomnia); PSG normal; MSLT <8min (longer than narcolepsy), <2 SOREMPs.

Differential diagnosis Narcolepsy, sleep apnoea syndromes, periodic limb movement disorder, or upper airways resistance syndrome.

Management As for narcolepsy (but naps do not help).

Hypersomnia not due to substance or known physiological condition

EDS due to underlying (undiagnosed) psychiatric disorder, e.g. bipolar II disorder, dysthymic disorder, SAD, undifferentiated somatoform disorder, adjustment disorder, personality disorder.

Prevalence May be the cause of up to 7% of hypersomnia referred to sleep centres. More common in women.

Clinical features Marked reported EDS, high Epworth Sleepiness Scale scores, sleep perceived as poor quality and non-restorative, excessive time spent in bed during both day and night ('clinophilia').

Diagnosis Careful history essential. PSG (not usually necessary): increased sleep latency, increased wake time after sleep onset, low sleep efficiency. MSLT usually normal.

Management Directed at the underlying psychiatric disorder.

Behaviourally-induced insufficient sleep syndrome

Persistently failing to obtain sufficient nocturnal sleep required to support normally alert wakefulness.

Prevalence Unknown, but may be the most common cause of hypersomnia in the general population, particularly amongst parents of young children, doctors, students, long-distance lorry drivers, and other occupations where unsociable long hours of work are commonplace.

Clinical features Periods of excessive sleepiness concentrated in the afternoon and early evening. Rest days usually characterized by late rising from bed and frequent naps. Associated reduced productivity, difficulty in concentration and attention, low mood or irritability, and somatic symptoms (usually gastrointestinal or musculoskeletal).

Diagnosis Made on history alone.

Management Directed towards scheduling increased time asleep, either at night or with regular short naps during the day.

---

1 Originally described by Willi Kleine in 1925 and subsequently by Max Levin in 1936, the eponym 'Kleine–Levin syndrome' was coined by Critchley and Hoffman in 1942.
2 Roth B (1976) Narcolepsy and hypersomnia: review and classification of 642 personally observed cases. *Schweiz Arch Neurol Neurochir Psychiat* **119**: 31–41.

Circadian rhythm sleep disorders 1: overview

Essence When an individual's sleep/wake schedule is not in synchrony with the sleep–wake schedule of their cultural environment or society, it may lead to complaints of insomnia or EDS, causing marked distress or interference with social or occupational functioning.

Subtypes (see Table 11.6)

Table 11.6 Classification of circadian rhythm sleep disorders (CRSD) with diagnostic codes

ICSD-2	ICD-10	DSM-IV-TR
Delayed sleep phase type	G47.21	327.31
Advanced sleep phase type	G47.22	
Irregular sleep-wake type	G47.23	
Non-entrained type (free running)	G47.24	
Circadian rhythm sleep disorder due to a medical condition	G47.20	
Other circadian rhythm sleep disorder	G47.20	
Jet lag type	F51.21	327.35
Shift work type	F51.22	327.36
Circadian rhythm sleep disorder due to a drug or substance	F11–19.x	292.85
Circadian rhythm sleep disorder due to alcohol	F10.x	291.82

Delayed sleep phase syndrome (DSPS)
The late appearance of sleep (typically around 02.00hr), but normal total sleep time and architecture, which may lead to complaints of sleep-onset insomnia and difficulty awakening at the desired time in the morning. Cause is unknown, although some cases are related to head injury, psychiatric disorder, or personality traits (e.g. schizoid, avoidant). Usually presents in adolescence, running a continuing course until old age. Individuals may adapt to the condition by taking evening or night jobs.

Advanced sleep phase syndrome (ASPS)
The opposite of DSPS, this syndrome leads to complaints of evening sleepiness, early sleep onset (e.g. 18.00–20.00hr), and early morning wakening. May be confused with depression (due to early morning wakening), particularly in elderly patients in whom the syndrome occurs more frequently.

Irregular sleep–wake pattern
Sleep occurrence and waking behaviour are very variable, leading to considerable disturbance of the normal sleep–wake cycle and complaints of

insomnia (inadequate nocturnal sleep and daytime somnolence/frequent napping). The idiopathic form is rare, and it is associated with Alzheimer's disease, head injury, developmental disorders, and hypothalamic tumours.

Non-entrained type (free running)
Rare occurrence of a greater than 24-hr sleep–wake period, leading to a chronic pattern of 1–2hr daily delays in sleep onset and wake times, with an 'in-phase' period every few weeks (free of symptoms). Associated with schizoid personality traits and may occur more frequently in blind individuals.

Jet lag type
Sleep disorder secondary to moving between time zones. Symptoms include varying degrees of difficulty in initiating or maintaining sleep, day-time fatigue, decrements in subjective daytime alertness and performance, feelings of apathy, malaise or depression, and somatic symptoms (GI upset, muscle aches, or headaches).

Shift work type
Symptoms of insomnia or excessive sleepiness occur as transient phe-nomena in most people working shifts. Adaptation to a change in shift-work schedule usually takes 1–2wks; however, rotating day/night shifts may present particular difficulties. Often sufferers consult with somatic complaints (general malaise, GI upset), rather than the underlying disorder of sleep.

Investigations
- Comprehensive history.
- Use of a 14-day sleep–wake chart.
- Actigraphy—objective measurement of the rest–activity cycle.
- Polysomnography is rarely needed.

Differential diagnosis
- Poor sleep hygiene.
- Depressive disorder.
- Misuse of drugs (particularly stimulants or sedatives) and alcohol. ICSD-2 codes this as 'CRSD due to drug or substance/alcohol'. *Note:* lifestyle factors are also clearly important.
- Physical conditions such as: dementia, head injury, other causes of brain damage or injury, and recovery from coma. ICSD-2 also codes this separately as 'CRSD due to medical condition'.

Circadian rhythm sleep disorders 2: management

General measures

These include education about the nature of sleep and establishing good sleep habits. This is particularly important for shift work sleep disorder in which alcohol, nicotine, and caffeine may be used to self-medicate symptoms. Other advice for shift-workers should emphasize maintenance of regular sleep and mealtimes whenever possible, use of naps to limit sleep loss, and minimization of environmental factors (noise, light, other interruptions) when sleeping during the day.

Chronotherapy

DSPS

- Establishing a regular waking time, with only 1hr variability at weekends and holidays, may help initially.
- If unsuccessful, '*phase-delay*'[1] methods may be employed to achieve a phase shift of the sleep–wake cycle. This involves:
  - Establishing a 27-hr day to allow progressive delay of the usual onset of sleep by about 3hrs in each sleep cycle.
  - Sleep should only be permitted for 7–8hrs, with no napping.
  - The disruption to the person's normal routine caused by undergoing this regime (which may take 5–7 days to complete) requires appropriate measures to be taken to ensure other family and work commitments are attended to.
- An alternative strategy is to advise the individual to remain awake at the weekend for one full night, and to go to bed the next evening 90mins earlier than usual.
  - Sleep periods should again be limited to 7–8hrs, with no napping.
  - The procedure can then be repeated each weekend until a normal bedtime is achieved.

ASPS

- Delaying sleep onset by increments of 15mins may be effective.
- Alternatively '*phase-advance*'[2] methods may be used:
  - The patient goes to bed 3hrs earlier each night until the sleep cycle is advanced back to a normal bedtime.
  - May be difficult to implement, particularly with elderly patients.

Light therapy[3]

This includes both the use of bright light (2500–10000lux) with UV rays filtered out, and light restriction. Bright light is assumed to suppress melatonin (which is sleep-promoting).

DSPS

Exposure to bright light is scheduled on waking to prevent morning lethargy, usually for 2hrs daily for 1wk, often with adjunctive light restriction after 16.00hr.

ASPS

Exposure to bright light is recommended 2hrs before scheduled bedtime, to delay this to a more sociable time. *Note:* evidence for the effectiveness of light therapy in other intrinsic circadian rhythm disorders of sleep (e.g. shift-work sleep disorders, jet lag) is lacking.

Medication

- The entrainment of circadian rhythms through the use of appropriately timed *short-acting BDZs*[4] (e.g. lormetazepam) has been advocated, particularly for the treatment of jet lag.
- *Melatonin*[5] (0.5–5mg) also appears capable of advancing the sleep phase and resetting the circadian rhythm in travellers with jet lag syndrome flying across five or more time zones, particularly in an easterly direction, and especially if they have experienced jet lag on previous journeys.

1 Czeisler CA, Richardson GS, Coleman RM, *et al.* (1981) Chronotherapy: resetting the circadian-clocks of patients with delayed sleep phase insomnia. *Sleep* **4**: 1–21.
2 Moldofsky H, Musisi S, and Phillipson EA (1986) Treatment of a case of advanced sleep phase syndrome by phase advance chronotherapy. *Sleep* **9**: 61–5.
3 Terman M, Lewy AJ, Dijk DJ. *et al.* (1995) Light treatment for sleep disorders: consensus report. IV. Sleep phase and duration disturbances. *J Biol Rhythms* **10**(135): 47.
4 Buxton OM, Copinschi G, Van Onderbergen A, *et al.* (2000) A benzodiazepine hypnotic facilitates adaptation of circadian rhythms and sleep–wake homeostasis to an eight-hour delay shift simulating westward jet lag. *Sleep* **23**(915): 27.
5 Herxheimer A and Petrie KJ (2002) Melatonin for the prevention and treatment of jet lag. *Cochrane Database Syst Rev* CD001520.

Parasomnias 1: overview

Essence
Parasomnias may be defined as undesirable physical and/or experiential phenomena accompanying sleep. They include unusual behaviours and motor acts, autonomic changes, and/or emotional-perceptual events. Sometimes these events occur when arousal is incomplete, or they are associated with REM sleep. Other episodes may arise during the transition from sleep to wakefulness, from wakefulness to sleep, or in transitions between sleep stages. They can usually be objectively diagnosed using PSG and successfully treated. Parasomnias are of academic interest as they may provide insights into the biological underpinnings of species-specific behaviours such as locomotion, exploratory behaviour, appetitive states (hunger, sexual arousal), fear and aggression, that may be released from control during sleep, itself a biological imperative.

Points to note
- The often 'bizarre' nature of the parasomnias frequently leads them to being misdiagnosed as psychiatric disorders, particularly if they appear temporally related to stressful situations.
- This may, in turn, lead to inappropriate treatment, with associated problems, including exacerbation of the parasomnia.
- Often there will be associated psychological distress or psychiatric problems secondary to the parasomnia.
- Rarely there may also be forensic implications, e.g. due to sleep-related violence (📖 p. 448), sexual activity (📖 p. 445) or even driving (📖 p. 445).

Classification of parasomnias
Parasomnias may be classified according to the sleep stages they occupy. ICSD-2 only classifies conditions under 'parasomnia' that are not included in other sections (see Table 11.7). Here, we list the differential according to sleep stages but discuss in detail those disorders included in ICSD-2.
- *Disorders of arousal/NREM sleep:* confusional arousals, sleepwalking, sleep terrors, nocturnal panic attacks.
- *Disorders associated with REM sleep:* REM sleep behaviour disorder (RSBD), recurrent isolated sleep paralysis, nightmare disorder, impaired sleep-related penile erections, sleep-related painful erections, REM sleep-related sinus arrest.
- *Sleep–wake transition disorders:* sleep-related dissociative disorders (see 📖 p. 448), exploding head syndrome (loud imaged noise or sense of violent explosion in the head on falling asleep or waking), sleep-related (hypnic) hallucinations, rhythmic movement disorder, sleep starts, sleep-talking, sleep-related leg cramps.
- *Miscellaneous (may occur in any sleep stage):* sleep-related eating disorder, sexsomnia, restless legs syndrome, periodic limb movements of sleep, sleep-related bruxism, sleep-related rhythmic movement disorder, sleep enuresis, sleep-related groaning.

Parasomnia overlap disorder[1]

Sometimes disorders of non-REM sleep (e.g. sleep walking, sleep terrors) may occur along with REM sleep behaviour disorder. 70% of cases are in young men (mean age 34yrs). Idiopathic cases, occurring at a younger age, are associated with other medical (brain injury, nocturnal paroxysmal atrial fibrillation), psychiatric (PTSD, depression, schizophrenia), or substance abuse (alcohol, amfetamine) disorders. There is no increased risk of psychiatric disorder.

Management Clonazepam (0.5–2mg nocte).

Table 11.7 Classification of parasomnias with diagnostic codes

ICSD-2	ICD-10	DSM-IV-TR
Confusional arousals	G47.51	
Sleepwalking	F51.3	307.46
Sleep terrors	F51.4	307.46
REM sleep behaviour disorder	G47.52	307.47
Recurrent isolated sleep paralysis	G47.53	
Nightmare disorder	F51.5	307.47
Sleep-related dissociative disorders	F44.9	300.15
Sleep enuresis	N39.44	307.6
Catathrenia (sleep-related groaning)	G47.59	
Exploding head syndrome	G47.59	
Sleep-related hallucinations	R29.81	
Sleep-related eating disorder	G47.59	307.50
Parasomnia, unspecified	G47.50	307.47
Parasomnia due to a drug or substance	F10–19.x	292.85

---

1 Schenck CH, Boyd JL, and Mahowald MW (1997) A parasomnia overlap disorder involving sleep-walking, sleep terrors, and REM sleep behavior disorder in 33 polysomnographically confirmed cases. *Sleep* **20**: 972–81.

Parasomnias 2: disorders of arousal/ NREM sleep

Confusional arousals ('sleep drunkenness')
- *Clinical features:* confusion during and following arousals from sleep, most typically from deep sleep in the first part of the night. Individuals appear disorientated, incoherent, hesitant and slow, but may walk about, get dressed, and even perform complex motor behaviours. Violence, assault, and even homicide may occur (rare: planning or premeditation is not possible).
- *Polysomnography:* arousal from NREM sleep, usually in first third of the night.
- *Prevalence:* almost universal in young children (under 5yrs), becomes less common in older childhood. Fairly rare in adulthood, usually occurring in the context of sleep deprivation, exacerbated by alcohol or other depressant drugs.
- *Associated disorders:* sleep-related breathing disorders, narcolepsy, idiopathic hypersomnia, encephalopathy.
- *Differential diagnosis:* acute confusional states, sleep terrors (evident autonomic arousal), sleepwalking (usually docile, not aggressive when challenged), and RSBD (evident dream enactment, see p. 446).
- *Management:*
  - Prevent the patient from falling into deep, prolonged NREM sleep: avoid sleep deprivation.
  - Restrict use of alcohol and other sedative drugs (illicit and prescribed).
  - Sleep hygiene measures (p. 426).

Sleep terrors (parvor nocturnes, incubus)
- *Clinical features:* sudden awakening with loud terrified screaming (the person may sit up rapidly) with marked autonomic arousal (tachycardia, tachypnoea, diaphoresis, mydriasis). Sometimes frenzied activity occurs—may lead to injury. Episodes usually last for 10–15min, with increase in muscle tone and resistance to physical contact. If wakened, individual appears confused and incoherent, but soon falls asleep, wakening next morning with no memory of the event. In children, usually occurs in the first third of the night. In adults, can occur at any time of night.
- *Polysomnography:* abrupt wakening out of N3 sleep is seen on EEG, with generation of alpha activity, usually in the first third of the night. Partial arousals out of N3, occurring up to 10–15 times in one night, are also seen even when a full episode is not recorded.
- *Prevalence:* children—3%, adults—1% (may be more common in males), evidence for heritability. Deep and prolonged N3 is a predisposing factor, precipitated by fever, sleep deprivation, and depressant medication.
- *Associated disorders:* as for sleepwalking.
- *Differential diagnosis:* nightmares, nocturnal epilepsy, nocturnal panic attacks.

- *Management:* reassure individual (and partner/parents) of the benign character of the disorder. If episodes are frequent (more than once a week), use similar methods as for sleepwalking.

Nocturnal panic attacks (NP)

- *Clinical features:* waking from sleep with no obvious trigger in a state of intense fear or discomfort, accompanied by cognitive and physical (autonomic) symptoms of arousal. Symptoms as for panic disorder (see 📖 p. 358). Avoidance of sleep may lead to delayed sleep onset and chronic sleep deprivation.
- *Polysomnography:* usually occurs in late N2 or early N3 sleep (particularly during the transition).
- *Prevalence:* lifetime prevalence may be 3–5% in non-clinical populations. NP is common among patients with panic disorder (44–71%).
- *Risk factors:* periods of sleep deprivation, withdrawal from alcohol/ drugs (esp. BDZs, antidepressants); mitral valve prolapse; stimulant use (including caffeine).
- *Aetiology:*
  - *Physiological*—respiratory drive dysregulation possibly due to extreme hypercapnia or chronic hyperventilation; heart rate variability during NREM sleep.
  - *Psychological*—increased discomfort related to relaxation, fatigue, and 'letting go' (possible fear of loss of vigilance); low-level somatic sensations of arousal or anxiety act like conditioned stimuli during sleep to elicit fear response and panic.
- *Associated disorders:* panic disorder, PTSD, depressive disorder, other anxiety and related disorders, alcohol and substance misuse.
- *Differential diagnosis:* panic attacks (*after* awakening), nightmares (during REM sleep), withdrawal syndromes (esp. BDZs), sleep terrors, sleep-related breathing disorders, sleep paralysis (see 📖 p. 447), nocturnal seizures, PTSD nightmares, anxiety due to nocturnal hallucinations.
- *Assessment:* full history, with an emphasis on possible comorbidity (i.e. other anxiety disorders), use of alcohol and drugs. Rating of severity using specific scales, e.g. Nocturnal Panic Screen[1] and self-monitoring using sleep diary. Additional formal assessment may be necessary for difficult cases and to exclude other treatable sleep disorders (e.g. sleep apnoea, nocturnal seizures).
- *Management:*
  - *Cognitive behavioural therapy*—most evidence as for panic disorder (see 📖 p. 362) including modification of maladaptive behaviours (e.g. sleeping with lights or TV on).
  - *Pharmacological*—little specific evidence (not systematically studied yet). Case reports support alprazolam or TCAs. Rational approach to prescribing as for daytime panic (📖 p. 362) and/or short-term use of hypnotics to help with 2° sleep avoidance.

---

1 Craske MG and Tsao JC (2005) Assessment and treatment of nocturnal panic attacks. *Sleep Med Rev* **9**: 173–84.

Parasomnias 3: sleepwalking and associated disorders of NREM sleep

Sleepwalking (somnambulism)

- *Clinical features:* complex, automatic behaviours (automatisms) (e.g. aimless wandering, attempting to dress or undress, carrying objects, eating [see ⌑ p. 448], urinating in unusual places, and, rarely, driving a car [see Box 11.3] or sexual behaviour [see Box 11.4]). Episodes often follow a period of sleep deprivation or increased stress. There is often a personal and/or family history of sleepwalking or other related disorders. Behaviours of variable duration usually occur 15–120min following sleep onset, but may occur at other times. Eyes usually wide open, glassy, and talk is incoherent with communication usually impossible. Injury may occur (e.g. falling down the stairs, exiting through a window). Activity never appears intentional or planned, and only rarely aggressive behaviour occurs. The person is usually easily returned to bed, falls back into normal sleep, and has no recollection of the episode the following morning. If awakened during the episode—confused and disorientated. Dream content (if present) is fragmented, without specific themes.
- *Polysomnography:* light, NREM sleep, with episodes sometimes preceded by hypersynchrony of generalized (non-epileptic) high-voltage delta waves.
- *Prevalence:* up to 17% in childhood (peak age 4–8yrs); 4–10% in adults. Familial forms do occur. Precipitants similar to confusional arousals.
- *Associated disorders:* sleep-related breathing disorders, PLMS, nocturnal seizures, medical/neurological disorders, febrile illness, alcohol use/ abuse, pregnancy, menstruation, psychiatric medication (lithium, anticholinergics), stress (no specific psychiatric illness).
- *Differential diagnosis:* confusional arousals, episodic wandering (N2 sleep, second half of the night), epileptic fugue states, and REM sleep behaviour disorder in the elderly.
- *Management:*
  • Reassurance.
  • Protect the patient from coming to harm (e.g. closing windows, locking doors, sleeping downstairs).
  • Relaxation techniques and minimization of stressors.
  • Sleep hygiene measures (⌑ p. 426).
  • Avoidance of sleep deprivation.
  • Medication (for patients with frequent episodes/high-risk behaviours: small night-time doses of a BDZ (e.g. diazepam 2–10mg, clonazepam 1–4mg), or low-dose sedating antidepressant at night.

Note: treatment of any concurrent psychiatric disorder does not control the parasomnia.

Box 11.3 Sleep Driving and the Z-drugs[1]

Sleep driving is regarded as a highly unusual variant of sleepwalking but may be confused with impaired driving due to misuse or abuse of sedative/hypnotic drugs when the driver may appear 'asleep'. The majority of case reports relate to the Z-drugs—especially zolpidem and zopiclone—and drivers have excessively high blood levels of z-drugs, failed to take the medication at the correct time or remain in bed for sufficient time and/or combined z-drugs with other CNS depressants/ alcohol. True sleep driving can be distinguished by the fact that sleep-walkers are completely unable to understand or interact with the police but can stand and walk unaided. In contrast, drivers under the influence of sedative drugs are still able to respond to the police but are unable to stand up or maintain balance. If in doubt, sleep studies may be indicated, especially if there are significant legal proceedings. Treatment of sleep driving is as for sleepwalking (see 📖 p. 444).

1 Pressman MR (2011) Sleep driving: sleepwalking variant or misuse of z-drugs? *Sleep Medicine Reviews* **15**: 285–92.

Box 11.4 The curious case of sexsomnia, 'sleepsex', or somnambulistic sexual behaviour[1]

Another rare sleepwalking variant, the sorts of sexual behaviour seen during sleep can include: explicit vocalisations (with sexual content), violent masturbation, and complex sexual activities including oral sex, and vaginal or anal intercourse. Sexual behaviour during sleep may be associated with injury to the subject or his/her bed partner, when it is a special form of sleep-related violence (see 📖 p. 448). Sexsomnia appears more common in men. There are sex differences in presentation with women almost exclusively engaging in masturbation and sexual vocalizations, whereas men are more likely to engage in sexual fondling and intercourse. It can be quite challenging to distinguish between typical sleepwalking and sexsomnia, but uniquely there is often involvement of a partner who is usually more than a witness. Most people with this disorder have a previous and/or family history of sleepwalking. PSG is necessary to confirm diagnosis and diagnoses associated with sexual behaviour during sleep include not only NREM sleep somnambulism but also RSBD and frontal lobe seizures. Treatment involves general measures of good sleep hygiene and addressing precipitating factors such as sleep deprivation, drug misuse, alcohol, stress, RLS, and OSA. If medication is being considered, evidence supports use of clonazepam (0.5–2mg nocte), sertraline, valproic acid and lamotrigine.

1 Anderson ML, Poyares D, Alves RSC, *et al.* (2007) Sexsomnia: abnormal sexual behaviour during sleep. *Brain Research Reviews* **56**: 271–82.

Parasomnias 4: disorders associated with REM sleep

REM sleep behaviour disorder (RSBD)[1]

- *Clinical features:* vivid, intense, action-packed, violent dreams (reported as 'nightmares'), dream-enacting behaviours (verbal and motor), sleep injury (ecchymoses, lacerations, fractures—of self and bed partner), general sleep disruption.
- *Polysomnography:* elevated submental EMG tone and/or excessive phasic submental/limb EMG twitching during REM sleep, in the absence of EEG epileptiform activity.
- *Prevalence:* a rare sleep disorder, more common in older males.
- *Associated disorders:* 50% of cases associated with neurological disorders, usually degenerative (e.g. Parkinson's disease), and narcolepsy (may be an early sign of neurological disease that manifests fully several years later—full neurological examination should be performed). Rarely associated with other psychiatric disorders, but may be induced or aggravated by psychiatric drugs (e.g. TCAs, MAOIs, high-dose SSRIs, SNRIs), cessation/misuse of REM-suppressing agents (e.g. alcohol, amfetamine, cocaine), or severe stress related to traumatic experiences.
- *Differential diagnosis:* sleepwalking, sleep terrors, nocturnal dissociative disorders, nocturnal epilepsy, obstructive sleep apnoea (where arousals from REM sleep associated with aggressive behaviour and vivid REM-related dreams), states of intoxication, malingering.
- *Management:*
  - Ensure a safe sleeping environment (for patient and sleeping partner).
  - Eliminate any factors that might be inducing or aggravating the condition (including treatment of any primary neurological, medical, or psychiatric disorder).
  - If symptoms persist and are problematic, clonazepam (0.5–1.0mg nocte) is the treatment of choice, effectively controlling both behaviours and dreams, with good evidence of long-term safety and sustained benefit. Alternatives include carbamazepine, melatonin, levodopa (L-dopa), and imipramine.

Nightmare disorder

- *Clinical features:* frightening dreams that usually awaken the sleeper from REM sleep, without associated confusion. May be preceded by a frightening or intense real-life traumatic event.
- *Polysomnography:* increased REM density, lasting about 10min, terminated by an awakening, usually in the second half of the night.
- *Prevalence:* common (occasional occurrence in ~50% of adults). Frequent nightmares (one or more a week) occur in about 1% of adults.
- *Differential diagnosis:* sleep terrors, REM sleep behaviour disorder, nocturnal panic attacks.

- *Management:* Treatment usually unnecessary. If episodes are frequent, distressing, or causing a major disturbance to the individual's carers or bed partner:
  - *General measures*—avoidance of stress, discontinuation of drugs that may potentially promote nightmares (see Box 11.5), principles of sleep hygiene (📖 p. 426),
  - Medication: REM-suppressing drugs (e.g. antidepressants). *Note:* sudden discontinuation may lead to exacerbation of the problem with REM-rebound.

Recurrent isolated sleep paralysis

- *Clinical features:* the frightening experience of being unable to perform voluntary movements either at sleep onset (hypnagogic or pre-dormital form) or awakening (hypnopompic or post-dormital form), either during the night or in the morning.
- *Polysomnography:* atonia in peripheral muscles (as in REM sleep) despite desynchronized EEG with eye movements and blinking (i.e. awake). H-reflex activity is also abolished during an episode (as in REM sleep).
- *Prevalence:* as an isolated phenomenon, reported to occur at least once in the lifetime of 40–50% of normal individuals (usually due to sleep deprivation). As a chronic complaint, however, it is much less common. Familial sleep paralysis (without sleep attacks or cataplexy) is exceptionally rare.
- *Differential diagnosis:* narcolepsy (occurs in up to 40% of cases), periodic hypokalaemia (in adolescents, following a high carbohydrate meal, and with low-serum potassium during the attack).
- *Management:*
  - Sleep hygiene (📖 p. 426), esp. avoidance of sleep deprivation, may help to prevent episodes.
  - Persistent problems may respond to REM-suppressant medication (e.g. clomipramine 25mg or an SSRI).

Box 11.5 Drugs associated with vivid dreams or nightmares

- Baclofen
- Beta-blockers (atenolol, propranolol)
- Clonidine
- Digoxin toxicity
- Famotidine
- Indometacin
- Methyldopa
- Nalbumetone
- Nicotine patches
- Pergolide
- Reserpine
- Stanozolol
- Verapamil
- Withdrawal (alcohol, BDZs, opiates, and other hypnotics)

1 Schenck CH and Mahowald MW (2002) REM sleep behavior disorder: clinical, developmental, and neuroscience perspectives 16 years after its formal identification in *Sleep*. *Sleep* **25**: 120–38.

Parasomnias 5: other presentations

Sleep-related eating disorder (SRED)[1]

First reported 1955; received very little attention until more recently. Sleep-related eating disorder is usually described in 20–30-yr-old women. Consists of recurrent episodes of involuntary eating and drinking during partial arousals from sleep.

- *Clinical features:* sometimes there may be particularly unusual consumption of inedible (pica) or even toxic substances such as raw meat, frozen pizza, or pet food. Sleep is disrupted and patients report often significant (sometimes unexplained) weight gain.
- *Polysomnography:* reports show multiple confusional arousals with or without eating, arising predominantly from N3 sleep, but also occasionally from N1, N2, and REM sleep.
- *Differential diagnosis:* can be either idiopathic or comorbid with other sleep disorders, e.g. sleepwalking, RLS-PLMS, OSA, narcolepsy, circadian rhythm disorders. Various medications associated with SRED, e.g. triazolam, zolpidem, olanzapine, and risperidone.
- *Management:* treatment is best directed at any comorbid sleep disorder and cessation of provoking medication. If pharmacotherapy is indicated, case reports suggest use of: topiramate, dopaminergics, clonazepam, and fluoxetine.

Sleep-related dissociative disorders[2]

First reported in 1976,[3] there is usually a history of repeated physical and/or sexual abuse in childhood and/or adulthood. Usually, there are also daytime states of dissociation too with self-harm behaviours.

- *Polysomnography:* complex and lengthy behaviours; appear to be re-enactments of previous abuse, occur during wakefulness after an episode of sleep.
- *Management:* treatment involves long-term therapy for the dissociative disorder which may require inpatient assessment. Night-time benzodiazepines may exacerbate the problem and are best avoided.

Sleep-related violence

Violence and sleep are commonly thought to be mutually exclusive, but in fact can co-exist (see Table 11.8). Key aspects of determining role of an underlying sleep disorder include:[4]

- *Presence of underlying sleep disorder:* solid evidence on PSG/video, history of previous episodes.
- *Characteristics of act:* on awakening or falling asleep, abrupt onset, brief duration, impulsive, senseless, without motivation, lack of awareness during event, victim was coincidentally present or was a possible arousal stimulus.
- *On return to consciousness:* perplexity, horror, no attempt to escape, amnesia for the event.
- *Presence of precipitating factors:* attempts to awaken the subject, intake of sedative/hypnotic drugs, prior sleep deprivation, not due to voluntary alcohol or drug intoxication.

Table 11.8 Disorders associated with sleep-related violence[1]

Disorder	State of occurrence	Clinical features	Circumstances of violence
Confusional arousal	Wake/NREM	Incomplete awakening, reduced vigilance, impaired cognition, amnesia	When being forced to wake from sleep
Sleepwalking	Wake/NREM	Like confusional arousals with complex motor activity	Incidental encounter or when approached
Sleep terror	Wake/NREM	Incomplete fearful awakening from NREM sleep	Linked to frightening dream
RSBD	Wake/REM	Acting out of dreams	Linked to dream content
Nocturnal paroxysmal dystonia	All sleep stages (esp. N2)	Bipedal automatisms, twisting of trunk/pelvis, vocalizations, posturing of head/limbs	Accidental or related to hyperkinetic features
Epileptic nocturnal wandering	All sleep stages (esp. N2)	Like sleepwalking, but more directed violence possible	Accidental or when approached/restrained
Confusional states	Awake	Variable	Variable
Dissociative disorder	Awake or wake/sleep	Variable, frequently wandering, amnesia	Self-harm, thrashing, assaults
Malingering	Awake	Variable (evident primary or secondary gain)	Variable

1 Mahowald MW, Bundlie SR, Hurwitz TD, *et al.* (1990) Sleep violence—forensic science implications: polygraphic and video documentation. *J Forensic Sci* **35**: 413–32.

1 Howell MJ, Schenck CH, and Crow SJ (2009) A review of nighttime eating disorders. *Sleep Med Rev* **13**: 23–34.
2 Schenck CH, Milner DM, Hurwitz TD, *et al.* (1989) Dissociative disorders presenting as somnambulism: polysomnographic, video and clinical documentation (8 cases). *Dissociation* **2**: 194–204.
3 Rice E and Fisher C (1976) Fugue states in sleep and wakefulness: a psychophysiological study. *J Nerv Ment Dis* **163**: 79–87.
4 Siclari F, Khatami R, Urbaniok F, *et al.* (2010) Violence in sleep. *Brain* **133**: 3494–509.

Sleep-related movement disorders

Essence Usually relatively simple, stereotyped movements disturbing sleep, and causing insomnia and EDS (see Table 11.9). Can also be a cause of sleep-related violence (see 📖 p. 449) and lead to harm to self or others.

Restless legs syndrome (Ekbom's syndrome)[1]

Unpleasant, often painful sensations in the legs, particularly on sleep onset. Significantly interferes with the ability to get to sleep. Usually idiopathic or familial. Exacerbated by caffeine, fatigue, or stress.

- *Prevalence:* ~10% general population, ♂ = ♀, greater in the elderly.
- *Associations:* PLMS, pregnancy, uraemia, rheumatoid arthritis, iron deficiency anaemia, folate deficiency, hypothyroidism, poliomyelitis, peripheral neuropathy (e.g. diabetes), chronic myelopathy, Parkinson's disease, drug-related (e.g. antidepressants; phenothiazines; lithium; Ca^{2+} channel blockers; withdrawal from barbiturates, other sedatives and opiates).
- *Differential diagnosis:* antipsychotic-induced akathisia, ADHD.
- *Investigations:* full history, examination, routine blood tests (polysomnography rarely needed).
- *Management:*
  - *General*—treat any secondary causes. Movement (walking, stamping) or stimulation of the legs (rubbing, squeezing, hot showers, hot packs, ointments).
  - *Medication*—possible agents include: clonazepam, cabergoline, levodopa, ropinirole, rotigotine (patch), pramipexole, opiates (oxycodone), clonidine, gabapentin (possibly other anti-epileptics), either alone or in combination.

Periodic limb movement (in sleep) disorder (PLMS)[1]

Periodic episodes of repetitive, stereotyped limb movements. Rare in children, common in over 60s (~34%). May be a feature in up to 15% of patients with insomnia. Movements usually reported by bed partner. Associated daytime somnolence. Polysomnography may aid diagnosis.

- *Differential diagnosis:* sleep starts (📖 p. 452), drug-related exacerbation (e.g. TCAs, lithium).
- *Management:* reassurance, remove exacerbating factors, clonazepam, levodopa.

Sleep-related leg cramps

Sensations of painful muscular tightness or tension, in the calf (or the foot), occurring during sleep, which awaken the sufferer.

- *Prevalence:* up to 16% of healthy individuals, more common in the elderly.
- *Associated problems:* excessive muscular activity, dehydration, diabetes, arthritis, pregnancy, and Parkinson's disease.
- *Differential diagnosis:* PLMS (painless), muscle spasm due to spasticity following stroke, other neurological causes of muscle spasticity.

- *Management:* only for severe, recurrent symptoms—heat, massage, muscle stretching; quinine sulphate (300mg nocte).

Sleep-related bruxism

Clenching and grinding of the teeth during sleep that can result in arousals. The activity may be severe or frequent enough to result in symptoms of temporomandibular joint pain, wearing down of the teeth, or severe injury to the tongue and mouth.

- *Management* General sleep hygiene measures, removal of exacerbating factors, occlusal splints/night-time bite guard, use of clonazepam.

Sleep-related rhythmic movement disorder

Stereotyped, repetitive movements involving large muscles, usually head and neck, typically immediately prior to sleep, sustained into light sleep. Common forms: head banging (*jactatio capitis nocturna*), head rolling, body rocking— movements may result in head injury.

- *Polysomnography:* rhythmic movement artefacts during light non-REM sleep, without evidence of epileptiform activity.
- *Prevalence:* common in young children (60% at 9mths), decline with age (25% at 18mths, 8% at 4yrs). More frequent in boys.
- *Associated problems:* developmental problems/psychopathology (older children).
- *Management:* unnecessary in most cases. Parents can be reassured that in the majority of infants the disorder will resolve by around the age of 18 months. If injury or social disruption occurs, medication may be used (e.g. low-dose BDZ or antidepressant).

Table 11.9 Classification of sleep-related movement disorders with diagnostic codes

ICSD-2	ICD-10	DSM-IV-TR
Restless legs syndrome	G25.81	
Periodic limb movement disorder	G47.61	
Sleep-related leg cramps	G47.62	
Sleep-related bruxism	G47.63	
Sleep-related rhythmic movement disorder	G47.69	
Other sleep-related movement disorder, unspecified	G47.60	
Sleep-related rhythmic movement disorder due to a drug or substance	F10–19	292.85
Sleep-related rhythmic movement disorder due to a medical condition		

---

1 Vignatelli L, Billiard M, Clarenbach P, *et al.* (2006) EFNS guidelines on management of restless legs syndrome and periodic limb movement disorder in sleep. *Eur J Neurol* **13**: 1049–65.

Isolated symptoms, apparently normal variants, and unresolved issues

Essence Conditions that sit on the borderline between normal and abnormal sleep (see Table 11.10). Rarely pathological, they may nonetheless become a focus of anxiety and a reason for consultation.

Long sleeper Sleep is normal in architecture and quality, but lasts longer than normal (i.e. >10hrs). The person may complain of EDS if they do not get their usual amount of sleep.

Short sleeper Someone who requires 5hrs or less of sleep/day. In children, short sleepers need ~3hrs less than the norm for their age.

Snoring Respiratory sounds that are disturbing to the patient, bed partner, or others, but not associated with either insomnia, EDS, or other sleep disorder (e.g. OSA).

Sleep-talking (somniloquy)

The common uttering of words or sounds during sleep, without subjective awareness, and speech generally devoid of meaning. Rarely, emotionally charged long 'tirades' occur with content related to the person's occupation or preoccupation.
- *Polysomnography:* brief partial arousal during non-REM sleep is usually seen on EEG in about 60% of cases. Less commonly, somniloquy may occur during REM sleep, if related to dream content or in association with another disorder of REM sleep.
- *Associated disorders:* confusional arousals, sleep terrors, RSBD, sleep-related eating disorder.
- *Management:* unless the problem is leading to disruption of sleep in a bed partner, or is a secondary symptom of other sleep pathology, treatment is rarely necessary.

Sleep starts (hypnic jerks)

Occur at sleep onset and present as sudden abrupt contractions of muscle groups, usually the legs, but sometimes also involving the arms, neck, or even the entire body. When wakened by jerks, an individual may have the feeling of falling in space ('siderealism'). Sometimes this feeling is so intense and frightening that it can lead to fear of going to sleep with subsequent sleep-onset difficulties.
- *Polysomnography:* occasional vertex waves, associated with muscular contraction.
- *Prevalence:* 60–70% (essentially a universal component of the sleep-onset process).
- *Differential diagnosis:* nocturnal myoclonic jerks (with evident epileptiform activity on EEG), fragmentary myoclonus (during non-REM sleep), nocturnal leg myoclonus/PLMS (often associated with restless legs syndrome), and the rare 'startle disease' or 'hyperekplexia'.

syndrome (myoclonus occurs following minor stimuli both during wakefulness and sleep).
• *Management:* treatment usually unnecessary. If there is significant interference with sleep—general measures (e.g. avoidance of stimulants such as caffeine, nicotine) or low-dose clonazepam at night.

Benign sleep myoclonus of infancy A disorder of myoclonic jerks that occur during sleep in infants, typically from birth to 6mths, resolving spontaneously.

Hypnagogic foot tremor and alternating leg muscle activation Occurs at the transition between wake and sleep or during light NREM sleep. PSG shows recurrent EMG potentials in one or both feet that are longer than the myoclonic range (>250ms).

Propriospinal myoclonus at sleep onset Recurrent sudden muscular jerks in the transition from wakefulness to sleep, which may be associated with severe sleep-onset insomnia.

Excessive fragmentary myoclonus Small muscle twitches in the fingers, toes, or corner of the mouth that do not cause actual movements across a joint. Often an incidental finding during PSG. Usually asymptomatic, but sometimes associated with EDS or fatigue.

Table 11.10 Isolated symptoms, apparently normal variants, and unresolved issues with diagnostic codes

ICSD-2	ICD-10	DSM-IV-TR
Long sleeper	R29.81	307.47
Short sleeper	R29.81	307.47
Snoring	R06.5	
Sleep-talking	R29.81	
Sleep starts, hypnic jerks	R25.8	
Benign sleep myoclonus of infancy	R25.8	
Hypnagogic foot tremor and alternating leg muscle activation	R25.8	
Propriospinal myoclonus at sleep onset	R25.8	307.47
Excessive fragmentary myoclonus	R25.8	307.47

Sleep disorders related to psychiatric disorders 1

Although unusual for psychiatric patients to present with a 1° sleep disorder, it is not uncommon for psychiatrists to have to deal with secondary problems of *insomnia* (not getting enough sleep or feeling 'unrefreshed') or *hypersomnia* (feeling excessively sleepy during the day or sleeping too much), in the context of a 1° psychiatric disorder, or as a consequence of medication. Equally, *sleep deprivation* may have its own psychological consequences, or may precipitate the onset of a psychiatric illness, particularly a manic episode.

Major affective disorders

Alterations in sleep are central symptoms in the mood disorders. Initial insomnia, frequent waking (for often prolonged periods), early morning waking, vivid or disturbing dreams, and daytime fatigue are frequently seen in major depressive disorder. These features are associated with changes in sleep architecture: shortened REM sleep-onset latency, increased REM density, reduced total sleep time, reduced sleep efficiency, increased awakenings, decreased N3 sleep (SWS), and a shift of N3 from the first NREM cycle to the second. Occasionally, hypersomnia may be a feature in atypical cases, bipolar affective disorder, and seasonal affective disorder. Episodes of mania may be characterized by marked insomnia and a decreased need for sleep associated with a much reduced total sleep time, reduction in N3 sleep and no consistent change in REM sleep.

Management
- Treat the primary disorder.
- *Initial insomnia*: use a more sedating antidepressant (e.g. TCA, trazodone, nefazodone, mirtazapine, agomelatine).
- *Hypersomnia*: use a more 'activating' antidepressant (SSRI, reboxetine, bupropion, MAOI, RIMA).

Note: most antidepressants are REM-suppressant and may exacerbate underlying primary sleep disorders (e.g. parasomnias and sleep-related movement disorders) either on commencement or cessation.

Anxiety disorders

Anxiety disorders commonly disrupt the normal sleep pattern leading to insomnia, which may be triggered by an acute stressful event. Symptoms include: initial insomnia, frequent waking, reduced total sleep time, and early morning waking.

Generalized anxiety Typically prolonged sleep-onset latency, increased stages N1 and N2, less N3, a smaller percentage REM, and increased or normal REM sleep latency.

Panic disorder
Sleep-related (nocturnal) attacks may occur with associated intense fear, feelings of impending doom, autonomic arousal, somatic symptoms, and fear of going to sleep (leading to avoidance behaviour, which may present as 'insomnia'), see 📖 p. 443. As many as 70% of patients with

panic disorder have difficulty with sleep-onset and maintenance insomnia, and often report sleep paralysis and hypnagogic hallucinations. Studies in non-depressed patients with panic disorder report normal sleep-onset latency and modestly reduced total sleep time and sleep. However, studies in patients with panic and comorbid major depression have report features typical of major depression, with substantially prolonged sleep onset latency, reduced total sleep time, sleep disruption, reduced N3, and early REM sleep onset.

PTSD

Sleep complaints almost universal in individuals diagnosed with PTSD; indeed, recurrent distressing dreams related to a traumatic event are a core feature of the disorder. Complaints include: nightmares, difficulties initiating and/or maintaining sleep (in 70–90%), sleep paralysis, RSBD. Sleep disturbance soon after the traumatic event is a risk factor for PTSD and more severe sleep symptoms in PTSD are associated with depression severity, suicidal tendencies, anxiety, and substance use. Studies report increased sleep-onset latency, decreased sleep efficiency, increased wakefulness after sleep onset, decreased total sleep time, reduction in N2 sleep, increased N1 sleep, and variable effects on REM (normal parameters vs. reduced REM latency and increased REM density).

Social phobia

Increased sleep-onset latency, awakening after sleep onset, and reduced total sleep time.

OCD

Sleep can become restricted due to engagement in compulsive behaviours. Sleep studies show decreased total sleep time, increased awakenings, shortened REM latency, reduced N3 sleep, and reduced sleep efficiency.

Management

- Treatment of the primary anxiety disorder will generally improve the patient's ability to initiate and sustain sleep.
- Most anxiolytics tend to be sedating, and it is usual to prescribe a higher dose at night.
- When less sedating drugs such as the SSRIs are used, additional treatment may be necessary to target persistent sleep problems (e.g. cognitive behavioural techniques, short-term use of hypnotics, or a small dose of a more sedating antidepressant at bedtime).
- Behavioural sleep interventions are effective in reducing night-time symptoms in PTSD, e.g. imagery rehearsal for chronic nightmares, stimulus control/sleep restriction for insomnia (see 📖 p. 427).
- Prazosin, an α_1-adrenergic receptor antagonist, has emerged as a promising treatment of PTSD-related sleep disturbance, including both nightmares and insomnia symptoms.

Borderline PD

Sleep architecture changes very similar to those seen in depresssion: reduced total sleep time, reduced sleep efficiency, reduced N3, increased N2, reduced REM latency, and increased REM density.

Sleep disorders related to psychiatric disorders 2

Schizophrenia

Patients with schizophrenia demonstrate increased nocturnal wakefulness and daytime somnolence. PSG shows sleep continuity disturbance, reduced N3, decreased REM latency, and increased REM sleep. It is often difficult to disentangle the effects of medication, active positive symptoms, persistent negative symptoms, and disorganized behaviour and some studies show relatively little change in sleep. Research has suggested an inverse relationship between SWS (N3)/sleep maintenance and brain ventricle size/negative symptoms in schizophrenia.

Management
- *EDS*: monitor effects of antipsychotic medication; adjust timing and dosage.
- *Insomnia*: general sleep hygiene measures, with emphasis on behavioural approach when 'disorganization' is central feature; judicious use of hypnotics or higher dose of sedating antipsychotic nocte.

Eating disorders

Patients with bulimia may report EDS, but sleep studies show very little change in sleep parameters. Studies in anorexia nervosa have been more contradictory due perhaps to the high rates of comorbidity with affective disorders and frequent family history of affective disorders in anorexia patients (hence, PSG similar to depression). In *severe* or untreated cases of anorexia nervosa, insomnia and frequent waking very common. Sleep studies show reduced total sleep time, decreased sleep efficiency, increased wakefulness after sleep onset, shortened REM latency, increased N1, and decreased N3 sleep, which normalize after weight is gained.

Management
- Treatment of the primary eating disorder to establish better eating behaviours and re-establish normal BMI.
- General principles for insomnia and EDS (see 🕮 p. 426).
- Possible use of SSRI or alternative antidepressant.

Dementia

Normal ageing is associated with increased sleep latency, reduced total sleep time, loss of NREM sleep, frequent arousals leading to fragmentation of nocturnal sleep, and an increase in daytime napping.
- Some sleep disorders (e.g. sleep apnoea syndromes, PLMS) occur more frequently in the elderly population.
- Dementia generally causes further increases in sleep latency, further reductions in total sleep time, and increased fragmentation of nocturnal sleep, in proportion to the severity of the illness.
- Disorders of normal circadian rhythm are also commonly seen, with a characteristic 'sundown syndrome' of confusion and agitation at bedtime (nocturnal agitated wandering).

Management
- General sleep hygiene measures (with an emphasis on establishing and reinforcing a normal 24-hr circadian cycle through the use of environmental cues, daily routine, avoidance of daytime napping, and regular activities).
- 'Sundown syndrome' may respond to low-dose antipsychotics (e.g. haloperidol, risperidone) or antidepressants (e.g. trazodone).

Alcohol use

Alcohol most probably exerts its sedative effects through a combination of GABA facilitation and glutamate inhibition. The acute effects of alcohol lead to reduced sleep latency, increased total sleep time, increased N3, mild suppression of REM sleep in first half of the night, and subsequent increased REM sleep in second half, associated with sleep disruption, intense dreaming, and even nightmares. Chronic effects of alcohol abuse include the loss of N3, sleep disruption, and significant insomnia. Withdrawal from alcohol is also associated with insomnia. Sleep architecture is disrupted, with increased sleep latency, reduced total sleep time, loss of N3, increased REM density and/or amount. 'Delirium tremens', with marked agitation, confusion, and hallucinations, is characterized by intense REM rebound.

Use of other recreational drugs

- *Nicotine:* this tends to cause initial insomnia, and may be associated with sleep disruption and increased REM sleep. Use of nicotine patches has been associated with vivid dreams and nightmares.
- *Cannabis:* hypnotic effects modulated by cannabinoid-1 receptors. Appear to be similar to the effects of benzodiazepines and alcohol, increasing NREM and suppressing REM sleep. Cessation may lead to problems of initial insomnia, sleep disruption and REM rebound.
- *Opiates:* although sleep is improved when opiates are used therapeutically for pain relief or in the treatment of restless legs, misuse is associated with generalized sleep disruption. Changes in sleep architecture include decrease in sleep efficiency, total sleep time, N3, and REM sleep. Withdrawal symptoms include insomnia, with fragmentation of sleep and disruption of normal sleep architecture, related to increased arousal and REM rebound.
- *Stimulants:* the effects of amfetamine and cocaine include reduced REM sleep, and increased sleep and REM latency. Xanthines (caffeine, theophylline) have similar effects, acting through adenosine receptors, directly interfering with the generation of sleep. Amfetamine derivatives, e.g. fenfluramine and MDMA (ecstasy) have a pharmacological action that is primarily serotonergic which may lead to both daytime sedation and disturbed sleep (due to periods of drowsiness and wakefulness), as well as a reduced duration of REM sleep. SWS may be increased during the withdrawal phase as a rebound phenomenon.

Psychiatric medication and sleep

Antidepressants

Sedating

- TCAs are usually sedative due to their anticholinergic effects. Amitriptyline, trimipramine, doxepin, imipramine, clomipramine are the most sedating and nortriptyline is the least sedating.
- Tetracyclic antidepressants (mianserin) and trazodone also have marked sedating properties, although these are less related to their anticholinergic properties and may be due to their $5-HT_2$ and histamine antagonism—properties shared by some of the newer antidepressants (e.g. mirtazapine)
- Agomelatine may promote sleep through melatonin (MT1/MT2) agonism.

Alerting

MAOIs, SSRIs, NARIs (reboxetine), DARIs (bupropion), SNRIs (venlafaxine, duloxetine) all tend to have alerting effects which may be useful in the treatment of hypersomnolence associated with 'atypical' depression, and should be taken in the morning or early afternoon.

Antipsychotic drugs

Most antipsychotics cause drowsiness and impaired performance. There is a great degree of variability even within groups of antipsychotics (see Table 11.11).

Table 11.11 Sedative effects of antipsychotics

Marked sedation	Moderate sedation	Mild sedation	Minimal sedation
Chlorpromazine	Asenapine	Flupentixol	Amisulpiride
Clozapine	Benperidol	Haloperidol	Aripiprazole
Levomepromazine	Droperidol	Paliperidone	
Pericyazine	Fluphenazine	Pimozide	
	Loxapine	Pipotiazine	
	Olanzapine	Quetiapine	
	Perphenazine	Risperidone	
	Promazine	Sulpiride	
	Thioridazine	Trifluoperazine	
	Zuclopenthixol		

Mood-stabilizing drugs

- *Lithium:* mildly sedating (increasing N3 and reducing REM).
- *Carbamazepine:* may cause drowsiness at start of treatment or when dose is being increased, but this is usually a transient effect.
- *Sodium valproate:* mild effects on sleep—less than carbamazepine.

Benzodiazepines and associated hypnotics

By definition, BDZs and barbiturates are sedating. Problems arise due to withdrawal insomnia on discontinuation, tolerance to the beneficial hypnotic effects after long-term use, and problems of dependence Newer hypnotics, such as the z-drugs, share the sleep-enhancing properties of the benzodiazepines, but may be less likely to cause rebound or dependence (see Table 11.12).

Table 11.12 Polysomnographic (PSG) effects of hypnotics

Drug	Acute effects	Withdrawal	Comments
Barbiturates	↑TST, N2, spindles ↓WASO, REM ↔ δ	↓TST	Rapid development of tolerance, withdrawal insomnia, daytime sedation
BDZs	↑TST, N2, spindles ↓SL, WASO, REM, δ	↓TST	Wide variation in onset and duration of action (see Table 11.2, 🕮 p. 427)
			Long T_{half} : EDS
			Short T_{half} : tolerance, withdrawal insomnia
Z-drugs	↑TST ↓SL ↔ δ, REM	↔ or ↑ WASO	No typical alteration of sleep architecture or withdrawal effects

BDZ = benzodiazepine; TST = total sleep time; WASO = waking after sleep onset; SL = sleep latency; δ = N3/slow wave sleep; EDS = excessive daytime somnolence

Psychostimulant drugs

Although very useful in the treatment of hypersomnia (particularly in narcolepsy), ADHD, and to suppress appetite, this group of drugs all tend to cause insomnia with fragmented sleep due to frequent awakenings (e.g. dexamfetamine, methylphenidate, methamfetamine, mazindol, pemoline, and modafinil) and should not be taken in the evening. Cessation, with the notable exception of modafinil, leads to increases in total sleep time and REM rebound.

Reproductive psychiatry, sexual dysfunction, and sexuality

Introduction

Of necessity this chapter is an amalgam of a number of areas in psychiatry that overlap but which are important subspecialties in themselves. They intersect with other medical specialties including gynaecology, obstetrics, urology, and general practice. Most services will be integrated with their medical counterparts as the assessment process necessitates a more holistic approach, even to the point where psychiatrists are employed in obstetric departments and offer a perinatal service for pregnant and post-partum women. It is true to say that research has formerly focused more on female reproductive psychiatry. This does not mean that men do not have their share of problems in this area, rather that the research base is relatively lacking at this point in time.

Mental health problems can arise at various milestones in an individual's physiological, psychological, and social development. It is important to include issues relating to normal physiological changes, hormonal factors, sexual orientation and its expression, and sexual function when consider-ing associated predisposing, precipitating, and perpetuating factors.

Other important considerations relate to side-effects and risks of the medications we prescribe for the treatment of mental disorders. These are covered in the therapeutic section of this Handbook—e.g. prescribing during pregnancy (☐ p. 968), prescribing during lactation (☐ p. 970).

It is also vital that psychiatrists are involved in assessing the presence or *absence* of psychiatric disorder when it comes to major life decisions, such as those generated by disorders of gender identity (☐ p. 484). The taboo associated with many of the topics covered in this section, even in the twenty-first century (and despite—or perhaps *because*—of the popular media) means that psychiatrists will often have an educative role. There are still many myths that need to be dispelled.

Equally, many psychiatrists have neither the theoretical framework nor the experience to deal competently with reproductive or sexual issues. Whilst this text can serve as an introduction to the topic and offers some signposts to management, there is no substitute for seeking expert advice when confronted with complex problems.

Menstrual-related disorders

Premenstrual symptoms

Characteristic physical signs and symptoms affect up to three-quarters of women with regular menstrual cycles. The most common presentations are abdominal bloating (present in 90% of women with any symptoms), breast tenderness, and headaches. These mild symptoms do not usually interfere with a woman's ability to function.

Management

Premenstrual symptoms that do not meet premenstrual syndrome (PMS) or premenstrual dysphoric disorder (PMDD) criteria are initially managed conservatively unless there is significant psychiatric comorbidity. This management involves a diet low in salt, fat, caffeine, and sugar; restriction of alcohol and tobacco; exercise; and measures to reduce stress. If there is failure to adequately respond to conservative management after 2–3mths, a trial of an SSRI may be considered.

Premenstrual syndrome (PMS) or tension (PMT)

For further details see 📖 p. 466.

Clinically significant PMS occurs in 20–30% of women with severe impairment, in about 5% including associated premenstrual dysphoric disorder (PMDD). PMS is characterized by the presence of both physical and behavioural symptoms that recur in the second half of the menstrual cycle, and often the first few days of menses. Most common behavioural symptoms are fatigue, labile mood, irritability, tension, depressed mood, increased appetite, forgetfulness, and difficulty concentrating (see Table 12.1). These symptoms must be severe enough to impair the patient's social and occupational functioning. Most common criteria used: University of California San Diego (UCSD) criteria for PMS.[1] Women with PMS have a higher incidence of affective and anxiety disorders and are at greater risk of having them in the future. The reason for this correlation is not yet known.

Premenstrual dyphoric disorder (PMDD)

For further details see 📖 p. 466.

PMDD is a research diagnosis in DSM-IV (coded as depressive disorder NOS) distinguished from PMS by the prominent presence of one or more marked affective symptoms: notably depressed mood, anxiety, affective lability, and/or irritability or anger. PMDD occurs in 2–8% of women with regular menstrual cycles. There is no evidence for cultural, ethnic, or socio-economic differences in prevalence.

Note: the criteria require behavioural symptoms only; the presence of physical symptoms is not required. PMDD may occur in the presence of other psychiatric disorders if it is not an exacerbation of these disorders.

Menopausal disorders

There is an increased incidence of anxiety and depression in peri- or post-menopausal women. This is not related directly to hormonal changes. Rather, patients presenting with mood-related problems around the menopause experience coincident psychosocial stressors,[2] and the changes in gonadal hormones may exacerbate pre-existing mood disorders.[3]

Assessment Exclude other causes of mood disturbance. Particular attention should be paid to past psychiatric history and current social history.

Management Evidence for HRT is inconclusive, although if mood symptoms are secondary to physical symptoms this may have a role (HRT may also augment effects of antidepressants).[4] Treatment is with standard approaches for depression/anxiety.

Table 12.1 Frequency of premenstrual symptoms[1]

Symptom	Frequency, % of cycles
Fatigue	92
Irritability	91
Bloating	90
Anxiety and/or tension	89
Breast tenderness	85
Mood lability	81
Depression	80
Food cravings	78
Acne	71
Increased appetite	70
Oversensitivity	69
Swelling	67
Expressed anger	67
Crying easily	65
Feeling of isolation	65
Headache	60
Forgetfulness	56
Gastrointestinal symptoms	48
Poor concentration	47
Hot flushes	18
Heart palpitations	14
Dizziness	14

[1]Mortola JF, Girton L, Beck L, *et al.* (1990) Diagnosis of premenstrual syndrome by a simple prospective reliable instrument. *Obstet Gynecol* **72**: 302.

1 Mishell DR (2005) *Epidemiology, and etiology of premenstrual disorders. Managing the spectrum of premenstrual symptoms, a clinician's guide*, pp. 4–9. San Antonio, Dannemiller Foundation/Med Pro Communications.
2 Cooke DJ (1985) Psychosocial vulnerability to life events during the climacteric. *Br J Psychiat* **147**: 71–5.
3 Sagsoz N, Oguzturk O, Bayram M, *et al.* (2001) Anxiety and depression before and after the menopause. *Arch Gynecol Obstet* **264**: 199–202.
4 Birkhauser M (2002) Depression, menopause and estrogens: is there a correlation? *Maturitas* **41** (Suppl. 1): S3–8.

Premenstrual disorders

Aetiology

Evidence supports a genetic vulnerability conferring increased sensitivity to normal changes in hormone levels throughout the menstrual cycle. This causes alterations in the normal cyclic ovarian steroid interactions with central neurotransmitters and neurohormones. Cyclic changes in ovarian steroids alone do not lead to PMS/PMDD. Most evidence supports involvement of the serotonergic system, endorphins and GABA, and the renin–angiotensin–aldosterone system. The autonomic and peripheral nervous systems may be involved in certain symptoms. Minimal or no evidence for: trace vitamin and element deficiencies, personality factors, and stress. Stress also has little effect on PMS severity, and PMS is more likely to cause stress than vice versa.

Morbidity

These disorders can extend over a woman's entire reproductive cycle, from approximately age 14 to 50. Symptoms are relatively constant between cycles, and can cause an aggregate total of years of disability over a lifetime. This negatively affects quality of life and can have both direct and indirect economic consequences.

Psychiatric consultation

For already diagnosed premenstrual symptoms this is rare unless emotional symptoms are marked and/or there are vegetative symptoms, suicidal ideation, or a frequent inability to function.

Differential diagnosis

Up to 40% of women presenting to a physician with presumed PMS have another mood disorder; many meet the criteria for a depressive or anxiety disorder.[1] PMDD can be a premenstrual exacerbation of an underlying psychiatric disorder or of a medical condition. Medical disorders such as migraine, chronic fatigue syndrome, and irritable bowel syndrome can have exacerbations prior to or during menses. Exclude perimenopause, gynaecological disorders (dysmenorrhoea, post-partum status, polycystic ovary disease, and endometriosis) and hypothyroidism and nutrient deficiencies (e.g. manganese, magnesium, B vitamins, vitamin E, and linoleic acid).

Investigations

- There are no specific tests diagnostic of premenstrual disorders. Prospective charting of daily symptoms for at least two menstrual cycles is essential to confirm the cyclical pattern.
- If menses are not regular and/or if they have length <25 days or >36 days referral should be made for a reproductive endocrine evaluation.
- For concomitant medical conditions consultation with a general practitioner or gynaecologist for a physical exam and exclusion of medical disorders as well as appropriate routine blood tests including TFTs may be warranted.

Assessment tools

Prospective Record of the Impact and Severity of Menstruation (PRISM), the Calendar of Premenstrual Experiences (COPE), and the Daily Record of Severity of Problems (DRSP). The DRSP is available online at ℜ http:// www.pmdd.factsforhealth.org/have/dailyrecord.asp.

Treatment of PMS and PMDD

First-line therapy

* Antidepressants are effective for PMDD, with fluoxetine the most studied. At a dose of 20mg/day the overall response is 60–75%. Other SSRIs and venlafaxine have also shown efficacy in placebo-controlled trials.
* Luteal phase therapy: therapy in the luteal phase alone, starting 14d prior to the expected next menses, and terminating with the onset of menses.

Second-line therapy

* Alprazolam (250–500mcg tid) for luteal phase depression.
* For severe PMDD, refractory to other treatment, refer to a specialist. Potential treatments include medical oophoriectomy with a GnRH agonist (e.g. leuprorelin, danazol). There are significant side-effects related to hypoestrogenism (e.g. hot flashes, long-term effects of oestrogen deficiency, osteoporosis, etc.). For patients who respond well, treatment can continue over the long term (>6mths) with continuous add-back of oestrogen (+ progesterone when indicated) to decrease and/or prevent these side-effects. For rare, refractory cases with severe disabling symptoms, surgical bilateral oophoriectomy may be considered.

Other promising possible treatments or adjuncts

* RCTs initially failed to demonstrate the effectiveness of OCP in treating PMS or PMDD. Newer placebo-controlled trials are showing that a 24-day (rather than 21-day) hormonal formulation is efficacious for PMDD.[2]
* Diuretics for severe oedema, e.g. furosemide, spironolactone; danazol for mastalgia.
* There is some evidence for the efficacy of pyridoxine (vitamin B6) (no more than 100mg/day), vitamin E, calcium, vitamin D, and magnesium.
* No evidence for multiple other treatment options including progesterone treatment, ginkgo biloba, evening primrose oil, essential free fatty acids.

1 Keenan PA, Stern RA, Janowsky DS, et al. (1992) Psychological aspects of premenstrual syndrome. I: Cognition and memory. *Psychoneuroendocrinol* **17**: 179–87.
2 Yonkers KA, Brown C, Pearlstein TB, et al. (2005) Efficacy of a new low-dose oral contraceptive with drospirenone in premenstrual dysphoric disorder. *Obstet Gynecol* **106**(3): 492–501.

Disorders associated with pregnancy

Anxiety/mood symptoms in normal pregnancy

Although there is usually an increase in symptoms of anxiety and depression during pregnancy, these are quite normal and usually related to 'adjustment' in the 1st trimester and 'fears' in the 3rd trimester. Unless there is a past history of psychiatric illness, there is no reported increase in the incidence of psychiatric disorders.[1]

Risk factors Family or personal history of depression; ambivalence about the pregnancy; high levels of neuroticism; lack of marital, family, or social supports.

Treatment Usually will focus on psychosocial interventions; specific psychiatric disorders should be identified and treated appropriately (see **Prescribing in pregnancy** 📖 p. 968).

Miscarriage and abortion[2]

There is an increase in psychiatric morbidity, with over 50% of women experiencing an adjustment disorder (grief reaction) with significant depressive symptoms. Chronic symptoms are rare, but risk is increased when there is a history of previous miscarriage or abortion, or where conflict is experienced related to religious or cultural beliefs.

Hyperemesis gravidarum[3]

Vomiting in pregnancy that is sufficiently pernicious to produce weight loss, dehydration, acidosis from starvation, alkalosis from loss of HCl in vomitus, and hypokalaemia. Occurs in 1–20/1000 pregnant women. Although psychological factors may be important in benign forms, these are now regarded as secondary rather than primary (i.e. *not* a somatoform disorder).

Complications Muscle weakness, ECG abnormalities, tetany, psychological disturbance, and more seriously (but rarely): oesophageal rupture, Wernicke's encephalopathy, central pontine myelinosis, retinal haemorrhage, renal damage, spontaneous pneumomediastinum, intrauterine growth retardation, and fetal death.

Associations Transient hypothyroidism (60% of cases), *H. pylori* infection.

Management Admission to hospital (~24%), parenteral fluid, electrolyte replacement, vitamin supplementation, anti-emetics or short-term steroids, diazepam (for nausea and associated distress).

Pseudocyesis[4]

A condition in which a woman firmly believes herself to be pregnant and develops objective pregnancy signs (abdominal enlargement, menstrual disturbance, apparent foetal movements, nausea, breast changes, labour pains, uterine enlargement, cervical softening, urinary frequency, positive pregnancy test) in the absence of pregnancy.

Differential diagnosis Possible medical disorders should be excluded (ectopic pregnancy, corpus luteal cyst, placenta praevia, pituitary tumour, pelvic tumour).

Aetiology Regarded as a somatoform disorder or variant of depression, it may present as a complication of postpartum depression or psychosis with amenorrhoea. It may be related to Couvade's syndrome in expectant fathers (see 📖 p. 90).

Treatment Tends to include supportive or insight-orientated psychotherapy and a trial of an antidepressant.

1 Klein MH and Essex MJ (1995) Pregnant or depressed? The effect of overlap between symptoms of depression and somatic complaints of pregnancy on rates of depression in the second trimester. *Depression* **2**: 308–14.
2 Clare AW and Tyrrell J (1994) Psychiatric aspects of abortion. *Ir J Psychol Med* **11**: 92–8.
3 Kuscu NK and Koyuncu F (2002) Hyperemesis gravidarum: current concepts and management. *Postgrad Med J* **78**: 76–9.
4 Small GW (1986) Pseudocyesis: an overview. *Can J Psych* **31**: 452–7.

Disorders related to childbirth

⚠ Always ask about thoughts of self-harm or harming the baby.

Despite the significant life event that pregnancy is, psychiatric admission and completed suicide are less common in pregnancy than at other times. There may be subclinical mild anxiety or mood disturbance, worse in the third and first trimesters. 10% risk of clinical depression in the first trimester associated with past history of depression, previous abortion, previous intrauterine loss, unwanted pregnancy. Third trimester depression may persist as post-partum depression. Avoid drug treatment in the first trimester.

Baby blues

Up to ¾ of new mothers will experience a short-lived period of tearfulness and emotional lability starting two or three days after birth and lasting 1–2 days. This is common enough to be easily recognizable by midwifery staff and requires only reassurance and observation towards resolution. There is weak evidence that it may be related to post-partum reductions in levels of oestrogen, progesterone, and prolactin (which do occur around 72hrs after the birth).

Postnatal depression (PND)

A significant depressive episode, temporally related to childbirth, occurring in 10–15% of women within 6mths post-partum (peak 3–4wks). The clinical features are similar to other depressive episodes, although thought content may include worries about the baby's health or her ability to cope adequately with the baby. There may be a significant anxiety component. 90% of cases last less than 1mth; 4% greater than 1yr. *Risk factors* Personal or family history of depression, older age, single mother, poor relationship with own mother, ambivalence towards or unwanted pregnancy, poor social support, significant other psycho-social stressors, severe 'baby blues', previous post-partum psychosis (no evidence for association with obstetric complications). *Management* Early identification and close monitoring of those 'at risk' (use of Edinburgh Postnatal Depression Scale in primary care setting—see Box 12.1); prevention by education, support, and appropriate pharmacological intervention; depressive episode treated in usual way with antidepressants and/or brief CBT, if severe or associated with thoughts of self-harm or harm to baby, may require hospital admission.

Postpartum psychosis

An acute psychotic episode, occurring following 1.5/1000 live births, peak occurrence at 2wks postpartum. *Aetiology* Unknown, but may relate to reduction of oestrogen (leading to DA super-sensitivity), cortisol levels, or postpartum thyroiditis. *Symptoms* 3 common clinical presentations: *prominent affective symptoms* (80%)—mania or depression with psychotic symptoms; *schizophreniform disorder* (15%); *acute organic psychosis* (5%). *Common features* Lability of symptoms; insomnia; perplexity, bewilderment, and disorientation; thoughts of suicide or infanticide. *Risk factors* Personal or family history of major psychiatric disorder; lack of social support; single parenthood; previous postpartum psychosis (30% risk of psychosis; 38% risk of PND). *Management* Prevention Identification, education, support, and treatment of 'at risk' individuals; **Treatment** Admission to hospital (specialist mother–baby unit if possible); for major affective disorder there is good evidence for ECT, mood stabilizers (esp. carbamazepine), and early use of antidepressants; psychotic symptoms should be treated with usual protocol (see 📖 p. 192).

Box 12.1 Edinburgh Postnatal Depression Scale (EPDS)[1]

As you have recently had a baby, we would like to know how you are feeling. Please UNDERLINE the answer which comes closest to how you have felt IN THE PAST 7 DAYS, not just how you feel today.

I have been able to laugh and see the funny side of things.
As much as I always could/Not quite so much now/Definitely not so much now/Not at all
I have looked forward with enjoyment to things.
As much as I ever did/Rather less than I used to/Definitely less than I used to/Hardly at all
* **I have blamed myself unnecessarily when things went wrong.**
Yes, most of the time/Yes, some of the time/Not very often/No, never
I have been anxious or worried for no good reason.
No, not at all/Hardly ever/Yes, sometimes/Yes, very often
* **I have felt scared or panicky for not very good reason.**
Yes, quite a lot/Yes, sometimes/No, not much/No, not at all
* **Things have been getting on top of me.**
Yes, most of the time I haven't been able to cope at all/
Yes, sometimes I haven't been coping as well as usual/
No, most of the time I have coped quite well/
No, I have been coping as well as ever
* **I have been so unhappy that I have had difficulty sleeping.**
Yes, most of the time/Yes, sometimes/Not very often/No, not at all
* **I have felt sad or miserable.**
Yes, most of the time/Yes, quite often/Not very often/No, not at all
* **I have been so unhappy that I have been crying.**
Yes, most of the time/Yes, quite often/Only occasionally/No, never
* **The thought of harming myself has occurred to me.**
Yes, quite often/Sometimes/Hardly ever/Never

Response categories are scored 0, 1, 2, and 3 according to increased severity of the symptoms. Items marked with an asterisk are reverse scored (i.e. 3, 2, 1, and 0). A total score of 12+ is regarded as significant.

Sexual dysfunction 1: general principles

A brief note on 'talking about sex'

Discussing sexual issues, particularly sexual dysfunction, may be embarrassing for the individual, and this is compounded if the clinician is also uncomfortable. Aside from experience of asking about these issues, a few general principles should be borne in mind.

- An empathic, non-judgemental, understanding approach is essential.
- Acknowledge the difficulty in talking about sexual problems.
- Reassure that such problems are common and are treatable.
- Avoid 'medical' terminology (or explain adequately any terms used).
- Start with general enquiries before moving on to more specific issues.
- Do not make *any* assumptions (esp. orientation, practices, experience, number of partners).
- Be aware of common sexual myths (see Box 12.2).

Defining sexual dysfunction

Despite disagreement about what constitutes 'normal', there is general consensus that sexual dysfunction is present when there are persistent impairments of normal patterns of sexual interest or response. Usually these manifest as lack or loss of interest/enjoyment of sexual activities, the inability to experience or control orgasm, or a physiological barrier to successful sexual intercourse. Criteria for a diagnosis of sexual dysfunction include:

- Inability to participate in a preferred sexual relationship.
- Presence of the sexual dysfunction on (almost) all occasions.
- Duration of at least 6mths.
- Significant stress or interpersonal difficulties.
- Not accounted for by a physical disorder, drug treatment (or use), or other mental or behavioural disorder.

Subclinical problems

Certain individuals will not meet strict criteria for a specific diagnosis, but nevertheless experience significant distress. Usually these problems are adjustment difficulties related to timing, frequency, and method of initiating sexual activity. Any treatment tends to be supportive (for the patient and their partner) and educative (sex education: see Box 12.4).

Box 12.2 Common sexual myths[1]

- Men should not express their emotions.
- All physical contact must lead to sex.
- Good sex leads to a wild orgasm.
- Sex = intercourse.
- The man should be the sexual leader.
- Women should not initiate sex.
- Men feel like sex all the time.
- Women should always have sex when her partner makes sexual approaches.
- Sex is something we instinctively know about.
- 'Respectable' people should not enjoy sex too much and certainly never masturbate.
- All other couples have 'great' sex, several times a week, have an orgasm every time, and always orgasm simultaneously.
- If sex is not good, there is something wrong with the relationship.

1 Adapted from Andrews G and Jenkins R (eds) (1999) *Management of mental disorders*, UK edn, vol. 2, Sexual Dysfunction, pp. 612–13. Sydney: World Health Organization Collaborating Centre for Mental Health and Substance Abuse.

Box 12.3 Common triggers for sexual problems

Psychological Relationship problems; life stressors; anxiety/depression; low self-esteem; sexual performance anxiety; excessive self-monitoring of arousal; feelings of guilt about sex; fear of pregnancy or sexually transmitted diseases (STDs); lack of knowledge about sexuality/'normal' sexual responses; previous significant negative sexual experience (esp. rape or childhood sexual abuse issues).
Environmental (Fear of) interruptions (e.g. from children, parents); physical discomfort.
Physical Use of drugs or alcohol; medication side-effects; pain or discomfort due to illness; feeling tired or 'run down'; recent childbirth.
Factors related to the partner Sexual attractiveness (gender, physical characteristics); evidence of disinterest, constant criticism, inconsideration, and inability to cope with difficulties (esp. sexual); sexual inexperience/poor technique; preference for sexual activities that are unappealing to the partner.

Sexual dysfunction 2: problems common to men and women

Sexual dysfunction is common in the general population with lifetime prevalence in young adults estimated as in Table 12.2.[1]

Table 12.2 Prevalence of sexual dysfunction in young adults

Problem	Male	Female
Reduced libido	30%	40%
Arousal difficulties	50%	60%
Reaching orgasm too soon	15%	10%
Failure to have orgasm	2%	35%
Dyspareunia	5%	15%

Lack or loss of sexual desire

Lack of pleasure in anticipating, or reduced urge to engage in, sexual activity. May be **primary** (always has been absent) or **secondary** (has declined recently), **situational** (specific settings or partners), or **total**. For a diagnosis, loss of desire ought not to be secondary to other sexual problems (e.g. dyspareunia or erectile failure).

Differential diagnosis Sexual aversion, lack of sexual enjoyment, depression, physical causes (chronic pain, endocrine disturbance, effects of drugs or alcohol).

Management
- Treat any primary cause found (physical, psychological, psychiatric).
- Establish the reasons for seeking help, provide information (e.g. common triggers (📖 p. 473).
- Address general relationship issues.
- Consider specialist referral (behavioural work, graded individual and couple exercises require experienced therapist (e.g. 'sensate focus' techniques, see Box 12.4).

Sexual aversion and lack of sexual enjoyment

Sexual aversion Strong −ve feelings, fear, or anxiety due to prospect of sexual interaction; of sufficient intensity to lead to active avoidance of sexual activity.

Lack of sexual enjoyment Lack of appropriate pleasure, despite normal sexual responses and achievement of orgasm.

Management Both conditions tend to be related to difficult and complex psychosocial factors, often stemming from a previous traumatic sexual experience (e.g. rape or molestation). For this reason, only a skilled, experienced therapist should attempt treatment. Where possible, refer to a specialist service. Establishing the reasons for seeking help may clarify sensible outcome goals.

Excessive sexual desire

Occasionally increased sexual drive may occur, presenting as a problem for individuals, partners (on whom 'unreasonable' demands are made), or carers (when sexual disinhibition occurs). Referred to as **nymphomania** (women) or **satyriasis** (men). Usually occurs in late teenage/early adulthood, secondary to a mood disorder (e.g. mania), in the early stages of dementia, associated with learning disability, secondary to brain injury, or as a side-effect of some drugs.

Management Treatment should address any 1° problem, general relationship issues. When the problem is persistent, specialist referral may be appropriate (for cognitive, behavioural, or, rarely, pharmacological therapy Box 12.4).

Box 12.4 'Sensate focus' (Masters and Johnson 1966)[1]

A series of specific exercises for couples (essentially a form of *in vivo* 'desensitization' to reduce sexual anxiety), initially encouraging each partner to take turns in paying increased attention to their own senses. There are a number of stages to a course of therapy:

Stage one The couple take turns to touch each other's body (with the breasts and genitals off limits), to establish an awareness of sensations (touching and being touched) and usually in silence (to avoid distractions). If sexual arousal does occur, they are not to proceed to intercourse. If any touch is uncomfortable, the partner being touched must let his or her partner know, either verbally or non-verbally.

Stage two Touching is expanded to include the breasts and genitals, still with an emphasis on awareness of sensations and not the expectation of a sexual response (intercourse and orgasm are still prohibited). A 'hand riding' technique is used (placing one hand on top of the partner's hand while being touched) to indicate more or less pressure, faster or slower pace, or change to a different spot.

Stage three The couple try mutual touching (not taking turns), to practise a more natural form of physical interaction. Intercourse is still off limits.

Stage four Mutual touching continues, moving to the female-on-top position without attempting penetration. The woman can rub the penis against her clitoral region, vulva, and vaginal opening regardless of whether or not there is an erection, still focusing on the physical sensations, and stopping or returning to non-genital touching if either partner becomes orgasm-orientated or anxious. In later sessions, she may progress to putting the tip of the penis into the vagina if there is an erection, and after completing a few sessions in this way, couples are usually comfortable enough to proceed to full intercourse.

1 Masters WH and Johnson VE (1966) *Human sexual response.* New York: Bantam Books.

1 Haas K and Haas A (1993) *Understanding human sexuality.* St Louis: Mosby.

Sexual dysfunction 3: problems specific to women

Failure of genital response

This is usually due to vaginal dryness or lack of lubrication, due to psychological factors (e.g. anxiety), physical problems (e.g. infection), oestrogen deficiency (esp. post-menopausal), or secondary to lack or loss of sexual desire.

Management

- General aims: increasing arousal levels during periods of sexual activity (see **Orgasmic dysfunction**), alleviating vaginal dryness (with use of lubricating gel, oestrogen replacement), and reducing factors that may inhibit arousal (see **Common triggers** 📖 p. 473).
- If problems persist, referral to a specialist should be considered.

Orgasmic dysfunction

The most common sexual complaint in women. Experience of orgasm is delayed or does not occur at all, despite normal sexual arousal and excitement. Individuals may consider this to be normal and not complain of dysfunction. Problems may be **primary** (never had an orgasm in any situation), secondary (previously able, but not currently), **situational** (problems only occur in certain situations), or **total** (in all situations). Complicating factors may include secondary lack or loss of sexual desire, other sexual dysfunctions, and relationship problems.

Management

- Complex cases should be referred to a specialist sex therapist.
- Less complex cases may respond to a directed self-help programme.[1] This usually includes directed masturbation, 'sensate focus' for couples, Kegel's pelvic floor exercises, and use of sexual fantasy.

Non-organic vaginismus

Penetration is impossible or painful due to blockage of the vaginal opening caused by spasms of the pelvic floor muscles. Usually related to anxieties or fearful thoughts—e.g. fear of pain on penetration, previous sexual assault, belief in premarital sex being wrong or sinful, childhood punishment for masturbation, general fear of sex (esp. the first experience of intercourse is likely to be painful or bloody), fear of pregnancy and painful labour. Vaginismus leads to pain during intercourse, thus reinforcing these beliefs.

Management

- Physical examination (to exclude vaginal obstruction due to a growth, a tumour, or the hymen).
- Vaginismus is best treated by an expert and management will include: education (to dispel myths and tackle misunderstandings or negative attitudes), relaxation techniques, and strategies to achieve penetration (e.g. self-exploration, Kegel's exercises, use of graded trainers, sensate focus exercises, involvement of partner, graded attempts at intercourse, reassurance for the partner; see Box 12.5).

Non-organic dyspareunia

Pain during intercourse that may be felt superficially (at the entrance of) or deep within the vagina.

Management

- Exclude physical causes of pain (e.g. infection, tender episiotomy scar, endometriosis, ovarian cyst).
- Provide information about ensuring adequate arousal, variation of intercourse positions to avoid 'deep' penetration.
- Relaxation techniques (including Kegel's exercises) and 'positive self-talk' may help reduce anxiety and ensure the woman feels 'in control'.
- Where deep pain is experienced *after* intercourse, this may be due to *pelvic congestion syndrome* (with symptoms similar to premenstrual syndrome) caused by accumulation of blood during arousal without occurrence of orgasm. Achieving orgasm (by intercourse, masturbation, or use of a vibrator) may help to alleviate this congestion.
- For complex cases, with vague or intermittent problems, associated secondary sexual or psychiatric problems, or when initial treatment is unsuccessful, referral to a specialist is indicated.

Box 12.5 Kegel's exercises

These are pelvic floor muscle exercises. The muscle can be identified by attempting to stop urine flow, and contraction of this muscle may need to be practised before voluntary control is mastered. The exercises should be practised for a few minutes every day. Repeat (a) and (b) ten times initially (building up to 30 times over 4–6 weeks) and (c) and (d) five times (building up to 20 times over 4–6 weeks).
(a) Breathing normally, quickly contract and relax the muscle.
(b) Breathing normally, contract the muscle for a count of three, and then relax.
(c) Inhale slowly, contracting the muscle for a count of three, hold for a count of three, then, exhaling slowly, relax to a count of three.
(d) With the muscle relaxed, bear down (as if trying to push something out of the vagina) for a count of three.

1 Heiman JR and LoPiccolo J (1988) *Becoming orgasmic*. London: Piatkus Books.

Sexual dysfunction 4: problems specific to men

Erectile failure (failure of genital response) Inability to develop or maintain an erection, leading to failure of coitus or sexual intercourse. **Subtypes** *Primary* Never been able to sustain an erection; *Secondary* Able to do so in the past; *Situational* Only successful under certain circumstances; *Total* Not under any circumstances. **Contributing factors** Moral/religious views on sex and masturbation; previous negative sexual experiences (may undermine sexual confidence and increase 'performance anxiety'); secondary to other sexual dysfunction (e.g. premature ejaculation); use of alcohol and drugs; stress and fatigue.

Management Physical assessment to exclude organic causes (disease or surgery affecting the blood supply of the penis, side-effects of drugs or medication); refer to expert on sexual problems if *primary, total, long-standing* (years), or not associated with obvious triggers. **General** Education (about physical and psychological factors that may contribute to erectile failure) and self-help exercises[1,2] (better if partner involved). **Physical** Sildenafil (Viagra); training in self-administration of papaverine or prostaglandin E_1 into the penis prior to intercourse; use of a vacuum constriction device; surgical implantation of semi-rigid or inflatable penile prostheses. *Note:* relapse common (~75%), usually related to clear triggers, and will improve naturally or through use of previously successful techniques. (Seeing this as a 'normal' situation may help relieve anxiety and reduce the sense of failure which might otherwise prolong problems further.)

Orgasmic dysfunction (or 'inhibited ejaculation') Relatively rare in men. Orgasm delayed/does not occur at all, despite normal sexual excitement and arousal. **Situational dysfunction** usually has a psychological cause (see **Common triggers** 📖 p. 473); **total dysfunction** may have a variety of causes.

Management Main aims: reducing 'performance anxiety', increasing arousal and physical stimulation, i.e. addressing any common triggers, relationship problems, associated feelings of anxiety or guilt, or memories of past traumatic/unpleasant sexual experiences. Education (dispelling myths, understanding 'normal' physiology, the effects of alcohol); use of sensate focus techniques. Persistent problems should be referred to an expert.

Premature ejaculation The inability to control ejaculation adequately for both partners to enjoy the sexual interaction. Ejaculation may occur immediately after penetration, or in the absence of an erection.

Differential diagnosis Delayed erection (prolonged stimulation needed to achieve adequate erection; short time to ejaculation); organic impairment (esp. pain); 'normal' rapid ejaculation in young or sexually inexperienced men (control is learned with practice); secondary to psychological stressors; transient problem following a period of reduced sexual activity.

Management Expert advice should be sought for complex cases or where there is associated orgasmic dysfunction/lack or loss of sexual desire.

Sympathetic partner is crucial to successful management. General education (specific issues of 'normal' time before ejaculation occurs). Reduction of 'performance anxiety' (as for **Orgasmic dysfunction**). Use of self-help guides.[2] Specific exercises may include: the 'stop–start' technique (see Box 12.6), the 'squeeze technique' (see Box 12.7), and sensate focus (see 📖 p. 475).

Non-organic dyspareunia Pain during intercourse in men; usually has a physical cause (e.g. urethral infection, scarring secondary to STD, tight foreskin) that can be directly treated. If psychological factors are the root cause, reassurance, education, and use of relaxation and cognitive techniques may be helpful. Complex cases require expert management.

Box 12.6 The stop–start technique (Semans' technique)

Developed by Masters and Johnson;[1,2] effective in up to 90% of cases of premature ejaculation.

Aims: To increase the frequency of sexual contact and increase the sensory threshold of the penis.

Setting: Best performed in the context of *sensate focus* exercises—to ensure non-genital areas are focused on first (less threatening for anxious individuals, allowing the recognition of sensations leading up to ejaculation, and may make the 'quality' of the sexual experience better), to limit the number of 'accidental' ejaculations (that may discourage couples early on), and increase good communication and cooperation.

Technique:
- Stimulation of the penis until high arousal (but not the ejaculation threshold) is achieved.
- Cessation of stimulation for a few minutes to allow arousal to subside.
- Repetition 4–5 times until ejaculation is permitted.

Box 12.7 Squeeze technique

If control does not develop using the 'stop–start' technique, this method may be used to inhibit the ejaculatory reflex:
- Stimulation of the penis until high arousal (but not the ejaculation threshold) is achieved.
- The man (or his partner) applies a firm squeeze to the head of the penis for 15–20 seconds. (Forefinger and middle finger are placed over the base of the glans and shaft of the penis, and the thumb applies pressure on the opposite side at the base of the undersurface of the glans.)

Note: this technique should be practised before high arousal occurs to establish how firmly the penis may be squeezed without causing pain.

1 Masters WH and Johnson VE (1966) *Human sexual response.* New York: Bantam Books.
2 Masters WH and Johnson VE (1980) *Human sexual inadequacy.* New York: Bantam Books.

1 Williams W (1985) *It's up to you.* Sydney: Maclennan and Petty.
2 Zilbergeld B (1980) *Men and sex.* London: Fontana.

Disorders of sexual preference 1: general aspects[1]

Essence

Disorders of sexual preference (the term used in ICD-10) or paraphilias (the term used in DSM-IV) are disorders in which an individual is sexually aroused by inappropriate stimuli. Other terms used include sexual deviation and perversion. There is some overlap between these disorders, sex offending, and inappropriate sexual behaviour, but the three are separate concepts. Homosexuality was previously included, but this is no longer the case.

Disorders of sexual preference are one of three broad types of sexual disorders. The others are gender identity disorders and sexual dysfunctions (see Table 12.3). In some cases two or more of these are present.

Definition

DSM-IV defines each paraphilia as at least 6mths of recurrent, intense, sexually arousing fantasies, sexual urges, or behaviours involving a particular inappropriate act or object. These fantasies, urges, or behaviours must cause clinically significant distress or impairment in social functioning. ICD-10 has less strict and less detailed criteria, referring to the particular object or act as being the most important source of sexual arousal or essential for satisfactory sexual response.

Classification

There are many different objects and acts that may be the focus of disorders of sexual preference. Most of the defined categories are extreme forms of behaviours that are common parts of 'normal' sexual activity. The classification systems in DSM-IV and ICD-10 are very similar (see Table 12.3). A disorder of sexual preference may be present in addition to other mental disorders.

Aetiology

Physiological factors These may include genetic factors, prenatal influence of hormones *in utero*, hormonal abnormalities in adults, and perhaps brain abnormalities.

Psychological theories These include absence of effective father with overprotective/close binding/intimate mother; failure of successful resolution of oedipal conflict; modelling and conditioning; masculine insecurity.

The various factors may lead to sexual deviation by (a) preventing normal sexual development and relationships, and/or (b) promoting deviant sexual interest.

Epidemiology

It is difficult to estimate the prevalence of these disorders as many individuals do not present for help and are unlikely to admit to sexually deviant arousal in surveys. Rates of sexual offending do not give a good approximation of rates of disorders of sexual preference, as these disorders represent one of many factors that may lead to such offending (see 📖 p681). There is probably a wide range of sexual practices in the 'normal' population. Disorders of sexual preference are more common in males than females (perhaps 30 times more common). From clinical samples, age of onset is usually between 16 and 20, and many individuals have multiple paraphilias, in series and/or in parallel.

Table 12.3 Classification of disorders of sexual preference

ICD-10	DSM-IV	Sexually arousing object or act
Fetishism	Fetishism	Non-living object (e.g. clothing, shoes, rubber).
Fetishistic transvestism	Transvestic fetishism	Cross-dressing (not few articles but complete outfit, perhaps with wig and make-up). Clear association with sexual arousal distinguishes from transsexual tranvestism. However, may be an early phase in some transsexuals.
Exhibitionism	Exhibitionism	Exposure of genitals to strangers.
Voyeurism	Voyeurism	Watching others who are naked, disrobing, or engaging in sexual acts.
Paedophilia	Paedophilia	Children (usually prebubertal or early pubertal). May be specified as attracted to males, females, or both, or as limited to incest.
Sadomasochism	Sexual masochism	Being humiliated, beaten, bound, or made to suffer.
	Sexual sadism	Psychological or physical suffering of others.
—	Frotteurism	Touching and rubbing against non-consenting person.
Other disorders of sexual preference	Paraphilia not otherwise specified	Includes telephone scatalogia (obscene phone calls), necrophilia (corpses), partialism (exclusive focus on part of body), zoophilia (animals), coprophilia (faeces), urophilia (urine), klismaphilia (enemas), autoerotic asphyxia (self-asphyxiation).
Multiple disorders of sexual preference	—	Many individuals manifest multiple disorders. Term 'polymorphous perversity' has been used. Most common combination is fetishism, transvestism, and sadomasochism.

---

1 Abel GG and Osborn CA (2000) The paraphilias. In: Gelder MG, Lopez-Ibor JJ, Andreasen NC (eds), *New Oxford textbook of psychiatry, Vol, 1*, pp. 897–913. Oxford: Oxford University Press.

Disorders of sexual preference 2: assessment and management[1]

Assessment

Why is the person presenting now?
- May present directly or at request of spouse when behaviour is discovered or starts to cause problems in relationships. Occasionally present as sexual dysfunction, with disorder of preference coming to light on further assessment.
- May present at own request, or more likely at request of court, prosecutor, or solicitor, after committing offence.

Is there another mental disorder?

Various psychiatric disorders may lead to release of sexually deviant behaviour, perhaps in individuals who have experienced fantasies but not acted on them previously. Particularly important to exclude in someone presenting for first time in middle age or later. So full psychiatric history, MSE, and perhaps neurological examination/investigation important.

Psychosexual assessment

Full psychosexual assessment essential in anyone presenting with sexual problems. Interviewer should put person at ease and be able to facilitate by being open, sensitive, and able to discuss sexual matters. Involvement of sexual partner in assessment (either at the same time or through another interview) is usually helpful. Following areas should be covered:
- *Sexual knowledge* and sources of information
- *Sexual attitudes* to self and others
- Age of onset and development of sexual interest, masturbation, dating, sexual intercourse
- *Relationship history*, including: age of self and partner, gender of partners, duration, quality, problems, abuse
- *Fantasy* (content/use/development)
- *Orientation*
- *Drive* (frequency of masturbation/intercourse) and *dysfunction* (specific inquiry about arousal, impotence, premature ejaculation)
- *Experience* (range of sexual behaviours with specific enquiry about paraphilias)
- *Current sexual practices*: mood, thoughts, visual images, material used, and conditions for arousal during both intercourse and masturbation (many men with paraphilias report 'normal' intercourse although at the time they are imagining deviant scenarios); where various forms of arousal are reported, estimate proportion of sexual practice devoted to each.

What does the person want from treatment?
- Do they want help at all or have they just come as they have been forced to (by spouse, courts, etc.)?
- Do they want to change the focus of their sexual arousal and/or desist from the overt behaviour?
- Do they want to adapt better to the behaviour without changing it?
- Are they motivated to engage in treatment?

Further investigations
Physical examination and investigations may be indicated, particularly if sexual dysfunction coexists. Penile plethysmography, polygraphy, and visual reaction times may be useful in assessing paraphilias.

Management
General issues
Treatment should not be imposed on people who do not want it. Patients should realize that treatment will take considerable effort on their part. The aims of treatment should be clear from the beginning. Broadly, there are three possible aims:
- Better adjustment without changing the behaviour.
- Desisting from overtly problematic behaviour but retaining 'deviant' arousal.
- Changing the focus of the arousal.

Where treatment is aimed at change, the following may need to be addressed:
- Encouraging development of 'normal' relationships.
- Addressing sexual inadequacy (perhaps using approaches similar to those for sexual dysfunction).
- Develop interests, activities, and relationships that will fill the time previously taken up by fantasizing about, preparing for, and taking part in the deviant activity.
- Decreasing masturbation to deviant fantasies and encouraging masturbation to more appropriate fantasies.

Specific treatment approaches
Physical treatments Neurosurgery and bilateral orchidectomy ('castration') of historical interest only. Various medications have been used: antipsychotics, oestrogens, progestogens, luteinizing hormone-releasing analogue, anti-androgens, and SSRIs. There is evidence for the efficacy of cyproterone acetate (an anti-androgen) and medroxyprogesterone acetate (a progestogen) in the treatment of hypersexuality and paraphilias. Recently, SSRIs have been used increasingly, and some use them first-line due to their relative lack of side-effects.

Psychodynamic psychotherapy Individual and group approaches have been used, ranging from sophisticated psychoanalysis to primarily supportive therapy.

Cognitive behavioural therapy Specific techniques may be used to decrease deviant (covert sensitization, aversive therapy, masturbatory satiation, biofeedback) and increase 'normal' arousal (orgasmic reconditioning, shaping, fading, exposure to explicit stimuli, biofeedback, systematic desensitization). Controversially used to treat homosexuality until the 1970s. Social skills training, assertiveness training, sexual education, and relapse prevention can also be helpful. Addressing cognitive distortions regarding sex, women, or children may also be important.

1 Brockman B and Bluglass R (1996) A general psychiatric approach to sexual deviation. In: Rosen I: (ed.), *Sexual deviation*, 3rd edn, pp. 1–42. Oxford: Oxford University Press.

Transsexualism 1: diagnosis

Transsexualism is a disorder of gender identity characterized by the desire to live and be accepted as a member of the opposite sex, usually accompanied by a sense of discomfort with one's anatomical sex. Transsexuals usually come to psychiatric attention, not because they wish to change these feelings, but in order to gain the psychiatrist's support for onward referral to specialist gender services with the eventual aim of gender reassignment +/- sex reassignment surgery (SRS).

Gender disorder specialists are usually specially trained psychiatrists who work as part of an extended team of specialists which may include gender surgery, endocrinology, psychology, specialist counsellors and speech therapy. There are few large specialist clinics within the UK and many areas are supported by smaller services which refer on to a larger regional service for surgical intervention. The aim of the gender disorder specialist is to make an accurate and appropriate diagnosis, to assess and treat comorbidities, and to provide ongoing support through the period of assessment, transition, and beyond.

Aetiology Primary cause not understood. Most transsexuals report that their gender dysphoria was present from early childhood. A range of explanatory models has been suggested but there is little evidence for one theory over another. Karyotype and phenotypic development is normal.

Epidemiology Estimated incidences are based on those who seek help for gender reassignment or gender dysphoria. Reported figures range widely between countries and cultures. In the UK male to female (MTF) 1 in 7500; female to male (FTM) 1 in 31 000. MTF to FTM ratio is 3–4:1 in most samples.

Diagnosis Transsexual identity should have been present for at least 2yrs, and must not be a symptom of another mental disorder, such as schizophrenia, or associated with any intersex, genetic, or chromosomal abnormality.

Differential diagnosis *Transvestism*—the wearing of clothing of the opposite sex without the purpose of sexual arousal, often described as a stress alleviating activity, not associated with the core belief of incorrect gender found in transsexuals; *fetishistic transvestism*—the wearing of clothes of the opposite sex for the purposes of sexual arousal but not associated with the ideal of living as the opposite sex; *dual role transvestism*—individual spends time split between male and female role without the desire to transition completely, they are clear regarding retaining biological sex persona and genitalia; *dysmorphobia*—focus of individual's dissatisfaction is with their primary or secondary sexual characteristics, the desire is for change or removal of genitalia rather than any wish to change gender; *third sex*—individual identifies self as a 'third' sex or 'neutral' sex, presents without identification with either gender and may request medical surgical help to remove sexual characteristics and function; *intersexed condition*—ruled out by normal karyotyping and normal primary and sexual characteristics for the birth sex; *schizophrenia*—occasionally associated with a delusion that the patient is the wrong sex or is changing sex.

Comorbidity Self-harming and suicidal gestures are seen and may be directed at underscoring the need for surgery. Genital mutilation is rare. Some MTF transsexuals work in the sex industry and have consequent increased risk of STDs and HIV infection. There is an increased incidence of other mental disorders including depression, personality disorders, obsessive–compulsive disorder, anorexia nervosa, conversion disorders, and coincidental psychosis.

Transsexualism 2: management

Assessment Many patients will arrive with their diagnosis ('I am a transsexual') and preferred treatment option (hormones and sex reassignment surgery) already fixed in their minds. The aim of assessment is to establish the diagnosis with certainty and to identify significant comorbidities and contraindications to treatment such as psychotic illness, major depression, substance misuse, and personality disorder. The majority of patients with confirmed diagnosis of transsexualism on initial psychiatric assessment will be referred on to specialist gender services.

- *History taking* Full psychiatric history with the addition of a detailed history of gender development, sexual history, and discussion of gender dissatisfaction.
- *Physical assessment* This may have already have been performed by the referring service or by GP or may be recommended following assessment—weight and BMI, cardiovascular status, evidence of abnormal clotting or thrombotic disease, additional number of blood tests may be required (including FSH, LH, sex hormone binding globulin, testosterone, dihydrotestosterone, oestradiol, prolactin, bone metabolic parameters, lipid profile). In biological males PSA and testicular examination should be considered, in biological females routine smear tests should be up to date.
- *Third party history/confirmation* Information from patients' families, employers, friends, and any other supportive persons is not only extremely helpful in determining diagnosis but can also be vital in recruiting support for the patient. Families of younger transsexual patients usually need support, guidance, and education if they are to cope with a child's transition.

Treatment

- *Psychological treatment* Treatments aimed at altering the core beliefs are ineffective in the majority of cases and are generally not welcomed by the patient. If the diagnosis of transsexualism is made then the psychiatrist's role is supervision of the transition, with liaison with the primary care and surgical teams and psychological support during the inevitable difficulties.
- *Real-life test* Most centres require a successful 'real-life test' of at least one year prior to consideration for surgery. During this time the patient undertakes to live full time and attempt to find employment in the new sex. Patients will change their name and 'come out' to friends and family.
- *Hormones (male to female)* Synthetic oestrogen (e.g. ethinylestradiol) and anti-androgen (e.g. finasteride or cyproterone acetate) treatment produces feminization effects including some breast and hip development, and skin softening, body fat redistribution, diminished libido and erectile function. There is no effect on voice pitch and speech therapy may be required to produce an acceptable female vocal pattern. Negative effects include increased risk of thromboembolic disease, abnormal liver function, increased risk of breast cancer, emotional dysregulation.

- *Hormones (female to male)* Testosterone treatment (via injection or gel) produces muscle development, male pattern hair growth, suppression of menstruation, some lowering of vocal pitch, growth of clitoris, increased aggression, increased libido. Negative effects: abnormal liver function, polycythaemia, artherogenic lipid profile increasing risk of cardiac disease, osteoporosis.
- *Surgery (male to female)* Sex reassignment surgery involves orchidectomy and penectomy with vaginoplasty using penile skin. The cosmetic results can be good, although candidates vary in their ability to be orgasmic post-surgery. Some patients may undergo breast augmentation, facial feminization procedures, and thyroid chondroplasty.
- *Surgery (female to male)* Sex reassignment surgery involves bilateral mastectomy, hysterectomy, and bilateral salpingo-oophorectomy. Phalloplasty is undertaken in less than half of patients as current techniques are neither cosmetically acceptable or functional for penetration.

Legal In the UK the Gender Recognition Act 2004 allows transsexual individuals to change their legal gender and be issued with a new birth certificate reflecting their current, rather than birth, gender. Evidence of the change of gender (which does not have to include sex reassignment surgery) is presented to a Gender Recognition Panel at least two years after transition to the new gender.

Prognosis No RCTs are available comparing SRS with other treatment. Cohort follow-up studies report >90% of patients reporting improvement following SRS on measures of psychological adjustment, absence of regret, and vocational adjustment. Specialist services report significant improvements in patients, general well-being and quality of life in those who have been appropriately assessed and supported. Reversion to former gender is very uncommon and is most likely in individuals where pre-assessment has been insufficient.

Chapter 13

Personality disorders

The concept of personality disorder

Essence

Personality describes the innate and enduring characteristics of an individual which shape their attitudes, thoughts, and behaviours in response to situations. We all recognize, amongst people we know well, some who manifest certain characteristics more than others: shyness, confidence, anger, generosity, tendency to display emotions, sensitivity, and being pernickety to name but a few. When these enduring characteristics of an individual are such as to cause distress or difficulties for themselves or in their relationships with others then they can be said to be suffering from *personality disorder* (PD). PD is separate from mental illness, although the two interact.

Definition

The following definition is based on ICD-10 and DSM-IV (both are very similar). PDs are enduring (starting in childhood or adolescence and continuing into adulthood), persistent, and pervasive disorders of inner experience and behaviour that cause distress or significant impairment in social functioning. PD manifests as problems in **cognition** (ways of perceiving and thinking about self and others), **affect** (range, intensity, and appropriateness of emotional response), and **behaviour** (interpersonal functioning, occupational and social functioning, and impulse control). To diagnose PD, the manifest abnormalities should not be due to other conditions (such as psychosis, affective disorder, substance misuse, or organic disorder) and should be out of keeping with social and cultural norms.

Development of the concept

The development of clinical concepts of conditions which would today be recognized as PD started in the early nineteenth century, at a time when the main two groups of mental conditions acknowledged by psychiatrists were insanity and idiocy. It became clear that there were individuals who were neither insane (i.e. suffering from delusions or hallucinations) nor clearly idiots, imbeciles, or morons (to use the then contemporary terminology for learning disability), but who nevertheless had abnormalities in their behaviour.

In 1801 Pinel described non-psychotic patients with disturbed behaviour and thinking as 'manie sans délire', while the term 'moral insanity' was introduced by Prichard in 1835. 'Moral' then meant 'psychological' (rather than the modern meaning concerning ethics), and amongst the patients described were people who had affective disorders as well as people who were personality disordered. Koch in 1873 described 'psychopathic inferiority', making the socially maladaptive nature of the disorder the key to diagnosis.

Kraeplin is reported as finding 'the classification of PD defeating'. Nonetheless, he attempted to find a place for the description of its subtypes within his evolving classification system. In 1921 he postulated that the PDs as they were then described were biologically related to the major psychotic and affective illnesses.

In 1927 Schneider introduced a classification system which can be seen as a forerunner of the current categorical approaches in DSM-IV and ICD-10. He did not use a spectrum concept, but saw PD as representing a pronounced and maladaptive variation of normal personality traits and used social deviance as a diagnostic marker for his ten subtypes.

The individual PD subtypes in use today derive from a number of different academic and theoretical backgrounds: antisocial (dissocial) PD from child psychiatric follow-up studies; borderline, histrionic, and narcissistic PDs from dynamic theory and psychotherapeutic practice; schizoid and anankastic PDs from European phenomenology; and avoidant PD from academic psychology. Notably absent from the list of academic sources is the psychological study of normal personality which has developed a trait model of normal personality along a varying number of axes (📕 p. 493).

Controversy

There is ongoing debate about the clinical usefulness, diagnosis, categorization and description of PD. A frequently repeated criticism of the present clinical concept has been the problem of tautology. That is, the same features displayed by a patient which suggest a diagnosis of PD are then 'explained' by the presence of that diagnosis. For example a patient may, among other features, display 'an incapacity to experience guilt' and 'a low threshold for discharge of frustration, including violence'. This may lead to an ICD-10 diagnosis of dissocial PD. It is then illogical to use that same diagnosis to 'explain' a subsequent episode of violence without remorse in that individual.

Some psychiatrists believe that psychiatry has *no* role in the treatment of people with PDs. They argue that:

- Personality is by definition unchangeable.
- There is no evidence that psychiatry helps individuals with PD.
- These people are disruptive and impinge negatively on the treatment of other patients.
- These people are not ill and are responsible for their behaviour.
- Psychiatry is being asked to deal with something that is essentially a social problem.

On the other hand there are those who believe that people with PD clearly fall within the remit of psychiatry, arguing:

- People with PD suffer from symptoms related to their disorder.
- They have high rates of suicide, other forms of premature death, and of other mental illnesses.
- There are treatment approaches which are effective.
- Their opponents are rejecting patients because they dislike them.
- The problem is not that these people cannot be helped but that traditional psychiatric services do not provide the type of approach and services that are necessary.

'Normal' personality

Psychologists have sought to conceptualize and describe the variations in normal personality. There are two main approaches: **nomothetic and ideographic**.[1] In general these approaches have developed separately from concepts of abnormal personality and PD.

Nomothetic approaches

Personality seen in terms of attributes shared by individuals. Two subdivisions: **type (or categorical) approaches** (discrete categories of personality); and **trait (or dimensional) approaches** (a limited number of qualities, or traits, account for personality variation). Type approaches dominate the description and classification of PD, but trait approaches are pre-eminent in modern personality psychology.

Type approaches These describe individual personality by similarity to a variable number of predefined archetypes. These may attempt to include all aspects of personality and behaviour—the 'broad' models—or they may describe one aspect of personality—the 'narrow' models. An example of the former is the humoral model of Hippocrates which described four fundamental personality types (choleric, sanguine, melancholic and phlegmatic); an example of the latter is the type A vs. type B model which describes groups of behaviours exhibited by people at higher and lower risk of cardiac disease.

Trait approaches These view a variable number of traits as continuous scales along which each person will have a particular position; the positions on all the traits represent a number of dimensions which describe personality. Examples include: *Eysenck's three-factor theory* (neuroticism, extraversion, psychoticism); *Costa and McCrae's five-factor model* (neuroticism, extraversion, openness, agreeableness, conscientiousness); *Cloninger's seven-factor model* (novelty-seeking, harm avoidance, reward dependence, persistence, self-directedness, cooperativeness, self-transcendence; originally only first 3 factors); *Cattell's sixteen-factor theory*. A consensus has emerged from personality questionnaire research and from lexical approaches that there are five fundamental traits (the 'big five') similar to those of Costa and McCrae. The heritability of personality traits in twin and adoptive studies has been found to be moderately large (about 30%).

Ideographic approaches

Unlike nomothetic approaches, these emphasize individuality and seek to understand an individual's personality by understanding that individual and their development rather than by reference to common factors. Examples are psychoanalytic, humanistic, and cognitive–behavioural approaches. The first two have little scientific validity and the last has compromised with trait theorists.

Is personality stable?

Are there traits which are persistent and predict a person's behaviour over time in a number of situations? Situationists have argued that the situation was a stronger determinant of behaviour than personality traits. However, more recent research has demonstrated the long-term stability of a number of personality traits and, perhaps unsurprisingly, most now agree that both the situation and personality traits are important in determining behaviour.

1 Deary I and Power M (1998) Normal and abnormal personality. In: Johnstone EC, Freeman CPL, and Zeally AK (eds) *Companion to psychiatric studies*, 6th edn, pp. 565–96. Edinburgh: Churchill Livingstone.

Classification of personality disorder

It is largely accepted that normal personality is best described and classified in terms of dimensions or traits. Although this also applies to PD, our current psychiatric classifications are categorical. The various categories of PD described in ICD-10 and DSM-IV have a number of origins: psychodynamic theory, apparent similarities between certain PDs and certain mental illnesses, and descriptions of stereotypical personality types. The various categories used come together in a piecemeal and arbitrary fashion and do not represent any systematic understanding or study of PD. The categorical classification of PD is psychiatric classification at its worst.

There are a number of important points to bear in mind when using standard categorical approaches in the diagnosis of PDs:

• Due to their heterogeneous origins, there is overlap between the criteria for some categories.
• It is more common for individuals to meet the criteria for more than one category of PD than to meet only the criteria for a single category.
• When making a diagnosis one should use all the categories for which a person meets the criteria.
• If a person meets criteria for more than one category, then they do not suffer from more than one actual disorder. A person has a personality and this may or may not be disordered. If it is disordered it may have various features which are rarely described adequately by a particular category.
• Clinically it is more important to understand and describe the specific features of a person's personality than it is to assign them to a particular category.
• The diagnosis of PD is a particular area where one may believe, wrongly, that one has a better understanding of a person by assigning them to a specific category (an example of 'tautology').[1]

ICD-10 and DSM-IV

The PD categories in ICD-10 and DSM-IV are set out in Table 13.1. The two schemes are similar, but there are categories that appear in one but not the other, and for some categories different terms are used. Each category has a list of features, a number of which should be present for the person to be diagnosed as manifesting that particular aspect of PD. DSM III (and subsequent editions) placed PD on a separate axis (along with other developmental disorders in axis II) from mental illness (axis I); see 📖 p. 1042.

---

1 Tautology (the restatement of the same information using different words) is a particular danger in psychiatry generally, and the diagnosis of PD in particular. For example, saying that someone has 'borderline' traits gives a gloss of understanding to the simple fact that a person repeatedly self-harms, without actually communicating any new information (except perhaps the 'therapeutic despair' of the psychiatrist!).

Table 13.1 ICD-10 and DSM-IV classifications of personality disorder

ICD-10	DSM-IV*	Description
Paranoid	Paranoid	Sensitive, suspicious, preoccupied with conspiratorial explanations, self-referential, distrust of others.
Schizoid	Schizoid	Emotionally cold, detachment, lack of interest in others, excessive introspection and fantasy.
(Schizotypal disorder classified with schizophrenia and related disorders)	Schizotypal	Interpersonal discomfort with peculiar ideas, perceptions, appearance, and behaviour.
Dissocial	Antisocial	Callous lack of concern for others, irresponsibility, irritability, aggression, inability to maintain enduring relationships, disregard and violation of others' rights, evidence of childhood conduct disorder.
Emotionally unstable– impulsive type	—	Inability to control anger or plan, with unpredictable affect and behaviour.
Emotionally unstable– borderline type	Borderline	Unclear identity, intense and unstable relationships, unpredictable affect, threats or acts of self-harm, impulsivity.
Histrionic	Histrionic	Self-dramatization, shallow affect, egocentricity, craving attention and excitement, manipulative behaviour.
—	Narcissistic	Grandiosity, lack of empathy, need for admiration.
Anxious (avoidant)	Avoidant	Tension, self-consciousness, fear of negative evaluation by others, timid, insecure.
Anankastic	Obsessive– compulsive	Doubt, indecisiveness, caution, pedantry, rigidity, perfectionism, preoccupation with orderliness and control.
Dependent	Dependent	Clinging, submissive, excess need for care, feels helpless when not in relationship.

*DSM-IV uses three broader clusters to organize the categories of personality disorder—cluster A (odd/eccentric)—paranoid, schizoid, schizotypal; cluster B (emotional/dramatic)—antisocial, histrionic, narcissistic, borderline; and cluster C (fearful/anxious)—avoidant, dependent, obsessive–compulsive. Although this may seem sensible, there is no particular validity to this clustering.

Psychopathy and 'severe' personality disorder

Psychopathy

The terms 'psychopathy', 'psychopathic PD', 'psychopathic disorder', and 'psychopath' have dominated much of the PD literature until relatively recently. In England and Wales the 2007 revision to the 1983 MHA has removed the description of 'psychopathic disorder' as one of the subcategories of mental disorder. The term should probably now be reserved for individuals meeting criteria as defined by the Psychopathy Checklist—Revised (PCL-R) as an extreme form of antisocial or dissocial PD (Box 13.1).

Psychopathy Checklist—Revised (PCL-R)[1]

In *The mask of sanity* Cleckley[2] described various features of psychopathy referring to cold, callous, self-centred, predatory, parasitic individuals. This concept has led to the development of the PCL-R, which measures the extent to which a person manifests the features of this prototypical psychopath. The items of the PCL-R are listed in Box 13.1. Psychopathy as defined by the PCL-R is strongly correlated with risk of future violence. It defines a narrower group of individuals than antisocial or dissocial PD, and individuals scoring highly commonly fulfil the criteria for antisocial, narcissistic, histrionic, paranoid, and perhaps borderline categories in DSM-IV.

Severe personality disorder[3]

The term 'severe personality disorder' is often used but has no clear meaning or definition. Severity of PD has been defined in various ways:
- In terms of severe impact on social functioning.
- By using the PCL-R cut-off and being synonymous with psychopathy.
- By defining severity as the presence of features fulfilling the criteria for multiple categories of DSM-IV or ICD-10 PDs (sometimes this is further defined by stating that the categories should be from at least two DSM-IV clusters, and perhaps that one must be from cluster B).

None of these approaches is entirely satisfactory, and each defines different but overlapping groups of individuals.

Box 13.1 Notes on the PCL-R

The items of the PCL-R cover the affective, interpersonal, and behavioural features of psychopathy. Assessment is based on a comprehensive records review and in-depth interview(s). Each item is rated 0 (absent), 1 (some evidence but not enough to be clearly present), or 2 (definitely present). There are detailed descriptions of each item in the coding manual. The summed score (out of 40) gives an indication of the extent to which a person is psychopathic and may be converted into a percentile using reference tables for different populations. In the USA a score of 30 or above is used as a cut-off to diagnose 'psychopathy'; in the UK this cut-off is 25 or above.

PCL-R items

1. Glibness/superficial charm
2. Grandiose sense of self-worth
3. Need for stimulation/proneness to boredom
4. Pathological lying
5. Conning/manipulative
6. Lack of remorse or guilt
7. Shallow affect
8. Callous/lack of empathy
9. Parasitic lifestyle
10. Poor behavioural control
11. Promiscuous sexual behaviour
12. Early behaviour problems
13. Lack of realistic, long-term goals
14. Impulsivity
15. Irresponsibility
16. Failure to accept responsibility for own actions
17. Many short-term marital relationships
18. Juvenile delinquency
19. Revocation of conditional release
20. Criminal versatility

1 Hare RD (1991) *The Hare psychopathy checklist-revised*. Toronto: Multi-Health Systems.
2 Cleckley H (1941) *The mask of sanity*. London: Henry Klimpton.
3 Tyrer P (2004) Getting to grips with severe personality disorder. *Crim Behav Ment Hlth* **14**: 1–4.

Aetiology of personality disorder

While there is no single, convincing theory explaining the genesis of PD, the following observations are suggestive of possible contributing factors.

Genetic

Evidence of heritability of 'normal' personality traits; some evidence of heritability of cluster B PDs; familial relationship between schizotypal PD and schizophrenia, between paranoid PD and delusional disorder, and between borderline PD and affective disorder. There is no good evidence for a relationship between XYY genotype and psychopathy.

Neurophysiology

'Immature' EEG (posterior temporal slow waves) in psychopathy; functional imaging abnormalities in psychopathy (e.g. decreased activity in amygdala during affective processing task); low 5-HT levels in impulsive violent individuals; autonomic abnormalities in psychopathy (slowed galvanic skin response).

Childhood development

Difficult infant temperament may proceed to conduct disorder in childhood and PD; ADHD may be a risk factor for later antisocial PD; insecure attachment may predict later PD (particularly disorganized attachment); harsh and inconsistent parenting and family pathology are related to conduct disorder, and may therefore be related to later antisocial PD; severe trauma in childhood (such as sexual abuse) may be a risk factor for borderline PD and other cluster B disorders.

Psychodynamic theories

Freudian explanations of arrested development at oral, anal, and genital stages leading to dependent, obsessional, and histrionic personalities; 'borderline personality organization' described by Kernberg (diffuse unfiltered reaction to experience prevents individuals from putting adversity into perspective leading to repeated crises); narcissistic and borderline personalities seen as displaying primitive defence mechanisms such as splitting and projective identification; some see antisocial personalities as lacking aspects of superego, but more sophisticated explanation is in terms of a reaction to an overly harsh superego (representing internalization of parental abuse).

Cognitive–behavioural theories

There are maladaptive schemata (stable cognitive, affective, and behavioural structures representing specific rules that affect information processing). These schemata represent core beliefs which are derived from an interaction between childhood experience and pre-programmed patterns of behaviour and environmental responses. Schemata are unconditional compared with those found in affective disorders (e.g. 'I am unlovable' rather than 'If someone important criticizes me, then I am unlovable') and are formed early, often pre-verbally.

Theories synthesizing cognitive–behavioural and psychodynamic aspects

The following are two quite similar models that underlie relatively recently introduced therapies for borderline PD.

Cognitive–analytical model (see 📖 p. 858) Borderline patients experience a range of partially dissociated 'self-states', which arise initially as a response to unmanageable external threats and are maintained by repeated threats or internal cues (such as memories). Abusive experiences in childhood lead to internalization of the harsh parental object leading to intrapsychic conflict which is repressed or produces symptomatic behaviours. Deficits in self-reflection, poor emotional vocabulary, and narrow focus of attention lead to incoherent sense of self and others.

Dialectical behavioural model (see 📖 p. 856) Innate temperamental vulnerability interacts with certain dysfunctional ('invalidating') environments leading to problems with emotional regulation. Abnormal behaviours which are manifested represent products of this emotional dysregulation or attempts to regulate intense emotional states by maladaptive problem-solving.

Epidemiology of personality disorder[1]

The measurement of the prevalence of PD of any type and of specific categories of PD in any population has a number of problems: in earlier studies PD and other mental disorders were mutually exclusive, not allowing for the recording of comorbidity; studies differ in the method used to make a diagnosis (interviews/case notes/informants; clinical diagnosis versus research instruments; emphasis on current presentation or on life history); and in some studies subjects were only allowed to belong to one category of PD.

Findings regarding PD of any type will be considered separately from findings related to specific PD categories (see Table 13.2).

Personality disorder of any type

- *Community:* rates of PD in the community have been found to be 2–18% (the generally accepted approximate is 10%). It is more prevalent in younger adults, and may be more prevalent in males.
- *Primary care:* of patients presenting with conspicuous psychiatric morbidity, 5–8% will have a primary diagnosis of PD. The rate of comorbid PD in patients with other primary diagnoses is 20–30%.
- *Psychiatric patients:* 30–40% of outpatients and 40–50% of inpatients have a PD, not usually as a primary diagnosis. A primary diagnosis of PD occurs in about 5–15% of inpatients.
- *Other populations:* 25–75% of prisoners have a PD. Antisocial PD is most prevalent, but many prisoners fulfil the criteria for more than one diagnostic category, and many personality disordered prisoners do not meet the criteria for the antisocial category.

1 Casey P (2000) The epidemiology of personality disorder. In: P Tyrer (ed.), *Personality disorders: diagnosis, management and course*, pp. 71–9. Oxford: Butterworth Heinemann.

Table 13.2 Specific categories of personality disorder

The prevalence rates of the categories of personality disorder (most studies have used DSM categories, so these are used here) in the general population are approximately:

DSM-IV	Prevalence (%)
Paranoid	0.5–3
Schizoid	0.5–7
Schizotypal	0.5–5
Antisocial	2–3.5
Borderline	1.5–2
Histrionic	2–3
Narcissistic	0.5–1
Avoidant	0.5–1
Dependent	0.5–5
Obsessive–compulsive	1–2

Relationship between personality disorder and other mental disorders

The current state of classification and understanding of the aetiology and pathogenesis of mental disorders is such that most psychiatric diagnoses are based on descriptive criteria. It is common to find that an individual meets the criteria for an axis I disorder along with a PD. At one extreme, both may be a manifestation of the same underlying condition; at the other, they may represent two completely separate aetio-pathogenic entities.

The relationship between PD and other mental disorders may be:

- *Mutually exclusive* Personality disorder cannot be diagnosed in an individual with another mental disorder. The personality pathology displayed is a manifestation of the other mental disorder, and giving a separate personality diagnosis has no purpose. This was the only approach possible prior to DSM-III's introduction of multi-axial diagnosis. This approach is not favoured by current classification systems, even where the two appear to be manifestations of the same condition.
- *Coincidental* In an individual, PD and another disorder may come together by chance. However, epidemiologically there is support for an association between PD and other mental disorders.
- *Associative* Both in individual cases and epidemiologically there are a number of reasons why the coexistence of PD and other mental disorders may be more than just coincidental:
  - Sharing common aetiology (but separate disorder).
  - Prodromal (part of the development of the axis I disorder).
  - Part of spectrum (a 'partial' manifestation of the axis I disorder).
  - Vulnerability (a separate disorder, manifestations of which make an individual more likely to suffer from an axis I disorder).

Problems in assessing personality in patients with other mental disorders

A number of problems may arise in the diagnosis of PD in people who appear to have axis I disorders:

- Underlying PD may be missed as assessment may focus on the current mental state disorder.
- PD may be misdiagnosed as axis I disorder and vice versa.
- In an individual with PD, an axis I disorder may be missed or misconstrued as being part of the PD.

In such cases it is important to remember that axis I pathology is common in people with PDs and any change in the presentation of a patient with PD may be due to this. Equally, it is important to base assessment of personality on information (preferably from a number of sources) on the premorbid functioning of an individual, rather than on their current functioning or just their own account of their previous functioning (their memory or interpretation of which may be coloured by their current mental state).

Comorbidity between personality disorders and other specific mental disorders[1]

Strong associations
- Avoidant PD and social phobia (possibly because they both describe a group of people with the same condition).
- Substance misuse and cluster B PDs.
- Eating disorders and cluster B and C PDs (particularly bulimia nervosa and cluster B).
- Neurotic disorders and cluster C PDs (it has been suggested that these individuals have a 'general neurotic syndrome').
- Somatoform disorders and cluster B and C PDs.
- Habit and impulse disorders and cluster B PDs (unsurprisingly).
- PTSD and borderline PD (this is not borderline PD redefined as chronic PTSD, but is probably due to the increased rate of life events and vulnerability of such individuals).

Moderate associations
- Schizotypal PD and schizophrenia (also a weaker association between schizophrenia and antisocial PD).
- Depression and cluster B and C PDs.
- Delusional disorder and paranoid PD.

Impact of personality disorders on manifestation, treatment, and outcome of other mental disorders

Although the concept of 'comorbid PD' may seem spurious from an aetio-pathological perspective, its presence has an impact on the presentation, treatment, and outcome of axis I disorders, and it is therefore useful to recognize such comorbidity from a clinical perspective.
- **Presentation** The presentation of axis I disorders may be distorted, exaggerated, or masked by the presence of an underlying PD.
- **Treatment and outcome** The presence of comorbid PD will usually make treatment more difficult and worsens the outcome of axis I disorders. This may be due to problems in the following areas: help-seeking behaviours, compliance with treatment, coping styles, risk-taking, lifestyle, social support networks, therapeutic alliance, alcohol and substance misuse.

Some contend that it is the presence of this comorbidity which makes it more likely for a person to fail to respond to standard primary care treatment approaches, therefore necessitating referral to psychiatric services.

1 Tyrer P (2000) Comorbidity of personality disorder and mental state disorders. In: Tyrer P (ed.), *Personality disorders: diagnosis, management and course*, pp. 71–9. Oxford: Butterworth Heinemann.

Assessment of personality disorder[1]

Potential pitfalls

There are a number of potential pitfalls in the assessment and diagnosis of personality disordered patients:

- Relying on diagnoses made by others (psychiatrists are notoriously poor at diagnosing PD).
- Failing to recognize comorbidity.
- Misdiagnosing PD as mental illness, and vice versa.
- Inadequate information.
- Negative countertransference (basing diagnosis on your negative reaction to a patient rather than on an objective assessment; transference and countertransference may be a part of this but negative feelings towards an individual should not be the primary basis for a diagnosis of PD).
- Applying ICD-10 or DSM-IV categories without a broader assessment of personality.

Making the diagnosis of personality disorder

- A clinical diagnosis of PD should be based on an accurate assessment of a person's enduring and pervasive patterns of emotional expression, interpersonal relationships, social functioning, and views of self and others *when they are not suffering from another mental disorder.*
- In many cases information from sources other than the patient will be essential. Potential sources of information include: clinical interviews (perhaps repeated); observation (usually repeated); previous records (medical, prison, school, social work); independent accounts (perhaps from several sources such as relatives and other professionals).
- Information from various areas of the *psychiatric history* (childhood and adolescence; work record; forensic history/other aggression or violence; relationship history; psychiatric contact/self-harm) will give an indication of a person's personality and whether it may be disordered.
- In addition, specific enquiry can be made regarding the following aspects of *personality*: interests and activities; relationships; mood/ emotions; attitudes (religious, moral, health); self-concept; coping with difficulties; specific characteristics or traits (perhaps based on PD categories); include both positive and negative aspects.
- In describing personality and PD, first the features of a person's personality should be described, then a decision should be made as to whether the degree of distress and disruption due to personality traits is such as to indicate the presence of PD, then the features that are pathological should be described. If one wants to make categorical diagnoses then the category or categories for which the criteria are met may be stated.

Instruments to assess personality disorder

There are a number of instruments available for assessing PD. Such instruments are mainly used in research, and are rarely seen in clinical practice. Most require training and some take a considerable amount of time to complete.

Self-report questionnaires Millon Clinical Multiaxial Inventory (MCMI), Personality Disorder Questionnaire (PDQ-IV), Wisconsin Personality Inventory (WISPI).

Structured clinical interviews with patient only Structured Clinical Interview for DSM-IV Personality Disorder (SCID-II), Diagnostic Interview for DSM-IV Personality Disorders (DIPD-IV).

Structured clinical interviews with informant only Standardized Assessment of Personality (SAP).

Structured clinical interviews with patient and/or informant Personality Assessment Schedule (PAS), Structured Interview for DSM-IV Personality Disorders (SIDP-IV).

Instruments assessing specific personality disorders Schedule for Interviewing Borderlines (SIB), Diagnostic Interview for Borderline Patients (DIB), Borderline Personality Disorder Scale (BPD-Scale), Psychopathy Checklist-Revised (PCL-R), Psychopathy Checklist-Screening Version (PCL-SV), Schedule for Schizotypal Personalities (SSP).

Diagnostic instruments including an assessment of antisocial personality disorder Diagnostic Interview Schedule (DIS), Feigner Diagnostic Criteria.

Functional assessment

The functional assessment of personality and associated problems has been proposed as a useful clinical approach which can produce a formulation identifying issues to be addressed in management.

- **List abnormal personality traits**—thoughts about self and others (e.g. identity problems, paranoia, grandiosity, magical thinking, exaggerating, suggestibility, preoccupation with death, obsessionality, self-esteem), feelings and emotions (e.g. depression, elation, mood instability, callousness, loneliness, anger, irritability), behaviour (e.g. stubbornness, quarrelsomeness, sadism, self-destructiveness, compliance, impulsivity, theatricality, attention-seeking), social functioning (e.g. social isolation, controlling others, dependence on others, mistrust of others, inviting rejection, forming unstable intense relationships, manipulating and using others), insight (including the ability to understand and integrate one's thoughts, feelings, and actions).
- **Describe associated distress and comorbid axis I disorders.**
- **Describe interference with functioning**—occupational, family and relationships, offending/violence.

1 Gunn J (2000) Personality disorder: a clinical suggestion. In Tyrer P (ed.), *Personality disorders: diagnosis, management and cause*, pp. 44–50. Oxford: Butterworth Heinemann.

Management of personality disorder 1: general aspects

It is generally felt that PD is resistant to specific psychiatric treatment. However, there is no good evidence to either refute or support this statement. Patients often present at a time of crisis and/or when they develop a comorbid axis I disorder. Although some may wish to, psychiatrists cannot avoid having to manage patients with PD.

Principles of successful management plans[1]

A successful management plan in PD is tailored to the individual's needs andjj explicitly states jointly agreed and realistic goals. The approach to these patients should be consistent and agreed across the services having contact with the patient. Plans should take a long-term view, recognizing that change, if it comes, will only be observable over a long period.

Possible management goals

Potential management goals include: psychological and practical support; monitoring and supervision; intervening in crises; increasing motivation and compliance; increasing understanding of difficulties; building a therapeutic relationship; limiting harm; reducing distress; treating comorbid axis I disorders; treating specific areas (e.g. anger, self-harm, social skills); and giving practical support (e.g. housing, finance, childcare).

Managing comorbid axis I disorders

It is important to recognize and treat comorbid axis I pathology in patients with PD. Standard treatment approaches should be used, taking into account aspects of the patient's personality (e.g. impulsivity and an antiauthoritarian attitude may lead to non-compliance with medication).

Understanding and managing the relationship between the patient and staff[2]

Rejection for treatment of patients with PD (even when they present with mental illness) is often due to the intense negative feelings these patients may engender, and the disruptive and uneasy relationships they form with those that try to help them. Just as they do in many of their interpersonal relationships, patients with PDs display disordered attachment in their relationships with staff (whether with individuals or with a service). When dealing with such patients this needs to be recognized, acknowledged, and managed. An acceptance of, and tolerance for, these difficulties needs to be combined with continuing commitment to the patient. However, patients, staff, and other agencies need to realize there are no instant solutions and that psychiatric services cannot take responsibility for all adverse behaviours.

Admission to hospital

Patients with PD benefit little from prolonged admissions to conventional psychiatric units. Admission to such units may be necessary when there is a specific crisis (usually in the short term) or when the patient presents with an axis I disorder. Longer-term admission for the treatment of PD could be undertaken in a therapeutic community. Involuntary long-term hospitalization of patients with PD primarily to prevent harm to others where there is little prospect of clinical benefit to the patient is ethically dubious.

Managing crises

Individuals with PD often present in crisis. This may follow life events, relationship problems, or occur in the context of the development of comorbid mental illness. In some cases the crisis may follow what appears to the outside observer to be a relatively minor or non-existent stressor. Where patients repeatedly present in crisis it can be helpful for the various professionals involved to plan what the response should be in such situations. A consistent response is important, but there should be sufficient flexibility to deal with changes in circumstances. For example, where a patient repeatedly presents with self-harm it may be appropriate for out-patient treatment to continue following any necessary medical treatment; however, if this patient presents threatening suicide following the death of a partner, then it may be appropriate to arrange admission to hospital. Other approaches to individuals presenting with threats of self-harm or of violence and to manipulative patients are covered on 📖 p. 994.

1 Davison SE (2002) Principles of managing patients with personality disorder. *Advances in Psychiat Treat* **8**: 1–9.
2 Adshead G (1998) Psychiatric staff as attachment figures. Understanding management problems in psychiatric services in the light of attachment theory. *Br J Psychiat* **172**: 64–9.

Management of personality disorder 2: specific treatments[1,2]

Medication[3]

The main indication for medication in patients with PD is the development of comorbid mental illness. There is no good evidence that medication has any effect on PD itself. The positive findings from studies have been short-term, and probably due to the effects of medication on comorbid disorders rather than on the PD itself. Bearing this in mind, the following have been suggested:

- **Antipsychotics** may be of some benefit in cluster B (particularly borderline) and cluster A (particularly schizotypal and perhaps paranoid) disorders.
- **Antidepressants** may be of benefit in impulsive, depressed, or self-harming patients (particularly borderline), and in cluster C (particularly avoidant and obsessive–compulsive) disorders.
- **Anticonvulsants and lithium** have been suggested where there is affective instability or impulsivity.

Therapeutic community

A therapeutic community is a consciously designed social environment and programme within a residential or day unit, in which the social and group process is harnessed with therapeutic intent. It is an intense form of psychosocial treatment in which every aspect of the environment is part of the treatment setting, in which interpersonal behaviour can be challenged and modified. The main principles are democratization, permissiveness, communalism, and reality confrontation. There are various interactions between patients and staff both individually and in groups, particularly in the daily community groups, which contribute towards achieving these principles. There is some evidence that such treatment is effective with some patients with PDs.

Dialectical behavioural therapy (DBT) (📖 p. 856)

Combination of individual and group therapy lasting at least 12mths. In stage 1, individual therapy focuses on a detailed cognitive–behavioural approach to self-harm and other 'therapy interfering' behaviours. Internal and external antecedents are explored, and alternative problem-solving strategies are developed. Group therapy focuses on tolerance of distress, emotional regulation and interpersonal skills. 'Mindfulness training' based on Eastern meditation techniques is a key part of this. In stage 2, patients are helped to process previous trauma, but only when stage 1 skills are developed. In stage 3, the focus is on developing self-esteem and realistic future goals. Another aspect of DBT is that patients may contact therapists by telephone between sessions to help them apply skills when difficulties arise. There is evidence that DBT may be an effective therapy for out-patients with borderline PD.

Cognitive analytic therapy (📖 p. 858)

May be appropriate for some patients with borderline PD. Aims to identify different 'self-states' and associated 'reciprocal role procedures' (patterns of relationships learned in early childhood). Patients are helped to observe and change thinking and behaviour related to these self-states. Countertransference helps provide useful information about 'reciprocal role relationships' either through identification with the patient or reacting to their projections. The aim is for patients to be able to recognize their various 'self-states' and to be aware of them without dissociating.

Psychodynamic therapy (📖 p. 840)

Classic Freudian or Jungian psychoanalysis is of no proven benefit for patients with PD, and is probably contraindicated in patients with severe PDs. However, psychodynamic concepts are extremely useful in understanding personality disordered patients and the reactions they provoke in others, including ourselves. Modified psychodynamic approaches for patients with borderline and narcissistic PDs have been developed.

Cognitive behavioural therapy (📖 p. 850)

Schema-focused therapy concentrates on identifying and modifying early maladaptive schemas and related behaviours. Patients are educated about schemas and led to expect that they will be difficult to change (for example, patients will distort new information to fit in with their existing schemas). 'Empathic confrontation' is used to help patients to repeatedly and persistently challenge their core beliefs about themselves and others. Issues related to interpersonal schemas may arise in the therapeutic relationship and be used as 'data' for dealing with these schemas.

There are other models used in cognitive behavioural therapy to treat PD, but all have in common: the goal-directed problem-solving approach; the teaching of specific skills; a longer timescale than the relatively brief length of therapy for most other disorders; emphasis on developing, maintaining, and utilizing the therapeutic relationship; a focus on underlying core beliefs (schemas) regarding self and others; and, a longer-term historical perspective in therapy as opposed to the here-and-now focus with many other disorders.

1 Davidson K and Tyrer P (2000) Psychosocial treatment in personality disorder. In Tyrer P (ed.), *Personality disorders: diagnosis, management and cause*, pp. 90–100. Oxford, Butterworth Heinemann.
2 Deary I and Power M (1998) Normal and abnormal personality. In Johnstone EC, Freeman CPL and Zeally AK (eds), *Companion to psychiatric studies*, 6th edn, pp. 565–96. Edinburgh: Churchill Livingstone.
3 Tyrer P (2000) Drug treatment of personality disorder. In Tyrer P (ed.), *Personality disorders: diagnosis, management and cause*, pp. 126–32. Oxford: Butterworth Heinemann.

Outcome of personality disorder[1]

Morbidity and mortality

High rates of accidents, suicide, and violent death, particularly where cluster B features are prominent. As mentioned already, there are high rates of other mental disorders.

Outcome of other disorders in patients with personality disorder

The outcome of mental illness and physical illness is worse in patients with PDs.

Persistence of personality disorder

Some contend that PD is by definition lifelong and therefore has a poor prognosis, but the evidence for this is far from conclusive.

Comparison between different age groups

Personality disorder is less prevalent in older adults than younger adults, particularly for cluster B disorders. In terms of 'normal' personality, compared with young adults the elderly are more likely to be cautious and rigid, and less likely to be impulsive and aggressive. However, cross-sectional studies looking at different age groups at one point in time tell us little about the development of personality in individuals over time.

Follow-up of individuals over time

Antisocial/dissocial Children presenting to child services with antisocial behaviour are 5–7 times as likely to develop antisocial PD as those presenting with other problems. May show some improvement in antisocial behaviour by fifth decade. However, may just change with time from 'overt' criminal behaviour to more 'covert' antisocial behaviour such as domestic violence and child abuse. There is contradictory evidence as to whether 'burnout' or 'maturation' in later life really does occur.

Borderline A third to a half of patients fulfilling the criteria for borderline PD do not have PD at all when followed up after 10–20yrs. About a third continue to have borderline PD and others have other predominating PDs. Poor prognostic indicators are severe repeated self-harm and 'comorbid' antisocial personality; a good prognostic indicator may be an initial presentation with comorbid affective disorder.

Schizotypal Generally have poorer prognosis than borderline patients. About 50% may develop schizophrenia.

Obsessional May worsen with age. More likely to develop depression than OCD.

Clusters There is some evidence that cluster A traits worsen with age, cluster B traits improve, and cluster C traits remain unchanged.

---

1 Tyrer P and Seivewright H (2000) Outcome of personality disorder. In Tyrer P (ed.), *Personality disorders: diagnosis, management and cause*, pp. 105–25 Oxford: Butterworth Heinemann.

Old age psychiatry

Psychiatric illness in older people and psychogeriatrics

Psychogeriatrics, or old age psychiatry, is a comparatively new specialty which has developed over the last 50yrs in response to demographic changes and the growth of geriatric medicine. It was inspired by the 'social psychiatry' movement and growing emphasis on the care and welfare of vulnerable sectors of the population.

Psychiatric illnesses in older people include:

• Pre-existing psychiatric disorders in the ageing patient.
• New disorders related to the specific stresses and circumstances of old age (e.g. bereavement, infirmity, dependence, sensory deficits, isolation).
• Disorders due to the changing physiology of the ageing brain, as well as psychiatric complications of neurological and systemic illnesses.

Psychiatric problems often coexist with physical problems, and treatment strategies need to take account of this (as well as the different pharmacokinetics of the older patient). Furthermore, the elderly are more likely to manifest physical symptoms of psychiatric disorder than younger adults. Cognitive assessment and physical examination are always essential parts of psychiatric management of the older person. Dementia is generally the main focus of interest in psychogeriatrics, but the discipline also concerns itself with depressive illness, paranoid states, and other late-onset problems.

Since older people are often dependent on others, consideration of the role and the needs of carers are important aspects of holistic care. Psychiatric care of the elderly interfaces with multiple services, both state and independent (e.g. social services, housing and welfare services, the legal system, charity organizations, and religious institutions).

The demographics of old age

In developed countries such as the UK, the elderly population has been increasing steadily over the last century. For example, in the UK the percentage of the population older than 65yrs was 5% in 1900, 15% in 2003, and is projected to be 24% in 2034.[1] This trend is largely attributed to the decline in infant mortality, control of infectious diseases, and improvement in sanitation, living standards, and nutrition as well as a declining birth rate. The implications of increasing elderly people in society are many, including a drop in the proportion of the working population, an increase in overall disability and health needs, and a corresponding increase in the need for both health and social services.

In terms of psychiatric disorders, it is well known that certain disorders increase in frequency with advancing age. For example, 5% of people older than 65yrs suffer from moderate to severe dementia and the prevalence increases to over 30% of those over 85yrs.[2] The prevalence of other disorders in people >65yrs is approximately: 1.1% for schizophrenia; 1.4% for bipolar disorder; and 12.5% for neurosis and personality disorder.[3]

Other research has shown a particularly high prevalence of mental disorder among elderly people in sheltered accommodation. Of the 80 000 persons in the UK who die in care homes annually, up to two thirds have some form of dementia. Up to two thirds of patients >65yrs in general hospital wards have psychiatric disorder; of these, 20% may suffer from delirium, 31% from dementia and 29% from depression at any one time.[4] Finally, it is regrettably also the case that psychiatric disorders are commonly either undiagnosed or misdiagnosed at primary care level. Having said this, research has demonstrated a marked improvement over the last decade in both diagnosis and management at this level.

The role of the old age psychiatrist[5]

- **Advocate** Together with various pressure groups, the old age psychiatrist is an active proponent of the interests of the elderly, whether it comes to sourcing funding or providing education to the public in an effort to dispel the stigma attached to ageing.
- **Teacher** An old age psychiatrist is well placed to provide education in both medical and non-medical contexts. Medical and nursing students, across-discipline specialists and trainees, school pupils, community forum and service organizers may all benefit from their expertise.
- **Health educationalist/promoter** Holistic care of the elderly includes both health education and preventative intervention.
- **Student** Psychogeriatrics is a major arena of new research, while the changing demography of ageing requires the old age psychiatrist to make academic forays into other disciplines such as sociology, history, and human geography.
- **Innovator** The relative infancy of the discipline means that individuals working in this area have had the opportunity to be creative and innovative in developing appropriate services.
- **Team player** The multidisciplinary nature of old age psychiatry means that the old age psychiatrist engages with professionals and lay people both in the community and in institutions.
- **'Missionary'** The concept and practice of psychogeriatrics originated in the UK and was spread to North America, Australia, and the rest of Europe by a core of zealots. A number of international organizations have formed and the global challenges for the twenty-first century include expanding the discipline within developing countries as well as finding new strategies for caring for the growing numbers of elderly people within the first world.

1 Butler R and Brayne C (1998) Epidemiology. In Butler R and Pitt B (eds), *Seminars in old age psychiatry*, pp. 16–27. London: Gaskell.
2 Jorm AF, Korten AE, and Henderson AS (1987) The prevalence of dementia: a quantitative integration of the literature. *Acta Psychiat Scand* **76**: 465–79.
3 Kay DW, Beamish P, and Roth M (1964) Old age mental disorders in Newcastle upon Tyne. I. A study of prevalence. *Br J Psychiat* **110**: 146–58.
4 Who Cares Wins (2005) RCPsych. http://www.rcpsych.ac.uk/PDF/WhoCaresWins.pdf
5 Jolley D (1999) The importance of being an old age psychiatrist. In Howard R (ed), *Everything you need to know about old age psychiatry*, pp. 107–19. Petersfield: Wrightson Biomedical Publishing Ltd.

Normal ageing[1]

Neurobiology of ageing

- The **weight** of the brain decreases by 5% between ages 30 and 70yrs, by 10% by the age of 80, and by 20% by the age of 90. There is a proportionate increase in **ventricular size** and size of the **subarachnoid space**.
- **MRI** shows changes affecting grey and white matter, reduction in volume prominent in the hippocampus, association cortices, and cerebellum.
- **CBF** in frontal and temporal lobes and thalamus decreases with age.
- There is some **nerve cell loss** in the cortex, hippocampus, substantia nigra, and Purkinje cells of the cerebellum, but less than was thought previously and reductions in dendrites and synapses are thought to be more important. The cytoplasm of nerve cells accumulates a pigment (**lipofuscin**), while there are also changes in the components of the cytoskeleton.
- **Tau protein** (links neurofilaments and microtubules) can accumulate to form **neurofibrillary tangles (NFTs)** in some nerve cells. In normal ageing NFTs are usually confined to cells of the hippocampus and entorhinal cortex.
- **Senile plaques** (extra-cellular amyloid and neuritic processes) are found in the normal ageing brain in the neocortex, amygdala, hippocampus, and entorhinal cortex.
- **Lewy bodies** (intracellular inclusions) occur normally and are confined to the substantia nigra and the locus coeruleus.
- **Hirano bodies** occur in new hippocampal pyramidal cells.
- **Amyloid deposits** (β-amyloid and A4 amyloid) may be widespread in superficial cortical and leptomeningeal vessels as well as patchy within the cortex.

Psychology of ageing

- **Cognitive assessment** is often complicated by physical illness or sensory deficits.
- **IQ** peaks at 25yrs, plateaus until 60–70, and then declines.
- **Performance IQ** drops faster than verbal IQ, which may be due to reduced processing speed or to the fact that verbal IQ depends largely on familiar 'crystallized' information while performance IQ involves novel, fluid information.
- **Problem-solving** deteriorates due to declining abstract ability and increasing difficulty applying information to another situation.
- **Short-term/working memory (WM)** shows a gradual decrease in capacity and this is worse with complexity of task and memory load.
- **Long-term memory (LTM)** declines, except for remote events of personal significance which may be recalled with great clarity.
- There is a characteristic pattern of **psychomotor slowing** and impairment in the manipulation of new information.
- Tests of well-rehearsed skills such as **verbal comprehension** show little or no decline.

Social problems of old age

With the breakdown of traditional family structures in many societies, increasing numbers of elderly live alone or in homes for the aged. Losses include: loss of status, loss of independence, and loss of spouse/partner. Most elderly have limited income and are unemployed. Increase in medical problems compounds the dependency and care needs. The elderly face variable degrees of isolation, marginalization, and stigmatization.

1 Bittles AH (2009) The biology of ageing. In Gelder M, Andreasen N, Lopez-Igor J, and Geddes J (eds), *New Oxford Textbook of Psychiatry*, pp. 15 007–110. New York: Oxford University Press.

Multidisciplinary assessment

Elderly people suffering from mental health problems often have a range of psychological, physical, and social needs. This implies that individual assessment, management, and follow-up requires collaboration between health, social, and voluntary organizations and family carers. Assessment of the older patient with mental illness includes the following:

- Full history from the patient, family, and carers.
- Full physical and neurological examination.
- MSE, including full cognitive assessment.
- Functional assessment (evaluation of ability to perform functions of everyday living).
- Social assessment (accommodation; need for care; financial and legal issues; social activities).
- Assessment of carers' needs.

The best place for performing an assessment is in the patient's home. A domiciliary visit has the advantage of being more convenient and relaxing for the patient and it provides the health carer with an opportunity to assess living conditions, social activities, and medications kept in the house. In addition, family members, neighbours, and carers may be available for interviewing. Historically, day hospital may then be involved in more complex cases, but these now tend to be replaced by intensive home assessment and treatment teams that can also lead to admission being avoided in some cases. Sometimes brief admission is indicated, especially if the elderly person has pressing physical or psychiatric needs or if support is unavailable (or desperately needs respite). Obviously a full assessment may involve doctors, nurses, occupational therapists, psychologists, social workers, voluntary workers, legal professionals, and others involved with the elderly.

In obtaining a thorough history it is important to allow the patient to tell their own story. One needs to enquire about the presenting problem and how it has evolved, whether it is a new or long-standing problem, and whether the individual has a personal or family history of mental problems. In addition, enquire about losses, social history, and social circumstances (housing, income, social activities, etc.), medical problems and medications, alcohol history, and presence or absence of family support and carers. It is particularly important to assess activities of daily living such as level of independence, ability to cook, shop, pay accounts, maintain the home, and cope with bathing, toilet, laundry, etc.

MSE needs to include an assessment of sight and hearing as well as determining the presence or absence of anxiety or mood symptoms, thoughts of suicide, abnormal beliefs or perceptions, and cognitive impairment. Cognitive assessment must include: orientation; memory; concentration and attention; language, praxis, and simple calculation; intelligence; insight; and judgement. An MMSE will incorporate these elements (see 📖 p. 70). There is a wide range of rating scales for assessing mental state, cognitive performance, activities of daily living, and carer burden—see Burns et al.[1] (2002) for an overview.

Key questions for carers include:[2]

- Relationship to the patient.
- Amount of care provided.
- Degree of stress they are under.
- What help they would accept.
- Understanding and knowledge of the patient's illness.
- What expectations they have from services.
- Their awareness of support or voluntary organizations.

1 Burns A, Lawlor B, and Craig S (2002) Rating scales in old age psychiatry. *Br J Psychiat* **180**: 161–7.
2 Butler R and Pitt B (1998) Assessment. In Butler R and Pitt B (eds), *Seminars in old age psychiatry*, pp. 1–16. London: Gaskell.

Specific aspects of psychiatric illnesses in the elderly 1: overview and neuroses

Overview

The range of psychiatric illnesses in the elderly is very similar to that in younger people. However, the individual factors that contribute to aetiology, clinical presentation, and management strategy differ due to the specific biopsychosocial conditions of old age. In order to grasp a full understanding of elderly psychopathology it is necessary to appreciate the physiological, psychological, and sociocultural factors unique to this age group. Disorders in the elderly may present with some 'classic' symptoms (common to adult psychopathology), but very often their clinical manifestation varies significantly due to the unique conditions of old age. The following pages focus on the 'unique' features of psychiatric illnesses in the elderly.

Neuroses

Prevalence Depression and anxiety are common in old age. There is no decline in their prevalence with advancing age, but of concern is the fact that there is a reduction in referrals to psychiatry. This may be due to increased acceptance of symptoms by the elderly or due to deficiencies in detection by health professionals. The estimated prevalence of neurotic disorders is 1–10% with a female predominance and roughly equal frequency of 'old' and 'new' cases.

Clinical features Non-specific anxiety and depressive symptoms predominate and hypochondriacal symptoms are often prominent. Obsessional, phobic, dissociative, and conversion disorders are less common. Factors such as physical ill health, immobility, and lack of social support may give rise to fear and lack of confidence about going out of the home—this has been termed 'space phobia'.

Aetiology Multiple factors may contribute to new neurotic symptoms in the elderly. Among these, major life events, physical illness, feelings of loneliness, impaired self-care, and 'insecure' personality style are most common.

Differential diagnosis Physical illness; acute or chronic organic brain disease; affective disorders.

Management

- The mainstay of treatment is to identify and manage aetiological factors. This obviously very often calls for social interventions and thus a multidisciplinary approach is essential.
- Counselling may be difficult especially where older people have had limited exposure to psychological methods but there is increasing evidence for the efficacy of CBT in the elderly.
- Antidepressants may be indicated for severe and disabling symptoms and are certainly preferable to BDZs.

Specific aspects of psychiatric illnesses in the elderly 2: mood disorders

Epidemiology Less than 10% of new cases of mood disorder occur in old age. Episodes occur more frequently and last longer. Studies suggest that mood disorders in the elderly have a worse prognosis and there may be a tendency towards chronicity. Gender differences in prevalence also diminish with advancing age. Prevalence of clinically significant **depression** is 10% for those >65yrs, with 2–3% being severe. Rates of depression differ depending on setting: 0.5–1.5% in the community; 5–10% of clinical out-patients; 10–15% of clinical inpatients with up to 30% of inpatients suffering from at least mild depression; 15–30% of those in residential and nursing homes. **Mania** accounts for 5–10% of mood disorders in the elderly.

Aetiology Positive family history becomes less relevant in older-onset mood disorder. Physical illnesses are associated in 60–75% of cases. Major life events are common, as is the lack of a confiding and supportive relationship. Older patients are less likely to complain as losses are 'expected'. Neuroimaging yields conflicting results and brain changes noted may relate to the normal ageing process. The strongest imaging evidence for brain changes is for mania in men.

Clinical features

There are no clear distinctions between the clinical presentation of depression in the elderly and that in younger people. However, some symptoms are often more striking:
- Severe psychomotor retardation or agitation occurs in up to 30% of depressed elderly patients.
- A degree of cognitive impairment has been detected in 70% (esp. with effortful tasks).
- Depressive delusions regarding poverty, physical illness, or nihilistic in nature, are common (e.g. Cotard's syndrome, 📖 p. 89).
- Paranoia is also common, while derogatory and obscene auditory hallucinations may occur.
- Classic symptoms may not even be evident and the patient may instead present with somatic, anxiety, or hypochondriacal complaints. A high index of suspicion is required when older patients present with these symptoms, especially abnormal illness behaviour.

Pseudodementia A minority of retarded depressed elderly present with 'pseudodementia' (i.e. marked difficulties with concentration and memory). Features suggestive of pseudodementia include: previous history of depression; depressed mood; biological symptoms; 'islands of normality'; exaggerated symptoms; poor effort on testing, frequent comments such as 'I can't be bothered', 'it's too difficult' to relatively easy tasks; response to antidepressant medication. For some this may herald/uncover the onset of a dementia syndrome and there is a proven association between depressive pseudodementia and later diagnosis of dementia.

Mania or hypomania present a similar clinical picture as in younger patients; however, they are more often followed by a depressive episode in older patients. There is usually a history of bipolar affective disorder. A first episode of mania in an elderly person requires careful screening for cerebral or systemic pathology (e.g. stroke or hyperthyroidism).

Differential diagnosis Dementia—difficult to distinguish and can occur together, if in doubt best to treat; **paranoid disorder**—depressive paranoia and delusions may be difficult to distinguish from psychoses; **stroke**—especially after left frontal CVA or 2° to the lability, reactive stress, organic apathy, ↓ motivation, or drug side-effects associated with stroke; **Parkinson's disease**—drug side-effects in treating may suggest depressive illness; **other physical disorders** e.g. infection, hypothyroidism, tumours, alcohol, drug side-effects. *Note:* full physical investigation is vital.

Management

- **Antidepressants** TCAs are not absolutely contraindicated in the elderly, but care must be exercised in prescribing. ECG and BP monitoring is important due to postural drops as well as other cardiac problems. First-line is probably SSRIs due to ↓side-effects and relative safety in OD. Others include: SNRIs such as venlafaxine; and, occasionally, moclobemide (delayed hypotension a problem). General rules include: low starting dose; gradual increases; longer maintenance periods (up to 2yrs); beware of suicide risk; consider lithium augmentation. Caution needs to be observed when considering changing/reducing/stopping long-term antidepressants in this group as this not uncommonly may precipitate a relapse even in persons who have been stable for years.
- **ECT** (📖 p. 284) First-line treatment for severe illness and specifically where there is marked agitation, life-threatening stupor, suicidality, or contraindications, failure, or excessive side-effects of drugs. ECT is generally safe and effective. Dementia is not a contraindication. Post-ECT confusion may be a problem, in which case treatments should be given at longer intervals.
- **Psychological treatments** Therapies include: CBT for depression; supportive psychotherapy; bereavement counselling.
- **Treatment of mania** Age-appropriate doses of antipsychotics may be used, in particular haloperidol and risperidone. Lithium is first-line in prophylaxis but lower dosages are indicated (levels: 0.4–0.8 mmol/L) and regular thyroid and renal checks (at least three monthly) are essential. Also note that levels may easily change in the presence of infection, dehydration, and use of other medications (e.g. diuretics). Levels should be taken at 10–14hrs after last lithium dose. Following increase in lithium dose, 5–7 days should be allowed for serum levels to stabilize.

Prognosis Generally prognosis is good, especially: onset <70yrs; short illness; good previous adjustment; absent physical illness; good previous recovery. Poor outcome is associated with: severity of initial illness; psychotic symptoms; physical illness; poor medication compliance; severe life events during follow-up period.

Specific aspects of psychiatric illnesses in the elderly 3: psychoses

Psychotic illness in the elderly may be classified as follows:
- 'Old psychosis'—the 'graduate' population.
- 'New psychosis'—late-life schizophrenia or late paraphrenia.
- Other conditions with paranoid and/or hallucinatory symptoms (Box 14.1)

Old psychosis

With the advent of antipsychotic drugs in the 1950s, there followed a progressive decrease in the numbers of long-stay patients with schizophrenia in institutions. Thus more and more ageing patients with chronic schizophrenia moved into the community, and in countries such as the UK and USA, many of these patients are increasingly referred to psychogeriatric services. Caution needs to be observed when considering changing/reducing/stopping long-term antipsychotic in this group as this not uncommonly may precipitate a relapse even in persons who have been stable for years. It is advisable that the patient have a psychiatric review and opinion in this regard.

New psychosis

Paraphrenia—a term coined by Emil Kraepelin in 1909; described a psychotic illness characterized by delusions and hallucinations, without changes in affect (although there may be reactive anxiety), form of thought, or personality.

Late paraphrenia—described by Roth and Morrisey in 1952; they noted that this type of illness was the most common form of psychosis in old age (defined as >60yrs).

Epidemiology—relatively rare condition; population studies estimate <1% prevalence. Approximately 10% of admissions to psychiatric wards for the elderly will have the condition. One study showed that when ICD-10 criteria were used, 60% of cases were classified as paranoid schizophrenia, 30% as delusional disorder, and 10% as schizoaffective disorder.[1] Gender distribution is estimated at 4–9:1 female:male predominance.

Aetiology

- **Genetics** The risk of schizophrenia in 1st-degree relatives is 3.4% in late paraphrenics, compared with 5.8% in young schizphrenics, and less than 1% in the general population.[2]
- **Premorbid personality** of people with late paraphrenia is characterized by poor adjustment and it is estimated that nearly 45% show lifelong paranoid and/or schizoid traits.
- **Sensory impairments** such as deafness, of onset in middle life, increases risk of late paraphrenia.
- **Social isolation** and major **life events** may also contribute.
- **Organic factors** Structural imaging demonstrates mild ventricular enlargement; cerebrovascular pathology is a common comorbid finding.

Clinical features Persecutory delusions are the most common symptom of late paraphrenia (roughly 90% of patients) and tend to relate to commonplace themes (such as neighbours spying, entering the patient's home, moving items etc.). Other common delusions include: referential, misidentification, hypochondriacal, and religious. Auditory hallucinations (typically third person) occur in approximately 75%, while visual (13%), somatic/tactile (12%), and olfactory (4%) hallucinations are not uncommon.[3] Schneiderian 1st-rank symptoms are common (46%), while negative symptoms, thought disorder, and catatonia are extremely uncommon. 10–20% may present with delusions only.

Treatment
- Relieve isolation and sensory deficits.
- Establish rapport and develop a therapeutic alliance (often difficult!).
- Exclude cognitive or medical disorders.
- Hospital admission is often required.
- Low-dose atypical antipsychotics preferred as elderly are very sensitive to side-effects, but non-compliance secondary to lack of insight is often an issue.

Box 14.1 Other conditions with paranoid or hallucinatory symptoms

These include the following conditions:
- **Secondary paranoid states**—due to organic disorders or substances (see 📖 p. 130)
- **Delirium** (see 📖 p. 790)
- **Dementia** (see 📖 p. 132)
- **Affective disorders** (see 📖 p. 520)
- **Schizoaffective disorder** (see 📖 p. 218)

Hallucinations of sensory deprivation In the elderly, complex visual hallucinations can occur as a non-specific phenomenon, 2° to visual impairment—sometimes referred to as Charles Bonnet syndrome. Hallucinations may be well-formed, containing animals, people, or scenes. May be partial or complete insight. Differential diagnosis includes: Lewy body dementia (📖 p. 140), acute confusional state (📖 p. 790). Reassurance may be adequate, but in some cases a small dose of antipsychotic medication may reduce distressing symptoms.

---

1 Howard R, Castle D, Wessely S, et al. (1993) A comparative study of 470 cases of early-onset and late-onset schizophrenia. Br J Psychiat **163**: 352–7.

2 Kay DWK and Roth M (1961) Environmental and hereditary factors in the schizophrenias of old age (late paraphrenia) and their bearing on the general problem of causation in schizophrenia. J Ment Sci **107**: 649–86.

3 Almeida O (1998) Late paraphrenia. In Butler R and Pitt B (eds), Seminars in old age psychiatry, pp. 148–63. London: Gaskell.

Other mental health problems in the elderly

Alcohol problems

With decreasing tolerance for alcohol in advancing age, there is a corresponding increase in risk of intoxication and adverse effects. Risk factors for late onset of alcohol problems include: female gender; higher socioeconomic class; physical ill-health; precipitating life events; neurotic personality; psychiatric illness.

Principles of management

- Prognosis is good if alcohol problems commence secondary to practical problems.
- Encourage and facilitate involvement in non-drinking social activities.
- In extreme cases consider need for supervision of finances.
- Orientate towards reducing physical problems.
- Moving to residential care may reduce social isolation.

Caution must be displayed when detoxing the elderly from alcohol with benzodiazepines. There may be comorbid cognitive impairment which makes the patient more susceptible to benzodiazepine precipitated deliriums (secondary to use of too high doses), rather than alcohol withdrawal delirium, and this should always be considered in the differential diagnosis of, especially elderly, persons with a non-resolving delirium in this context.

Drug abuse

Generally, illicit substance abuse is not a significant problem in the elderly although with changing demographics this may become an increasing problem in the future. However, misuse of prescription drugs such as benzodiazepines, opiates, and analgesics frequently becomes a problem in this age group. Dependence on these medications may result from careless prescription of long-term treatments for common problems of ageing such as insomnia and arthritis. With the best of intentions, doctors sometimes believe that it is 'cruel' to withdraw patients from these medications, especially if the patient has been using the drug for years and is advanced in age. Underlying this belief is the common clinically evidenced precipitation of difficult to treat anxiety states. However, it is important to consider whether withdrawal may actually enhance quality of life by diminishing chronic side-effects such as depression.

Sexual problems

Factors influencing the sexual life of younger adults are relevant to older people too (e.g. social stresses, illness, and side-effects of medications). In addition, the elderly may experience added problems related to the specific physiological changes that accompany ageing. Dementia sufferers may become sexually demanding as part of the disinhibition that frequently characterizes this disorder. Health carers may fail to detect sexual problems experienced by older people as a sexual history is commonly overlooked. This may result from incorrect assumptions that carers often make regarding sexuality in this age group. The client too may assume that his or her sexual dysfunction is a 'normal' aspect of ageing. Some practical remedies are: hormone replacement therapy; vaginal lubricants and topical oestrogen; and, of course, sildenafil (Viagra).

Personality problems

Personality traits often become more prominent and rigid in old age; in particular, traits such as cautiousness, introversion, and obsessionality. Paranoid traits may intensify, especially in situations where there is increasing social isolation. In some cases increasing paranoia may be mistaken for a paranoid psychotic state such as delusional disorder. Psychopathy is said to burn out with advancing age and criminal behaviour is uncommon in the elderly. Roughly 5–10% of older people exhibit features of personality disorder and these individuals often come to the attention of health services when they are residents in homes for the elderly. Since personality disorder is by definition lifelong, any significant change in personality needs explanation. Both organic and functional brain disorders may manifest as 'a change in personality'. Personality problems are often the cause of **Diogenes syndrome**—also called senile squalor syndrome—in which eccentric and reclusive individuals become increasingly isolated and neglect themselves, living in filthy, poor conditions. They are often oblivious to their condition and resistant to help, necessitating intervention.

Suicide

Old age is a risk factor for suicide and it is estimated that approximately 20% of all suicides are of the elderly. There is a male predominance of 2:1 in this age group, as suicide rates tend to increase with age in men and decrease with age in women. The rate of elderly suicides declined markedly during the 1960s due to the detoxification of the mains gas supply.

Predictive factors for suicide in the elderly
- Increasing age.
- Male.
- Physical illness (35–85% cases).
- Social isolation.
- Widowed or separated.
- Alcohol abuse.
- Depressive illness, current or past (80% cases).
- Recent contact with psychiatric services.
- Availability of means.

Self-harm

Self-harm is relatively uncommon with older people, accounting for only 5% of cases. Gender distribution is roughly equal. An apparent parasuicide in this age group is much more likely to be a failed suicide and thus all parasuicides should be taken very seriously. It is important to exclude depression and also personality disorder as 90% have a depressive illness. Also 60% are physically ill; 50% have been previously admitted to a psychiatric hospital; and 8% go on to complete a suicide within 3yrs of a parasuicide.

Issues of elder abuse[1,2]

In recent decades the unfortunate problem of elder abuse has become increasingly recognized. It is often overlooked and requires an integrated response from multiple disciplines and agencies, including health and social services, the criminal justice system, and government. The need for a unified multidisciplinary approach cannot be emphasized enough as a fragmented response is fraught with problems.

Types of elder abuse Elder abuse is an all-inclusive term representing all types of mistreatment or abusive behaviour towards older adults. This mistreatment can be an act of commission (abuse) or omission (neglect), intentional or unintentional, and of one or more types:
- Physical, sexual, verbal, or psychological abuse.
- Physical or psychological neglect.
- Financial exploitation.

The abuse or neglect results in unnecessary suffering, injury, pain, or loss and leads to a violation of human rights and a decrease in the quality of life.

Epidemiology of elder abuse Occurs in both domestic and institutional settings:
- **Domestic settings** Approximately 4–6% of elderly people report incidents of abuse or neglect in domestic settings. The most common forms of abuse are verbal abuse and financial exploitation by family members and physical abuse by spouses. Gender distribution (of victims) is equal and economic status and age are unrelated to risk of abuse. Importantly, elder abuse is under-reported—450 000 older adults in domestic settings were abused, neglected, or exploited in the USA during 1996, of which only 70 000 were self-reported.
- **Institutional settings** No data exists for the extent of abuse within institutional settings. However, one survey of nursing home staff in a US state disclosed that 36% of staff had witnessed at least one incident of physical abuse in the preceding year, while 10% admitted having committed at least one act of physical abuse themselves.

Explaining elder abuse The main risk factors for elder abuse are: dependency and social isolation of the victim; carer has mental or substance misuse problems; absence of a suitable guardian. Factors vary according to the type of abuse; for example, dependency is a risk factor for financial or emotional abuse, but not necessarily for physical abuse. Also the causes of spouse abuse may differ from the causes of abuse by adult offspring.

An integrative response to elder abuse Prevention is the best approach and a number of measures have proved effective: training and support of carers; reducing isolation of elders; respite care; CPN visits; etc. Responding to abuse effectively requires a multidisciplinary approach and a proactive system of assessment of suspicious cases (a number of assessment instruments have been developed).[3,4] There may now also be legislation available to allow assessment and intervention, e.g. The Adult Support and Protection (Scotland) Act 2007.

1 Payne BK (2002) An integrated understanding of elder abuse and neglect. *J Crim Just* **30**: 535–47.
2 Wolf RS (1999) Suspected abuse in an elderly patient. *Am Fam Physician* **59**: 1319–20.
3 Fulmer T (2003) Elder abuse and neglect assessment. *J Gerontolog Nurs* **29**: 8–9.
4 Reis M (1998) Validation of the indicators of abuse (IOA) screen. *Gerontologist* **38**: 471–80.

Psychopharmacology in the elderly[1,2]

Pharmacokinetics The physiological changes associated with ageing mean that the older patient's system handles drugs quite differently from that of a younger individual.

- *Absorption* generally remains the same, although there are reductions in gastric pH and mesenteric blood flow.
- *Distribution* of drugs is altered, however: reduced body mass, body water, and plasma proteins, together with increased body fat cause increased levels of free drug and longer half-lives (especially of psychotropics).
- *Drug metabolism* is reduced due to decreased blood flow to the liver and loss of efficiency of liver microsomes.
- *Excretion* is reduced with the drop in renal clearance that accompanies old age. Thus drug effects are generally prolonged and cumulative and the risk of toxicity is high.

Pharmacodynamics Technology such as PET is enlightening our understanding of the direct effects of drugs in the CNS. Specific differences in these effects in the elderly include:

- **Dopaminergic system**—there are fewer DA cells in the basal ganglia; thus there is increased sensitivity to the EPSEs of neuroleptics (not dystonias).
- **Cholinergic system**—there is a normal reduction in cholinergic receptors with advancing age.
- **Noradrenergic system**—NE levels decrease with age, which may cause this age group to become increasingly vulnerable to mood disorders.
- **Narcotics and sedative hypnotics**—there is increased sensitivity to sedatives in the elderly due to a reduction in the number of available receptors.

The implications of these changes are that elderly patients are more sensitive to almost all drugs used in psychiatry. See Box 14.2.

Box 14.2 General principles of prescribing include:

- Start with a very low dose.
- Increases should be made slowly.
- Maximum efficacy is often achieved at significantly lower doses than in younger adults.
- Beware of dangerous side-effects such as postural hypotension, arrhythmias, and sedation.
- The elderly are particularly sensitive to EPSEs and anti-cholinergic side-effects.
- Beware of drug interactions due to common problem of polypharmacy in the elderly.
- Atypical neuroleptics are generally better tolerated than conventionals.
- SSRIs, SNRIs, and NARIs are generally safer than TCAs; while MAOIs and lithium may be useful in resistant depression.
- Monitor lithium therapy closely as levels can fluctuate easily and long-term effects on thyroid and renal function are not infrequent.
- Always consider suicide risk as old age is a risk factor for suicide.

1 Baldwin R and Burns A (1998) Pharmacological treatments. In Butler R and Pitt B (eds), *Seminars in old age psychiatry*, pp. 247–65. London: Gaskell.
2 Gareri P, Falconi U, De Fazio P, *et al.* (2000) Conventional and new antidepressant drugs in the elderly. *Progr Neurobiol* **61**: 353–96.

Services for the elderly[1,2]

Services for the elderly are organized differently according to government policies and availability of resources. In principle though, the ideal service should plan to:
- Maintain the elderly person at home for as long as possible.
- Respond quickly to medical and social problems as they arise.
- Ensure co-ordination of the work of those providing continuing care.
- Support relatives and others who care for the elderly at home.
- Promote liaison between medical and social and voluntary services.

Primary care services At the primary care level GPs, health visitors, community nurses, and health workers will deal with most of the problems of elderly people.

Acute and long-term hospital services Elderly patients often require admission for acute assessment and treatment, respite care, or long-term care. Services may be situated within general medical wards for the elderly or within specialized old age psychiatry units. The advantage of acute services being located in general hospitals rather than in psychiatric hospitals is that a range of associated specialist services (such as old age medicine, neurology, and radiology) is often more readily available.

Day and outpatient care Ideally a service should have outpatient facilities for the assessment, treatment, and follow-up of mobile elderly patients with mental health problems. Sometimes these clinics offer a specialist service such as the 'memory clinic'. Day-care services may take the form of a general or psychiatric day hospital, and local authorities often provide day centres and social clubs for functional and social support.

Community psychiatric nurses (CPNs) CPNs provide a vital link between primary care and specialist services. They often perform assessments on patients after receiving a referral from a GP. They also monitor treatment in collaboration with GPs and the psychiatric services. In addition, they take part in the organization of home support for the demented elderly.

Informal carers These are the unpaid relatives, neighbours, or friends who care for the elderly person at home. Demographic changes and the move to community care have increased the burden on carers. Informal carers are twice as likely to be women. Carers often suffer considerable stress, especially where the patient is suffering from advanced dementia. Relieving carer burden is a challenge for any service. Active involvement of medical and social personnel, as well as provision of education and respite, are important aspects of carer support.

Domiciliary services These include; home helps; meals at home; laundry and shopping services; emergency call systems. In some countries such as the UK, local authorities provide these services; however, in many others these services are either privately engaged, obtained from voluntary organizations, or are unavailable.

Residential and nursing care In most countries the local authorities take responsibility for providing old people's homes and other sheltered accommodation. These range in standard from large crowded institutions to small independent units and, ideally, they need to balance individual privacy with involvement in outside activities. In many communities private homes are available, but financial constraints put these out of the reach of the majority of older people. In planning residential care for the elderly, authorities need to provide for a wider range of accommodation: a small supported unit with 2 or 3 people may be ideal for the still independent and mobile individual; while larger homes with nursing support are required for those who are more dependent, with a number of physical and/or psychiatric needs.

1 Wertheimer J (1997) Psychiatry of the elderly: a consensus statement. *Int J Geriat Psychiat* **12**: 432–5.
2 Gelder M, Gath D, Mayou R, *et al.* (1996) *Oxford textbook of psychiatry*, 3rd edn. Oxford: Oxford University Press.

The end of life, living wills, and withdrawal of active treatment

The end of life Managing a patient's final weeks or days and ensuring that their death is a 'good death' is a challenge that has only recently been addressed in our health services and training programmes.[1] Many health professionals have never received any guidance regarding their involvement in this common and extremely important phase of people's lives. Contemporary palliative services stress the following components in providing a 'good death':

- A multidisciplinary approach
- Ability to 'diagnose dying'
- Communication with patient and family
- Provision of adequate physical support (e.g. analgesia, hydration)
- Minimize unnecessary interventions
- Establish a non-resuscitation plan
- Psychological, social, cultural, and spiritual support

Living wills A living will is an advance directive (usually written and witnessed), also referred to as an anticipaitatory care plan, made by an individual regarding their preferences for future treatment during a terminal illness. Usually the person specifies the degree of irreversible deterioration after which they want no further life-sustaining treatment. They may also give clear instructions refusing certain medical interventions. If a health professional is asked to assist someone in drawing up a living will, the following issues should be considered:

- the patient should be fully informed about the illness and treatment options;
- the patient should be mentally competent;
- the patient should be reflecting his/her own views, free from influence.

The health carer is required to abide by the living will, although basic care (i.e. analgesia, catheter, fluids) should be provided in all cases. (The BMA has a code of practice entitled **Advance Statements about Medical Treatment**). The Mental Capacity Act 2005 (covering England and Wales) allows for 'advance decisions' (p. 876) in case of future incapacity.

If a patient lacks capacity, and information about a written or verbal advance refusal of treatment is recorded in their notes or is otherwise brought to your attention, you must bear in mind that valid and applicable advance refusals must be respected. A valid advance refusal that is clearly applicable to the patient's present circumstances will be legally binding in England and Wales (unless it relates to life-prolonging treatment, in which case further legal criteria must be met). Valid and applicable advance refusals are potentially binding in Scotland and Northern Ireland, although this has not yet been tested in the courts.

Withdrawal of treatment[2,3] The active or passive involvement of a carer in hastening an individual's death is highly controversial and morally complex. There are differing degrees of involvement that should be distinguished:

- Withdrawal of active interventions such as medications, blood transfusion, etc. This is an accepted aspect of palliative care and draws little debate.
- Withdrawal of life-sustaining treatment such fluids, food, etc. This is equivalent to 'allowing a patient to die'. Since the current emphasis is on preserving human dignity rather than preserving life, this is morally acceptable for many and should not be considered euthanasia.
- Active intervention which hastens or precipitates the patient's death— euthanasia. This is distinguishable from homicide in that the patient has either consented to the assisted death or is unable to (e.g. comatose) and the intervention is regarded as a 'mercy killing'.

That time of year thou mayst in me behold
When yellow leaves, or none, or few, do hang
Upon those boughs which shake against the cold,
Bare ruin'd choirs, where late the sweet birds sang.
In me thou see'st the twilight of such day
As after sunset fadeth in the west;
Which by and by black night doth take away,
Death's second self, that seals up all in rest.
In me thou see'st the glowing of such fire,
That on the ashes of his youth doth lie,
As the death-bed whereon it must expire
Consum'd with that which it was nourish'd by.
This thou perceiv'st, which makes thy love more strong,
To love that well which thou must leave ere long.

Shakespeare: Sonnet 72

1 Ellershaw J and Ward C (2003) Care of the dying patient: the last hours or days of life. *Br Med J* **326**: 30–4.

2 Hermsen MA and ten Have HA (2002) Euthanasia in palliative care journals. *J Pain Sympt Manag* **23**: 517–25.

3 Sharma BR (2003) To legalize physician-assisted suicide or not?—a dilemma. *J Clin Foren Med* **10**: 185–90.

Substance misuse

The psychiatry of substance misuse

The subspecialty of substance misuse is concerned with the assessment and treatment of patients with problems arising from the misuse of harmful or addictive substances. These include: (1) alcohol, (2) illegal or 'street' drugs, (3) prescription and over-the-counter medicines, and (4) volatile chemicals. The resultant problems include both mental and physical illnesses and family, housing, employment, and legal difficulties. Both psychological and pharmacological interventions are used in treatment, which may include detoxification and substitute prescribing.

The majority of medical interventions in patients with substance use problems are undertaken by GPs. In areas where there are no substance misuse specialists, more complex cases are seen by general psychiatrists, with management of the acute medical problems, including overdose and withdrawals, treated in the general hospital. All psychiatrists will have ample opportunity to see and develop skills in treating patients with substance misuse.

Around the UK there is variable service provision for drug and alcohol misuse. Some services will restrict themselves to the primary substance misuse, while others will address all mental health needs. Specialists tend to work alongside voluntary and non-medical treatment agencies, many of which provide a good and vital service. Strong links between psychiatry/substance use services and non-medical agencies should be fostered.

Drug treatment services within the health care system make up only one part of the wider range of centrally and locally funded and volunteer services for problem drug users. Within the health service the majority of service provision is within primary care, who will have a variable degree of experience of (and enthusiasm for) such work. The availability of specialist services will vary by area and setting (e.g. rural/urban) and may range from the special interest of an individual psychiatrist or GP, to a specialist service with support staff and dedicated facilities. Local pharmacists can also be a useful resource in supervising consumption of substitute drugs.

Non-health care provision will also vary by setting, though may include: advice shops offering leaflets and education about drugs and harm reduction strategies; self-help groups, some adhering to an Alcoholics Anonymous (AA)-style 'twelve-step approach', usually involving peer support from ex-users; and residential rehabilitation facilities, offering detoxification and abstinence programs. The practitioner working in the field of drug misuse should develop an awareness of these services and their referral criteria and encourage a collaborative and co-ordinated approach to patient management.

The skills required for those working in the field of substance misuse are:

- *Knowledge of the psychiatric symptoms and syndromes associated with substance misuse* This includes the effects of substance misuse on the brain, in causing psychiatric symptoms, and the effects of substance misuse on pre-existing mental and physical illness.
- *Knowledge and understanding of the influence of psychological and social factors on substance misuse and relapse.*
- *Experience of interviewing and counselling methods* Skills in interviewing and motivating patients who may have very ambivalent feelings about changing their behaviour.
- *Experience of available pharmacological and psychological treatment methods* An area undergoing constant development, where there is a need to keep abreast of changes in evidence.
- *Awareness of the culture and pattern of drug use within a community* Patterns of drug use change over time, and the types and strengths of drugs available in a community will also change dynamically. Information from police and the voluntary sector can be helpful here.
- *Willingness to be involved with other agencies* Valuable work in the field of substance misuse is done by agencies outside the health care system. Practitioners should attempt to understand the work of these agencies, and refer to them where appropriate.
- *Understanding of the natural history of substance misuse/addiction* Substance misuse disorders can be chronic, and at times lifelong, with a relapsing/remitting course (like many psychiatric conditions). Taking a long-term approach is therefore essential.
- *Ability to consider health in its wider context* Substance misuse gives rise to health risks beyond the effect of the drug (e.g. drink driving deaths, HIV infection). In addition, it is a community problem leading to lost productivity, crime, road accidents, violence, and family break-up.
- *Consideration of change beyond change in an individual patient* Patterns of substance misuse in a society are susceptible to political manipulation (e.g. licensing hours, decriminalization, legalization, availability of treatment services). One role of substance misuse specialists is to understand these factors and to present the case for political change.

A non-judgemental approach. Sometimes there is a perception that drug or alcohol users are 'difficult' patients to treat. Bear in mind GMC guidelines direct that it is *'unethical for a doctor to withhold treatment from any patient on the basis of a moral judgement that the patient's activities or lifestyle may have contributed to the conditions for which treatment was being sought'*.

Note: for the purposes of this chapter, we refer to alcohol misuse and drug misuse separately and refer to them collectively as substance misuse. Alcohol is of course a drug and should be thought of as such, but we believe this terminology to be clearer and more understandable to patients.

Substance use and misuse

'Humankind cannot bear very much reality' T.S. Eliot

'The urge to escape, the longing to transcend themselves, if only for a few minutes, is and always has been one of the principal appetites of the soul.' Aldous Huxley

People in all cultures, at all times throughout history, have sought out mood or perception-altering substances. 25% of adults smoke; 90% drink alcohol; 33% have lifetime experience of one illegal drug (mostly cannabis). Society's attitude to substance use and to those with substance use problems has varied, from prohibition and condemnation to tolerance and treatment. Within British society at the moment caffeine use is legal and accepted; alcohol and tobacco use are accepted with legal limitations; and other substances have severe legal limitations—some available only on prescription, others not at all. Despite this, the harmful effects of alcohol dwarf those of other drugs.

Many of the abused substances subsequently described have been used in their naturally occurring form throughout history (e.g. the chewing of coca leaves by Peruvian Indians). There has been a tendency for the development of more potent drug preparations which contain a higher concentration of the active ingredient (e.g. freebase cocaine), and the development of routes of administration which produce more rapid and intense effects (e.g. IV use). This has generally been associated with an increase in the attendant problems.

Patients presenting with drug misuse problems represent only a small percentage of those who take drugs. Little is known about the non-presenting drug users. Their numbers may be hinted at by community surveys, but they are otherwise poorly studied. It is clear, however, that the normal route from use of to abstinence from a substance is the individual deciding to discontinue use and then doing so, without medical consultation or help.

Reasons given for substance use are varied, and may change over the course of a patient's life. They include: a search for a 'high'; a search for a repeat of initial pleasurable effects; cultural norm in some subcultures; self-medication for anxiety, social phobia, insomnia, symptoms of psychotic illness, and to prevent development of withdrawal symptoms. There is evidence for increased vulnerability to substance use in those with a family history of substance misuse, and the role of environmental stressors in perpetuating use cannot be underplayed.

The pattern of risks associated with substance use varies with the substance taken, the dose and route of administration, and the setting. They include: acute toxicity; behavioural toxicity (e.g. jumping from height due to believing one can fly); toxic effects of drug contaminants; secondary medical problems; secondary psychiatric problems; risk of development of dependency; and negative social, occupational, marital, and forensic consequences.

Substance misuse disorders

Acute intoxication The pattern of reversible physical and mental abnormalities caused by the direct effects of the substance. These are specific and characteristic for each substance (e.g. disinhibition and ataxia for alcohol, euphoria and visual sensory distortions for LSD). Most substances have both pleasurable and unpleasant acute effects; for some, the balance of positive and negative effects is situation-, dose-, and route-dependent.

At-risk use A pattern of substance use where the person is at increased risk of harming their physical or mental health. This is not a discrete point but shades into both normal consumption and harmful use. At-risk use depends not only on absolute amounts taken but also on the situations and associated behaviours (e.g. any alcohol use is risky if associated with driving).

Harmful use The continuation of substance use despite evidence of damage to the user's physical or mental health or to their social, occupational, and familial well-being. This damage may be denied or minimized by the individual concerned.

Dependence The layman's 'addiction'. Encompasses a range of features initially described in connection with alcohol abuse (📖 p. 542), now recognized as a syndrome associated with a range of substances. Dependence includes both physical dependence (the physical adaptations to chronic, regular use) and psychological dependence (the behavioural adaptations). In some drugs (e.g. hallucinogens), no physical dependence features are seen.

Withdrawal Where there is physical dependence on a drug, abstinence will generally lead to features of withdrawal. These are characteristic for each drug. Some drugs are not associated with any withdrawals; some with mild symptoms only; and some with significant withdrawal syndromes. Clinically significant withdrawals are recognized in dependence on alcohol, opiates, nicotine, BDZs, amfetamines, and cocaine. Symptoms of withdrawal are often the 'opposite' of the acute effects of the drug (e.g. agitation and insomnia on BDZ withdrawal).

Complicated withdrawal Withdrawals can be simple, or complicated by the development of seizures, delirium, or psychotic features.

Substance-induced psychotic disorder Illness characterized by hallucinations and/or delusions occurring as a direct result of substance-induced neurotoxicity. Psychotic features may occur during intoxication and withdrawal states, or develop on a background of harmful or dependent use. There may be diagnostic confusion between these patients and those with primary psychotic illness and comorbid substance misuse. Substance-induced illnesses will be associated in time with episodes of substance misuse, will occur more readily with specific substances (e.g. cocaine) and may have atypical clinical features (e.g. late first presentation with psychosis, prominence of non-auditory hallucinations).

Cognitive impairment syndromes Reversible cognitive deficits occur during intoxication. Persisting impairment (in some cases amounting to dementia) caused by chronic substance use is recognized for alcohol, volatile chemicals, BDZs, and, debatably, cannabis. Cognitive impairment is associated with heavy chronic harmful use/dependence and shows gradual deterioration with continued use and either a halt in the rate of decline, or gradual improvement with abstinence.

Residual disorders Several conditions exist (e.g. alcoholic hallucinosis, 📖 p. 568; persisting drug-induced psychosis, 📖 p. 604; LSD flashbacks, 📖 p. 586) where there are continuing symptoms despite continuing abstinence from the drug.

Exacerbation of pre-existing disorder All other psychiatric illnesses, especially anxiety and panic disorders, mood disorders, and psychotic illnesses may be associated with comorbid substance use. Although this may result in exacerbation of the patient's symptoms and a decline in treatment effectiveness, it can be understood as a desire to self-medicate (e.g. alcohol taken as a hypnotic in depressive illness) or escape unpleasant symptoms (e.g. opiates taken to 'blot out' derogatory auditory hallucinations). Sometimes there is debate about whether there is, for example, a primary mood disorder with secondary alcohol use or vice versa. Careful examination of the time course of the illness may reveal the answer. In any case, it is advisable to address substance misuse problems first, as this may produce secondary mood improvements and continuing substance misuse will limit antidepressant treatment effectiveness.

The dependence syndrome

This is a clinical syndrome describing the features of substance dependence. It was described initially by Edwards and Gross[1] as a provisional description of alcohol dependence, but may be applied to the description of drug dependence. These features form the core of both ICD-10 and DSM-IV descriptions of substance dependence.

- **Primacy of drug-seeking behaviour** Also called 'salience' of drug use. The drug and the need to obtain it become the most important things in the person's life, taking priority over all other activities and interests. Thus drug use becomes more important than retaining job or relationships, remaining financially solvent and in good physical health, and may diminish moral sense leading to criminal activity and fraud. This diminishes the 'holds' on a person's continued use. If he rates drug use above health, then stern warnings about impending illness are likely to mean little.
- **Narrowing of the drug-taking repertoire** The user moves from a range of drugs to a single drug taken in preference to all others. The setting of drug use, the route of use, and the individuals with whom the drug is taken may also become stereotyped.
- **Increased tolerance to the effects of the drug** The user finds that more of the drug must be taken to achieve the same effects. They may also attempt to combat increasing tolerance by choosing a more rapidly acting route of administration (e.g. IV rather than smoked), or by choosing a more rapidly acting form (e.g. freebase cocaine rather than cocaine hydrochloride). In advanced dependence there may be a sudden loss of previous tolerance; the mechanism for this is unknown. Clinically, tolerance is exhibited by individuals who are able to display no or few signs of intoxication while at a blood level in which intoxication would be evident in a non-dependent individual.
- **Loss of control of consumption** A subjective sense of inability to restrict further consumption once the drug is taken.
- **Signs of withdrawal on attempted abstinence** A withdrawal syndrome, characteristic for each drug, may develop. This may be only regularly experienced in the mornings because at all other times the blood level is kept above the required level.
- **Drug taking to avoid development of withdrawal symptoms** The user learns to anticipate and avoid withdrawals (e.g. having the drug available on waking).
- **Continued drug use despite negative consequences** The user persists in drug use even when threatened with significant losses as a direct consequence of continued use (e.g. marital break-up, prison term, loss of job).
- **Rapid reinstatement of previous pattern of drug use after abstinence** Characteristically, when the user relapses to drug use after a period of abstinence, they are at risk of a return to the dependent pattern in a much shorter period than the time initially taken to reach dependent use.

1 Edwards G and Gross MM (1976) Alcohol dependence: provisional description of a clinical syndrome. *Br Med J* **1**: 1058–61.

Stages of change and harm reduction

Stages of change

A model for understanding motivation and action towards change in harmful patterns of drug use was proposed by Prochaska and DiClemente.[1] Motivation is regarded as a prerequisite for and a precursor to action towards abstinence or more controlled drug use. This model can be used when trying to tailor treatments to the individual.

- **Pre-contemplation** The user does not recognize that problem use exists, although this may be increasingly obvious to those around them.
- **Contemplation** The user may accept that there is a problem and begins to look at both the positive and negative aspects of continued drug use.
- **Decision** The point at which the user decides on whether to continue drug use or attempt change.
- **Action** The point of motivation, where the user attempts change. A variety of routes exist by which change may be attempted, which may or may not include medical services.
- **Maintenance** A stage of maintaining gains made and attempting to improve those areas of life harmed by drug use.
- **Relapse** A return to previous behaviour, but with the possibility of gaining useful strategies to extend the maintenance period on the user's next attempt.

Harm reduction

Harm reduction is a method of managing drug users in which it is accepted that steps can be taken to reduce the mortality and morbidity for the user without necessarily insisting on abstinence from drugs. This approach gained currency during the 1980s in an attempt to halt the projected AIDS epidemic. The majority of patients will present before abstinence is a realistic or achievable goal for them. Optimum care for this group of patients will involve engaging them with the service, exploring and encouraging motivation to change, and suggesting harm reduction strategies. Examples of such strategies include:

- Advice directed at use of safer drugs or routes of administration.
- Advice regarding safer injecting practice (📖 p. 583).
- Advice regarding safe sex.
- Prescription of maintenance opiates (substitution prescribing) or BDZs.
- Assessment and treatment of comorbid physical or mental illness.
- Engagement with other sources of help (e.g. social work, housing).

Drug misuse is a community problem. Some aspects of harm reduction include consideration of reduction of morbidity to the community more generally. Prescription of methadone may reduce criminality in a dependent individual, with consequent community benefit. Equally, there is a responsibility with the prescriber to consider the potential for community harm via leakage and accidental overdose when monitoring the prescription of any drug.

1 Prochaska JO and DiClemente CC (1986) Towards a comprehensive model of change. In Miller WR and Heather N (eds), *Treating addictive behaviours: processes of change*, pp. 3–27. New York: Plenum Press.

Alcohol misuse

In the UK, roughly 93% of men and 87% of women drink alcohol. Minimal alcohol consumption can of course be pleasurable, socially enjoyable, and associated with health benefits (reduction in deaths from coronary artery disease). There is a tendency to view most people as normal drinkers and a subset as vulnerable to the development of alcohol problems. In fact on a population level, increasing the overall alcohol consumption (e.g. by reducing the real price of alcohol) tends to increase the total number of problem drinkers.

Alcohol consumption in the community is roughly normally distributed with a long 'tail' to the right. The distinction between normal and heavy drinking is arbitrary. On both a population and individual level, increased consumption is associated with increased risk of harm of all kinds. However, the fact that normal drinkers heavily outnumber heavy drinkers means that, despite their lower rates of problems, greater numbers of alcohol-related problems occur in normal rather than heavy drinkers. This gives rise to the so-called 'prevention paradox'—that to significantly reduce overall alcohol related morbidity we must look to reduce problems in normal rather than heavy drinkers. This applies more to problems such as drink driving and drink-related trauma rather than to medical complications of heavy use such as liver cirrhosis.

The term 'alcoholic' is often used by patients themselves and is the preferred term of Alcoholics Anonymous. It has unfortunately acquired a pejorative meaning to the general public, and images of the 'down and out' or 'skid row' alcoholic, drinking strong drink from brown paper bags, have damaged this word's use in clinical contexts. It is not used in DSM-IV or ICD-10 where the preference is to make the diagnosis of alcohol dependence or harmful use (abuse in DSM-IV).

A history of alcohol use

Alcohol has been used in all societies throughout recorded history, with documentary evidence of brewing and wine making as early as 3000 BC. The intoxicating effects of alcohol were most probably discovered independently in many cultures around the time of the evolution of agriculture, possibly on noting fermentation in fruit. Ancient peoples produced alcoholic beverages from a wide variety of materials including fruits, berries, honey, corn, barley, wheat, sugar cane, and potatoes. The use of alcohol by individuals has been variously regarded, from complete tolerance through to outright prohibition.

Alcohol has always had a place in the lifestyles and formal rituals of many peoples around the world. It was used as an intoxicant in religious rituals, as a celebration, as a gift, as a greeting, and to mark births and deaths. For almost as long as alcohol use is recorded there are recorded attempts at control on its use by the authorities. In AD 92 the Roman emperor Domitian attempted to restrict wine production and its distribution and sale. Similar restrictions were attempted at various times by other leaders, sometimes accompanied by moral disapproval of drinking or drunkenness in particular. In medieval Britain, ale was a staple part of the diet and was consumed in huge quantities, while drunkenness, particularly among the clergy, was frowned upon by the Christian churches. Consumption of wine, however, continued to play a role in Christian worship. After initially preaching moderation, Mohammed later forbade the use of alcohol to followers of his religion, possibly as a way of differentiating his converts from the Christians around them.

The process of natural fermentation of alcohol by yeasts can produce beverages of up to 13% proof: above this concentration the yeast dies. Stronger concentrations of alcohol are produced by the process of distillation which was discovered in the Middle East in 1000 AD. Public consumption of distilled liquor became prevalent in the eighteenth century and the accompanying social problems together with the conservative attitudes of the emerging Protestant clergy led to a developing moral disapproval of alcohol consumption.

In the mid-eighteenth century, as part of a continuing military and trade dispute with France, the British government imposed heavy taxes on French wine imports and encouraged the distillation of cheap domestic spirits—in particular, gin. This change in the drinking practice in the general population from low- to high-strength alcohol produced significant alcohol-related problems in the general public, immortalized in the lithographs of the 'gin palaces' by George Cruikshank. In an effort to control the problem the government passed laws to restrict the time and place at which alcohol could be sold and began to levy increasing taxes on distilled spirits. This had the positive effect of reducing consumption but the negative effect of introducing a government interest in continuing consumption. The late eighteenth-century writings of Benjamin Rush describe habitual drunkenness as a 'disease of the mind'.

Eighteenth-century America saw the development of an increasingly widespread temperance movement (those signing a pledge 'TA' for total abstinence becoming known as teetotallers). The temperance movement lobbied for a complete ban on alcohol consumption, and succeeded in 1921 following the passing of the 18th amendment to the US Constitution which provided for prohibition. The period of 11 years until the repeal of prohibition in the 21st amendment did indeed see a reduction in social problems and mortality; however, its unpopularity, widespread flouting of the law, and the flourishing of illegal activity in gangsterism led to its repeal.

Today, in most Western countries, alcohol use is widely tolerated and socially accepted. Interestingly, moral disapproval of drinking during pregnancy and drinking while driving a motor vehicle has resulted in substantial decreases in these activities. Despite improvement in these limited areas, most Western countries have seen an increase in absolute consumption and alcohol-related medical harm compounded by an increasing passion for drug misuse.

Alcohol as a drug

Preparations The active ingredient in alcoholic drinks is ethyl alcohol which makes up a variable percentage of the volume. The flavour of drinks comes from 'congeners'—the additional organic substances derived from the brewing materials.

Pattern of use Of all drugs, alcohol has the widest range of patterns of use, ranging from yearly light consumption to continuous consumption throughout the waking hours.

Drug actions The effects of alcohol on the CNS were traditionally described as being due to non-specific effects on neuronal cell wall fluidity and permeability. It is now believed that in addition to these general effects there are neurotransmitter-specific effects, including: enhancement of GABA-A transmission (anxiolytic effects), release of dopamine in the mesolimbic system (euphoriant and 'reward' effects), and inhibition of NMDA-mediated glutaminergic transmission (amnesic effects). Ethyl alcohol is oxidized by alcohol dehydrogenase (ADH) to acetaldehyde, which in turn is oxidized by acetaldehyde dehydrogenase (ALDH) to carbon dioxide and water. 98% of alcohol metabolism takes place in the liver. Approximately 1 unit (or 8g) of alcohol can be metabolized per hour. Illicitly brewed alcohol may contain methanol, which is broken down to formaldehyde, which has marked toxic effects on the retina.

Acute effects Alcohol is absorbed rapidly from mouth, stomach, and small intestine, and from a single consumption maximum blood levels are obtained in ~60min. Absorption is slowed by the presence of food in the stomach and is speeded up by taking effervescent drinks. Alcohol is hydrophilic and is widely distributed throughout the body organs including the brain, placenta, lungs, and kidneys. Blood alcohol concentration (BAC) is consistent throughout the body with the exception of fat and can be estimated from breath samples. In normal drinkers BAC correlates with the subjective and the observable CNS effects of alcohol. Heavy drinkers may have a high BAC with limited outward signs of intoxication due to the development of tolerance. Because of their different body fat distribution, women will have a higher BAC than men following the same oral intake. Initial symptoms of alcohol intoxication are subjective elevation of mood, increased socialization, and disinhibition. Continuing consumption, intended to prolong these effects, can lead to lability of mood, impaired judgement, aggressiveness, slurred speech, unsteady gait, and ataxia.

Societal factors The prevalence of alcohol-related harm increases with the mean population consumption. This mean consumption is increased by increased availability of alcohol, increased societal tolerance of drinking, decreased restrictions on the sale of alcohol, and a decreased 'real price' of alcohol. Price is the most influential factor in demand, the real price of a pint of beer or bottle of whisky having dropped considerably since the war. Where societies forbid all alcohol consumption (e.g. prohibition America, Islamic counties), there is a decrease in alcohol-related problems but an increase in the level of personality abnormality in those who continue to drink.

Risk factors Heavy drinking is more common in men, in lower socio-economic groups, in those with lower educational levels, and in the young. Some professions are also associated with heavy drinking and drink-related harm. These include drinks industry workers (easy availability and effect of heavy drinkers seeking out jobs here); travelling salesmen (boredom, periods away from home, acceptance of drinking on the job); doctors (stress, freedom from direct supervision, reluctance to seek help with incipient problems).

Genetics First-degree relatives of alcoholics have double the risk of alcohol problems themselves. Significantly higher rates in identical compared with fraternal twins (although not 100% concordance). Children of alcoholics have increased risk of development of alcohol problems themselves even when adopted into families without alcohol problems. A metabolically relatively inactive form of ALDH is common in Southeast Asian people, leading to accumulation of acetaldehyde and an unpleasant 'flushing' reaction in affected individuals who take alcohol. This may account for the significantly lower rate of alcohol problems found in affected individuals. No causative genes for alcoholism have been identified and it is expected that it will show polygenic inheritance. Problem drinkers contain a significant subgroup of individuals with dissocial personality traits which predisposes to alcoholism, and is itself heritable.

Medical complications Acute toxicity occurs at levels over 300mg% (see 📖 p. 566), with clouding of consciousness and coma, risk of aspiration, hypoglycaemia, and acute renal failure. Associated with a wide range of chronic medical problems (📖 p. 574).

Psychiatric complications Harmful use and dependent use (📖 p. 566) distinguished by the presence of withdrawals on abstinence; withdrawals may be complicated by seizures and development of an acute confusional state—delirium tremens (📖 p. 558); acute alcohol-induced amnesia; alcoholic hallucinosis (📖 p. 568); alcohol-induced delusional disorder (📖 p. 568); Wernicke–Korsakoff syndrome (📖 p. 572); pathological jealousy (📖 p. 569); alcohol-related cognitive impairment and alcoholic dementia (📖 p. 568); alcohol misuse is also associated with development of, or exacerbation of, anxiety/depressive symptoms and with deliberate self-harm and suicidal behaviour.

Interventions Advice and 'brief interventions' regarding safer drinking patterns in those with 'at risk' or harmful use (📖 p. 566); strategies towards encouraging and maintaining abstinence in those with dependency and those with established medical or psychiatric damage; medically managed detoxification (📖 p. 560); psychological and pharmacological support of abstinence or changed drinking pattern (📖 pp. 562–5).

Screening for alcohol problems

Diseases related to alcohol abuse are common, significant, and amenable to improvement by early detection and intervention. Screening is therefore indicated. There are low rates of detection in primary care and hospital settings, which may be improved by increased vigilance, increased awareness of alcohol problems, awareness of routes of referral, asking routine alcohol-screening questions (e.g. CAGE—see Box 15.1), paying special attention to at-risk groups. Many patients give reasonably accurate drinking histories if asked, although some may underestimate consumption. A combination of clinical history, screening measure, and a biomarker is the optimal approach to detection.

Disorders suggesting underlying alcohol abuse Hepatitis; cryptogenic (i.e. medically unexplained) cirrhosis; seizures—particularly late onset; gastritis; anaemia; unexplained raised MCV or deranged LFTs; cardiomyopathy; accidents, particularly repeated and poorly explained; TB; head injury; hypertension persisting despite apparently adequate treatment; treatment resistance in other psychiatric conditions; impotence in men.

Breath testing Blood alcohol concentration (BAC) measures recent alcohol consumption, in mg alcohol per 100mL blood (mg%). Correlates well with breath alcohol measured by breathalyser (see Table 15.1). Useful in assessing recent drinking (e.g. in supervised detox regimes) and as an objective measure of intoxication (e.g. in A&E). Discrepancy between high BAC and lack of apparent intoxication suggests tolerance. This measurement is dependent on adequate technique, and reasonable co-operation from the patient.

Blood tests Elevated red cell mean corpuscular volume (MCV), gamma glutamyl transferase (γ-GT), and carbohydrate-deficient transferrin (CDT) are markers for excess alcohol consumption. They are best used to monitor consumption in patients at follow-up. Not sensitive/specific enough for routine screening purposes.

- **MCV** Sensitivity 20–50%, specificity 55–100%. Remains raised for 3–6 months due to 120-day lifespan of RBC. False positive in B12 and folate deficiency.
- **γ-GT** Sensitivity 20–90%, specificity 55–100%. Raised for 2–3wks. Other LFTs are less specific for alcoholic-related liver damage. False positive in liver diseases of other cause, obesity, diabetes, smoking, and medication (e.g. anticonvulsants), and may remain raised in chronic alcoholic liver disease despite abstinence.
- **CDT** Sensitivity 70%, specificity 95%. Increased levels in response to heavy drinking (7–10 days), 2–3wks to return to normal, can be used to monitor relapse. More expensive than γ-GT and not available in all areas.

Urinary tests Urinary ethyl glucoronide (an alcohol metabolite) has been proposed as a measure of alcohol intake, being sensitive to ingestion of 1 or 2 drinks, remaining elevated for several days. It has still to be used routinely, though has been used in forensic settings.

Hair testing Testing of hair for ethyl glucoronide or fatty acid ethyl esters has been proposed as a method for detecting alcohol use over prior months, though requires further research and validation.

Box 15.1 CAGE questionnaire

A brief screening questionnaire for identification of at-risk drinking:
C: Have you ever felt you should **C**ut back on your drinking?
A: Has anyone ever **A**nnoyed you by criticizing your drinking?
G: Have you ever felt **G**uilty about your drinking?
E: Have you ever had a drink early in the morning as an **E**ye-opener?
More than two positive responses suggests possible at-risk drinking and should prompt further assessment.
Note: the '**Cage +2**' adds two additional questions:
  1. What is the most alcohol you have drunk in a single day?
  2. What is the most alcohol you have drunk in a single week?

Table 15.1 Breath and blood alcohol levels

Breath alcohol reading (mcg%)	BAC (mg%)
0.35	80
0.52	120
0.70	160
0.87	200
1.05	240
1.40	320
1.75	400

A breathalyser allows an objective measurement of the breath alcohol and hence an approximation of the BAC. Breath alcohol reading should form part of the routine assessment of a patient presenting with alcohol problems and of patients in follow-up (e.g. supervised detox), rather than being prompted by suspicion of inaccuracy of oral report.

Assessment of the patient with alcohol problems

Patients with a primary alcohol problem, or where it is thought that alcohol consumption is a contributory factor in their presentation, should have a more detailed assessment of their alcohol use, in addition to standard psychiatric history and MSE.

Lifetime pattern of alcohol consumption Age at first alcoholic drink. Age when began to drink regularly. Age when first drinking most weekends. Age when first drinking most days. When did they first begin to drink more than their peers? When (if ever) did they first feel they had an alcohol problem? Pattern of drinking throughout life until present—describe periods of abstinence and more heavy drinking and the reasons for these (including environmental/psychosocial stressors).

Current alcohol consumption Describe a current day's drinking. When is the first drink taken? What types of drink are taken and in what setting? What is the total number and volume of drinks taken in a day? Some patients find it hard to describe a typical day or easy to over-rationalize recent heavy consumption. Ask them to describe the previous day's drinking, then the day before that, etc., until a pattern emerges. Describe a typical and a 'heavy' day's drinking.

Signs of dependence Do they experience withdrawals in the morning or when unable to obtain alcohol? Have they ever drunk more alcohol as way of relieving withdrawals? Are they having to drink more to get the same intoxicating effect? Do they no longer get 'drunk' at all? Do they find it difficult to stop drinking once started? Have they tried and failed to give up, and if so why? Do they have episodes of 'lost' memory/'blackouts'?

Physical/mental health Have they been told of any physical health problems due to drinking? Have they previously been told to stop drinking by a doctor? Any previous or current psychiatric diagnoses?

Problems related to alcohol Have they missed days at work, or had warnings about poor performance, or lost a job as a result of alcohol? Are there relationship difficulties or a relationship breakdown due to drinking? Are there financial problems? Have they been in trouble with the police or do they have outstanding charges against them?

Previous treatment attempts Describe the nature and type of previous treatments. Describe the subsequent return to drinking. Describe any periods of abstinence since the development of the drinking problem. How were they maintained and what ended them?

Family history Drinking problems in parents and extended family. Quality of relationships in past and present. Childhood environment.

Attitude to referral Why have they attended the appointment today? Do they feel they have an alcohol problem and if so will they accept help for it? What sort of help do they want and are there types of treatment they will not accept? What stage of change are they at (pre-contemplative, contemplative, decision, action)?

Patient goals What (if anything) do they want to change about their drinking? What pattern of drinking do they aspire to?

Physical examination Note general condition; evidence of withdrawals including tremor in hands or protruded tongue; degree of facial capilliarization; stigmata of liver disease (palpable liver edge, jaundice, spider naevi, ascites, palmar erythema); evidence of peripheral neuropathy; ataxia of gait; breath alcohol reading.

Blood testing FBC, LFTs, other blood tests as indicated on history/ examination.

Cognitive testing Although not generally indicated until 4wks of abstinence, it is helpful to get a feel for the patient's level of cognition, especially if there is a suggestion they may be experiencing delirium, or have significant alcohol-related brain damage.

Giving drinking advice

There are a variety of situations where the doctor will be called on to give 'safe drinking' advice: individuals whose histories reveal evolving risky drinking patterns; patients with comorbid psychiatric illness; and individuals with alcohol problems who are attempting controlled drinking rather than abstinence.

There is a wide variety of types of alcoholic drink, each of a different 'strength', (i.e. percentage alcohol by volume; see Table 15.2). It is the amount of alcohol taken, rather than the type of drink, which contributes to physical/mental health effects—avoiding spirits or other drinks perceived as 'strong' will not protect from health risks if the absolute amount of alcohol is above safe limits.

Sensible drinking Men should drink no more than 21 and women no more than 14 units/wk of alcohol. There should be at least two non-drinking days per week. The amounts should be spread over several days, not drunk all at once. Amounts should not be 'saved up' from a light week and drunk on top of the following week's allowance. The amounts quoted are not 'safe' amounts, but represent levels of drinking not associated with significant risks to health. In some situations (e.g. driving, operating machinery) the 'safe amount' is zero. Some individuals (e.g. previously alcohol-dependent, chronic medical conditions, pregnant) should not drink at all.

Brief interventions for hazardous and harmful drinking

Low intensity, short interventions, based predominantly at primary care level, to reduce hazardous drinking. Techniques include presenting patients with screening results, identifying risks, giving medical advice, assessing the patient's goals/commitment and working collaboratively to support the patient.

Techniques of controlled drinking Patients who are seeking advice about avoiding potential alcohol problems and those individuals who are seeking to change from 'at-risk' or harmful drinking patterns to controlled drinking patterns may find a selection of the following strategies helpful:

- Set a weekly and daily alcohol limit and keep to it.
- Do not drink alone.
- Do not drink with individuals who drink heavily themselves.
- Pace drinking, matching the consumption of a light or slow drinker.
- Don't buy rounds.
- Alternate soft and alcoholic drinks. Drink with a meal.
- Rehearse what to say if offered a drink that you don't want.
- Plan alternative, enjoyable non-drinking activities to replace drinking periods (e.g. cinema, sports).

Table 15.2 Amounts of alcohol in common drinks

The amount of alcohol in drinks is measured in units. One unit contains ~8 grams of alcohol. In alcoholic drinks where the percentage of alcohol by volume is given, the number of units = volume in L x % alcohol. Numbers of units in common drinks are given below. In calculating numbers of units in an alcohol history, remember that home measures of drinks are usually more generous than those in pubs.

Drink	Alcohol % by volume	Measure	Alcohol units
Beer and stout	4.0	Pint	2.0
Continental lager	5.0	440ml can	2.2
Strong lager	9.0	440ml can	4.0
Normal cider	4.5	Pint 1L	2.5 4.5
Strong cider	8.4	1L	8.4
Wine	9–14	125ml glass 750ml bottle	1.5 6.8–10.5
Gin/vodka/ rum	37.5	25ml measure 700ml bottle	1 26.3

Planning treatment in alcohol misuse

Patients presenting with alcohol problems often display marked ambivalence about whether there is even a problem, let alone about the need for change. This reflects both the perceived positive as well as negative roles alcohol plays in their lives and the memory of previous failure or difficulties in attempting change. The aim in counselling such patients is to guide them in making their own decision towards change, or if change is not likely or possible now, to guide them towards harm reduction and considering the possibility of future change.

Motivational interviewing This is a technique aimed at enabling a patient to move through the stages of change (📖 p. 544) to the point where action can be contemplated. It is based on the principle that: 'people believe what they hear themselves say'. The interviewer aims to aid the patient in explaining why they should change their behaviour and how this will be achieved.
- Therapist does not take a directive or prescriptive role but expresses interest and concern for the patient's problems and explores the consequences of their behaviour.
- Uses open-ended questions, reflective listening and summarizing with identification of discrepancy between individual statements.
- Aids the assessment of the pros and cons of current behaviour, avoiding confrontation or direct challenge.
- Emphasizes patient's own perceptions of degree of risk rather than telling them about risks which they may not believe.
- Encourages personal responsibility and patient's choice of treatment options.

Planning interventions The initial assessment interview forms the beginning of intervention. Its aims are to gather and impart information, promote the possibility of positive action, and to plan treatment. The ongoing therapeutic relationship aims to maintain purpose, monitor progress, aid self-monitoring and self-awareness. The process of planning treatment should proceed along the following lines:
- Make diagnosis (alcohol dependence, harmful, or at-risk use).
- Assess stage of change (📖 p. 544).
- Decide with patient the goal of intervention:
- **Continue current drinking pattern** In some patients there will be no need for change at all. In others there will be a clear history of alcohol problems but the patient presents as 'pre-contemplative' regarding change. In these cases give harm-reduction advice and 'leave the door open' to further assessment and help rather than alienating the patient.
- **Change to safer drinking pattern** Many individuals will be able to modify risky or harmful drinking patterns given appropriate advice and help (perhaps monitored by a 'drinking diary', which is later reviewed).
- **Attempt abstinence from alcohol** In some individuals the only safe course is to aim to abstain from alcohol completely.
- For abstinence in a dependent drinker, consider the need for and setting of detox (📖 p. 560).

Plan support methods and follow-up (📖 p. 562).
- At follow-up contact, review progress, emphasize changes made, review mental health.
- Anticipate and deal with relapse if it occurs.

Abstinence vs. controlled drinking The decision to try for controlled drinking rather than abstinence is one for individual patient choice. The doctor should offer suitable advice.
- **Factors suggesting possibility of success of controlled drinking:** previous prolonged periods of controlled drinking, alcohol misuse primarily in context of other mental disorder which has responded to treatment, otherwise stable lifestyle, absence of drinking problem in family and friends.
- **Factors against controlled drinking:** previously alcohol-dependent, previous failure at controlled drinking, comorbid mental illness, comorbid drug use, established organ damage, risk of job loss/ marriage loss.

Relapse Alcohol misuse is a chronic illness and many patients will 'fall off the wagon' several times before achieving long-standing change. The possibility of relapse should be anticipated with the patient and appropriate strategies should be in place to deal with it (e.g. early review).

Causes of relapse: ambivalent motivation, insufficient support, novel events, over-confidence, mental illness, environmental stressors.

Counselling families The family of a patient with alcohol problems may contact you directly to ask for advice regarding their relative.
- Patient's relatives sometimes request that their relative be detained in hospital 'to stop them drinking'. The Mental Health Acts in the UK specifically do not allow detention of patients solely for reason of drug or alcohol dependency.
- Aim to encourage and reward moves by the drinker to achieve change in their drinking pattern, while avoiding rewarding and hence reinforcing drinking, but avoiding confrontation or ultimatums.
- Sometimes continued family involvement, despite their best intentions, serves only to support the drinker in their chosen lifestyle. In this case the family may have to be aided to step back (AA call this 'disengaging with love').

Prognostic factors There is ~3.6-fold excess mortality cf. age-matched controls. Of 100 45-yr-old patients at 20yrs follow-up: 40% dead, 30% abstinent, 30% problem drinking. **Positive factors** Motivated to change; supportive family or relationship; in employment; treatable comorbid illness (e.g. anxiety disorder, social phobia); accepting of appropriate treatment goal; AA involvement. **Negative factors** Ambivalent about change; unstable accommodation or homeless; drinking embedded into lifestyle (e.g. limited pursuits outside alcohol, all friends are drinkers); repeated treatment failures; cognitive impairment.

Alcohol withdrawal syndromes

In a patient with alcohol dependence, stopping alcohol completely or substantially reducing the usual amount causes the development of characteristic withdrawal syndromes. These syndromes should be anticipated, and prophylaxis considered in any patient:

- With a history of dependence.
- Who has previously experienced withdrawal syndromes.
- Who has consumed more than 10 units of alcohol on a daily basis for the previous 10 days.
- Currently experiencing withdrawals.

Uncomplicated alcohol withdrawal syndrome

- Occurs 4–12hrs after the last alcoholic drink.
- Features—coarse tremor, sweating, insomnia, tachycardia (pulse >100), nausea and vomiting, psychomotor agitation, and generalized anxiety.
- Occasionally, transitory visual, tactile, or auditory hallucinations or illusions.
- There may be increasing craving for alcohol both in itself and as a relief from withdrawal symptoms.
- Symptoms increase in severity in rough proportion to the habitual alcohol consumption, peaking at 48hrs and lasting 2–5 days, with symptoms being more prolonged in heavier drinkers.

Alcohol withdrawal syndrome with seizures

- In 5–15% of cases withdrawals are complicated by grand mal seizures occurring 6–48hrs after the last drink.
- If seizures occur only during withdrawal they do not signify the development of idiopathic epilepsy.
- Predisposing factors: previous history of withdrawal seizures, idiopathic epilepsy, history of head injury, hypokalaemia.

Delirium tremens

Acute confusional state (📖 p. 790) secondary to alcohol withdrawal. A medical emergency requiring inpatient medical care.

- Occurs in ~5% of episodes of withdrawal. Onset 1–7 days after the last drink with a peak incidence at 48hrs.
- Risk is increased by severe dependence, comorbid infection, and pre-existing liver damage.
- In addition to the features of uncomplicated withdrawal there is:
  - Clouding of consciousness.
  - Disorientation.
  - Amnesia for recent events.
  - Marked psychomotor agitation.
  - Visual, auditory, and tactile hallucinations (characteristically of diminutive people or animals—'Lilliputian' hallucinations).
  - Marked fluctuations in severity hour by hour, usually worse at night.
  - In severe cases: heavy sweating, fear, paranoid delusions, agitation, suggestibility, raised temperature, sudden cardiovascular collapse.

- Reported mortality of 5–10%. It is most risky when it develops unexpectedly and its initial manifestations are misinterpreted (e.g. in a patient not known to be alcohol-dependent developing symptoms post-operatively).
- Differential diagnosis: hepatic encephalopathy, head injury, pneumonia, acute psychotic illness, acute confusional state with other primary cause.

Management of alcohol withdrawal

Detoxification (detox) is the medical management of withdrawal symptoms in a patient with substance dependence. Alcohol detox involves: psychological support; medication to relieve withdrawal symptoms (usually via a reducing BDZ regime); observation for development of features of complicated withdrawal; nutritional supplementation; and integration with follow-up. Detox may be carried out as inpatient or, with support, in the community. The need to medically manage the complications of alcohol withdrawal can also arise in an unplanned fashion (e.g. in an alcohol-dependent patient in police custody or following emergency surgery). Most of the problems of alcohol use are related to inability to maintain abstinence, rather than to the initial problems of withdrawal.

Detox procedure

- Decide on setting.
- Assess need for BDZ-reducing regime.
- Consider need for other medications.
- Provide verbal and written advice.
- Inform GP of the plans.
- Give the patient a contact in case of emergency.
- Decide on explicit follow-up after detox.

Setting

Outpatient detox

- Treatment of choice for most uncomplicated alcohol-dependent patients, with comparable completion rates to inpatient detoxification and comparable percentage remaining abstinent at 6mths.
- Where there are doubts about compliance or concerns about drinking 'on top of' the prescribed drug, the patient should be seen daily in the morning and breathalysed before dispensing that day's and the following morning's supply of the drug.

Indications for inpatient detox

- Past history of complicated withdrawals (seizures or delirium).
- Current symptoms of confusion or delirium.
- Comorbid mental/physical illness, polydrug misuse, or suicide risk.
- Symptoms of Wernicke–Korsakoff syndrome ([] p. 572).
- Severe nausea/vomiting; severe malnutrition.
- Lack of stable home environment.

Reducing regime

BDZs are prescribed in alcohol withdrawal to ameliorate unpleasant withdrawal symptoms (e.g. tremor, anxiety) and to reduce the risk of withdrawal seizures. They are prescribed in a rapidly reducing regime in order to avoid the development of secondary, iatrogenic dependence, while covering the period of maximum risk (see Table 15.3).

- Many units prefer chlordiazepoxide to diazepam for outpatient use as it has lower abuse potential.
- Diazepam is often preferred for inpatient use as it is faster acting, allowing dose titration against effect, and can be given parenterally. Preferred in those with history of alcohol withdrawal seizures.

Indications for prescribing a reducing regime
• Clinical symptoms of withdrawal.
• History of alcohol dependence syndrome.
• Consumption is greater than 10 units/day over the previous 10 days.

Not required if
• <10 units daily.
• No history of withdrawals/drinking to avoid anticipated withdrawals.
• BAC = 0 and no withdrawal symptoms.

Symptom monitoring
Review patients regularly to assess withdrawals. Continuing symptoms should be managed by increasing the next day's planned dosages, rather than increasing the length of the course or relying on 'PRN' dosage.

Table 15.3 Benzodiazepine withdrawal regime
Suggested outpatient reducing regime using chlordiazepoxide.

	On waking	Midday	Early evening	At bedtime
Day 1	—	30mg	30mg	30mg
Day 2	20mg	20mg	20mg	20mg
Day 3	20mg	10mg	10mg	10mg
Day 4	10mg	10mg	—	20mg
Day 5	10mg	—	—	10mg

Other medications
• **Anticonvulsants** BDZs in sufficient dosage are the most effective anticonvulsants in alcohol withdrawal. Other oral drugs (e.g. phenytoin, carbamazepine) do not reach therapeutic level until after the time of maximal risk.
• **Antipsychotics** Where hallucinations or delusions develop they can usually be managed by temporarily increasing the BDZ dose. Addition of an antipsychotic (e.g. haloperidol 5–10mg orally up to tds) should be considered if this fails. Antipsychotics reduce seizure threshold; with sufficient BDZ cover this should not be a concern.
• **Supplementary vitamins** Where there are symptoms suggestive of Wernicke–Korsakoff syndrome or evidence of malnourishment give parenteral B vitamins (📖 p. 572). In other patients give a 4-wk course of 100mg thiamine, tds, in addition to multivitamins (mineral deficiencies, e.g. magnesium, are commonly seen in this group, and can predispose to withdrawal seizures).
• **Other psychotropics** While many patients withdrawing from alcohol complain of anxiety and/or depressive symptoms, many will be directly 2° to alcohol use/withdrawal. Do not treat with psychotropics until patient has been assessed when abstinent from alcohol. Generally speaking, do not start new psychotropics at this time.

Maintenance interventions in alcohol misuse 1: psychological methods

In planning treatment in alcohol problems, attention should be focused not only on achieving, but also on maintaining change. Many patients find the initial change (e.g. moving to abstinence or controlled drinking) surprisingly easy, but find it difficult to maintain change in the longer term. Alcohol misuse is a chronic illness characterized by relapse and in dependent drinkers there is the tendency for dependent drinking patterns to recur rapidly on abstinence. For this reason, maintenance interventions should support change, and in every patient, relapse should be anticipated and strategies to deal with it should be in place.

Individual counselling In addition to monitoring agreed change, individual counselling can address the following:
- Social skills training (e.g. 'saying no').
- Problem-solving skills.
- Relaxation training.
- Anger management.
- Cognitive restructuring.
- Relapse prevention.

In selected patients there may be a role for more formal psychotherapies.

Group support Variety of group methods both within the health service and in the voluntary sector. Variable local provision. Most widespread and best known is AA (see Box 15.2).

Pharmacological support (📖 p. 564).

Residential abstinence In selected patients, time in a residential facility may offer a period of abstinence which is unachievable 'outside', allowing interventions in physical and mental health and a chance to plan social change to permit continued abstinence on discharge. A variety of facilities exist, usually outside health care provision; some offer detoxification, while others will only accept patients following detox. Most residential rehabilitation centres will utilize group therapies, and follow the '12-step' approach, advocated by Alcoholics Anonymous (📖 p. 563). Residential rehabilitation is used in patients where home environment is unsupportive of abstinence and there has been failure of previous treatment options.

Advice to all patients regarding relapse Returning to drinking is the most common outcome in patients (and some consider relapse as pathognomonic of addiction). The stages of change model (📖 p. 544) considers relapse to be at the beginning of a further process of change, but with increased knowledge as to future strategies to combat relapse. A relapse can be motivated by over-confidence or forgetting gains. A 'slip' does not mean a full-blown relapse is inevitable and all patients should have strategies to deal with relapse discussed and agreed 'ahead of time'.

Box 15.2 Alcoholics Anonymous (AA)

Alcoholics Anonymous (AA) is the best known and the most widespread of the voluntary self-help organizations for problem drinkers. It was founded in 1935 in the USA by Bill Wilson and Dr Bob Smith, themselves both problem drinkers. Currently there are 73 000 groups in the UK and 788 000 groups worldwide. Associated organizations are Al-Anon (for relatives of problem drinkers); Al-Ateen (for teenage children of problem drinkers); and Narcotics Anonymous (NA) (for addicts of illicit drugs).

AA views alcoholism as a lifelong, incurable disease whose symptoms can be arrested by lifelong abstinence. Many other groups will use a variant of the AA model '12-step' programme. AA is a useful and effective intervention in many problem drinkers and all patients should be informed about AA and encouraged to consider attendance.

An AA meeting will generally follow a standard routine: there will be 10–20 people in each group, only first names are used; a rotating chairman will introduce himself with 'my name is X, and I am an alcoholic', then will read the AA preamble; a number of speakers are called from the floor who give an account of their stories and recovery if possible, leading to general discussion; the meeting ends with a prayer and is followed by informal discussions and contact between new members and sponsors who may offer emotional and practical support and perhaps a phone number. Open meetings are held where friends, family, and interested professionals can attend. Closed meetings are for AA members only. (See **Useful resources** for AA contacts in the UK and Ireland 📖 p. 1014.)

The '12 steps'
1. We admitted we were powerless over alcohol—that our lives had become unmanageable.
2. Came to believe that a power higher than ourselves could restore us to sanity.
3. Made a decision to turn our will and our lives over to the care of God as we understood him.
4. Made a searching and fearless moral inventory of ourselves.
5. Admitted to God, to ourselves, and to another human being the exact nature of our wrongs.
6. Were entirely ready to have God remove these defects of character.
7. Humbly asked Him to remove our shortcomings.
8. Made a list of the persons we had harmed, and became willing to make amends to them all.
9. Made direct amends to such people wherever possible, except when to do so would injure them or others.
10. Continued to take personal inventory, and when we were wrong promptly to admit it.
11. Sought through prayer and meditation to improve our conscious contact with God as we understood Him, praying only for knowledge of His will for us and the power to carry that out.
12. Having had a spiritual awakening as a result of these steps, we tried to carry this message to alcoholics and to practise these principles in our affairs.

Maintenance interventions in alcohol misuse 2: pharmacological methods

Aversive drugs

Disulfiram

Action Irreversible inhibition of acetaldehyde dehydrogenase (ALDH) which converts alcohol to carbon dioxide and water. If alcohol is taken, there is a build-up of acetaldehyde in the bloodstream causing unpleasant symptoms of flushing, headache, nausea and vomiting, and tachycardia. There is also recent evidence to suggest it may block dopamine B hydroxylase, increasing dopamine and decreasing noradrenaline.

Indication Can act as a helpful adjunct to therapy and allow the patient's relatives/employers to regain confidence in their ability to remain abstinent (evidence for increased efficacy with supervised administration).

Dose Prescribe once abstinence achieved. Starting dose: give loading dose of 800mg and then reduce over 5 days to 100–200mg daily or 200–400mg on alternate days.

Side-effects Halitosis and headache. Rare reports of psychotic reactions and hepatotoxicity.

Notes
- Patients should be counselled as to the nature and purpose of the drug and the likely side-effects if they drink.
- It is no longer recommended to give an alcohol 'challenge' to a patient newly started on disulfiram.
- Compliance is increased if the taking of the drug is monitored by another person (e.g. spouse).

Anti-craving drugs

Acamprosate

Action Believed to act through enhancing GABA transmission in the brain. Has been found to reduce alcohol consumption in animal models of alcohol addiction, with possible neuroprotective effects. Patients taking it report diminished alcohol craving. In RCT, cohort treated with acamprosate showed an increased percentage remaining abstinent and a doubling of time to first relapse. The majority of trials have been conducted with adjunctive psychosocial treatments, and therefore these should accompany treatment.

Indications Patients who wish to remain abstinent from alcohol.

Dose Once abstinence achieved: 666mg tds. Can be started at the end of detoxification.

Side effects GI upset, pruritus, rash, altered libido. (Generally well tolerated.)

Notes
- Discontinue if patient returns to regular drinking or relapses more than once while on the drug.
- Has no role in assisting with controlled drinking.
- Has no aversive action if alcohol is taken (though can be used in conjunction with disulfiram).
- Has no addictive potential itself.

Naltrexone

Action Antagonizes the effects of endogenous endorphins released by alcohol consumption. It is believed that this diminishes both the desirable 'high' experienced on taking alcohol and the loss of control reported by most dependent drinkers.

Indications In motivated subgroups of alcohol-dependent patients it appears to be effective in reducing total alcohol consumed and number of drinking days.

Dose Once abstinence achieved, give 25mg od initially, maintenance 50mg od.

Side effects GI upset, feeling anxious/'on edge', headache, fatigue, sleep disturbance, flu-like symptoms.

Notes
- Does not have an aversive or dependence-producing effect.
- Not currently licensed in the UK for treatment of alcohol dependence.

Alcohol misuse disorders 1

Acute intoxication The symptoms of alcohol intoxication will vary depending on the blood alcohol concentration (BAC), individual alcohol tolerance, and to some extent the setting in which the alcohol is taken. In general, as BAC rises from mild intoxication (BAC <100mg%) to moderate intoxication (BAC 100–200mg%) to severe intoxication (BAC >200mg%) a characteristic syndrome of acute intoxication is observed. Initial symptoms are elevated mood, disinhibition, and impaired judgement, followed by slurred speech, unsteady gait, nystagmus, ataxia, aggressiveness, lability of mood and impaired concentration, and eventually sopor and coma.

At-risk drinking There are reported benefits to health (lowered risk of coronary artery disease and strokes) associated with low levels of alcohol consumption as compared with those who are abstinent (the 'J-shaped curve'), though this remains a contentious area. Above this low level, health risks increase with increasing alcohol consumption. It is therefore arbitrary at which point drinking is considered 'at risk'. Patient and situational factors are important (e.g. any alcohol consumption while driving or in pregnancy carries increased risks; for patients with established alcohol-related organ damage any consumption is risky).

Harmful drinking (DSM-IV—alcohol abuse) Non-dependent drinking which continues despite established harm to the patient's physical or mental health secondary to the alcohol consumption. ICD-10 diagnosis considers only physical and mental health harm, not harm related to social sanction.

Alcohol dependence Harmful use of alcohol + established dependence syndrome (📖 p. 542). Usually daily, stereotyped drinking pattern with increased tolerance, withdrawal features on abstinence, and 'relief drinking' (i.e. further drinking to alleviate the effects of withdrawals).

Pathological intoxication ('mania à potu') This is a medically and legally disputed syndrome which was not included in DSM-IV due to lack of empirical evidence. It is described as an idiosyncratic reaction to a small amount of alcohol characterized by severe agitation, belligerence, and violent behaviour followed by collapse, profoundly deep sleep, and amnesia for the events which followed the alcohol consumption. It is a dubious diagnosis which is mainly sought after by defence lawyers, as most legal systems do not regard normal self-induced intoxication as a valid defence. There is of course a strong association between alcohol and violent crime. Careful re-examination of the history will usually demonstrate that significant quantities of alcohol have been consumed.

Alcohol-induced amnesia ('blackouts' or 'palimpsest') This term refers to transient amnesic episodes related to periods of intoxication. Characteristically the patient will report a 'gap' in their memory lasting several hours with global or partial amnesia for their actions during that time. The patient's behaviour as reported by witnesses is usually characteristic of their normal behaviour when intoxicated. This amnesia seems to be a failure of recall rather than initial registration and represents a reversible form of brain damage. Its occurrence is not predictive of longer-term cognitive impairment. It occurs in the later stages of a drinking career, if at all, and tends to recur once established. Two forms are described:

- *'En bloc'*—dense amnesia with well demarcated start and finish points.
- *Partial*—episodes with indistinct start and end point with islands of preserved memory and variable degrees of recall.

There is some degree of state-dependent recall in blackouts and a return to intoxication may aid recall. Because of the potential confusion of the term 'blackout' with periods of loss of consciousness, the term '*alcoholic palimpsest*' is to be preferred.

Alcohol misuse disorders 2

Alcoholic hallucinosis This is a substance-induced psychotic illness (defined in ICD-10), which is a rare complication of prolonged heavy alcohol abuse. The sufferer experiences hallucinations—usually auditory—in clear consciousness and while sober. The auditory hallucinations may begin as elemental hallucinations (e.g. bangs or murmurings) before, with continued alcohol use, being experienced as formed voices, most usually derogatory in nature. There may be secondary delusional elaboration. The nature of hallucinations tends to worsen during periods of alcohol detoxification, and at times, when intoxicated with alcohol.

- **Differential diagnosis** Transitory hallucinatory or illusionary experiences while intoxicated, delirium tremens, psychotic illnesses.
- **Course** In ~95% of patients there is rapid resolution of these symptoms on ceasing alcohol consumption but the symptoms rapidly recur on restarting drinking. In ~5% there are prolonged symptoms (<6mths after abstinence) and an emergence of more typical schizophrenic symptomatology.
- **Management** Persisting symptoms may be treated with anti-psychotic medication (bearing in mind the medical comorbidities seen in this population).

Alcohol-induced psychotic disorder with delusions Long recognized, but only recently included in DSM-IV. Development of persecutory or grandiose delusions after long history of heavy drinking. No other features of delirium tremens. Resolves on abstinence.

Delirium tremens (📖 p. 558)

Alcohol-related cognitive impairment/alcohol-related brain damage (ARBD)

The classification of alcohol-related cognitive impairment is unclear, with both ICD-10 and DSM-IV viewing it as a number of discrete entities, as opposed to a continuum. ICD-10 describes amnesic disorder (F10.6), dementia (F10.73), and other persisting cognitive disorder (F10.74), DSM-IV-TR using the terms alcohol-induced persisting amnestic disorder and alcohol-induced persisting dementia. It is worth noting that the DSM-IV-TR categories ignore the possibility of slow recovery over 1–2yrs in this patient group.

The majority (50–60%) of heavy drinkers display some degree of cognitive impairment on cognitive testing while sober. There is impairment in short-term memory, long-term memory recall, new skill acquisition, executive function, relative preservation of language ability and mildly impaired visuospatial function. IQ (measured by the WAIS) is generally preserved (in comparison with pre-morbid IQ, measured using the NART). CT/MRI examination of the brains of heavy drinkers reveals cortical and subcortical atrophy. White matter loss is prominent, which correlates with neuropathology findings. Degree of structural abnormality poorly correlated with degree of functional impairment. In all patients with alcohol-related brain damage (including those with 'alcohol dementia' and Korsakoff syndrome), a significant amount of medical comorbidity is seen, including small vessel disease, repetitive head injuries, and comorbid alcohol liver disease. The neurotoxic effects of alcohol on the brain are exacerbated significantly by thiamine deficiency, and there is evidence to suggest earlier onset in women. Abstinence from alcohol use has been shown to correlate with functional improvement and MRI improvement at 1yr.

The term alcohol dementia is used at times, describing a generalized dementia syndrome, in which there is intellectual decline and more pronounced neuropsychological deficits. The changes correlate with total lifetime drinking and length of drinking history.

Wernicke–Korsakoff syndrome (📖 p. 572)

Pathological jealousy (Othello syndrome)

This is a monosymptomatic delusional disorder (see 📖 p. 220) seen most commonly secondary to current or previous alcohol abuse. The form is a primary delusion in which the content is that the patient's spouse or partner has been or is being unfaithful. Delusional evidence may be provided to back up this belief and the patient may go to great lengths to obtain 'evidence' (e.g. following her, planting tape recorders, examining discarded clothing). There is a significant association with violence and even homicide towards the supposedly unfaithful partner.

Management
- Abstinence from alcohol with addition of antipsychotic medication.
- It may be necessary for the couple to separate and advice to this effect may have to be given to the at-risk partner.

Psychiatric comorbidity

Anxiety and depressive disorders Symptoms such as generalized anxiety, panic attacks, and low mood are very frequently reported in alcohol abusers. Many patients with alcohol problems also merit diagnoses of depressive illness (~50%) or anxiety disorder (~75%). The phenomenology of these disorders is similar to that found when the disorders occur in isolation. The difficulty is deciding the sequence of events, as in some cases the alcohol problem is secondary to the patient 'self-medicating' with alcohol in order to relieve primary anxiety or depressive symptoms. Nonetheless, chronic alcohol use will act as a direct depressant, its secondary effects will produce depressogenic life events (e.g. loss of job) and alcohol-related effects such waking at 04.00hr due to withdrawal, or weight loss related to nausea may masquerade as, or mask, biological depressive features.

Patients may emphasize the primacy of the mood or anxiety features and seek their resolution before tackling the alcohol problem. Generally a primary mood or anxiety disorder diagnosis should not be made in the presence of continuing alcohol misuse and psychological or pharmacological treatment for mood disorder is unlikely to be effective. The correct course is to initiate detox if indicated and to reassess mood/anxiety symptoms after 4wks of abstinence, treating residual symptoms at this point. Only a minority will require formal treatment. An undiagnosed depressive illness preceding the alcohol problem is more common in women. Alcohol problems can also arise as a result of self-medication of agoraphobia and social phobia.

Suicide Classically quoted as lifetime risk of 10–15% in dependent drinkers. Now estimated at ~4% lifetime risk of suicide in those with alcohol problems. Psychiatric comorbidity is important, as is social isolation, physical ill health, and repeated failed attempts at abstinence.

Schizophrenia High rates of alcohol and substance use found in schizophrenic patients (~50%). Increased risk of violence, EPSEs, TD, non-compliance, relapses, and rehospitalizations. Alcohol is an easily available temporary treatment for some of the distressing symptoms of psychotic illness.

Drug misuse Comorbid alcohol and drug misuse can be to enhance effects (e.g. euphoriant effect of alcohol and cocaine combined) or to minimize unpleasant side-effects (e.g. alcohol to relax after taking stimulants), or as a substitute when the primary drug is unavailable. Comorbid drug misuse is associated with poorer outcome. Some comorbidity can have an iatrogenic component where there is mixed abuse or substitution of BDZs for alcohol. This can result from inappropriate prescribing of anxiolytics, misdiagnosis of alcohol problems as anxiety disorders, and repeated unsupervised withdrawals with hoarding of tablets. Aim to limit new prescriptions, review diagnosis in patients with treatment-resistance anxiety disorders, and avoid short-acting BDZs (e.g. lorazepam).

Wernicke–Korsakoff syndrome

Wernicke encephalopathy and Korsakoff psychosis represent the acute and chronic phases of a single disease process—Wernicke–Korsakoff syndrome—which is caused by neuronal degeneration secondary to thiamine deficiency, most commonly seen in heavy drinkers.

Wernicke encephalopathy

Clinical features Acute onset of tetrad of: (1) acute confusional state; (2) ocular signs (ophthalmoplegia, nystagmus); (3) ataxic gait. Associated features of: peripheral neuropathy, resting tachycardia, and evidence of nutritional deficiency. Ophthalmoplegia is most commonly 6th nerve palsy (paralysis of lateral gaze). Triad only seen in 10% of cases, confusion in ~80% of cases.

Aetiology Occurs secondary to thiamine (vitamin B_1) deficiency. Heavy drinkers are especially vulnerable due to poor intake (alcohol is calorie-rich but vitamin-poor), reduced absorption, and impaired hepatic storage. Other rare causes of thiamine deficiency are starvation, post-gastric resection, anorexia nervosa, and hyperemesis gravidarum.

Pathology Haemorrhages and secondary gliosis in periventricular and periaqueductal grey matter involving the mamillary bodies, hypothalamus, mediodorsal thalamic nucleus, colliculi, and tegmentum of midbrain.

Treatment

- Give high potency parenteral B_1 replacement—IV *Pabrinex*®, 2 ampoules by influnce over 30min twice daily for 3–7 days. Specialist use. (*Note:* associated with allergic reactions; facilities for treatment of anaphylaxis must be available, though recent evidence suggests negligible risk with recent preparations.) Avoid carbohydrate load until thiamine replacement is complete (i.e. do not rehydrate with glucose solutions prior to thiamine).
- Treat immediately diagnosis is made or strongly suspected. In addition, consider treating all those at high risk (alcohol-dependent patients with poor nutrition) prophylactically with parenteral vitamins.
- All patients with symptoms of Wernicke encephalopathy and those at high risk should have parenteral vitamins as in *Treatment*. All other patients undergoing detox, or being assessed for alcohol problems, should receive oral replacement—thiamine 100mg tds for 1mth.
- Assess and treat for alcohol withdrawal syndrome (🔲 p. 558).

Prognosis

- Untreated the acute phase lasts ~2 weeks with 84% of cases developing features of Korsakoff psychosis. Mortality of ~15% in untreated cases.
- With treatment, the ophthalmoplegia and confusion resolve within days, but the ataxia, neuropathy, and nystagmus may be prolonged or permanent.

Korsakoff syndrome

Clinical features Absence or significant impairment in the ability to lay down new memories, together with a variable length of retrograde amnesia. Working memory (e.g. ability to remember a sequence of numbers) is unimpaired as is procedural and 'emotional' memory. Thus the affected individual may be able to go with a psychologist to an interview room, perform adequately on working memory testing, show evidence of a new skill (e.g. mirror writing) they practised the day before, and yet later have no memory of ever having been in that room or having seen that psychologist before (although, on returning to the room, they may be more relaxed on subsequent occasions, due to state-related emotional memories). Confabulation for the episodes of amnesia may be prominent. Other neuropsychological deficits associated with ARBD may be seen.

Aetiology Most commonly due to thiamine deficiency, secondary to heavy alcohol use. Rarer causes are head injury, post-anaesthesia, basal/temporal lobe encephalitis, carbon monoxide poisoning, and thiamine deficiency secondary to other causes. It should be remembered that Korsakoff syndrome is not invariably preceded by Wernicke encephalopathy, and can present in a 'chronic' form.

Pathology Pathological features are those of Wernicke encephalopathy. The presumed mechanism is disconnection of a mamillothalamic pathway crucial for memory formation.

Treatment
- Continue oral thiamine replacement and multivitamin supplementation for up to 2yrs.
- Treat psychiatric comorbidity (e.g. depression)
- OT assessment, cognitive rehabilitation within an appropriate setting, acknowledging that some patients improve and may progress to independent living. Therefore, these patients will require continuous assessment of their functioning, bearing in mind that improvement occurs in approximately 50% of those presenting with Korsakoff syndrome.

Prognosis
- 20% of cases show complete recovery, and 25% significant recovery over time, with the remainder largely unchanged.
- The degree of functional impairment is directly related to the degree of memory impairment which may be incompatible with independent living.

Medical complications of alcohol misuse

Hepatic

- **Alcoholic liver disease (ALD)** is the most common cause of liver damage in the developed world. Presents as fatty change, alcoholic hepatis, and, finally, as cirrhosis.
  - Fatty change seen in >90% of heavy drinkers, can emerge after single heavy bout, may be asymptomatic, or may present as lethargy, malaise, painful and swollen liver, and obstructive jaundice. Reverses with abstinence.
  - Alcoholic hepatitis—40% of heavy drinkers.
  - Cirrhosis—up to 30% of heavy drinkers after 10–30yrs. Predisposed to by genetic variation (reduced alcohol oxidation and increased acetaldehyde accumulation), female sex (less first-pass metabolism and lower body water content for alcohol dispersal), comorbid hepatitis B or C infection.

Gastrointestinal

- Gastritis/gastric erosions with consequent haematemesis.
- Metaplasia of lower third of the oesophagus (Barrett's oesophagus).
- Mallory–Weiss oesophageal tears secondary to vomiting.
- Peptic ulceration.
- Chronic diarrhoea.
- Chronic pancreatitis (alcohol is most common cause) with chronic fluctuating abdominal pain and steatorrhoea.

Cancers

- Hepatocellular, oesophagus, stomach, mouth, tongue, and pharynx.

Cardiovascular

- Hypertension.
- Dilated cardiomyopathy.
- Cardiac arrhythmias (esp. atrial fibrillation).
- CVA.
- Non- or very light drinkers have higher risk than light drinkers even after controlling for smoking, hypertension, etc. (i.e. 'the J-shaped curve' for mortality); no specific drink type (i.e. not red wine); mechanism may be increase in protective HDL and reduced platelet adhesion.

Respiratory

- Tuberculosis.
- Klebsiella and streptococcal pneumonia.
- Increased vulnerability is related to decreased immunity, poor nutrition, and self-neglect.

Neurological
- Wernicke–Korsakoff syndrome (📖 p. 572).
- Peripheral neuropathy.
- Central pontine myelinolysis (pseudobulbar palsy + quadriplegia).
- Marchiafava–Bignami disease (corpus callosum degeneration).
- Cerebellar degeneration.
- Optic atrophy.
- Alcoholic myopathy.

Genitourinary
- Erectile problems.
- Hypogonadism in men.

Other
- Foetal alcohol syndrome (📖 p. 756).
- Gout.
- Osteoporosis.
- Impaired absorption and diminished intake of specific vitamins and food overall.
- Contribution to accidents, particularly RTA.
- Exacerbating factor in violent crime and assaults.
- Diminished compliance with treatment for other medical and psychiatric disorders.

Illegal drugs

In the UK, community surveys indicate that one third of adults have tried illegal drugs in their lifetime, with 10% having used them in the previous year. The rates for those aged under 25 are higher, with 50% lifetime use and 33% in the previous year. At all ages males have higher rates of drug use than females ($\male$:$\female$ = 3–4:1). Cannabis is the most commonly used illegal drug, while community rates for the other drugs of abuse are low. Users show a variable pattern of consumption with episodic and situational use for drugs with low dependence potential and a tendency to continuous dependent use for more 'addictive' drugs. Among some users, particularly those in the dance scene, polydrug use is the norm with individuals consuming more than 10 different drugs. Use of illegal drugs is commoner in the young, in the lower socio-economic classes, and in those with psychiatric illness. At any one time <33% of dependent users will be in contact with treatment services; mean length of dependent use before seeking help is 9yrs.

There are as many patterns of drug use as drug user, and individual patient assessment is mandatory; nonetheless a number of patterns of use of illegal drugs can be recognized:

- **Experimental use** Use of drug in order to explore effects. Common among young and heavily driven by drug availability and drug use among peers. Very common for 'softer' drugs (e.g. cannabis, volatile chemicals), rarer for more 'hard' drugs (e.g. heroin).
- **Situational use** Drug use limited to certain situations (e.g. parties, raves). Mainly drugs with stimulant/hallucinogenic properties.
- **Recreational use** Regular, but non-dependent use. May be limited in time by period of life (e.g. ending at the end of university life) or may progress to dependent use.
- **Polydrug use** Non-dependent use of variety of drugs. One drug may be taken to potentiate the effects of another or to manage unpleasant after-effects of drug use. Risks can be additive or multiplicative.
- **Dependent use** Use of a drug for which a dependence syndrome (🕮 p. 542) has developed. Continued use may be motivated more by the desire to avoid withdrawals than by positive drug effects which may have diminished due to the development of tolerance. Tendency is for the use of the dependent drug to predominate, with other drugs being taken only if the primary drug is unavailable.
- **Dual diagnosis** Drug users who also suffer from a major mental illness. An important group for therapeutic intervention.

Categories of drugs of abuse

- **Opiates:** e.g. heroin, dihydrocodeine, methadone, codeine, buprenorphine, pethidine.
- **Depressants:** e.g. BDZs, barbiturates, alcohol, GHB.
- **Stimulants:** e.g. amfetamines, cocaine, MDMA.
- **Hallucinogens:** e.g. LSD, PCP, mushrooms, ketamine.
- **Others:** e.g. cannabis, volatile substances, anabolic steroids.

Street slang associated with drug misuse

Table 15.4 Drug 'street names'

Street drug name	Conventional name
Acid	LSD
Adam	MDMA
Angel dust	PCP
Billy	Amfetamine
Blow	Cannabis
Brown	Heroin
C, Charlie, Coke	Cocaine
Crack	Freebase cocaine
Dope	Cannabis
Downers	Depressant drugs
E, Ecstasy, Eccies	MDMA
GBH, grievous bodily harm	GHB (gammahydroxybutyrate)
Gear	Heroin
Grass, hash	Cannabis
Jellies	Temazepam
Marijuana	Cannabis
Mushies	Psilocybin mushrooms
Poppers	Volatile nitrates
Roids	Anabolic steroids
Roofies	Rohypnol®
Skag	Heroin
Skunk	Potent form of cannabis
Smack	Heroin
Snow	Cocaine
Special K	Ketamine
Speed	Amfetamine
Sulph	Amfetamine
Uppers	Stimulant drugs
Vallies	Diazepam
Vitamin K	Ketamine
Whizz	Amfetamine

Table 15.5 Drug slang terms

Slang term	Meaning
Backtrack	Allow blood to flow back into IV syringe and then re-inject
Chasing	Consume heroin by heating on foil and inhaling the fumes
Cold turkey	Withdrawal symptoms (referring to the piloerection)
Cooking up	Melting down heroin prior to injection
Fix	The required regular dose of drug in a dependent user
Gouching	Apparent somnolence following heroin use
Jag up	To inject drugs IV
Juggling	Selling drugs to finance one's own dependency
Junkie	An individual dependent on a drug
Mainline	To inject drugs IV
Nodding, on the nod	Apparent somnolence following heroin use
Rattling	Suffering from withdrawals
Score	Obtain drugs
Script	Legitimate prescription for drugs
Shooting gallery	Place where individuals meet to use drugs IV
Skin popping	To inject drugs subdermally
Sorted	Having obtained sufficient drug for one's own needs
Spliff	Cannabis cigarette
Tab	Dose of LSD impregnated onto paper
Works	Syringe and needles

Opiates/opioids

The opiates are a group of chemicals derived from the opium poppy (*papaver somniferum*); synthetic compounds with similar properties are called opioids. They have potent analgesic properties and as such have wide legitimate uses in medicine. They are widely abused for their euphoriant and anxiolytic properties. Heroin is the most frequently abused opiate.

Heroin Illicit heroin is sold as a brown or white powder in 'bags' or 'wraps', costing £50–£100/g, with a typical dependent user taking 0.25–2.0g/day. It is most commonly consumed by smoking ('chasing'), but is also taken orally, occasionally snorted, and parenterally by IV, IM, or subcutaneous routes. Street supplies are of variable purity (25–50% by volume); occasionally, a particularly pure batch is associated with a series of deaths and ODs from users used to a less concentrated form.

In common with other opiates, heroin binds to specific receptors for which there are endogenous ligands (endorphins). There are overall cortical inhibitory effects with diminished pain sensation. After consumption, effects are virtually immediate with euphoria amounting to ecstasy, intense relaxation, and untethering from worries and cares.

Although recreational use is not unknown, the tendency is for progression to dependent use and this is the most usual pattern by the time of presentation to treatment services. An established dependent user may move from smoking to occasional or regular IV use to potentiate effects. Users develop tolerance with regular use and there is cross-tolerance to other opiates. Dependent patients may describe limited euphoriant effects, with the drug being mainly taken to avoid unpleasant withdrawals.

Acute medical problems associated with heroin use by any route include nausea and vomiting, constipation, respiratory depression, and loss of consciousness with aspiration (the cause of many fatalities). Injected use adds risks of local abscesses, cellulitis, osteomyelitis, bacterial endocarditis, septicaemia, and the transmission of viral infections (hepatitis B and C, HIV). Opiate dependency develops after weeks of regular use and is associated with an unpleasant (but not generally medically dangerous) withdrawal syndrome (📖 p. 596).

Interventions Give harm reduction advice to users who continue to use opiates: do not use opiates while alone; do not use in combination with other drugs; avoid IV route; if injecting, give safe injecting advice (Box 15.3). Consider managed detox (📖 p. 598) or transfer to maintenance prescribing (📖 p. 598) in established dependence.

Other opiates/opioids These include dihydrocodeine, morphine, methadone, pethidine, buprenorphine, and codeine. They may be taken in their pre-prepared tablet or liquid form or prepared for injection. Their acute and chronic risks are similar to heroin.

Box 15.3 Safer injecting advice

If using heroin it is safest to avoid IV use which has the greatest risk of overdose and other complications. If using heroin IV:

• Use new sterile needles and syringes on each occasion (give details of local needle exchange services if available)
• Use sterile water (water from running cold kitchen tap is closest)
• Never share needles, syringes, spoons, or filters with another user
• Rotate injection sites
• Avoid injecting into neck, groin, or breast
• Avoid injection into infected areas
• Ensure that the drug is completely dissolved before injecting
• Always inject with, not against, the blood flow
• Do not take heroin while alone

It is safest to use new sterile needles and syringe on each occasion. Failing this, rather than use dirty equipment, flush both needles and syringes several times with thin bleach, then several times with clean water.

Depressants

Drugs of this group produce their effects by generalized or specific cortical depression. They include the BDZs, alcohol, and the barbiturates. They can be taken for their pleasurable anxiolytic and relaxant properties alone, or as a way of counteracting unpleasant side-effects of other drugs of abuse (e.g. to 'come down' after stimulant use).

Benzodiazepines A class of chemicals initially synthesized in the 1950s. Largely replaced barbiturates in clinical practice as they did not cause fatal respiratory depression. They have therapeutic uses as anxiolytics, hypnotics, anticonvulsants, and muscle relaxants. Problems of dependency arising from long-term use became recognized in the 1980s leading to a fall in their legitimate prescription, but did nothing to diminish their popularity as drugs of abuse. All BDZs have similar effects and are distinguished by their length of action: short-acting (e.g. temazepam, oxazepam), medium-acting (e.g. lorazepam, alprazolam), long-acting (e.g. diazepam, nitrazepam, chlordiazepoxide).

Benzodiazepines are taken orally, or less commonly by injection. There is hepatic metabolism to active compounds, some with long half-lives. They enhance GABA transmission and produce marked anxiolytic and euphoriant effects. Tolerance develops rapidly (with cross-tolerance to all drugs in the benzodiazepine group), so requiring increasing doses to achieve similar effects.

Acutely they cause forgetfulness, drowsiness, and impaired concentration and co-ordination with consequent risk of accidents. Use by injection is associated with the same infective risks as IV heroin (📖 p. 581). An additional problem seen in IV benzodiazepine users is limb ischaemia secondary to intravenous use of melted tablet contents. Chronic use is associated with impaired concentration and memory and depressed mood, all of which are more severe in the elderly. Benzodiazepine dependency develops after 3–6wks of regular use. There is a withdrawal syndrome (📖 p. 600) which can be complicated by seizures and delirium.

Interventions Harm reduction advice to user as for opiates (📖 p. 580), specifying safe injecting advice (📖 p. 581) if using via IV route. Consider managed detox or transfer to maintenance prescribing (📖 p. 600) in established dependence.

Flunitrazepam (Rohypnol)® A short-acting potent BDZ seen particularly in dance settings with intoxicant and (probably apocryphal) aphrodisiac effects. As it can produce impaired judgement and anterograde amnesia and is tasteless in solution it has been implicated in cases of 'date rape'.

Gamma-hydroxybutyrate (GHB) A synthetic compound originally developed as an anaesthetic which is a probable intrinsic neurotransmitter. Particularly seen in dance settings usually in combination with other drugs or alcohol. Produces a sense of dissociation, euphoria, and intoxication. Taken as liquid, 5–10mg dosage with effects coming on in 15–30min and lasting several hours. Side-effects of nausea and vomiting, seizures, and respiratory depression. Usually taken episodically, but a cohort of patients is increasingly seen with consumption of the drug multiple times daily, with consequent physical dependence. Withdrawal from established dependence can present as a medical emergency, and is associated with delirium, severe behavioural disturbance, psychotic features, autonomic instability, and occasionally acute renal failure. Such patients will usually require joint psychiatric and medical management. Drug treatment of these withdrawals is via reducing benzodiazepine regime as per alcohol withdrawal (higher doses usually required), with the addition of regular baclofen given as a reducing regime, starting at 20mg five times daily, reducing over the subsequent week.

Barbiturates Group of compounds used as hypnotics/anxiolytics in clinical practice prior to the introduction of the benzodiazepines. Now rarely prescribed and rarely seen as drugs of abuse. They act by facilitating GABA neurotransmission. There is rapidly increasing tolerance to their anxiolytic effects in regular use but not to the associated respiratory depression.

Stimulants

These drugs potentiate neurotransmission and increase cortical excitability, producing effects of increased alertness and endurance, diminished need for sleep, and a subjective sense of well-being. They include cocaine (and crack cocaine), amfetamines, 3,4,-methylenedioxymethamfetamine (MDMA or ecstasy), and caffeine.

Cocaine The mild stimulant/euphoriant effects of the chewed leaves of the coca shrub have been known to the people of South America for thousands of years, but in its refined form cocaine is a potent and highly addictive drug. Cocaine hydrochloride is refined to a white powder which may be inhaled ('snorted') or dissolved and injected. The main route of intake is by inhalation as it undergoes rapid 'first pass' liver metabolism. The user forms the powder into 'lines' and inhales via rolled paper tube (classically, a high denomination banknote). Each line contains ~25mg cocaine. Freebase ('crack') cocaine (produced by alkalinization, which produces the hydrochloride-free ion form) has a lower vaporization temperature than the hydrochloride and can be smoked. In terms of rapidity of action and peak blood levels this compares with IV use.

Cocaine acts as a local anaesthetic at the mucous membranes. It has widespread effects in potentiating dopaminergic, serotinergic, and noradrenalinergic neurotransmission by blocking neurotransmitter reuptake. Its actions begin a few minutes after consumption. There is increased energy, increased confidence, euphoria, and diminished need for sleep, but with rapid fall-off in effects due to rapid metabolism, leading to repeated use. There are very intense effects from freebase cocaine use with rapid and intense 'high' with subsequent dysphoria. Cocaine is usually taken in an opportunistic way, sometimes in association with other stimulant drugs.

Acute harmful effects include arrhythmias, intense anxiety, hypertension → CVA, acute impulsivity, and impaired judgement. Chronic harmful effects include necrosis of nasal septum, fetal damage ('crack babies'), panic and anxiety disorders, persecutory delusions, and psychosis. It is not associated with classical dependence but a minority of users will consume in a regular 'compulsive' pattern.

Interventions Harm reduction advice (including safe injecting advice, 📖 p. 581, if appropriate). No role for substitute prescribing in managing withdrawal or for maintenance prescribing.

Amfetamines A group of compounds synthesized in the late nineteenth century with current legitimate uses in child psychiatry (📖 p. 628) and in narcolepsy (📖 p. 432). Sold as 5mg tablets or as white powder (£10 per gram). The powder may be swallowed, inhaled, or dissolved and injected. Use is usually situational or recreational, although very regular use with dependence is recognized. There is chemical similarity to noradrenaline and dopamine, producing similar pharmacological effects to cocaine, but its slower metabolism gives a longer duration of action.

Acute harmful effects include tachycardia, arrhythmias, hyperpyrexia, irritability, post-use depression, and quasi-psychotic state with visual, auditory, and tactile hallucinations. Dependency is not seen but marked psychological addiction occurs, particularly in situations associated with drug use. Anxiety and depressive symptoms are frequently seen in users; their proper assessment requires a period of abstinence.

Interventions Harm reduction advice (including safe injecting advice, if appropriate). No role for substitute prescribing in managing withdrawals. Very limited role for maintenance prescribing of dexamfetamine sulphate in the management of chronic, primary, heavy IV users (specialist instigation only).

MDMA (ecstasy) This compound was synthesized in 1914. Initially, was occasionally used as an adjunct to psychotherapy. Initially legal, it became widely used in the mid-1980s in association with house, rave, and techno music. It is taken orally as 50–200mg tablet. A typical pattern of use is two or more tablets taken at weekends.

MDMA causes serotonin release and blocks reuptake. It has structural similarities to mescaline and amfetamine, therefore has both hallucinogenic and stimulant properties, these effects appearing ~30mins after ingestion. The initial 'rush' period of intoxication lasts ~3hrs and is characterized by a feeling of increased camaraderie and 'closeness' to others, a pleasurable agitation relieved by dancing, and decreased fatigue.

Acute harmful effects include increased sweating, nausea and vomiting, and diminished potency despite increased libido. Deaths have occurred associated with dehydration and hyperthermia (a toxic reaction similar to serotonin syndrome appears to exist [📖 p. 960]). Chronic harmful effects include possible neurotoxicity, hepatotoxicity, and possible chronic cognitive impairment. There is tolerance to its effects but dependence does not occur. 'Hangover' effects develop 24–48hrs after ingestion including fatigue, anorexia, and depressed mood (which may be severe).

Interventions Harm reduction advice regarding maintaining hydration and avoiding overheating during use. No role for substitute prescribing in managing withdrawal or for maintenance prescribing. For all stimulant drugs there may be a problem of assessing other aspects of mental state, particularly affective and psychotic features while chaotic use continues. In selected patients, inpatient assessment will be indicated to allow this.

Hallucinogens

Hallucinogens (or psychedelics) are a heterogeneous group of natural and synthetic substances which produce altered sensory and perceptual experiences. They include: lysergic acid diethylamide (LSD), phenylcyclidine (PCP), magic mushrooms, ketamine, mescaline, 2,5-dimethoxy-4-methyl-amfetamine (DOM), and dimethyltriptamine (DMT).

Lysergic acid diethylamide (LSD) A compound synthesized by Hofman while working at Sandoz pharmaceuticals in 1944. He reported the hallucinatory experiences that followed his initial, accidental ingestion. The drug also occurs naturally in seeds of the Morning Glory plant. It became strongly associated with 1960s culture when its use was at its peak. There was early experimentation with its role in psychotherapy but there is no current legitimate use. It is very soluble and intensely potent (effective dose ~250 micrograms). It is sold impregnated onto paper, in tablets, or as a powder.

LSD is an indolealkylamine with structural similarity to serotonin. There are direct and indirect effects on serotinergic and dopaminergic transmitter systems. It is not now thought to provide a good model for endogenous psychosis. Its actions are very markedly situation- and expectation-dependent. Effects develop 15–30mins after ingestion and last up to 6hrs. There is initial euphoria; a sense of detachment; a sense of novelty in the familiar and a sense of wonder at the normal; visual distortions and misperceptions; synaesthesia; and distorted body image. Somatic effects include dizziness and tremors.

Acute harmful effects are behavioural toxicity (i.e. harm related to acting on beliefs such as having the ability to fly) and 'bad trips' (i.e. dissociation, fear of incipient madness, frightening perceptions). There is no risk of overdose and physiological dependence and withdrawals do not occur. Chronic harmful effects include flashbacks (🕮 p. 96) even many years after consumption, post-hallucinogenic perceptual disorder, persistent psychosis, and persistent anxiety/depressive symptoms.

Interventions Harm-reduction advice directed towards maintaining a safe environment during use and avoiding behavioural toxicity—do not use alone, use accompanied by non-user if possible. For all hallucinogens, acute psychotic features should in general be managed by admission, maintenance of a safe environment, symptomatic treatment of agitation (e.g. with benzodiazepine), with expectation of resolution. Continuing psychotic features should be managed as for acute psychosis (🕮 p. 192).

Phenylcyclidine (PCP) An hallucinogen rarely seen in the UK except as a contaminant of other drugs. May be smoked, snorted, taken orally, or, more rarely, parenterally. There is direct binding to opioid and aspartate excitatory receptors as well as serotonergic and cholinergic effects producing acute effects of confusion, visual sensory distortions, aggression, and sudden violence (which may be severe). Intoxication may give way to longer psychotic states.

Magic mushrooms About a dozen varieties of hallucinogenic mushrooms grow in the UK, the best known being the Liberty cap (*Psilocybe semilanceata*). They may be eaten raw or cooked, dried or prepared as a drink. Possession and consumption of mushrooms is not an offence unless they have been processed or prepared for illicit use. Small doses cause euphoria, while larger doses (>25 mushrooms) cause perceptual abnormalities similar to LSD. They are not associated with dependence or withdrawal features and tolerance develops quickly, making continuous use unlikely. Harmful effects include nausea and vomiting, dizziness, diarrhoea and abdominal cramps, behavioural toxicity, and risk of accidental consumption of toxic fungi.

Ketamine A compound structurally similar to phencyclidine used as a veterinary anaesthetic and in battlefield surgery. It is a unique anaesthetic as it does not produce reticular activating system (RAS) depression, instead it prevents cortical awareness of painful stimuli. It is taken illicitly as a sniffed powder, mean dose ~100mg. Small amounts lead to a sense of dissociation, larger amounts to LSD-like synaesthesia and hallucinations, associated with nausea, ataxia, and slurred speech. Rare late effects are flashbacks, psychosis, and amnesic syndromes.

Other drugs

Cannabis The most commonly used illegal drug, with only a small minority of its users ever using another illegal drug. Used for centuries as a pleasurable mind-altering substance and as a medication for a wide variety of ailments. Clinical trials are underway to clarify its role in the treatment of chronic pain. Its illegal use is of interest to psychiatrists because of its association with other drugs of abuse (as a 'gateway drug') and because of its exacerbating effect on chronic psychotic illnesses.

Cannabis is produced from the dried leaves, flowers, stems, and seeds of the weed *Cannabis Sativa*. It may be distributed as herbal material ('grass' or marijuana), as a resin ('hash'), or as cannabis oil. Cannabis may be smoked in cigarettes, alone, or mixed with tobacco; the resin form may be eaten directly or incorporated into foodstuffs (e.g. cakes). These various forms contain at least 60 psychoactive cannaboids, the most important of which is 9-δ-tetrahydrocannabinol (THC). The dried herb contains ~5% THC by weight; resin ~10%; and cannabis oil ~15%.

Usage pattern is very variable, from infrequent situational use to daily heavy use; the latter at highest risk of harmful effects and most likely to take other drugs. There is a specific cannabinoid receptor and a naturally occurring agonist at this receptor—'anandamide'. The role of this endogenous system has yet to be defined. In addition, cannabis shows both weak opiate-like and weak barbiturate-like effects. The drug is metabolized to active and inactive metabolites and their absorption into fat means that urine tests remain positive for up to 4 weeks after regular use has ceased.

The effects of intoxication are apparent within minutes if the drug is smoked, peaking in ~30min and lasting 2–5hrs. The effects of orally consumed cannabis are slower to begin and more prolonged. The immediate effects include mild euphoria ('the giggles'), a sense of enhanced well-being, subjective sense of enhanced sensation, relaxation, altered time sense, and increased appetite ('the munchies'). Physically there is mild tachycardia and variable dysarthria and ataxia.

Acute harmful effects include mild paranoia, panic attacks, and accidents associated with delayed reaction time. Cannabis is normally smoked with tobacco, therefore all of the health risks associated with tobacco will also apply. The tendency of cannabis smokers to inhale deeply and to retain the smoke in the lungs for as long as possible will exacerbate this risk. There are no reports of fatal overdose. Chronic harmful effects include dysthymia, anxiety/depressive illnesses, the disputed *amotivational syndrome* (possibly representing a combination of chronic intoxication in a heavy user and a long half-life). The drug is not usually associated with physical dependency but there is a mild but characteristic withdrawal syndrome in the previously heavy regular user who stops suddenly, consisting of insomnia, anxiety, and irritability. Cannabis use can precipitate an episode of or relapse of schizophrenia. In addition, in regular users it is associated with dose-related paranoid ideation and other psychotic features.

Interventions As an illegal drug there are no set guidelines on safe use. Clinical experience suggests that irregular use can be free from major problems. Abstinence is indicated in those with major mental illness and continuing cannabis use may expose those recovering from more serious drug problems to dealers and the drugs subculture.

Volatile substances

Simple hydrocarbons such as acetone, toluene, xylene, and butane have intoxicant properties. These chemicals are found in a variety of common products including glue, lighter fuel, paint stripper, fire extinguishers, aerosols, paints, petrol, correcting fluid, and nail varnish remover. They are rapidly absorbed when inhaled or by sniffing propellant gases or aerosols. They cause non-specific increased permeability of nerve cell membranes and produce euphoriant effects, disinhibition, slurred speech and blurred vision, and visual misperceptions.

Acute harmful effects include local irritation, headache, cardiac arrhythmias, acute suffocation by bag or laryngeal oedema, unconsciousness, aspiration, and sudden death. Chronic harmful effects include liver and kidney damage, memory/concentration impairment, and probable long-term cognitive impairment. There is a withdrawal syndrome similar to alcohol in very heavy regular users.

Interventions Education of users and 'at risk' groups. Most use will be experimental with few going on to regular use. Legal controls on substance availability.

Anabolic steroids

These prescription-only medicines (e.g. nandrolone and stanozolol) have limited legitimate uses in the treatment of aplastic anaemia and osteoporosis. They can be abused by athletes and body builders seeking competitive advantage or, more rarely, for their euphoriant effects alone. They produce increased muscle mass and strength, with increased training time and reduced recovery time as well as euphoriant effects and a sense of increased energy levels. (Other drugs misused by athletes include levothyroxine, growth hormone, diuretics, erythropoietin, and amfetamine.)

Use of anabolic steroids is associated with physical health problems including hypertension, hypogonadism, gynaecomastia, amenorrhoea, liver damage, impotence, and male pattern baldness; and with mental health problems including acute emotional instability (sometimes known as 'roid rage'), increased aggressiveness, persecutory/grandiose delusions, depressive illness, and chronic fatigue. If injected they can also be associated with infection risks (📖 p. 582). There is no withdrawal syndrome.

Interventions Education of risks through coaches, teachers, etc. Effective monitoring of individual sports with out-of-season testing.

Legal highs

Heterogeneous group of psychoactive substances that are not controlled under the Misuse of Drugs Act, and are therefore legal to possess. It should be noted that a significant number of these drugs are regulated under the Medicines Act, and it is against the law to sell, supply, or advertise them for human consumption. They are broadly sold over the

Internet and specialist shops. They can consist of plant-based and synthetic compounds, with variable effects. A good example is that of mephadrone ('meow-meow' or 'M-CAT'), a cathenone that acts as a stimulant, with equivalent psychiatric sequelae. A difficulty encountered with these drugs is that synthesis occurs at a rate quicker than regulation, although regulatory bodies are changing practice to reflect this.

Assessment of the drug user

In most cases an assessment of a patient's history of drug use will form part of a routine psychiatric interview. In addition, all doctors should consider the possibility of, and be prepared to ask about, comorbid drug misuse when interviewing patients for other reasons. The more detailed assessment described here is appropriate for patients in whom drug use is the primary focus of clinical concern and who are being assessed for entry into a treatment programme. The detailed assessment of a patient with drug use problems will usually be carried out over more than one consultation. There are only a few circumstances (such as an opiate-dependent patient presenting as an acute medical emergency), where treatment should be considered before full assessment. History should cover the following topics:

Background information Narne, address, next of kin, GP, names of other professionals involved (e.g. social worker, probation officer).

Reasons for consultation now Why has the drug user presented now (e.g. pressure from family, pending conviction, 'had enough', increasing difficulty injecting)? What does the user seek from the programme? In females, is there a possibility of pregnancy?

Current drug use Enquire about each drug taken over the previous 4wks. Describe the frequency of use (e.g. daily, most days, at weekends); and the number of times taken each day. Record the amount taken and the route. Ask the user about episodes of withdrawal. Include alcohol, tobacco, and cannabis. If there is IV use, inquire about needle or other equipment sharing.

Lifetime drug use Record the age at first use of drugs and the changing pattern of drug use until the most recent consultation. Enquire about periods of abstinence or stability and the reasons for this (e.g. prison, relationship, treatment programme).

Complications of drug use Overdoses—deliberate or accidental. History of cellulitis, abscesses, or phlebitis. Hepatitis B and C and HIV status if known.

Previous treatment episodes Timing, locus, and type of previous drug treatment. How did the treatment attempt end? Was the treatment helpful?

Medical and psychiatric history All episodes of medical or psychiatric inpatient care. Contact with hospital specialists. Current health problems. Relationship with GP.

Family history Are there other family members with drug or alcohol problems? Family history of medical or psychiatric problems.

Social history Current accommodation. How stable is this accommodation? Sexual orientation and number of sexual partners. Enquire about safe sex precautions. Describe the user's relationships—sexual, personal, and family. Note how many of these individuals currently use drugs.

Forensic history Previous or pending convictions. Periods of imprisonment. Enquire about continuing criminal activity to support drug use (remind the patient about confidentiality).

Patient's aims in seeking treatment What is the patient's attitude to drug use? What treatment options do they favour?

MSE Observe for history or objective signs of depressed mood or suicidal thoughts or plans. Inquire directly about generalized anxiety and panic attacks (a benzodiazepine user may be self-medicating a neurotic condition). Inquire directly about paranoid ideas and hallucinatory experiences and the directness or otherwise of their relationship with drug use.

Physical examination General condition. Weight. Condition of teeth. Signs of IV use (examine particularly arms for signs of phlebitis, abscess, or old scarring). Examine for enlarged liver. Signs of withdrawals on assessment.

Urine screening This is essential. Several specimens should be taken over several weeks. Repeated absence of evidence of a drug on screening makes its dependent use unlikely (see Table 15.6). Occasionally, testing errors do occur so do not take action (e.g. stopping maintenance prescription) on the basis of the results of a single sample.

Blood testing FBC, LFTs, discuss with patient the need for HIV and hepatitis screening.

Table 15.6 Urine drug testing

Substance	Duration of detectability
Amfetamines	48hrs
Benzodiazepines	
Ultra short-acting (e.g. midazolam)	12hrs
Short-acting (e.g. triazolam)	24hrs
Intermediate-acting (e.g. temazepam)	40–80hrs
Long-acting (e.g. diazepam)	7 days
Cocaine metabolites	2–3 days
Methadone (maintenance-dosing)	7–9 days (approximate)
Codeine/morphine	48hrs
(Heroin is detected in urine as the metabolite morphine)	
Cannabis	
Single use	3 days
Moderate use (4 times per week)	4 days
Heavy use (daily)	10 days
Chronic heavy use	21–27 days
Phencyclidine (PCP)	8 days (approximate)

Planning treatment in drug misuse

The longer-term goal of treatment will be eventual abstinence from drugs, but this may not be an achievable short or medium-term goal in an individual case. Immediate treatment aims are therefore: to reduce drug-related mortality and morbidity; to reduce community infection rates; to reduce criminal activity, including the need for drug users to sell to others to finance their own habit; to optimize the patient's physical and mental health; and to stabilize where appropriate on an alternative substitute drug.

Make diagnosis Confirm drug use (history, signs of withdrawals, urine testing). Assess presence and extent of dependence. Assess severity of current problems and risk of future complications. Explore social, relationship, and medical problems. Assess stage of change (p. 544 and motivation. What are the short-term and medium-term aims of treatment?

Consider need for emergency treatment Where there is evidence of psychotic illness or severe depressive illness the patient may require inpatient assessment.

Engage in service Treatment of drug misuse cannot be carried out through 'one-off' interventions. Patients should be engaged in the service by empathic and non-judgemental interviewing, availability of the service close to the point of need, and ability of the service to respond to change in a previously ambivalent patient. Substitute prescribing will be a strong motivator for engagement in some patients, but should always also have a role in helping the patient achieve some worthwhile change.

Decide treatment goals and methods After assessment and diagnosis the doctor should discuss with the patient their thoughts about treatment options given the patient's drug history and local treatment availability. The doctor may have strong feelings about the appropriateness of a certain treatment but this will not be successful unless the patient agrees. Plans may include:

- **Return to dependent use as previously** Where individuals present in withdrawals, without other medical, surgical, or psychiatric reasons for admission, and where there is no history of complicated withdrawal, and where there has been no previous involvement in treatment services, it is inappropriate to prescribe. The individual should not receive replacement medication. They should be offered the opportunity to attend for further assessment.
- **Counselling and support** For non-dependent drug use, particularly episodic use, this may be the appropriate course. Give drug information and harm-reduction advice, possibly coupled with referral to a community resource.
- **Detoxification** (p. 598, p. 600) Where there is drug dependence and the patient wishes abstinence, then a plan for detox is considered. This may be community-based, with psychological support, symptomatic medication, or reducing substitute medication, or as an inpatient. Consideration should be given to support after detox. How is abstinence to be maintained?

- **Supported detox without prescription** Some individuals can withdraw from drugs of dependence without use of a prescription. This may occur particularly where other changes in a person's life (e.g. change of area, break from dependent partner) facilitate abstinence. Unsupported detox without any medical help is frequently reported by users.
- **Supported detox with symptomatic medication** Here, in addition to the support mentioned here, the individual is prescribed other, non-replacement drugs to ameliorate withdrawal symptoms (e.g. lofexidine in opiate withdrawal).
- **Conversion to substitute drug with aim of detox** Here the aim is to convert the individual's drug use from street-bought to prescribed, then, from a period of stability, attempt supervised reduction in dose, aiming towards abstinence.
- **Conversion to substitute drug with aim of maintenance** Here the aim again is to convert from street to prescribed drugs, with stabilization via maintenance prescribing in the medium term. In a dependent user who does not feel that they can move to abstinence in the short term, maintenance prescribing to suitably selected patients is useful and associated with overall health benefits.

Address other needs The drug treatment service should consider part of its role as being a gateway to other services which the drug user may require but be reluctant or unable to approach independently. Patients with social, financial, or physical health needs should have these explored and the need for referral considered. Do not make such referrals without the knowledge and agreement of the patient. Review psychiatric symptoms which have been attributed to drug use to assess their resolution. Consider 'in-house' or specialist psychiatric treatment of residual anxiety/depressive symptoms.

Substitute prescribing 1: principles

Withdrawal syndromes Any drug consumed regularly and heavily can be associated with withdrawal phenomena on stopping, even if not a classical withdrawal syndrome. The severity of withdrawal symptoms experienced by individual patients does not correlate well with their reported previous consumption and so it is best to rely on objective evidence of withdrawal severity. Clinically significant withdrawal phenomena occur in dependence on alcohol, opiates, and benzodiazepines and are occasionally seen in cannabis, cocaine, and amfetamine use. In general, drugs with short half-lives will give rise to more rapid but more transient withdrawals. Detoxification refers to the process of managed withdrawal from drugs of dependence which can be aided by psychological support, symptomatic prescribing, or by prescription of reducing doses of the same or similar drug.

Substitute prescribing In many circumstances the management of a drug user will include prescription of substitute medication. This may be to enable *detoxification* from a dependent drug, or *maintenance prescribing*—a move from unstable street use to prescribed dependent use to facilitate change now with abstinence later. The prescription of a drug should not occur in isolation, but should be part of a comprehensive management plan, previously agreed with the patient and with relevant members of the multidisciplinary team. Prescribing for drug users should be guided by local procedures and practice, by the Home Office document *Drug misuse and dependence—guidelines on clinical management*, and by the *British National Formulary* (see Box 15.4).

Substitute prescribing may have the following indications

- To acutely reduce or prevent withdrawal symptoms. Where detoxification is planned, a first step can be the conversion of all opiate or BDZ use to a single prescribed drug, which can then be reduced in a planned manner. Short-term prescription of a substitute drug may also be indicated to alleviate symptoms of withdrawal complicating the assessment of a dependent patient presenting with a medical or surgical emergency.
- To stabilize drug intake and reduce secondary harm associated with street drug use. In patients who are not considering detox in the short term, substitute prescribing can be a means of harm reduction (e.g. by reducing risk of accidental overdose [OD] or by changing from IV to prescribed oral use). In addition, having a stable, legitimate supply can reduce the need to resort to criminal activity to fund drug use, reducing the secondary, wider social harms of drug use.
- To begin a process of change in drug-taking behaviour. A major aim in substitute prescribing is to fully supply the dependent drug and to move the patient away from extra, recreational drug use and chaotic, polydrug misuse. After stabilization, the user should be encouraged to discontinue contact with dealers and friends who continue to use drugs in a chaotic fashion.
- To provide an incentive to continued patient contact and involvement with treatment services.

Substitute prescribing should only be considered where:
- There is objective evidence of current dependence. This should include a history of daily consumption, description of withdrawal symptoms, history of drug seeking to relieve or prevent withdrawals, and consistent presence of the drug on urine screening.
- The patient displays realistic motivation to change their drug use in a way which would be aided by prescription (e.g. to cease IV heroin use on instigation of oral methadone prescription).
- The doctor believes the patient will co-operate with the prescription and that circumstances exist to allow adequate monitoring.

Assessing need for substitute medication
Before prescribing substitute medication for detoxification or mainte-nance, the treating doctor should positively confirm dependence via:
- Positive history of daily use with features of dependence syndrome.
- Presence of drug in two urine specimens at least 1wk apart.
- Objective evidence of withdrawal features at assessment.

Box 15.4 Requirements for a controlled drug prescription

- The prescription may be printed but must be signed by hand.
- States patient's name, age, and current address.
- Gives name, concentration, and type of preparation required (e.g. methadone, 1mg in 1mL, sugar-free suspension).
- States required dose and frequency.
- States total quantity of drug to be dispensed in both words and figures (not required for temazepam).
- Clearly signed and dated.

Substitute prescribing 2: opiates

Opiate detoxification

Opiate withdrawal In an opiate-dependent individual, withdrawal symptoms appear 6–24hrs after the last dose and typically last 5–7 days, peaking on the 2nd or 3rd day. The withdrawal following discontinuation of the longer-acting methadone is more prolonged with symptoms peaking on the 7th day or so and lasting up to 14 days. *Symptoms of opiate withdrawal:* sweating; dilated pupils; tachycardia; hypertension; piloerection ('goose flesh'); watering eyes and nose; yawning; abdominal cramping; nausea and vomiting; diarrhoea; tremor; joint pains; muscle cramps.

Symptomatic medication Several non-opiate, oral medications are effective in ameliorating symptoms of opiate withdrawal. Unlike opiates, they are not liable to abuse or diversion to the black market.
- *Lofexidine* Alpha-adrenergic agonist. Starting dose: 200micrograms bd, increased in 200–400-microgram steps up to maximum of 2.4mg daily given in 2–4 divided doses. Measure baseline BP and monitor BP while raising dose (risk of symptomatic hypotension). 10-day course, withdraw over 2–4 days.
- *Loperamide* For treatment of diarrhoea. 4mg initial dose with 2mg taken after each loose stool for up to 5 days. Maximum daily dose: 16mg.
- *Metoclopramide* For nausea and vomiting. 10mg dose, up to maximum of 30mg daily.
- *Ibuprofen* For headaches and muscle pains. 400mg dose, up to maximum of 1600mg daily.

Substitute prescribing Several opiates are used in detoxification regimes. Where it is planned to continue prescribing on a maintenance basis, currently methadone is the drug of choice.
- *Methadone* Long-acting synthetic opiate. Its half-life is 24hrs and it is therefore suitable for daily dosing (which can be supervised) (see Table 15.7). At daily dose >80mg it produces near saturation of opiate receptors, minimizing the 'reward' of further consumption. It is prescribed as a coloured liquid, unsuitable for IV use, at concentration 1mg/1mL. A sugar-free form is available. Licensed for use in opiate withdrawal and maintenance.
- *Buprenorphine* A partial opiate agonist. Licensed for treatment of drug dependence. Available in once-daily sublingual preparation. 8mg ~ = 30mg methadone. Believed to produce less euphoria at higher doses than methadone. Abuse potential, as tablet can be prepared for injection.
- *Dihydrocodeine* Short-acting opiate. Not licensed for use in drug dependence. Occasional use in reduction regimes in patients already on a stable dose of street dihydrocodeine or in final stages of dose reduction in patients on doses of methadone <15mg daily. Need for 2–4 times daily doses means that all dosages cannot be supervised.

Opiate maintenance

In maintenance prescribing, the aim is to prevent under-dosing (risk of use of street opiates, withdrawal symptoms) and overdosing (sedation, more drug available than required with diversion to the black market). There is research evidence that a methadone script reduces street usage, criminality, and drug-related mortality. For outpatient initiation of methadone maintenance, arrange to review the patient in the morning with them having consumed no opiates for the previous 24hrs. Assess withdrawals and dispense methadone as follows:

- None or mild → no prescription. Review following day.
- Moderate (aches, dilated pupils, yawning) → 10–20mg methadone.
- Severe (vomiting, piloerection, hypertension) → 20–30mg methadone.

Review after 4hrs and repeat dose if severe withdrawals continue, up to 30mg. Review daily over the first week with dose increments of 5–10mg daily if indicated. Methadone reaches a steady state 5 days after the last dose change. Arrange regular review after first week, making subsequent increases by 10mg on each review up to ~120mg. Stabilization may take up to 6 weeks to achieve. For maintenance monitoring, see 📖 p. 602.

Dose reduction After stabilization and complete abstinence from street opiates, a decision should be made as to whether the aim is dose reduction or maintenance prescribing. Rapid reduction regimes reduce the dose over 14–21 days (perhaps using the drugs outlined in *Symptomatic medication* 📖 p. 598, as adjuncts). Usually reduction is more gradual. Slow reduction is over 4–6 months, reducing by ~5–10mg each fortnight. In reduction regimes, make the largest absolute cuts at the beginning and make smaller, more gradual cuts as the total dose falls (i.e. aim to keep the percentage drop in dose similar). In general do not carry out reduction against the wishes of the patient as it is better to carry on a maintenance script rather than return to street use. Occasionally 'tread water' then restart reduction.

Opiate relapse prevention In previously dependent opiate users who have successfully completed detox, the opiate antagonist *naltrexone* may be used as an aid to relapse prevention. Taken regularly it will prevent the rewarding, euphoric effect of opiate consumption.

Naltrexone Prescribed to aid abstinence in formerly dependent patients who have been drug free for >7 days. Starting dose 25mg, increased to 50mg daily. Total weekly dose of 350mg may be divided and given 3 days/wk (e.g. to aid compliance, or to enable supervision), give 100mg Monday and Wednesday and 150mg on Friday. Naltrexone is also used in specialist inpatient facilities to facilitate rapid detox over 5–7 days.

Table 15.7 Converting opiate dose to methadone dose

Drug	Daily dose	Methadone equivalent
Street heroin	0.5mg–1g	50–80mg
Morphine	10mg	10mg
Dipipanone (Cyclizine)®	10mg/30mg	4mg
Dihydrocodeine	30mg	3mg
Pethidine	50mg	5mg
Codeine phosphate	30mg	2mg

Substitute prescribing 3: benzodiazepines

Benzodiazepine detoxification

Benzodiazepine withdrawal Chronic BDZ use leads to development of dependence, with a characteristic withdrawal syndrome. The symptoms appear within 24hrs of discontinuing a short-acting benzodiazepine, but may be delayed for up to 3 weeks for the longer-acting preparations. *Symptoms of benzodiazepine withdrawal:* anxiety; insomnia; tremor; agitation; headache; nausea; sweating; depersonalization; seizures; delirium.

Substitute prescribing As for opiates, BDZ substitute prescribing should only be undertaken where there is clinical evidence of dependence, a clear treatment plan, and suitable patient monitoring in place. Substitute prescribing in BDZ dependency uses the long-acting *diazepam*. In prescribing for patients with BDZ dependency, convert all BDZ doses to diazepam using Table 15.8. The aim is to find the lowest dose which will prevent withdrawal symptoms (which may be well below the amount the patient has been taking). Divide the daily dose to avoid over-sedation.

Benzodiazepine maintenance

Unlike methadone maintenance in opiate dependency, there is no evidence that long-term BDZ prescription reduces overall morbidity. There is evidence that long-term prescription of >30mg diazepam daily is associated with harm. New prescriptions should be for 30mg or less with patients already on higher doses reduced to this amount.

Dose reduction Cut dose by ~1/8th of total dose each fortnight. For low dose 2.5mg fortnightly; for high dose 5mg fortnightly. Review and halt or temporarily increase if substantial symptoms re-emerge. If patient is also opiate-dependent and on methadone, keep methadone stable while reducing benzodiazepine.

Table 15.8 Conversion to equivalent diazepam dose

Drug	Dose
Diazepam	5mg
Nitrazepam	5mg
Temazepam	10mg
Chlordiazepoxide	15mg
Oxazepam	15mg
Loprazolam	500micrograms
Lorazepam	500micrograms
Lormetazepam	500–1000micrograms

Monitoring of maintenance prescribing

Detoxification and stabilization on maintenance medication are often followed by rapid relapse despite successful completion. It is important to build monitoring of compliance into treatment strategies from the beginning.

Review Regular review of all patients on maintenance prescription is indicated at least monthly. At each review:

- Is dose sufficient? Is there evidence of withdrawals? Obtain feedback from pharmacist/community nurse.
- If dose insufficient? Consider small weekly increases in dose. Stop if evidence of intoxication.
- Confirm use of illegal drugs via history, urine testing, and observation of evidence of IV use.
- Plan movement towards goals.
- Consider intervention in mental health/other issues.
- Consider need for period of increased supervision.

Supervision of substitute prescribing The aim of supervised consumption is to ensure that the drug is being used as prescribed.

- Supervised consumption usually for initial minimum period of 3mths, taking into account work and childcare issues.
- Consider ongoing supervised consumption (e.g. in pharmacy).
- Once-daily dosing with daily pick-up of drugs.
- No more than 1wk's prescription at a time.
- Advice re children and methadone.
- Close liaison with pharmacist and GP.
- Thorough and clear records should be kept.
- No replacement of 'lost' prescriptions.

Discontinuing a failing treatment Where there is persistent non-compliance with treatment and where attempts to improve compliance or modify treatment goals have failed then the maintenance should be discontinued.

- Discontinue via reduction regime.
- Offer involvement with other services.
- Inform GP and pharmacist.

Psychotic illnesses and substance misuse

The association of substance misuse and psychotic features is a common and problematic one in clinical practice. The key to management is accurate diagnosis. Psychotic symptoms represent underlying psychiatric abnormality in this group of patients as in any other. There is not a general finding of 'low-grade' psychotic features in substance users and apparent psychotic features should not be attributed to effects of substance use without further inquiry.

Psychotic features during drug intoxication Substances with hallucinogenic or stimulant activity can produce psychotic features during acute intoxication. This is not consistent and varies by drug dose and setting. These are characterized by a rapidly changing pattern of symptom type and severity and include visual and other hallucinations, sensory distortions/illusions, and persecutory and referential thinking. They are characteristically rapidly fluctuating hour by hour and show resolution as the drug level falls.

Psychotic features during withdrawal In patients with physiological dependency on alcohol, BDZs, or cocaine, withdrawals may be complicated by delirium in which variable psychotic features may be prominent. These will occur in the context of the general features of delirium (🕮 p. 790). There may be fluctuating visual or tactile hallucinations and poorly formed persecutory delusional ideas.

Residual psychotic illness (drug-induced psychosis) In some individuals, psychotic features continue after the period of acute intoxication and withdrawals has passed. These may be symptomatically more typical of primary psychotic illness and, once established, should be treated as for acute episodes of schizophrenia (🕮 p. 192).

Genuine comorbidity Many individuals with primary psychotic illnesses will misuse substances. In addition to the intrinsic risks of substance misuse, this carries risks in this group of diminished treatment compliance, risk of disinhibition leading to violence, and exacerbation of the primary illness. In view of the sometimes obvious (to others) causal link between drug use and relapse it is worth asking why patients persist in substance use. Reasons include:

- Endemic drug use within patient's environment (e.g. home or social setting) or within other individuals with mental health problems.
- As means of self-medicating distressing positive and negative symptoms (which may be improved by addressing these symptoms directly).

Legal issues related to drug and alcohol misuse

Fitness to drive It is the patient's responsibility to inform the DVLA of any 'disability likely to affect safe driving'. The DVLA regards drug misuse as a disability in this context. Group 1 licences cover motor cars and motorcycles, group 2 licences cover HGVs and buses. Decisions regarding licensing are made on a case-by-case basis; however, the DVLA's current guidelines are as follows:

- **Alcohol misuse:** loss of licence until 6-months (group 1) or 1-year (group 2) period of abstinence or controlled drinking has been achieved with normalization of blood parameters.
- **Alcohol dependence:** loss of licence until 1-year (group 1) or 3-year (group 2) period of abstinence, with normalization of blood parameters. Consultant referral and support may be required.
- **Dependency/persistent use of cannabis, amfetamines, MDMA, LSD, and hallucinogens:** loss of licence until 6-mth (group 1) or 1-yr (group 2) period of abstinence. Medical assessment and urine screening may be required.
- **Dependency/persistent use of heroin, morphine, cocaine, methadone:** loss of licence until 1-yr (group 1) or 3-yr (group 2) period of abstinence. Independent medical assessment and urine screening prior to relicensing. A favourable consultant report may be required for group 1 and will be required for group 2. Subject to annual review and favourable assessment, drivers complying fully with a consultant-supervised methadone maintenance programme may be licensed.

Travel abroad Patients receiving a methadone prescription can travel abroad with a supply. If travelling for less than 3 months and carrying less than 3 months' supply, a personal import or export licence is not required. However, it is advised that a letter is obtained from the prescribing doctor or drug worker, which should confirm the patient's name, travel itinerary, names of prescribed controlled drugs, dosages, and total amounts of each to be carried. This advice applies only to the right to take the drug out of the UK and return with any surplus. Travellers are advised to contact the embassy or consulate of the destination country prior to travel to ensure that import of methadone is allowed under local laws: countries' regulations vary widely. If travelling for more than 3 months and for more detailed information, see http://www.homeoffice.gov.uk/.

Registration of drug addicts Compulsory registration of all drug addicts to the Home Office register of addicts ceased in 1997. Since then data have been collected on a regional basis via the anonymized regional drug misuse databases. Details regarding supply of forms in each area can be found in the *BNF*.

Drug testing and treatment orders (DTTOs) A form of community sentence introduced in the UK in 2000. The court makes an order requiring offenders with drug problems to undergo treatment and follow-up with a drug treatment service. This may be part of another community order or a sentence in its own right. The sentencing court monitors compliance via mandatory urine testing. Sentence plans may change in response to individual progress or problems. May last 6mths to 3yrs.

Child and adolescent psychiatry

Introduction

Child psychiatry is an enormously stimulating and varied area of psychiatric practice. Practitioners see children and their families throughout their development and with a multitude of presentations, from anorexia to autism, depression to drug misuse and parenting problems to psychosis. Child psychiatrists make use of multiple psychotherapeutic approaches, as well as drug treatments. The multifactorial nature of children's difficulties means that multidisciplinary and multi-agency working are the norm. The links between childhood disorder and the later development of adult mental disorder are becoming more apparent and there is the opportunity to make a real positive difference to a child's development and future.

What is CAMHS?

The term CAMHS (Child and Adolescent Mental Health Services) is used in two different ways. One includes all services that contribute to the mental health care of children and young people; the other applies specifically to specialist child and adolescent mental health services, provided in Tiers 2, 3, and 4 (see **The tier concept of CAMHS**). The remit of specialist CAMHS has expanded recently to provide services up to the eighteenth birthday, and in some areas to transfer care of learning disabled children into CAMHS from learning disability services.

The tier concept of CAMHS

- Tier 1 CAMHS is provided by professionals whose main role and training is not in mental health, for example GPs, health visitors, paediatricians, social workers, teachers, youth workers, and juvenile justice workers.
- Tier 2 CAMHS is provided by specialist mental health professionals with training in child development, working primarily alone, rather than in a team. Their role may include direct contact with young people, consultation to Tier 1 and training.
- Tier 3 services are provided by a multidisciplinary team who see young people with more complex mental health problems.
- Tier 4 services are very specialized services in residential, day patient, or outpatient settings for children and adolescents with severe and/or complex problems requiring a combination or intensity of interventions that cannot be provided by Tier 3 CAMHS.

The role of the multidisciplinary team

Child and adolescent (C&A) mental health care exemplifies the relevance of and need for a multidisciplinary approach. The professional groups represented in a team vary but may include psychiatry, psychology, nursing, family therapy, child psychotherapy, social work, and occupational therapy. Additionally a newer group of primary mental health workers has been developed, largely operating at Tier 2 but linking with Tier 3 CAMHS. For medically trained professionals who are used to 'leading the team', C&A work may be at first a little bewildering. As young people are embedded within family, social, and educational systems, their problems must be understood and treated from a holistic perspective which draws on the various models available within the team, of which the medical and psychiatric perspective is one.

CAMHS in context

There is an emphasis on specialist CAMHS being part of a child-centred integrated network of services (including other health providers, education, social care, and criminal justice) which work together to meet the needs of the child. Even when CAMHS are not directly involved in a child's care, through consultation it can be useful to have a mental health perspective in thinking about the child.

> The barb in the arrow of childhood suffering is this: its intense loneliness, its intense ignorance.
>
> Akhenaton (1354 BC), Egyptian king

> If there is anything we wish to change in the child, we should first examine it and see whether it is not something that could better be changed in ourselves.
>
> Carl Gustav Jung (1875–1961)

Assessment 1: principles

The biopsychosocial approach

Understanding and managing successfully the mental and behavioural problems of children depends upon the thoughtful consideration of all the biological, psychological, and social factors that may play a role in the generation of symptoms. It is important to remember that several factors may interact in a dynamic two-way fashion, giving rise to symptoms. The 'biopsychosocial approach' is useful at all stages of the evaluation and intervention provided to a child.

Children and families

When a young person comes into contact with mental health services they are more likely to have been referred for help than to have sought help themselves. This is important to remember, since 'the patient' may have no say in their referral and this may have implications for the therapeutic relationship. In addition, one is rarely dealing with the young person alone—they are usually dependent upon caregivers, whether they are parents or other adults. Thus one is commonly confronted by a room full of people who may have differing experiences and interpretations of the young person's problems and of what is needed to improve the situation. The professional in this situation needs to be aware of the various dynamics and be vigilant in remaining objective and non-partisan, while engaging with each family member. It is important to bear in mind that although the family has come hoping for help, they may also have feelings of failure or guilt related to their child's problems which one must be sensitive to.

Who should attend the assessment

Flexibility is important when assessing children and their families. Usually it is advisable to invite the child along with whoever lives in the family home. The standard 'nuclear family' is far less common nowadays with single parent and reconstituted families, kinship care, and professional foster care featuring prominently. It is helpful to find out who is in the room with you at the start of the assessment. Older adolescents may live away from home, perhaps alienated from their families. Thus sensitivity to individual circumstances is mandatory. Sometimes it is helpful for other people to attend, e.g. the social worker, where this would aid in understanding a family's difficulties, facilitate joined-up working, or support the family in attending and using the appointment.

Communication

A number of factors influence how one communicates with the family members in the room, including: the level of the child's development; the presence of mental or physical disorder, e.g. autistic spectrum disorder, deafness; and the language spoken (an interpreter may be required). Developing skills for communicating well is essential for making a good assessment.

Assessment 2: practice

Starting the interview with the family

- Introduce yourself and clarify who is in the room with you.
- Allow the family to settle by explaining the purpose and duration of the appointment. If a one-way screen is in use explain this.
- Discuss confidentiality and the limits of this, particularly in relation to child protection.
- Identify who will be sent copies of any letters produced following the assessment. It is common practice for letters to be copied to families if they wish this.
- Provide age-appropriate toys and drawing materials to younger children.
- Establish 'rules', e.g. all toys are put away at the end of the session.

Taking a history

- Throughout the history, facilitate each person's participation.
- Obtain a description of the problem as each person sees it.
- Obtain the family history and construct a genogram. This is useful in gathering information about family members' relationships, upbringings, and mental and physical health.
- Enquire about school, hobbies, and peer relationships.
- Take a developmental history for each child in the family.
- Particularly with adolescents, enquire about substance use and forensic activity.
- What has already been tried and have any other agencies been involved?
- Often there will be aspects of the history which either the child or the adults are unwilling to discuss in front of the other. It is important to allow individual time for a full history to emerge, while remembering that people often either know or suspect these secrets.

Mental state and observations

- Observe family functioning and interactions. Note patterns of communication, degree of warmth, power dynamics, alliances, etc.
- The mental state examination follows a similar pattern to that for adults, but with allowance for the child's level of development. It will be difficult to conduct a formal mental state examination on children under age 12, but one can comment on observable aspects, e.g. levels of activity and attention; physical and mental level of development; mood and emotional state; quality of social interaction; response to boundary setting.
- Sometimes it is appropriate to carry out physical examination at this interview—e.g. low weight anorexia—usually have a parent/other chaperone present.

Interview with the child alone

- It is usually helpful to offer to meet with the child alone, particularly for adolescents for whom greater independence is developmentally appropriate. Establishing rapport and gaining the child's confidence are primary objectives of the first interview. Young children should be invited to play, draw, etc.
- Clarify confidentiality and exceptions to this again with the child, using age-appropriate language.
- Begin with subjects well away from the presenting problem (e.g. interests and hobbies, friends and siblings, school, holidays).
- Progress to enquiring about the child's view of the problem, worries, fears, sleep and appetite, mood, self-image, peer and family relationships, experiences of bullying or teasing, abuse, persistent thoughts, fantasy life, abnormal experiences, suicidal thoughts, etc. (It may take more than one interview to obtain a full picture.)

Gathering other information

- Obtain consent to contact school for a classroom observation, meeting, or report from teachers.
- Consult other caregivers, health professionals who have treated the child, social agencies that have been involved with the child and/or family, and educational psychology if involved.
- Consider using rating scales (e.g. Connor's Questionnaire, Moods and Feelings Questionnaire, CY-BOCS, K-SADS as indicated).
- It will sometimes be appropriate to request other assessments, e.g. speech and language, occupational therapy, neuropsychology, educational psychology, or to arrange physical investigations, e.g. haematology, chromosome studies, EEG, CT.

Formulation of the problem

- Consider the problem in terms of biological, psychological, and social aspects, and identify predisposing, precipitating, perpetuating, and protective factors.
- Use this along with a risk assessment to develop a management plan. Involvement of the family in this, and in its execution, is likely to be beneficial.

Consent/capacity/legislation

- An assessment of a young person's capacity, and ability to give consent, is important. Details of this vary across the UK.
- It is important to familiarize yourself with legislation around capacity and consent/refusal of treatment, as well as Mental Health and Children's Acts (if applicable) in your jurisdiction.

Development

An understanding of normal child development is essential to assessing and working with children. Differentiating 'normal' from 'abnormal' can be difficult in young people since they are subject to developmental change and thus 'normality' evolves and varies according to differing age. Furthermore, what is normal may vary according to the family, social, religious, and cultural environment. Models of normal childhood experience and behaviour that are based solely on the norms of a particular society may be completely inappropriate in a different context. Having said this, there are a number of core 'norms' that transcend societal barriers, and likewise there are a number of mental disorders that have been shown to exist worldwide.

Assessing development

In assessing a child's development it is helpful to consider the following areas which show significant changes during development:

- 'Theory of mind' is the ability to attribute beliefs, knowledge, and desires to oneself, and to understand that other people also hold beliefs, knowledge, and desires which may differ from one's own. This allows the child to understand concepts such as deception, that others may hold different beliefs, and distinguishing fantasy from reality. The pre-school child will rarely acknowledge their own or others' thinking. It is not until around age 10 that an awareness of different types of cognitive processes, e.g. memory, reasoning, comprehension, develops.
- Emotional development involves the skills of emotion differentiation, acceptable expression of emotion, and emotional containment/concealment. Emotional and social development are closely linked.
- Social development including type of play (solitary, parallel, co-operative), friendships, social skills, and popularity.
- Cognitive development involves a number of mental processes including understanding, believing, calculating, reasoning, inference, and conceptualizing.
- Physical development including the acquisition of motor and language skills.
- Moral development.

Adolescence

Adolescents deserve a special mention as their greater physical maturity can lead one to have adult expectations of them. Adolescence is not just a blend of childhood and adulthood; it is a stage with unique biological and social characteristics of its own. Adolescence is a relatively new social phenomenon, since the age of puberty has steadily dropped while education has become prolonged over the last few centuries. This means that, particularly in the developed world, individuals achieve physical and sexual maturity before they assume adult roles. Different sociocultural influences will inevitably also shape the normal adolescent presentation.

Biological factors defining adolescence include the achievement of sexual maturity as well as the physical and cognitive changes resulting from hormonal shifts which allow the development of new abilities. Social development is also accelerated with stronger peer relationships and influence. These physical, cognitive, and social changes lead to the achievement of autonomy. Adolescence is also a time of identity formation which involves experimentation and which can lead to conflict with authority. Abnormal adolescent development is characterized by inability to adjust to these physical, sexual, and social changes, or by impaired development in these areas.

I would there were no age between ten and three-and-twenty, or that youth would sleep out the rest; for there is nothing in the between but getting wenches with child, wronging the ancientry, stealing, fighting.

Shakespeare: *The Winter's Tale,* Act III Scene 3

Resilience

Definition

'Resilience refers to the process of, capacity for, or outcome of, successful adaptation despite challenging or threatening circumstances.' Masten et al. 1990.

'A resilient child can resist adversity, cope with uncertainty and recover more successfully from traumatic events or episodes.' Newman 2002.

Factors promoting resilience

- **Child:** easy temperament and good nature; female gender prior to, and male gender during, adolescence; higher IQ; good social skills with peers and adults; feeling of empathy with others; sense of humour; attractiveness to others; awareness of strengths and limitations.
- **Family:** warm and supportive parents; good parent–child relationship; parental harmony; a valued social role, e.g. helping siblings; where parental conflict exists, a close relationship with one parent.
- **Environment:** supportive extended family; successful school experiences; valued social role, e.g. job, volunteering, helping neighbour; a close relationship with an unrelated mentor; membership of religious or faith community; extra-curricular activities.

The importance of resilience

Children with mental health problems usually have historical and current adversities which are affecting their functioning. They will also have qualities in themselves, their families, or their environment which promote resilience—their ability to 'bounce back' from adversity. The identification and promotion of these qualities during assessment and management enhances the formulation and recognizes resources the child and family can draw on.

Resilience is also important in understanding those children who do not develop psychopathology despite significant stress and adversity. This has relevance for Tier 1 CAMHS preventative work, as the promotion of resilience factors in children may prevent or inhibit the development of mental disorder, e.g. emotional health cognitive behavioural therapy programmes delivered on a whole class basis in schools.

Attachment

Attachment refers to the strong emotional bond that exists between a child and a caregiver. It develops through appropriate, sensitive parental responses to the child's behavioural cues. It allows the child to develop understanding of his 'inner world' and how to understand the world around him. It is the foundation for safe separation and development of autonomy, and establishes beliefs about the value and reliability of relationships in the child's mind. The effectiveness of parental attunement permanently influences the hypothalamic–pituitary–adrenal axis and thus the baseline around which stress responses are modulated. This has lifelong implications for emotional and behavioural regulation and mental health. Early satisfactory care is particularly important.

Types of attachment

- *Secure:* child values relationships and is confident of self-worth.
- *Insecure avoidant:* child appears emotionally independent, does not value relationships.
- *Insecure anxious:* self-worth depends on approval of others. Values relationships but sees them as unreliable. Develops strategies for achieving attention.
- *Insecure ambivalent:* values relationships but is cautious about their safety.
- *Disorganized:* neither effectively self-sufficient nor able to use relationships.

Attachment styles are not fixed and can coexist. Parental attunement and style heavily influence attachment.

Considering attachment in the psychiatric interview

In addition to observations of the child's interactions with parents/caregivers during the assessment interview, also consider:

- Factors that can affect parental attunement, e.g. parental mental illness, LD, substance misuse, social chaos, domestic violence.
- Child's experiences, e.g. significant separations, change of carers, abuse.
- Enquire about: understanding of 'inner world' (e.g. pain, hunger, satiety); outside world (e.g. social norms, awareness of danger, stress regulation); explorative behaviour (e.g. inquisitiveness, cognitive and motor skills); and understanding of relationships (e.g. benefits, communication, empathy).
- Disordered attachment can closely resemble other disorders, e.g. ADHD, autism spectrum disorder (ASD). Furthermore, it increases the risk of many mental disorders developing.

Management of attachment problems

Management is primarily aimed at improving attachment and therefore requires comprehensive assessment to determine what is required for attachment needs to be met. This may include health, social care, and education agencies.

- Build on strength and resilience in child and parent.
- Provide appropriate support and education to parent. This could include behavioural management work, support groups, respite care, and help with parental mental health problems.
- Work with child may be helpful, e.g. reduce stress, increase emotional awareness, and reduce temper. It is important to remember that individual work with the child will be far less influential than the successful modification of primary relationships in improving attachment, and the consequent emotional and behavioural problems.
- Support and liaison with school.
- Treat mental disorder, e.g. ADHD, PTSD, depression.
- If the child's needs cannot be met, even with all support, it may be in the child's best interests to be accommodated away from the family home.

Reactive attachment disorder

This disorder reflects a disturbed pattern of social relatedness, is diagnosed before age 5yrs, and may manifest as either *inhibited* or *disinhibited* subtypes. It represents the severe end of the spectrum of disordered attachment.

An approach to behavioural problems

Children, and to a lesser extent adolescents, often present with behavioural problems rather than complaints of stress or depression. They may not have the necessary level of development to recognize and then express these feelings; and they are often brought to services rather than referring themselves, therefore it is the observable problem, i.e. the behaviour, that is presented.

Differential diagnosis of various behavioural 'symptoms'

Common behavioural presentations include hyperactivity, inattention, separation problems, moodiness, peer/social problems, aggression/oppositionality, sexually inappropriate behaviour, regressed behaviour, somatization, tantrums, and rituals.

Since individual 'symptoms' can occur in more than one disorder, it is worth considering a differential diagnosis for the presenting behavioural symptom. It is also extremely important to differentiate a clearly maladaptive behaviour from one that is developmentally or situationally appropriate. 'Normal' behaviours also include those that form part of the child's expected testing and experimentation of the world.

Assessment of behavioural disorders—general principles

- **Identify the problem behaviour/s**—obtain a full description (from parents, child, teachers, etc.) of the problem behaviour/s. This should include the evolution of the behaviour, a chronology of the child's typical daily activities, the setting in which the behaviour occurs, its effects on family, school, relationships, etc. and attitudes of others to the behaviour/s. It is always appropriate to speak to the child alone (if possible) to establish his/her views, desires, and mental state.
- **Determine the parental strategy**—it is important to find out how the parents deal with the behaviour/s. *Do they agree with each other?* This also includes information about their expectations, philosophy of parenting, interpretation of the behaviour/s, moral, religious, and cultural views on parenting, etc. How do the parents react or respond to the behaviour/s? How do they discipline or punish? What do they tolerate? Are they permissive or restrictive? Are they over-protective or uninvolved? Do they feel empowered or impotent, helpless, and incompetent as parents? How do they manage their frustrations, anger, etc.? What coping mechanisms do they have?
- **Family history and dynamics**—as well as gathering a full family history of health, psychiatric problems, social and cultural circumstances, and support structures, it is also important to assess parental and sibling relationships, the presence of any significant stressors or losses, and how the problem behaviour interacts with family dynamics.
- **Social behaviour**—the evolution of the child's social behaviour, including social developmental, attachment behaviour, imaginary play, reading of social cues, relationships, and language use.
- **School behaviour**—attendance, changes in school, separation issues, performance, peer and teacher interactions and responses, friendships, bullying, etc.

- **Child's health and development**—pregnancy, birth, and developmental milestones. Was the child planned, wanted? How did siblings react? How did parents and siblings cope? Any post-partum problems? Was any professional support required? Also, child's temperament, illnesses, treatment, etc.
- **Direct observation of parent–child interaction**—during the interview it is important to note how the child behaves and how parents respond and interact with the child. If siblings can be present their behaviour and interactions can also be evaluated. A home and/or school visit may add additional information about the behaviour in these settings.
- **Collateral information**—teachers, extended family, and social services may be able to provide important input, and permission should be sought to contact and involve them where appropriate.

Management

This will be informed by the assessment, but generally it is useful to help the child and family understand the thoughts and feelings contributing to the behaviour. This aids in both reducing negative interpretations of the behaviour and in helping to change the problem behaviour. More specific management issues are addressed under topic headings.

Conduct disorders

The conduct disorders are characterized by a *repetitive* and *persistent* pattern of antisocial, aggressive, or defiant behaviours that violate age-appropriate societal norms. Conduct disorders can be divided into conduct disorder (CD) and oppositional defiant disorder (ODD).

Conduct disorder

Epidemiology Commoner in boys and in urban populations. Prevalence 5–7% in UK.

Clinical features Aggression/cruelty to people and/or animals, destruction of property, deceitfulness, theft, fire-setting, truancy and running away from home, and severe provocative or disobedient behaviour. These behaviours result in significant impact on family and peer relationships, and schooling. ICD-10 requires 1 or more feature at a marked level for over 6mths; DSM-IV requires 3 or more over 12mths, with 1 in last 6mths.

Aetiology/associations
- **Social disadvantage:** poverty, low socio-economic class, overcrowding, homelessness, social isolation, high community rates of deviancy, truancy, unemployment.
- **Parenting:** parental criminality, parental psychiatric disorder and substance misuse, inconsistent and critical parenting style, parental conflict, teenage pregnancy, single parenthood.
- **Child:** low IQ, neurodevelopmental problems, brain damage, epilepsy, difficult/under-controlled temperament, attachment problems, and poor interpersonal relationships.

Comorbidity ADHD; learning difficulties (especially dyslexia); substance abuse; depression; anxiety disorder; autism spectrum disorders (ASD).

Differential diagnosis adjustment disorder; ADHD; ASD; normal child (but parents/teachers have unrealistic expectations); PTSD; anxiety disorder; learning difficulty; psychosis; subcultural deviance.

Course and outcome
- Persistent disorder, particularly where onset is younger.
- Around half will receive a diagnosis of antisocial personality disorders as adults. Substance misuse, mania, schizophrenia, OCD, major depressive disorder, and panic disorder are also seen in adult life. There is an increased risk of early death, often by violent and sudden means.
- Increased risk of social exclusion, poor school achievement, long-term unemployment, criminal activity, and poor interpersonal relationships including those with their own children.

Assessment
- See family and child.
- Obtain a full history with collateral from school, social worker, and legal system.
- Identify causal, risk, and protective factors.
- Assess for comorbidity and make a diagnosis.
- Formulate the problem and establish management plan.

Management of CD

This will be planned on a case-by-case basis, and is likely to require multi-agency communication and co-operation. Possible components include:

• Parent management training (📖 p. 667). NICE recommends group-based parent-training/education programmes in children aged 12yrs or younger, e.g. Webster–Stratton incredible years programme, positive parenting programme (Triple P). It sets out criteria that such programmes should demonstrate. Individual-based programmes are recommended only in situations where there are particular difficulties in engaging with the parents, or a family's needs are too complex to be met by group programmes.
• Functional family therapy.
• Multi-systemic therapy—family-based, including school and community. Highly resource-intensive, but good outcomes (Box 16.1).
• Child interventions—social skills, problem-solving, anger management, confidence building.
• Treat comorbidity.
• Address child protection concerns.

Oppositional defiant disorder (ODD)

Essence An enduring pattern of negative, hostile, and defiant behaviour, without serious violations of societal norms or the rights of others. Behaviour may occur in one situation only (e.g. home) and tends to be most evident in interactions with familiar adults or peers.

Epidemiology More common in boys and in childhood rather than adolescence. Prevalence 2–5%.

Outcome A quarter show no symptoms later in life but many progress to CD and/or substance abuse.

Management Same management principles as for CD (see above).

Box 16.1 Prevention strategies and policy implications

• **Pre-school child development programmes**—identifying parents and families at risk and instituting home visits and support.
• **School programmes**—identify children at risk and institute classroom enrichment, home visits, and parent and teacher training.
• **Community programmes**—identify children and adolescents through their involvement with social agencies and institute interventions such as enhanced recreation programmes, parent training, and adult mentoring of youth.
• **Social and economic restructuring** to reduce poverty and to improve family and community stability.

Attention deficit hyperactivity disorder (ADHD)

ADHD is characterized by the three core symptoms of inattention, hyperactivity, and impulsiveness. DSM-IV recognizes 3 subtypes: *a combined subtype* where all 3 features are present, *an inattentive subtype* (ADD), and *a hyperactive-impulsive subtype*. The DSM-IV definition of severe combined-type ADHD is similar to the ICD-10 definition of *hyperkinetic disorder*. Symptoms should be at developmentally inappropriate levels, be present across time and situations for at least 6mnths, and starting before age 7. 5% of UK school children would meet DSM-IV ADHD diagnostic criteria, 1% would meet criteria for ICD-10 hyperkinetic disorder. It is at least 4 times commoner in males.

Aetiology 80% of cases are genetically inherited and risk of ADHD in siblings is 2–3 times increased. Rates are increased in low birth-weight babies and babies born to mothers who used drugs, alcohol, or tobacco during pregnancy, following head injury, and in some genetic and metabolic disorders.

Differential diagnosis Age-appropriate behaviour in active children; attachment disorder; hearing impairment; learning difficulty; a high IQ child insufficiently stimulated/challenged in mainstream school; behavioural disorder; anxiety disorder; medication side-effects (e.g. antihistamines).

Comorbidity ADHD is highly comorbid with 50–80% of children having a comorbid disorder, including: specific learning disorders, motor-co-ordination problems, autism spectrum disorder, tic disorders, CD, ODD, substance abuse, anxiety, depression, bipolar disorder.

Clinical features of ADHD

- *Inattention* Careless with detail, fails to sustain attention, appears not to listen, fails to finish tasks, poor self-organization, loses things, forgetful, easily distracted, and avoids tasks requiring sustained attention.
- *Hyperactivity* Most evident in structured situations, fidgets with hands or feet, leaves seat in class, runs/climbs about, cannot play quietly, 'always on the go'.
- *Impulsiveness* Talks excessively, blurts out answers, cannot await turn, interrupts others, intrudes on others.

Problems associated with ADHD

- Short-term: sleep problems, low self-esteem, family and peer relationship problems, reduced academic achievement, and increased risk of accidents.
- Longer term: development of comorbid problems (see **Comorbidity**), reduced academic and employment success, increased criminal activity, and antisocial personality disorder. ADHD symptoms may persist into adulthood (20–30% with full ADHD syndrome and ~60% with 1 or more core symptoms). Impulsivity–hyperactivity remits early, while inattention often persists. Studies show a pattern of psychopathology,

cognition, and functioning in adults similar to that in children and adolescents. A poorer prognosis is associated with social deprivation, high expressed emotion, parental mental illness, predominantly hyperactive-impulsive symptoms, CD, learning difficulty, language disorder.

Assessment

- Interview family and child.
- Observe child, preferably in more than one situation, e.g. clinic and school.
- Collateral information from school, other involved parties.
- Rating scales may be useful, e.g. Connor's rating scale, Strengths and Difficulties Questionnaire (SDQ).
- Screen for comorbidity.
- Physical examination including neurological examination.

Management

- Psycho-education.
- Medication (📖 p. 628).
- Behavioural interventions, e.g. encouraging realistic expectations, positive reinforcement of desired behaviours (small immediate rewards), consistent contingency management across home and school, break down tasks, reduce distraction.
- School intervention.
- Treat comorbidity.
- Evidence base for dietary changes and fish oils poor at present.
- Voluntary organizations, e.g. ADDISS—Attention Deficit Disorder Information and Support Service.

🔊 Controversy of ADHD

The concept of ADHD has been criticized as medicalizing a social problem. It is said to be over-diagnosed and that it undermines parents. The long-term benefits of medication remain unclear. Nevertheless, there is recognition that symptoms can continue into adult life and that untreated, there are poor outcomes. Children and their families, who have experienced a good response to medication, usually want to continue with it despite long-term uncertainty.

Useful links:

- **NICE CG72** (http://guidance.nice.org.uk/CG72) Clinical Guideline – due for review 2014
- **RCPsych** (http://www.rcpsych.ac.uk/healthadvice/problemsdisorders/adhdinadults.aspx) A useful leaflet that can help signpost newly diagnosed adults.
- **ADDISS** (http://www.addiss.co.uk) Information and resources about **ADHD** for parents, sufferers, teachers and health professionals.
- **Adders** (http://www.adders.org) Attention Deficit/Hyperactivity Disorder online information.
- **UK Adult ADHD Network** (http://www.ukaan.org) Professional body that supports the NICE clinical guideline 72 and looks to establish clinical services for adults in the UK.

Drug treatment of ADHD

The currently available drug treatments for ADHD are symptomatic—they treat the core symptoms but do not cure them. 70% of affected children will show symptomatic response to medication, as demonstrated by: increased on-task behaviour; reduced fidgeting, finger-tapping, and interrupting; reduced impulsiveness; increased performance accuracy; reduced aggression; improved compliance; improved parent–child interactions; and improved peer status.

Commonly prescribed drugs

Methylphenidate A central nervous system stimulant licensed for treatment of ADHD in children over 6yrs. Available as an immediate-release preparation lasting around 4hrs (Ritalin®), and as modified release preparations lasting 8 or 12hrs (Equasym XL®, Concerta XL®, Medikinet XL®). Modified release preparations have the advantage that medication does not need to be administered at school. *Side-effects:* abdominal pain; nausea and vomiting; dry mouth; anxiety; insomnia; dysphoria; headaches; anorexia and reduced weight gain. Growth suppression may be a long-term outcome of high doses over long periods—growth monitoring is advised.

Atomoxetine (Strattera®) A non-stimulant NE reuptake inhibitor licensed for the treatment of ADHD. Taken once daily, providing 24-hr cover. May take up to 6wks to have a full effect. *Side-effects:* anorexia; dry mouth; nausea and vomiting; headache; fatigue; dysphoria.

Dexamfetamine A central nervous system stimulant licensed for the treatment of ADHD in children whose symptoms are refractory to other drugs. Side-effects are similar to those of methylphenidate.

Principles of prescribing in ADHD (NICE[1])

- The diagnosis of ADHD should be based on a comprehensive assessment conducted by a psychiatrist or a paediatrician with expertise in ADHD. It should also involve the child, parents, and carers, and the child's school, and take into account cultural factors in the child's environment.
- Multidisciplinary assessment, which may include educational or clinical psychologists and social workers, is advisable for children who present with indications of significant comorbidity.
- Drug treatment of ADHD should form part of a comprehensive treatment programme. A comprehensive treatment programme should involve advice and support to parents and teachers, and could include specific psychological treatments. While this wider service is desirable, any shortfall in its provision should not be used as a reason for delaying the appropriate use of medication.
- Drug treatment of ADHD should only be initiated by psychiatrists or paediatricians with expertise in ADHD, but continued prescribing and monitoring may be performed by GPs, under shared-care arrangements with specialists.
- The choice of drug should be guided by: the presence of comorbid conditions; the different adverse effects of the drugs; specific issues regarding compliance identified for the individual child or adolescent; the potential for drug diversion and/or misuse; the preferences of the

child or adolescent and/or his parent or guardian. If there is a choice of more than one appropriate drug, the drug with the lowest cost is prescribed.

- Caution is required in prescribing for children and young people with epilepsy, psychotic disorders, or a history of drug or alcohol dependence.
- Careful titration is required to determine the optimal dose level and timing. The drug should be discontinued if improvement of symptoms is not observed after appropriate dose adjustment.
- Children should receive regular monitoring. When improvement has occurred and the child's condition is stable, treatment can be discontinued at intervals, under careful specialist supervision, in order to assess both the child's progress and the need for continuation of therapy.

Adults with ADHD

ADHD tends to improve with age but can continue into adulthood. Over-activity often lessens, but impulsivity, poor concentration and risk-taking can worsen. Problems arise with work, education, family and social inter-actions. Comorbid depression, anxiety, low self-esteem, and drug misuse are common. Adults presenting with symptoms of ADHD in primary care or general adult psychiatric services, who do not have a childhood diag-nosis of ADHD, should be referred for assessment by a mental health specialist trained in the diagnosis and treatment of ADHD or a specialist service, if locally available. The most recent NICE Guideline (CG72) makes a number of recommendations regarding the management of adults with possible ADHD. Drug treatment for adults with ADHD should always form part of a comprehensive treatment programme that addresses psy-chological, behavioural and educational or occupational needs. None of the currently available drug treatments are licensed for initiation in adults, although atomoxetine is licensed for continuation treatment into adult-hood. It would be unusual to stop other effective treatments just because an individual has turned 18 yrs old. Most guidelines suggest methylpheni-date as first line treatment for adults provided it is not contraindicated. The need for long term medication should be closely monitored and reviewed at least annually. Specific guidance on dosing can be found in NICE CG72 and the BNF (4.4 CNS stimulants and drugs used for attention deficit hyperactivity disorder).

Autism spectrum disorders (ASD)

Autism spectrum disorders are a group of lifelong developmental disorders characterized by their effect on social and communication skills as well as by a restricted, stereotyped, repetitive repertoire of interests and activities. The spectrum ranges from clear-cut autism, to subtle variants, to traits found in the normal population and includes the diagnoses of autism, Asperger's syndrome, and pervasive developmental disorder not otherwise specified (PDD-NOS). Although 80% of individuals with childhood autism have learning disability, about 80% of the population with autism spectrum disorders are of normal intellectual ability. (For a more detailed description of autism and other PDDs see Chapter 18, **Learning disability**, 🕮 pp. 758–61).

Clinical features

Difficulties with social relationships

- Few or no sustained relationships.
- Persistent aloofness or awkward interaction with peers.
- Unusually egocentric with little concern for others or awareness of their viewpoint and limited empathy or sensitivity.
- Lack of awareness of social rules.

Problems in communication

- Odd voice, monotonous and perhaps at an unusual volume talking at (rather than to) you with little awareness of your response.
- Language is superficially good, but too formal, stilted, or pedantic and with difficulty in catching any meaning other than the literal.
- Impassive appearance with few gestures and abnormal gaze (i.e. limited non-verbal communicative behaviour).
- Awkward or odd posture and body language.

Absorbing and narrow interests

- Obsessively pursued and unusually circumscribed interests.
- A set approach to everyday life that may include unusual routines or rituals; change is often upsetting.

Comorbidity Depression; anxiety; bipolar disorder; psychosis; learning disability; OCD; ADHD; tic disorders; dyspraxia; impaired cognition in various domains, e.g. perception, executive functioning; visual/auditory impairment; epilepsy.

Assessment—key areas

- History of problems, eliciting difficulties in the domains (see **Clinical features**, 📖 p. 630).
- Level of distress and impairment in all aspects of life.
- Comorbidity.
- Cognitive ability.
- Impact on parents/carers and sources of support.
- Obtain information from as many sources as possible.
- Referral for specialist assessment, especially speech and language. Also educational psychology (via school), occupational therapy, and physiotherapy as indicated.
- Observation of child.
- Consider use of diagnostic tools, e.g. Autism Diagnostic Interview—Revised (ADI-R); Diagnostic Interview for Social and Communication Disorders (DISCO); Developmental Dimensional and Diagnostic Interview (3di).
- Medical investigation as appropriate, e.g. karyotyping, DNA, fragile X analysis, audiological examination, investigation for recognized aetiologies, e.g. tuberous sclerosis.

In practice, the diagnosis is made by a variety of professionals including psychiatrists, paediatricians, speech and language therapists and psychologists. While a multidisciplinary approach to all cases is ideal, this is particularly important in complex cases.

Management

Effective management will be informed by thorough assessment of the individual child and family's needs and is likely to involve more than one agency.

- Information (verbal and written) and support regarding the diagnosis.
- Liaison with education services re appropriate support and school placement. The educational psychologist is well suited to provide advice in this area.
- Parenting programmes specific to ASD.
- Adaptation of the child's environment, activities, and routines, e.g. visual timetabling.
- Communication interventions.
- Treat comorbidity—be aware that ASD may alter treatment approach and prognosis.
- Risperidone may be used for short-term treatment of significant aggression—monitor weight.
- Melatonin may help sleep disturbance where behavioural measures have failed.
- Wider family/sibling support including respite care, eligibility for benefits, and social work assistance.
- Inform about additional sources of information and support, e.g. National Autistic Society.

(Gilles de la) Tourette's syndrome

Essence A developmental neuropsychiatric disorder characterized by multiple motor and one or more vocal tics, present for at least a year, causing distress and impaired function.

- Motor tics often begin between the ages of 3 and 8, a few years before the onset of vocal tics.
- Typically, tics vary over time with more complex tics emerging after some years.
- Severity of tics waxes and wanes, with exacerbations often related to fatigue, emotional stress, and excitement.
- Tic severity usually peaks in early adolescence with most showing marked reduction in severity by the end of adolescence.
- Coprolalia is strongly associated in the public mind with this disorder, but is actually uncommon, and not required for diagnosis.

Epidemiology $\male : \female$ = 3:1. Prevalence is approximately 4–6/1000 in European and Asian populations.

Aetiology Thought to involve interaction of genetic and environmental factors. Multiple vulnerability genes implicated. Association with psychosocial stress well-known, and heightened HPA axis and NE system reactivity demonstrated. Other possibilities include gestational and perinatal insults, exposure to androgens, heat, fatigue, and post-infectious autoimmune mechanism (see PANDAS 🕮 p. 649).

Comorbidity OCD and ADHD common; depression, anxiety, learning difficulties, ASD, migraines. Associated problems include sleep difficulties, poor impulse control, and disruptive behaviours.

Key aspects of assessment
- Assess degree of interference with child's family, school, and social life.
- Careful perinatal, developmental, family, and medical history.
- Screen for associated difficulties.

Management
- Psychoeducation for child and family, and lifestyle adjustment: what tics are, realistic expectations, stress reduction, caffeine reduction.
- Close liaison with school and educational interventions.
- Treat comorbidity. SSRIs may be helpful in comorbid OCD. Methylphenidate is no longer contraindicated in comorbid ADHD.
- Behavioural interventions—habit reversal training looks promising. Consists of awareness training, self-monitoring of tics, relaxation training, competing response training and motivational techniques.
- If tics are severe and impairing, consider medication, e.g. antipsychotics, A-adrenergics. Beware tendency of tics to wax and wane regardless of treatment.
- Information and support can be gained from the Tourette Syndrome Association.

Other tic disorders

- Tics are sudden, rapid movements or vocalizations which occur in bursts. Tics are often under partial voluntary control and can be suppressed for brief periods.
- They are frequently associated with antecedent sensory phenomena including inner tension and premonitory urges, and tic performance may result in fleeting relief.
- Younger children may not experience these phenomena, or describe their tics as controllable.

Chronic motor or vocal tic disorder More common than Tourette's syndrome, with a better long-term outcome.

Transient tic disorder Motor and/or vocal tics are present transiently for less than one year. Occurs in at least 5% of children.

Language, learning, and motor co-ordination disorders

Speech and language delay and disorder

A distinction is drawn between speech and language delay and disorder. Delay indicates that speech and language acquisition is occurring at a slower rate, but in the expected sequence. Disorder implies that speech and language development is not following the usual sequence, suggesting specific difficulties in an aspect of the language system that is impacting on the child's overall language development.

Disorders include specific speech articulation disorder, expressive language disorder and receptive language disorder. Both delay and disorder are commonly multifactorial in aetiology. They can impact on a child's learning and literacy, social development, and emotional well-being and may initially present with behaviour problems. Assessment by a speech and language therapist is indicated.

Learning disorders

Generally, the educational psychologist is ideally placed to identify and advise on the management of these disorders. However, it is not unusual for the first presentation of these disorders to be to CAMHS as behavioural problems.

Reading disorder ('dyslexia')

Difficulty with reading, in most cases involving a deficit in phonological–processing skills. 4% of school-age children. Male predominance. There is often a family history of dyslexia. 20% have comorbid ADHD or CD Management includes 1:1 remedial teaching, and parent involvement improves long-term outcome.

Disorder of written expression

Often coexists with dyslexia and manifests as difficulties with spelling, syntax, grammar, and composition. Occurs in 2–8% of school-age children with a 3:1 male predominance. Difficulties may first emerge with the shift from narrative to expository writing assignments.

Mathematics disorder

Female predominance and occurs in 1–6% of school-age children. Often associated with visuospatial deficits and attributed to right parietal dysfunction.

Developmental co-ordination disorder (DCD)

- DCD and dyspraxia are generally held to be synonymous and refer to an impairment of, or difficulties with, the organization, planning and execution of physical movement with a developmental rather than acquired origin.
- It can be comorbid with disorders of learning and behaviour. Over half have attention difficulties, of which a minority will meet criteria for a diagnosis of DAMP: this disorder features **D**eficits in **A**ttention, **M**otor control, and **P**erception and there are overlaps with ODD and ASD.
- Can impact on self-esteem, family and peer relationships and school life.
- DCD prevalence 6%, commoner in males. Premature and low birth-weight babies at increased risk.
- First presentation may be to CAMHS with behavioural difficulties. More usually seen in paediatrics and primary care. Assessment and input from occupational therapy and physiotherapy may be necessary.

Enuresis

The normal variation in the age of acquisition of bladder control makes it difficult to demarcate disorder. By age 5, only 1% children have troublesome daytime wetting. Nocturnal enuresis, however, continues to affect 15–22% of boys and 7–15% of girls at the age of 7yrs. Primary (never dry) and secondary (previously dry) types are distinguished. Enuresis can impact on self-esteem, family and peer relationships and restrict activities. There is a reduction in rates of enuresis with time but a small minority will continue to experience problems into adult life.

Aetiology Nocturnal enuresis has a strong genetic component. Both psychosocial and pathophysiological associations have been demonstrated. Diurnal enuresis is more likely to be associated with structural and functional disorders of the urinary tract; and less likely to predict that other family members will have shown enuresis.

Management The majority of children will be managed in primary care, or by specialist enuresis clinics in the UK. Referrals to CAMHS are usually reserved for cases where enuresis is part of a wider disturbance of emotion and behaviour, or where serious psychological consequences have developed in an enuretic child.

- Careful assessment will inform management.
- Psychoeducation of child and parents.
- Treat organic causes, e.g. structural abnormality, infection.
- Nocturnal enuresis: there is robust evidence to support use of enuresis alarms. 'Night lifting', reward systems (e.g. star charts), and medication—desmopressin, imipramine, oxybutynin—may also be helpful.
- Diurnal enuresis: body alarms, watch alarm to remind child to use toilet, medication, specific psychological approaches, e.g. anxiety management if related to fear of toilet.
- ERIC (Enuresis Resource and Information Centre: ♒ http://www.eric.org.uk) provides information and resources to improve childhood continence. Website and helpline. Includes enuresis and encopresis.

Encopresis

Again, determining what is abnormal is problematic, but soiling more frequently than once a month after the fourth birthday is regarded as an elimination disorder if it is not attributable to a general medical condition. Primary and secondary forms are recognized as for enuresis. Constipation and soiling are common presentations to paediatrics, with only a small minority being referred to CAMHS. These latter children tend to have significant psychological problems in addition to soiling—association with emotional abuse. There can be considerable impact on self-esteem, family and peer relationships, and social activities. Most soiling will cease by age 16.

Types of soiling
- 95% present with functional constipation with retention and overflow. Both physical (persistent faecal loading leading to loss of sensation of rectal filling, anal fissure) and psychological (toilet fears, fear of painful defecation) factors may be relevant.
- Never toilet trained.
- Frightened to use the toilet.
- Deliberately depositing faeces in inappropriate places.

Management
As most cases are likely to have multifactorial causes, a comprehensive biopsychosocial assessment is necessary to guide management. Possible elements of treatment include:
- Lifestyle changes, e.g. adequate fluid and dietary fibre.
- Education of child and family, and assistance to view child more positively.
- Medical management, e.g. laxatives.
- Behavioural approaches, e.g. star charts.
- Family therapy, e.g. Sneaky Poo—a narrative therapy approach that helps to unite the family against the problem of soiling, which is personified as the character 'Sneaky Poo'.

Other behavioural disorders

Sleep disorders

Classified as for adult sleep disorders (see 📖 p. 414). The main syndromes that manifest in children and adolescents are: **nightmare disorder** (📖 p. 446); **sleep terror disorder** (📖 p. 442); and **sleepwalking disorder** (📖 p. 444). Management is the same as for adults.

Feeding and eating disorders of infancy and early childhood[1]

Pica This is a common condition where there is persistent (>1mth) eating of non-nutritive substances at a developmentally inappropriate age (>1yr). Common substances are: dirt, stones, hair, faeces, plastic, paper, wood, string, etc. It is particularly common in individuals with developmental disabilities and may be dangerous or life-threatening depending on the substance ingested. Consequences may include toxicity, infection, or GIT ulceration/obstruction. Typically occurs during 2nd and 3rd years of life, although young pregnant women may exhibit pica during pregnancy. Hypothesized causes include: nutritional deficiencies; cultural factors (e.g. clay); psychosocial stress; malnutrition and hunger; brain disorders (e.g. hypothalamic problem).

Rumination This is the voluntary or involuntary regurgitation and rechewing of partially digested food. Occurs within a few minutes postprandial and may last 1–2hrs. Regurgitation appears effortless and is preceded by belching. Typical onset 3–6mths of age, may persist for several months and then spontaneously remit. Also occurs in older individuals with LD. May result in weight loss, halitosis, dental decay, aspiration, recurrent respiratory tract infection (RTI), and sometimes asphyxiation and death (5–10% of cases). Causes include: LD; GIT pathology; psychiatric disorders; psychosocial stress. Treatment includes physical examination and investigations; behavioural methods; nutritional advice.

1 Ellis CR (2006) *Childhood habit behaviors and stereotypic movement disorder*. Medscape. ℅ http://www.emedicine.com.

Anxiety disorders: overview

Anxiety and fear are an inherent part of the human condition and in times of danger are often adaptive. As a result of changing developmental and cognitive abilities during childhood, the content of normal fears and anxieties shifts from concerns about concrete external things to abstract anxieties. Anxiety disorders are characterized by irrational fear or worry causing significant distress and/or impairment in functioning and their relative prevalence reflects this shift in content. Thus specific disorders appear more common during specific stages of development.

Epidemiology Anxiety disorders are among the most common psychiatric disorders in youth. Prevalence rates range from 5–15% with 8% requiring clinical treatment. Age of onset varies for each disorder. Separation anxiety disorder and specific phobia usually have onset in early childhood, generalized anxiety disorder occurs across all age groups, while obsessive–compulsive disorder, social phobia, agoraphobia, and panic disorder tend to occur in later childhood and adolescence.

Aetiological factors Genetic vulnerability; temperament that exhibits 'behavioural inhibition' (timidity, shyness, and emotional restraint with unfamiliar people or situations); insecure attachment; stressful or traumatic life events; high social adversity; over-protective/critical/punitive parenting.

Organic causes of anxiety *Medical conditions:* hyperthyroidism; cardiomyopathy; arrhythmias; respiratory and neurological diseases. *Substances:* alcohol; caffeine; cocaine; amfetamines; cannabis; SSRIs; LSD; ecstasy; etc.

Presentation of anxiety in children and adolescents

- Particularly in children, it is difficult to obtain a history of cognitive, emotional, and physical symptoms. Often somatic symptoms are the only feature that the child will be able to readily describe. Nevertheless, with sensitive questioning, fears and worries can be elicited.
- Behavioural presentations include overactivity, inattention, sleep disturbance, separation difficulty, regression, school refusal, social withdrawal, aggression, ritualistic behaviours, and somatization.

General principles of management

- Use ABC (antecedents, behaviour, consequences) approach to help child and family understand what happens when the child feels anxious.
- Show how others' reactions are influencing anxiety.
- Stress reduction including relaxation.
- Psychoeducation re anxiety, e.g. connection between physical, cognitive, and emotional components.
- Age-appropriate CBT approaches.

Separation anxiety disorder

Characterized by increased and inappropriate anxiety around separation from attachment figures or home, which is developmentally abnormal and results in impaired functioning. It occurs in about 3.5% of children and 0.8% of adolescents.

Causes Genetic vulnerability; anxious, inconsistent, or over-involved parenting; and regression during periods of stress, illness, or abandonment.

Symptoms Anxiety about actual or anticipated separation from or danger to attachment figure; sleep disturbances and nightmares; somatization; and school refusal.

Comorbidity Depression; anxiety disorders (panic with agoraphobia in older children); ADHD; oppositional disorders; learning disorders; and developmental disorders.

Normal separation anxiety Separation anxiety is a normal feature of development. Anxiety in a 2-yr-old who is being separated from his/her parent into the care of a stranger is normal since, at this developmental stage, the child may perceive the attachment figure as the only source of safety. On the other hand, disabling separation anxiety in a 7-yr-old is considered abnormal since the child has achieved a level of cognitive development at which he/she should have learned that many non-attachment figures might be considered 'safe'.

Generalized anxiety disorder

Essence Characterized by developmentally inappropriate and excessive worry and anxiety on most days about things not under one's own control. Severe enough to cause distress and/or dysfunction. Affected children are often perfectionist and self-critical. Most common anxiety disorder of adolescence with approximately 4% prevalence in this group. More common in females during adolescence. Only one-third seek treatment.

Symptoms Excessive worry; restlessness, irritability, and fatigue; poor concentration; sleep disturbances; muscle tension. In *children*: somatic symptoms (headache; stomach pains or 'irritable bowel'; rapid heartbeat; shortness of breath); nail biting and hair pulling; and school refusal.

Comorbidity Very high rates—up to 90%. Other anxiety disorders, depression, conduct disorders, and substance abuse are most common.

Management

- Good evidence for the use of CBT. This can be individual, group, or family-based, and it may be especially beneficial for parents to be involved in children under 11 or when parental anxiety is high.
- Psychoeducation regarding the nature and treatment of anxiety disorders along with supportive listening and clarification.
- The formulation may indicate the use of other psychosocial approaches.
- Although not supported by research evidence, use of SSRIs may be considered.

Panic disorder/agoraphobia

Essence Recurrent, unexpected **panic attacks** are the hallmark of this disorder, together with a period during which the child is concerned about having another attack and the possible consequences of an attack, and exhibits significant behavioural changes related to the attacks. These latter features are referred to as **anticipatory anxiety**. The first attack must be uncured. A panic attack is described as a discrete period of increased fear peaking at about 10min and lasting about 30min to 1hr.

Symptoms Sweating, flushing, trembling, palpitations and tachycardia, chest pain, shortness of breath and choking, nausea and vomiting, dizziness, paraesthesia, depersonalization and derealization, and a fear of dying. *Note:* in **young children** somatic symptoms predominate rather than classic symptoms. Agoraphobia may or may not coexist with the disorder, but is usually present. The essential feature is anxiety about being in a situation in which escape would be difficult or help unavailable should a panic attack occur. This leads to avoidance of places or situations and may result in school refusal and separation anxiety.

Epidemiology Panic disorder has an estimated prevalence of 3–6% and is more common in females post-puberty. Peak onset is 15–19yrs.

Comorbidity Depression, substance abuse, and other anxiety disorders (especially social phobia) are most common.

Management As for generalized anxiety disorder.

Social phobia, simple phobias, and selective mutism

Social phobia

Essence Extremely common and often undiagnosed. It is characterized by marked fear of one or more social or performance-related situations where the person is exposed to scrutiny and in which embarrassment may occur. Exposure to social situations usually causes an anxiety reaction (may be a panic attack) that is distressing. Thus situations are either avoided or endured with discomfort. This may lead to agoraphobia and in severe cases school refusal.

Epidemiology Social Phobia (SP) is most common in adolescents with an estimated prevalence of 5–15% as opposed to only 1% in children. It is more common in girls and the average age of onset for both genders is 12yrs. Family studies demonstrate a 2x increased risk for SP in the relatives of SP probands, while twin studies show a 3x increased risk in monozygotic twins.

Comorbidity High rates of other anxiety disorders (especially GAD, simple phobia, and panic disorder) in approximately 30–60% cases, with mood disorders (20%) and substance abuse also frequent comorbidly.

Prognosis Although the prognosis for treated SP is fair to good, comorbid conditions may persist and hinder educational and social progress. Those who experience symptoms in 2 or more situations have a poorer outcome than those experiencing symptoms in a single situation only.

Management
- Good evidence for the use of CBT exists. This can be individual, group, or family-based, and it may be especially beneficial for parents to be involved in children under 11 or when parental anxiety is high.
- SSRIs should be considered where CBT alone has failed.
- Psychoeducation regarding the nature and treatment of anxiety disorders along with supportive listening and clarification.
- The formulation may indicate the use of other psychosocial approaches.

Simple phobias

Essence Excessive fear of an object or situation with distress and phobic avoidance. There may be anticipatory anxiety and exposure can precipitate a panic attack.

Aetiology Probable interaction of genetic influence, inhibited temperament, parental influence and specific conditioning.

Epidemiology Very common (10% in some studies); $♀:♂ = 2:1$.

Comorbidity Depression; substance abuse.

Subtypes Animal phobias; natural environment phobias (especially 5–10-yr-olds); blood/infection/injury phobias; situational phobias (e.g. lifts, closed spaces); other.

Management
- Involve family and, if appropriate, others, e.g. teacher.
- CBT including desensitization, modelling, contingency management, relaxation training, self-statements.

Selective mutism (SM)

Essence A consistent failure to speak in social situations in which there is an expectation for speaking (e.g. at school) despite speaking in other situations. It has been considered both as an anxiety and an oppositional disorder.

Epidemiology Rare, affecting 3–8/10 000 in the UK, unlike extreme shyness which is common in the first year at school. Slightly commoner in girls.

Comorbidity Many children who develop SM have premorbid speech and language problems. Comorbidity with developmental delay/disorder, communication disorder, elimination disorders, and anxiety disorders observed.

Management Difficult to treat. There is a small evidence base for the use of behavioural therapy, CBT, SSRIs, and individual psychotherapy. Involve family and school in treatment.

Post-traumatic stress disorder[1,2]

Essence A syndrome characterized by a triad of symptoms: intrusive re-experiencing of a traumatic event; avoidance; and hyperarousal. Recognized in children since the 1980s. Symptoms variable in young children, but similar to adult pattern in older children (see 🕮 p. 390).

Traumatic event Requires exposure to a situation or event which is catastrophic or highly threatening.

Epidemiology Prevalence varies according to age, but develops in approximately 3–6% of children exposed to a trauma. Most exposed do not develop the disorder and those that are affected usually have a pre-existing vulnerability (i.e. 'an unnatural response to an unnatural event').

Clinical presentation in young children
Identification of PTSD in children presents particular problems, but can be improved by asking the child directly about their experiences. Do not rely solely on caregiver's history.
   Scheeringa criteria:[3]
- Compulsive repetitive play representing part of the trauma and failing to relieve anxiety.
- Recurrent recollections of the event.
- Nightmares, night terrors, and difficulty going to sleep.
- Constriction of play.
- Social withdrawal.
- Restricted affect.
- Loss of acquired developmental skills, especially language regression and toilet training.
- Decreased concentration and attention.
- New aggression.
- New separation anxiety.

Depression is common in older children and adolescents.
   Note that post-traumatic stress symptoms which do not meet criteria for a diagnosis can still be highly disabling and deserve attention in their own right.

Comorbidity Common in PTSD with depression, anxiety disorders, and substance abuse frequent in adolescents. Behavioural disorders common in young children. See Box 16.2 for NICE guidelines on treatment of PTSD.

Box 16.2 NICE guidance on treatment of PTSD in children and adolescents[1]

Interventions in the first month after a trauma
Offer trauma-focused CBT to older children with severe post-traumatic symptoms or with severe PTSD in the first month after the event.

Interventions more than 3mths after a trauma
- Offer children and young people a course of trauma-focused CBT adapted as needed to suit their age, circumstances, and level of development. (This should also be offered to those who have experienced sexual abuse.)
- For chronic PTSD in children and young people resulting from a single event, consider offering 8–12 sessions of trauma-focused psychological treatment. When the trauma is discussed, longer treatment sessions (90min) are usually necessary.
- Psychological treatment should be regular and continuous (usually at least once a week) and delivered by the same person.
- Do not routinely prescribe drug treatments for children and young people with PTSD.
- Involve families in the treatment of children and young people where appropriate, but remember that treatment consisting of parental involvement alone is unlikely to be of benefit for PTSD symptoms.
- Inform parents (and where appropriate, children and young people) that apart from trauma-focused psychological interventions, there is no good evidence for the efficacy of other forms of treatment, such as play therapy, art therapy, or family therapy.

1 ✇ http://publications.nice.org.uk/post-traumatic-stress-disorder-ptsd-cg26

1 Perrins S, Smith P, and Yule W (2000) The assessment and treatment of post-traumatic stress disorder in children and adolescents. *J Child Psychol Psychiat* **41**: 277–89.
2 Yule W (2001) Posttraumatic stress disorder in the general population and in children. *J Clin Psychiat* **63**(Suppl. 17): 23–8.
3 Scheeringa MS and Gaensbauer TJ (2000) Post-traumatic stress disorder. In Zeanah CH (ed), *Handbook of infant health*, pp. 369–81. New York: Guilford Press.

Obsessive–compulsive disorder (OCD)

Essence (see 📖 p. 376) OCD is characterized by recurrent obsessions and/or compulsions that cause impairment in terms of time (>1hr/day), distress, or interference in functioning.

Epidemiology Prevalence in adolescents 1–3.6%. May occur as early as 5yrs of age and mean age of onset is 10yrs. Male predominance (3:2) in childhood, with equal gender distribution in adolescence. Mild *subclinical* obsessions and compulsions are common in the general population (4–19%) and disorder merges with normality. This is a persistent disorder which is often veiled in secrecy—mean delay to presentation is 2yrs.

Aetiology Genetic and non-genetic factors probably equally important. Only 15% have clearly identifiable precipitating factor.

Clinical features
- *Obsessions:* intrusive, repetitive, and distressing thoughts or images. Common themes: contamination, harm coming to others, sexual, aggressive, religious.
- *Compulsions:* repetitive, stereotyped, unnecessary behaviours. Common rituals include washing, checking, repeating, ordering, reassurance seeking. Rituals may involve parents and are part of normal development, especially in 3–7-yr age group. More likely to be OCD if the rituals or thoughts distress the child, they take up a lot of time and if they interfere with the child's everyday life.
- Multiple obsessions and compulsions common.
- Poor insight commoner in child cases.

Differential diagnosis Normal developmental rituals; Tourette's/tic disorder; depression; ASD; eating disorder; psychosis.

Comorbidity 70% have at least one comorbid disorder. Includes other anxiety disorders, ADHD, ODD, Tourette's syndrome, autistic spectrum disorders and mood disorders.

Assessment
- Family and individual assessment where possible.
- Young person may be reluctant to discuss aspects of obsessions/compulsions.
- Children's Yale–Brown Obsessive Compulsive Scale may be useful both as rating scale and to obtain clear picture of obsession/compulsion.
- Screen for comorbidity.

Treatment

- Consider guided self-help for mild impairment in first instance.
- If more severely affected, offer developmentally appropriate CBT and ERP (exposure response prevention) in group or individual format. Involve family where possible in planning and process of treatment, and school, etc., as necessary.
- Following multidisciplinary review, consider SSRI in addition to CBT and ERP if no response. Monitor closely and advise of delay in onset of action of up to 12wks. After remission continue medication for 6mths then gradually withdraw.
- If SSRI fails, consider change to different SSRI/clomipramine. Need ECG prior to clomipramine treatment.
- In specialist settings, augmentation with antipsychotic may be appropriate.
- Consider inpatient care in most severe cases associated with major impairment and distress unresponsive to outpatient care. Also where there is significant self-neglect or suicide risk.
- Absence of comorbidity and good insight increase chances of successful outcome.

PANDAS[1] (paediatric autoimmune neurological disorder associated with streptococcus) An autoimmune syndrome associated with OCD and/or tic disorder, with pre-pubertal onset, characterized by episodic exacerbations of symptoms in association with evidence of Group A beta haemolytic streptococcal infection.

1 Swedo SE, Leonard HL, Garvey M, et al. (1998) Pediatric autoimmune neuropsychiatric disorders associated with streptococcal infections: clinical description of the first 50 cases. Am J Psychol **55**: 264–71.

Eating disorders

Eating disorders in children and adolescents include anorexia nervosa, bulimia nervosa, and their variants characterized by disturbed or inadequate eating patterns associated with abnormal preoccupation with weight and shape. Many children present with clinically significant disorder which does not fit diagnostic criteria. Children and adolescents may also present with other types of clinical eating disturbance, including:

• *Food avoidance emotional disorder:* food avoidance and weight loss unaccounted for by other psychiatric disorder and in the absence of abnormal cognitions about weight/shape. They know that they are underweight, would like to be heavier, and may not know why they find this difficult to achieve. Often have other medically unexplained symptoms. Can result in serious weight loss.
• *Selective eating characterized by long-standing restriction of types of food eaten:* rarely harmful but can result in social difficulties.
• *Pervasive refusal:* a rare disorder defined as 'a profound and pervasive refusal to eat, walk, talk or engage in self-care'[1]. Likely to require prolonged inpatient treatment.
• Eating disturbance may also be a feature of other disorders, e.g. depression, OCD; or part of a physical disorder where there is a psychological component to presentation.

Anorexia nervosa (AN)

Essence Self-induced weight loss associated with abnormal beliefs and preoccupation regarding weight and/or shape. ICD-10 and DSM-IV criteria are used (🕮 p. 398), but the 'weight criterion' of BMI <17.5 is problematic in children and adolescents who are still developing. A suggested alteration by the Royal College of Psychiatrists Eating Disorders Special Interest Group is BMI below the 2nd centile.

Epidemiology Prevalence 0.3% in adolescent females. Lower rates in boys and pre-pubertally.

Assessment
• Family and individual—often secrecy around behaviour.
• Eating—intake, weight control measures, attitude to weight/shape.
• Assessment of factors contributing to and maintaining disorder, e.g. acute life stress, obesity, parental weight concerns, peers, psychological factors such as perfectionism and personal ineffectiveness.
• Comorbidity and risk.
• Full physical assessment and investigations as appropriate, e.g. bloods, ECG, bone density, ovarian ultrasound scan (USS).
• Motivation to change.

Management

Involves physical, psychological, educational, and social aspects and will usually require a multidisciplinary approach.

• Treatment should normally involve whole family and the effects of AN on other family members should be recognized.
• Restoration of healthy weight allowing further growth and development, and treatment of physical complications.
• Provide education on nutrition and healthy eating. Carers should be included in any dietary education or meal planning.
• Patients should be offered family interventions that directly address the eating disorder, and also individual sessions to provide support, improve motivation, and address core maladaptive thoughts, attitudes, and feelings.
• Treat comorbidity. Note psychological symptoms often improve with weight gain.
• The balance of responsibility for treatment between parents and young people will vary according to the age of the young person. Nevertheless, where young people refuse necessary treatment, parental right to override this must be considered, as well as use of Mental Health Act legislation.
• Where the young person is at serious risk, e.g. through physical compromise or suicidality, or is not progressing in outpatient treatment, specialist inpatient or day patient care in age-appropriate settings should be considered.
• Liaison with school, e.g. graded return if has been absent.
• Relapse prevention.

Bulimia nervosa

Essence Disorder characterized by recurrent binges and purges, sense of lack of control and morbid preoccupation with weight and shape. Rarely occurs pre-pubertally, much commoner in girls, often comorbid with depression. Usually of normal weight.

Management

• Work with family to establish clear structures and boundaries. Strike a balance between individual work and family work.
• Adolescents with bulimia nervosa may be treated with CBT adapted as needed to suit their age, circumstances and level of development, and including the family as appropriate.
• Address physical health concerns, e.g. due to frequent vomiting.
• No clear evidence to support drug treatments in this age group, but fluoxetine could be a useful adjunct in older adolescents.

---

1 Lask B, Britten C, Kroll L, *et al.* (1991) Children with pervasive refusal. *Arch Dis Child* **66**: 866–9.

Depression in children and adolescents

Epidemiology 12-mth point prevalence 1% pre-pubertal, 3% post-pubertal. No sex difference pre-pubertal, commoner in females thereafter.

Risk factors include Female, post-pubertal, parental history of depression, personally undesirable life events resulting in permanent change of interpersonal relationships in friends or family, past history of depressive symptoms, high trait levels of neuroticism or emotionality, ruminative style of thinking.

Aetiology Stress-vulnerability model useful in understanding development of depression. Vulnerability (genes, endocrine, early family factors) interacts with social stressors (poverty, family discord, etc.) to provoke depression at time of life stress.

Clinical features
- *Mood changes:* unpleasant mood—may not be described as sadness but as 'grumpy', 'irritable', or 'down'; also anhedonia.
- *Thought changes:* reduced self-esteem, confidence, concentration, and self-efficacy. Hopelessness, guilt, indecisiveness. Suicidal thoughts must be taken seriously. Rarely psychotic symptoms.
- *Physical/behavioural changes:* reduced energy, motivation, self-care. Fatigue, apathy, withdrawal, appetite and sleep change, aches and pains, self-harming and suicidal behaviour.
- Results in impairment of functioning—school, social, family, etc.

Course
- *Recovery:* 10% at 3mths, 50% at 1yr, 70–80% at 2yrs. Treatment shortens duration of illness.
- 30% recurrence within 5yrs. 3% risk of suicide over next 10yrs. Chronic/recurrent illness significantly impairing in all aspects of life.
- 20% will later manifest bipolar disorder.

Comorbidity 50–80% meet criteria for additional non-depressive disorder including conduct disorder/ODD, separation anxiety, OCD, ADHD, eating disorder, other anxiety disorders.

Differential Medical conditions; substance misuse; adjustment disorders; other psychiatric disorders.

Assessment
- Family and individual interviews. Assess whether depression is present, contributing factors to development and maintenance, presence of comorbidity, suicide risk.
- Collateral from teachers, GP, social services, etc.
- Consider use of rating scales, e.g. Moods and Feelings Questionnaire.
- Physical examination and laboratory investigations as indicated.

Treatment (NICE)

Mild depression—usually at Tier 1 or 2

- Up to 4wks of 'watchful waiting'—stay in contact with family.
- If symptoms continue offer 2–3mths of individual non-directive supportive therapy, group cognitive behavioural therapy (CBT), or guided self-help (GSH).
- If unresponsive refer for Tier 2/3 review and treat as for moderate–severe.

Moderate–severe depression—Tier 2–4

- Offer individual CBT, interpersonal therapy, or family therapy for at least 3mths as a first-line treatment.
- If unresponsive after 4–6 sessions multidisciplinary review and consider alternative/additional psychological therapy and pharmacotherapy.
- If unresponsive after further 6 sessions, comprehensive multidisciplinary review and consider alternative psychotherapy including child psychotherapy.
- Consider inpatient treatment if child/young person is at high risk of suicide, serious self-harm and self-neglect, or when required intensity of treatment (or supervision) is not available elsewhere, or for intensive assessment.

Pharmacotherapy/ECT

Ensure that full discussion of rationale, delayed onset of action, time course and need to take regularly along with risks/benefits of drug takes place with family, and provide written information. Monitor for side-effects and benefits. There is limited evidence that all SSRIs/atypical antidepressants (including fluoxetine) may increase the risk of suicidal ideation and/or behaviour and increase the risk of discontinuation of treatment because of adverse events. Fluoxetine is the only antidepressant with a favourable risk:benefit ratio and should be prescribed first. Start at 10mg daily, increase if necessary to 20mg after 1wk. Second-line recommendations are sertraline or citalopram. TCAs, venlafaxine, and St John's wort are not recommended. Medication should be continued for at least 6mnths after remission then phased out over 6–12wks. In psychotic depression consider augmentation with atypical antipsychotic. Only consider ECT for young people (12–18yrs) with very severe depression and either life-threatening symptoms or intractable and severe symptoms that have not responded to other treatments.

Relapse and remission

Monitor for 1yr regularly for first episode or 2yrs for recurrent episode. If at high risk of relapse consider follow-up psychotherapy as prevention, or to promote child and family's identification and management of early warning signs.

Suicide and self-harm in young people

This section should be read alongside 📖 p. 784 in the liaison chapter.

Epidemiology Overall increase during the twentieth century, suicide now represents the third cause of death in adolescents (12% of mortality in this group). Completed suicide is commoner in males, however suicide attempts and deliberate self-harm (DSH) are commoner in females and include self-poisoning, cutting, and burning.

Two important points:
- Completed suicide is only the tip of the iceberg of suicidal behaviour/ideation.
- There is a very strong association between depression and suicidality. The combination of mood disorder, substance misuse, and conduct problems is particularly high risk.

Factors increasing risk of completed/attempted suicide
- Persistent suicidal ideas.
- Previous suicidal behaviour.
- High lethality of method used and ongoing availability of lethal method.
- High suicidal intent and motivation, e.g. planning, stated wish to die.
- Ongoing precipitating stresses, e.g. interpersonal conflict, legal problems.
- Mental disorder: mood disorders, psychosis, substance misuse, conduct disorder, anxiety disorders, PTSD, eating disorders.
- Poor physical health.
- Psychological factors: impulsivity, neuroticism, low self-esteem, hopelessness.
- Parental psychopathology and suicidal behaviour.
- Physical and sexual abuse.
- Disconnection from major support systems, e.g. school, family, work.

Prevention

General measures include:
- Screening and treating psychiatric disorders.
- Crisis lines/access to help.
- Education of parents, the public, and the media.
- Intervene in cluster situations (e.g. several suicides in a school).
- Reduce access to means, e.g. limits on paracetamol purchase.

Self-harm

Presentation with self-harm may indicate psychiatric disorder or significant psychosocial problems. Many risk factors for self-harm are shared with those for suicide.

Among adolescents who deliberately harm themselves, the factors that are most likely to be associated with a higher risk of later suicide include:

- Male gender.
- Older age.
- High suicidal intent.
- Psychosis.
- Depression.
- Hopelessness.
- Having an unclear reason for the act of deliberate self-harm.

Management

Parents have a responsibility to ensure the safety of their child. They should be involved in the assessment and management planning. Sometimes young people will ask us not to tell parents about their suicidal thoughts and acts. One should discuss this with them and try to persuade them otherwise, but ultimately one must inform the parents if risk is present. This exception to confidentiality should have been explained at the start of the assessment.

Management may involve the participation of several agencies: child and adult medical and mental health services; social services; police; education; non-statutory agencies.

- Usually admission to an age-appropriate medical ward to allow both medical treatment and a full psychosocial assessment.
- Mental health and risk assessment by a specially trained staff member with ready access to psychiatric opinion.
- A minority will need inpatient psychiatric care. This should be in an age-appropriate unit.
- It is usually appropriate to refer on to the local CAMHS if the family agrees to allow a fuller assessment and ongoing management.
- Where assessment reveals abuse issues, these need to be tackled according to local procedure.

Bipolar disorder in children and adolescents

Epidemiology BPD is rare in prepubescent children; prevalence in adolescents is approximately 1%. Familial factors are important with a 4 times greater risk of mood disorder in offspring of parents with BPD.

Presentation

Will depend on the phase of the disorder. See 📖 p. 652 for depression. A hypomanic/manic child may present as overactive, full of self-belief, grandiose, and challenging of authority. They are often irritable and can become aggressive or violent. Poor concentration affects school performance. Over-spending, sexual disinhibition and risk-taking behaviour may feature. Psychotic symptoms may be present. Mixed affective states are also recognized.

Diagnosis

NICE recommends (🔗 http://www.nice.org.uk/CG38):
- That adult criteria are used but (i) mania must be present, (ii) euphoria must be present most days, most of the time (for 7 days), and (iii) irritability is not a core diagnostic criterion.
- Do not diagnose solely on the basis of a major depressive episode in a child with a family history of bipolar disorder, but follow up such children carefully.
- For older or developmentally advanced adolescents, use adult criteria.
- Do not diagnose bipolar II (📖 p. 315) in younger adolescents or children.

Differential diagnosis

- ADHD or conduct disorder. Seek history of clear-cut episodes of elated mood, grandiosity, and cycles of mood. Mood cycles may also help distinguish BPD from schizophrenia.
- Substance misuse.
- Organic causes.
- Sexual, emotional, and physical abuse may manifest as disinhibition, hypervigilance, or hypersexuality.

Comorbidity ADHD (70%), substance abuse (40%), ODD (40%), anxiety disorders (30%), Tourette's syndrome (8%), bulimia nervosa (3%).

Outcome Early onset BPD has a poor outcome with 50% showing long-term decline in function. There is commonly a family history, suggesting that this is a highly genetic form of BPD. The course is often chronic and less responsive to treatment, with atypical and rapid-cycling features especially difficult to treat. Suicide risk is high with rates of completed suicide approximately 10%.

Assessment: key areas

- Individual and family.
- Thorough developmental history, family history mood disorder, pattern of mood changes.
- Comorbidity.
- Impact of disorder on life—family, friends, school, etc.
- Collateral information from school, etc.
- Physical examination and appropriate investigations.
- Level of risk—suicide, exploitation, violence.
- Capacity/consent/legislation.

Management

- Involve parents or carers in developing care plans so that they can give informed consent, support treatment goals, and help ensure adherence.
- Consider inpatient or day patient admission to age-appropriate services, or more intensive community treatment, for patients at risk of suicide or other serious harm.
- **Acute mania**: consider antipsychotic, valproate (not girls), or lithium. Before starting (and thereafter) check height, weight, and prolactin levels. Start at lower doses than for adults. If inadequate response to antipsychotic can add valproate or lithium.
- **Depression**: if mild, monitor and support. If moderate to severe, offer psychological therapy first. If no response at 4wks consider fluoxetine starting at 10mg daily. If this fails, consider sertraline or citalopram. Consider augmentation with antipsychotic if psychotic symptoms present.
- **Long term**: need for long-term treatment? Consider atypical antipsychotic that is associated with less weight gain and does not increase prolactin levels. As second-line, consider lithium for female patients and valproate or lithium for male patients.
- Psychological interventions include: psychoeducation and support to individual and family; more formal therapy, e.g. motivational interviewing, CBT; family therapy.
- Education and vocational training including school liaison, additional support, etc.
- Voluntary organizations and support groups.

Psychosis

Psychosis in adolescence is uncommon, and very uncommon in children. Diagnosis is on the basis of standard ICD-10 or DSM-IV criteria (□ p. 178).

Psychosis in children and adolescents

Psychotic illnesses are rare in young children and present a particular challenge in both diagnosis and management. Very young children under 6yrs have preoperational cognitions and thus 'reality testing' is blurred by a range of normal fantasy material. Imagined friends, transient hallucinations under stress, and loose associations may all occur within the normal spectrum of development.

Differential diagnosis There are many causes of apparent psychotic symptoms in children and adolescents. This means that the assessment of a child with symptoms requires extreme care and thoroughness.

Possible explanations include:

- Normal experience.
- Organic conditions (e.g. TLE, thyroid disease, brain tumour, Wilson's disease, and substance misuse disorders).
- Mood disorders.
- PDD/autism.
- OCD.
- Schizophrenia.
- Language disorders.
- Dissociative disorders.
- Culture-bound syndromes.

Schizophrenia

Clinical features

- More often insidious than acute onset.
- Associated with poor premorbid function with developmental delays.
- Below average IQ.
- Negative symptoms often precede positive, and are prominent.
- Comorbidity common—conduct and developmental problems, substance misuse.
- Strong family history of schizophrenia/psychosis.
- Poorer outcome than adult-onset schizophrenia. Poor premorbid functioning, negative symptoms, 'disorganized' clinical presentation, and greater duration of untreated psychosis predict worse outcome.

Assessment: key areas

- Good engagement important.
- Detailed developmental history.
- History from multiple informants including family and school.
- Negative symptoms.
- Screen for comorbidity.
- Risk assessment.
- Physical examination and medical investigations.
- Consider use of rating scale, e.g. K-SADS.

Management

- In-, day- or outpatient care? Will depend of complexity, level of risk, likely engagement/concordance, likely effect on child of being away from family. Care should be in age-appropriate setting. Early intervention in psychosis services that have emerged across the UK, often extending down into the adolescent age group—their input may be very useful.
- Medication—atypical antipsychotics favoured over typicals. Side-effects still often problematic. Clozapine useful in treatment resistance. Age-specific evidence base limited. BDZs or antipsychotics may be useful in managing acute behavioural disturbance not responsive to non-pharmacological measures.
- Supportive, psychoeducational and specific psychotherapeutic individual work, e.g. CBT, social skills training.
- Family support, education, and therapeutic work as appropriate.
- Manage comorbidity.
- Ongoing risk assessment and management.
- Educational/vocational input, e.g. reintegration package to school, specialist education provision, supported college/work placements.
- Awareness of consent/capacity/legal issues. Varies across UK.
- Voluntary sector—National Schizophrenia Fellowship, MIND.
- Access to benefits, etc.
- Thoughtful and measured transition to adult services.

Substance abuse in children and adolescents

Substance abuse is increasingly common in young people. It affects 13% of adolescents referred to mental health services. The characteristics of use and the approach to management can be different to those in adults. Comorbidity is common: conduct problems, depression and other emotional disorders, ADHD, eating disorders. Types of use include:

- Experimentation/exploration—usually social, about adventure.
- Social use—social acceptance important.
- Emotional/instrumental use—for the 'high' or to suppress unpleasant feelings and deal with stress.
- Habitual use—salience, tolerance, and negative consequences on life become prominent.
- Dependence—full dependence syndrome (📖 p. 542).

Assessment: key areas

- Involve family where possible.
- Substance—types, routes, quantity, cost, context.
- Consequences of use—family, friends, development, education, employment, physical and mental health, criminal activity.
- Attitude to referral—Prochaska's theory of change.
- Link with other agencies, e.g. social services, education, youth justice.
- Risk—to self, others, child protection.

Management

- Brief interventions may be sufficient for young people with less severe substance misuse problems. Developmental stage and shorter history means rapid changes can be made.
- More severe problems are addressed by co-ordination of multiple agencies, e.g. mainstream CAMHS, social and education services.
- Structured treatment by specialist young people's substance misuse treatment services is recommended for under-18s who have significant substance misuse problems (normally polydrug and alcohol misuse). This could include harm reduction interventions, psychosocial treatments (motivational therapies, cognitive behavioural treatments, family-based supports and treatment) and occasionally pharmacological interventions. Again this occurs in the context of interventions to address all of the young person's health, social, family, and educational needs, and therefore involves multiple agencies. The involvement of a young person's family or those with parental responsibility is considered good practice and may be required with regard to consent.

Child abuse 1: general issues[1]

In recent decades there has been growing awareness that the abuse of children can take many forms. All forms of child abuse involve the elements of power imbalance, exploitation, and the absence of true consent. They may concern acts of commission or acts of omission. Over recent times, domestic violence and parental substance misuse have been recognized as situations which should prompt concern for the protection of children from abuse.

Categories of abuse

Physical abuse includes hitting, shaking, throwing, poisoning, burning or scalding, drowning, suffocating or otherwise causing physical harm to a child. (Includes Munchausen syndrome by proxy—see Box 16.3.)

Neglect is the persistent failure to meet a child's basic physical/psychological needs, likely to result in serious impairment of the child's health and development. Includes failure to provide adequate: food, clothing, shelter and supervision; protection from harm or danger; and access to appropriate medical care. Also includes substance misuse during pregnancy.

Emotional abuse persistent emotional maltreatment resulting in severe and persistent effects on the child's emotional development. Includes denigration or rejection, emotional neglect, developmentally inappropriate expectations, repeated separations and mis-socialization of the child. Other types of abuse are likely to result in emotional abuse.

Sexual abuse involves forcing or enticing a child into sexual activity. This may include penetrative and non-penetrative physical acts, and non-contact activities such as involving children in looking at or producing sexual images, watching sexual activities or encouraging children to behave in sexually inappropriate ways.

> ### Box 16.3 Munchausen's syndrome by proxy: factitious or induced illness syndrome (FIIS)
>
> - Part of a factitious syndrome that is manifest by a person feigning or inducing illness in a child (or others) in order to obtain medical attention.
> - A form of child abuse in that it subjects the child to emotional abuse, unnecessary medical procedures, hospitalization or other treatments that are harmful to the child.
> - Can be very difficult to detect as the perpetrating (and colluding) adult/s often deny and disguise their behaviour.
> - It is essential for professionals to be alert to it, especially where a child repetitively presents for medical attention.
>
> *Undetected, this form of abuse can result in very serious consequences (including fatality) for the child.*

---

1 Adapted from HM Government (2006) *What to do if you're worried a child is being abused.* London: HMSO.

Child abuse 2: the duty of care

All practitioners have a duty to safeguard and promote the welfare of children. It is important to remain alert to the possibility of abuse or neglect. The assessment of risk, and interventions to protect children, require a multidisciplinary and multi-agency approach. In general, the duty to patients, including that of confidentiality, is overridden by the duty to protect children.

Referrals regarding possible abuse will usually be made to social services or the police.

Making a child protection referral

- **Know how to access your local multi-agency Child Protection Procedures and follow them.**
- It is good practice to discuss the referral with the child, as appropriate to their age and understanding, and with their parents, to seek agreement to the referral unless such discussion would place the child at risk of significant harm. It is not necessary to have agreement to make the referral.
- Ensure that you carefully document all concerns, discussions, decisions made and reasons for these decisions.
- Discuss the situation with a senior colleague.
- Follow up oral communications in writing.
- Have as much information regarding the child and your concerns available as possible.
- Do not do anything which may jeopardize a police investigation, e.g. asking a child leading questions, or attempting to investigate the allegations of abuse.

Child abuse—where does CAMHS fit in?

- Being alert to abuse, responding to concerns expressed by individuals and families, and making a child protection referral.
- Involvement in multi-agency discussion and planning for the child.
- Post-abuse work with children and families (abusing and non-abusing).

Psychiatric outcome of chronic abuse

Children who are abused have an extremely high rate of psychiatric disorders, both during the abuse and later on.

Some of the most common disorders associated with previous abuse:
- PTSD
- Dissociative disorders
- Conversion disorders
- Borderline personality disorder
- Depression
- Paraphilias
- Substance abuse.

The looked-after-child (LAC)

'Looked after' is the term used to describe all children in public care, including those in foster or residential homes, and those still with their own parents but subject to care orders. The majority have become 'looked after' because of abuse or neglect.

Outcomes for LAC

On leaving care, young people have significantly poorer outcomes in terms of education, employment, and physical and mental health. Teenage pregnancy, homelessness, and involvement in crime as both victim and perpetrator are increased.

Mental health of LAC

These children have often experienced many risk factors for development of mental disorder: abuse or neglect, family dysfunction, parental ill-health or substance misuse, changes of carer, high socio-economic disadvantage, discrimination and trauma. Attachment is likely to have been disrupted.

Common presentations include conduct disorder, depression, anxiety disorders, substance misuse, ADHD, and ASD-like difficulties.

Working with LAC

This requires multi-agency co-operation as multiple needs must be met.

- A stable and secure environment for the child where his physical, emotional, and social developmental needs are met is fundamentally important.
- Even if a change of environment is unavoidable, continuity in the form of attending the same school, retaining the same workers is desirable.
- Support to the child's carers—social services, CAMHS, and other agencies may all play a role.
- Individual CAMHS work with the child can be helpful in the context of these needs being met. It is very unlikely to be of benefit while the child remains in an insecure or harmful environment.

'The test of the morality of a society is what it does for its children.'

Dietrich Bonhoeffer (1906–1945)
German Protestant theologian and anti-Nazi activist

Prescribing in children and adolescents[1,2]

Principles

- They are not small adults! This is particularly important in regard to the dynamics and kinetics of drugs. Some drugs are metabolized faster while others more readily cross the blood–brain barrier. Susceptibility to side-effects also varies with age (e.g. children are more likely to develop dystonias and less likely to develop akathisia with neuroleptic treatment).
- Medication should be considered as just one component of treatment—it should be accompanied by psychological, social, and educational interventions.
- Drugs are often prescribed for symptoms rather than syndromes (e.g. stimulants for hyperactivity symptoms in a variety of disorders).
- Drug trials in children are problematic both ethically and practically, so there is inadequate data regarding safety and efficacy for many psychotropics. Thus clinicians are often faced with ethical decisions regarding the use of drugs not licenced for use in these age groups.
- The decision to prescribe needs to take into account both the young person's and parents' attitudes to medication, and to consider issues of consent and capacity.

---

1 For an interesting historical review see Zito JM, Derivan AT, Kratochvil CJ, *et al.* (2008) Off-label psychopharmacologic prescribing for children: history supports close monitoring. *Child and Adolescent Psychiatry and Mental Health* **2**: 24. Available online: ℘ http://www.capmh.com/content/2/1/24
2 Riddle MA, Kastelic EA, and Frosch E (2001) Pediatric psychopharmacology. *J Child Psychol Psychiat* **42**: 73–90.

Family therapy (FT)

Family therapy (FT) originated in the 1950s and has been influenced by many schools of thought since then, including psychodynamic theory, general systems theory, social constructionism, and feminist approaches. FT approaches differ in many ways, but all recognize the interrelatedness of the person with the problem and their family members, and the role of the family in problem resolution.

Indications

FT can be useful wherever there are difficulties in family relationships which are impacting on a family member's mental health. This may be as the main treatment, or concurrently with other treatment modalities, e.g. individual therapies, medication.

Key elements of some FT models

Structural FT Clear rules govern family organization—hierarchies, subsystems, boundaries. Distortion of these produces symptoms. Therapist takes directive stance to change family behaviours, and thereby their beliefs.

Strategic FT Family transactions are key. The problem is serving an interpersonal function for some members, so family is ambivalent about change. Therapist takes strategic stance and gives family tasks.

Milan Systemic FT Emphasis on family beliefs and meanings, no objective truth. Several techniques—reframing, hypothesizing, neutrality, curiosity. Team behind screen. Therapist takes 'not-knowing', non-expert stance.

Brief Solution Focused FT Collaborative; focus on exceptions, solutions, and competence of family. Use of goals and scales.

Narrative FT Problems relate to unhelpful, dominant, inaccurate narrative about life. Unique outcomes, differing from dominant narrative, are explored allowing a new, more helpful narrative to emerge. Therapist non-expert.

Many FT practitioners will use eclectic approaches, often incorporating teams. Reflecting teams put family in observer position of hearing their conversation with the therapist discussed, allowing new perspectives to emerge.

Duration

Extremely varied. Treatment can be as short as 1 or 2 sessions or take 12–24-weekly sessions or more. It is usually shorter than forms of long-term psychotherapy like psychodynamic psychotherapy.

Recommended further reading

Carr A (2006) *Family therapy: concepts, process and practice.* Chichester: John Wiley and Sons.

Parent management training

Parent management training (PMT) has until very recently been described as a group of treatment procedures in which parents are trained to modify their child's behaviour. More recent definitions of PMT encompass its broader power in improving the communication within families. PMT is not simply about generically changing a child's behaviour, which is achieved mostly by improving the quality of communication within the family. More importantly, PMT helps foster meaningful mutual understanding within the families, and helps create an environment that fosters healthier psychological development for children.

The treatment is conducted primarily with the parents (both parents when possible, but it can be conducted only with one parent or caregiver). PMT can be offered as its own therapeutic intervention, as one component of family therapy, or can be combined with pharmacological treatments (as in the case of children with ADHD). Significantly, the therapist works only with the parents, and therefore all the changes in a child's behaviours are mediated by the changes in the ways that parents/caregivers communicate with their children. Typically PMT is offered in 8–25-weekly sessions. It can be offered in very different settings: from school meetings to paediatricians' offices, or can even be integrated into psychiatric practice.

Techniques

- The main goal of PMT is to help parents promote prosocial behaviours and decrease deviant behaviour for their children. To accomplish that, the parents are trained to identify and conceptualize their children's problem behaviours in new ways. Hands-on practices/rehearsals are typically part of the training.
- Parents are taught to use positive reinforcement contingently, frequently, and immediately when children demonstrate 'good' behaviours.
- Mild punishment can also be used, but harsh or severe punishments are usually discouraged.

Indications

- PMT is the main component of the treatment of children with oppositional behaviour disorder. It is helpful in the treatment of ADHD.
- It has been recognized more recently to also be very helpful in the treatment of children with anxiety disorders.
- Its preventive potential has also been demonstrated, as PMT decreases the chance of children evolving with delinquent and antisocial behaviours when their parents receive the intervention.

Forensic psychiatry

Introduction

The word 'forensic' derives from the Latin *forensis* (the forum or court). The scope of forensic psychiatry can be broadly defined as those areas where psychiatry interacts with the law. Although all psychiatrists may be involved, from time to time, in forensic work, forensic psychiatrists in the UK are specifically involved in the assessment and management of mentally disordered offenders and other patients with mental disorders who are, or have been potentially or actually, violent. Provision of forensic services varies across the country and forensic psychiatrists work in a variety of settings (e.g. high-security hospitals; medium-secure units; low-secure wards and sometimes open wards; outpatients, day hospitals, and within community teams; prisons).

This chapter on forensic psychiatry concentrates on mentally disordered offenders. Mental health legislation, incapacity legislation, and other non-criminal legal matters are covered in Chapter 21; see also Table 17.1. The practice of forensic psychiatry is dependent on legislation, the criminal justice system, and local service provision. Hence, although some aspects have fairly wide applicability (e.g. the relationship between mental disorder and offending), many aspects (e.g. legal provisions for mentally disordered offenders) are specific to a particular jurisdiction. We have tried to cover the main legal jurisdictions of the British Isles—England and Wales, Scotland, Northern Ireland (NI), and the Republic of Ireland (RoI)—in some detail.

Table 17.1 Abbreviations used to refer to legislation

MHA 1983	Mental Health Act 1983
MH(NI)O 1986	Mental Health (Northern Ireland) Order 1986
MH(CT)(S)A 2003	Mental Health (Care and Treatment) (Scotland) Act 2003
CP(S)A 1995	Criminal Procedure (Scotland) Act 1995

Other legislation will be referred to in full, or abbreviations used in tables or boxes will be explained where they arise.

The criminal justice system[1,2,3]

The criminal justice process

The following outlines the chain of events that may happen following the commission of an offence:

Offence reported to police → police record offence → police investigate offence → police find suspect → police charge suspect → report to prosecutor → decision of prosecutor to prosecute → initial court appearance (remanded on bail or in custody) → trial → conviction → sentence (community, prison, fine, discharge, mental health disposal).

Most offenders will not go through all these stages (e.g. by pleading guilty an offender may go from initial court appearance directly to sentencing). At various stages there may be specific provisions for mentally disordered offenders (see 📖 p. 712 for overview and 📖 p. 714 for details).

Prosecution

- *England and Wales*—Following report by police, *Crown Prosecution Service* decides whether individual should be prosecuted; headed by *Director of Public Prosecutions*; service divided into areas and further into branches each headed by *Chief Crown Prosecutor*. Some minor offences prosecuted by police.
- *Scotland*—*Lord Advocate* responsible for prosecuting serious crimes; heads the *Crown Office* in Edinburgh; most work carried out by 'advocates-depute'. *Procurators fiscal* prosecute less serious crime locally.
- *NI*—Department of the *Director of Public Prosecutions* for NI. Director discharges his functions under the superintendence of the Attorney General.
- *RoI*—Director of Public Prosecutions responsible for prosecution.

Criminal courts

England and Wales

- *Magistrates Court* All adult defendants appear here first for decision to remand on bail or in custody; hear all summary (minor) cases and some indictable (serious) cases; maximum sentence 6mths' imprisonment; magistrates are mainly lay justices of the peace with legally qualified stipendiary magistrates in some urban areas.
- *Crown Court* Deals with more serious indictable offences—cases are committed by the Magistrates Court for trial and/or sentencing; deals with appeals from Magistrates Court; 6 regions or 'circuits'; trials heard by judge and jury (12 adults); sentencing by judge.
- *Youth Court* Juvenile offenders (10–17yrs); magistrates with special training hear cases; serious cases committed to Crown Court.
- *Court of Appeal (criminal division)* Usually 3 judges; hears appeals by defendant against conviction or sentence; hears appeals by the Crown against sentence; can increase or reduce sentence.
- *Queen's Bench Division of the High Court (Divisional Court)* Appeals on points of law and procedure.
- *UK Supreme Court* Established by the Constitutional Reform Act 2005 and assumed the judicial functions of the House of Lords in 2009.

Highest appeals court in the UK for civil matters and in England and Wales for criminal matters.

Scotland

- *District Court* Minor cases heard by lay justices of peace (maximum sentence 60 days' imprisonment) or (only in Glasgow) stipendiary magistrates (similar powers to sheriff).
- *Sheriff Court* 6 sheriffdoms, each headed by Sheriff Principal; summary (sheriff alone) or some solemn (sheriff and jury) cases heard; maximum sentence 12mths' (summary) or 5yrs' (solemn) imprisonment.
- *High Court of Justiciary (criminal trials)* Hears serious cases; judge and jury (15 adults); unlimited sentencing powers; Edinburgh, Glasgow, and on circuit in other towns and cities.
- *High Court of Justiciary (Court of Criminal Appeal)* Highest court of criminal appeal in Scotland. Cases heard by 3 or more judges; no appeal to UK Supreme Court.

NI

- Essentially as for England and Wales.
- *Diplock Courts* (judge sitting alone) for indictable scheduled (mainly terrorist) cases.

RoI

- *District Court* Legally qualified justices; summary (up to 6mths' imprisonment) and some indictable (up to 12mths' imprisonment) cases heard.
- *Circuit Court* Cases heard by judge and jury; indictable cases and appeals from District Court.
- *Central Criminal Court (High Court)* Cases heard by High Court judge and jury; serious indictable cases.
- *Special Criminal Court* Only scheduled offences (mainly terrorist cases); cases heard by 3 judges.
- *Court of Criminal Appeal* 1 justice of the Supreme Court and 2 of the High Court hear appeals from Circuit, Central Criminal, and Special Criminal Courts.
- *Supreme Court* Chief Justice and High Court justices hear appeals from the Court of Criminal Appeal.

1 Grounds A (1995) The criminal justice system. In Chiswick D and Cope R (eds), *Seminars in practical forensic psychiatry*. London: Gaskell.
2 Bailey S (1990) Lawyers, legislation, the administration of the law and legal aid. In Bluglass R and Bowden P (eds), *Principles and practice of forensic psychiatry*. Edinburgh: Churchill Livingstone..
3 Nicholson G (1990) The courts and law in Scotland. In Bluglass R and Bowden P (eds), *Principles and practice of forensic psychiatry*. Edinburgh: Churchill Livingstone.

Crime

A crime is an act that is capable of being followed by criminal proceedings. It is a man-made concept defined by the rules of the state and modified by legislation, therefore there are differences between countries and across time in the same country. Age of criminal responsibility: England and Wales, and NI—10yrs; Scotland—12yrs; RoI—7yrs.

Classification of crime

- **Crimes against the person** Offences of interpersonal violence: minor assault, homicide; sexual offences: indecent exposure, rape; robbery
- **Crimes of dishonesty** Burglary; theft and handling stolen goods; fraud and forgery
- **Criminal damage** Property damage; arson
- **Car crime**
- **Drug crime** Use, possession, supplying
- **Other**

Crime rates Table 17.2 shows the annual number of officially recorded crimes in the countries of the British Isles. From the British Crime Survey only about half of crime is reported to the police (and officially recorded), of which between 25 and 50% is cleared up by the police (conviction rates for sexual offences are significantly lower at 6–8%).

- Theft, burglary, criminal damage, and car crime are the most common.
- Violent crimes are uncommon; sex offences and robbery are rare.

Who commits crimes? Young males aged 10–20yrs account for 50% of crime. Females ~20% of offenders. Peak age: males 14–17yrs; females 12–15yrs.

What are the 'causes' of crime? The following factors are associated with offending. They interact, and causality cannot be assumed.

- **Genetic factors** MZ more concordant than DZ twins for officially recorded and self-reported offending. In adoption studies children are more similar to biological than adoptive parents.
- **Intelligence** Low intelligence associated with offending.
- **Personality** Impulsivity and lack of empathy with victims.
- **Family** Childhood factors linked to later offending: poor parental supervision, erratic/harsh discipline, marital disharmony and parental separation, parental rejection, low parental involvement, antisocial parents, and large family size. Offenders who marry non-offending spouses reduce their rate of offending.
- **Peers** Most delinquent acts are committed with others. Offending with others versus alone decreases with age. Close relationship between delinquent activities of friends. Offenders are unpopular in non-offending groups, but popular in offending groups.
- **Schools** No clear evidence that school factors influence offending. The following are not related to delinquency rates: age and state of buildings, number of children, amount of space, pupil/teacher ratio, academic emphasis, teacher turnover, number of outings. High punishment and low praise associated with delinquency—but is this cause or effect? Alternative placements and approaches to disruptive

and delinquent pupils may reduce delinquency compared with mainstream education.

- **Socio-economic deprivation** Poverty and poor housing associated with later offending. Employment protective.
- **Ethnicity** Higher rates of offending in Afro-Caribbean than in white males. Lower rates in Asian males. Is association due to socio-economic deprivation, discrimination, different rates of arrest?
- **Alcohol and substance misuse** Linked with antisocial behaviour, impulsivity, poor behaviour control, and directly to criminal acts (e.g. acquisitive crime to fund habit). Major indicator of risk in forensic populations.

Table 17.2 Crime statistics for the British Isles

The following table is based on offences officially recorded by the police for 2001 (Scotland and RoI) and 2001–2 (England and Wales and NI). Different jurisdictions use different categories and definitions so compari-sons between jurisdictions should be made very cautiously. Numbers of crimes with percentage of total for that jurisdiction in parentheses.

	England and Wales	Scotland	NI	RoI
Violence against the person	650154 (11.7)	19523 (4.6)	26104 (18.8)	3876 (4.5)
Sexual offences	49612 (0.9)	5987 (1.4)	1431 (1.0)	1939 (2.2)
Robbery	121375 (2.2)	4228 (1.0)	2222 (1.6)	2880 (3.3)
Theft	2267055 (41.0)	169454 (40.0)	41720 (30.0)	45652 (52.7)
Burglary	878535 (15.9)	44868 (10.7)	17143 (12.4)	24015 (27.7)
Fraud and forgery	317399 (5.7)	17410 (4.1)	8619 (6.2)	3492 (4.0)
Criminal damage	1064470 (19.3)	94924 (22.5)	39953 (28.8)	1407 (1.6)*
Drug offences	121332 (2.2)	36175 (8.6)	1108 (0.8)	2380 (2.7)
Total	5527082 (100.0)	421093 (100.0)	138786 (100.0)	86663 (100.0)

*Only arson for RoI

Homicide

Definition Homicide is the killing of a person by another.

Types of homicide

Legal classification:
- **'Lawful':** *Justifiable* (e.g. on behalf of State); *excusable* (e.g. accident).
- **'Unlawful':** *Murder*—mandatory life sentence; *manslaughter/culpable homicide*—discretion in sentencing (imprisonment, community, mental health disposal, discharge); *infanticide*—(not in Scotland) sentencing as for manslaughter; *death by dangerous driving*.

The traditional 'psychiatric' classification:
- **'Normal' homicides**—no psychiatric disorder
- **'Abnormal' homicides**—psychiatric disorder

However, this is determined by whether the individual was found insane, convicted of infanticide, or found to be of diminished responsibility—therefore it is really a legal classification (Box 17.1).

Homicide rates 882 recorded homicides in England and Wales in 2001–2,106 in Scotland (2001), 55 in NI (2001–2), 74 in RoI (2001). Rates per million population/yr for 1997–9: England and Wales 15, Scotland 20, NI 31, RoI 13.5, European Union average 17.0, USA 62.6, South Africa 564.9.

Victims of homicide Usually male (70%); 60–80% known to offender; 30–50% related or partner; 15% children (highest risk under 1-yr-old) usually killed by parent (75%); less than 5% parent (matricide > patricide); 40–50% of females killed by partner or ex-partner; males more commonly killed by acquaintances (25% England and Wales, 60% Scotland) and strangers (37% England and Wales, 20% Scotland).

Perpetrators of homicide Predominantly male (80–90%); using sharp implement (most common 30–40%), kicking/punching, strangulation (more common with female victims), or blunt force; anger, jealousy, revenge, or threat of separation are usual motives; often involving alcohol, or sometimes drugs.

Mental disorder and homicide Minority of homicide offenders are mentally disordered. Alcohol and drug dependence most common, then personality disorder. Schizophrenia, delusional disorder, and depression may be relevant in a few cases. England and Wales: 5–10% of cases result in diminished responsibility, infanticide, or insanity; half of these result in a hospital disposal. Scotland: 4% of cases result in hospital disposal.

Psychiatric assessment in homicide cases As with other offences need to assess mental state both currently and at time of offence. In most jurisdictions murder carries a mandatory punishment (life imprisonment in the main jurisdictions of the British Isles). To achieve a hospital disposal the offender has to be found insane or of diminished responsibility (does not apply in Ireland). See 🕮 p. 722.

Homicide inquiries In England and Wales independent inquiries following homicides committed by people in contact with mental health services have been mandatory since 1994. They have been criticized for being inefficient, costly, misleading, unsystematic, and unjust. A systematic national approach has been made in the National Confidential Inquiry.[1] The main issues to be highlighted include: need for training in risk assessment and management; better means of documentation and recording, particularly *risk* information; addressing non-compliance and disengagement from services; managing comorbid alcohol and drug misuse; access to help for families at times of concern; appropriate use of mental health legislation; policies on management of personality disorder; addressing stigma; culture of blame.

Box 17.1 Legal aspects of homicide in different jurisdictions

England and Wales

Murder Offender of sound mind and discretion, and had malice aforethought (intent to cause death or grievous bodily harm). Intent assumed if reckless, knowing that death or serious harm was virtual certainty.

Manslaughter Homicide unlawful, but circumstances do not meet full criteria for murder or there are certain mitigating factors, such as:
(1) immediate severe provocation
(2) abnormality of mind (diminished responsibility under section 2 (1) Homicide Act 1957; see 📖 p. 723)
(3) suicide pact (section 4 (1) Homicide Act 1957).

Infanticide (see 📖 p. 722)

Scotland

Murder Homicide committed with wicked recklessness or intent.

Culpable homicide Equivalent of manslaughter. Provocation, diminished responsibility are recognized, but no legal category for suicide pacts.

No officially recognized crime of *infanticide*, such cases are usually prosecuted as culpable homicide.

NI

Murder, manslaughter, infanticide—as for England and Wales.

RoI

Murder defined as an intentional act to kill (narrower than England and Wales definition). The concept of diminished responsibility was introduced into Irish law under the Criminal Law (Insanity) Bill 2002.

Manslaughter, infanticide—as for England and Wales.

---

1 Appleby L (2000) Safer services: conclusions from the report of the National Confidential Inquiry. *Adv Psychiat Treat* **6**: 5–15.

Violence 1: theoretical background[1,2]

Definition Violence is an act that causes injury or harm. The term may cover a range of acts from the killing of another person to verbal abuse, and may also be used to cover acts causing damage to property including arson. In this section the focus is on acts of physical assault on others. Property damage and arson are considered on 📖 p. 688, and sexual offences on 📖 p. 682.

Types of aggression Various types have been described in terms of the determinants, biological substrate, goals, and characteristics of the aggressive act. Broadly they fall into three groups:

- **Instrumental aggression** Aggression as a means to attain a goal, usually planned and not associated with increased arousal (e.g. violence used to carry out a robbery or control the victim of a sexual assault). A related term from animal studies is *predatory aggression*—aggression used by predatory animals when hunting food (aka *interspecific aggression*). *Sadistic aggression* is a form of instrumental aggression used to achieve sexual and/or emotional pleasure through control and/or inflicting harm on a victim.
- **Expressive aggression** (aka *affective aggression*, *reactive aggression*, *hostile aggression, angry aggression, fear-induced aggression, irritable aggression, indiscriminate aggression*). Aggression with the primary goal of harming the victim in response to feelings of hostility towards the victim; emotional arousal in the perpetrator (due to fear, frustration, anger, resentment) and usually impulsive (although may be planned) (e.g. violence in response to discovery of infidelity or in response to being threatened). A related term from animal studies is *defensive aggression*—aggression used when threatened.
- **Aggression seen in social interactions** (a form of expressive aggression, aka *intraspecific aggression*) e.g. intermale aggression, territorial aggression, and maternal aggression.

Although some acts of aggression clearly fall into one of these, many combine features of both, e.g. aggression may be used to subdue the victim of a sexual assault (instrumental) and also as an angry reaction to the victim striking back (expressive).

Theories of aggression

- **Biological** Ethological studies of lower animals suggest aggression functions to ensure population control, selection of the strongest for reproduction and social organization; low levels of 5-HT activity and cholesterol associated with aggression; modest genetic contribution; limbic and frontal areas important in determining aggression; testosterone may facilitate aggression.
- **Psychodynamic** *Freud*: aggression initially seen as response to frustration, later as an instinct; hostile character traits may be caused by fixation at/regression to oral or anal stage. *Ego psychologists*: aggressive instinct needs to be sublimated or displaced. *Neo-Freudians*: emphasized sociocultural origins of aggression. *Attachment theory*: emphasizes early relationships and the impact of their disruption on adult interaction.

- **Learning theory** Rewarding/reinforcing contingencies important, leading to the development and maintenance of aggressive responses to certain stimuli or in order to attain goal (material gain, escape from aversive stimulus). *Frustration aggression hypothesis:* frustration leads to aggression depending on the perceived value of the blocked goal and the degree of frustration (depends on degree of prior reinforcement or punishment); punishment may inhibit aggression, but may itself be frustrating or provide model for aggression. *Observational learning* (modelling).
- **Cognitive** Learning theories seen as too simple and cognition important; cognitive distortions about victims may facilitate aggressive behaviour; appraisal of arousal and context important in determining occurrence of aggression; causal attributions and moral evaluations of self and others may facilitate or reduce aggression.
- **Social** *Social structure theory:* poor socio-economic standing stifles pursuit of financial and social success, so seek success through deviant methods. *Social process theory:* socialization process through contact with institutions and social organizations steers individual towards violence. *Neutralization theory:* neutralization of personal beliefs and values as person drifts between conventional and offending behaviour. *Social control theory:* direct (e.g. through punishment) and indirect (e.g. through social affiliation) control prevents violence. *Labelling theory:* an original deviant act (primary deviance) results in stigmatization and labelling, leading to hostility, alienation, and resentment in the individual and further deviant behaviour (secondary deviance).

1 Mackintosh J (1990) Theories of violence. In Bluglass R and Bowden P (eds), *Principles and practice of forensic psychiatry*, Edinburgh: Churchill Livingstone.
2 Gunn J (1993) Non-psychotic violence. In Gunn J and Taylor P (eds), *Forensic psychiatry: clinical, legal and ethical issues*. Oxford: Butterworth-Heinemann.

Violence 2[1,2]

Causes of a violent act

Violent acts involve a perpetrator, a victim, and contextual factors. There will usually be an interplay between factors related to these three. Many of the background factors associated with offending generally (see 📖 p. 674) are associated with violence, although violent offenders are usually young adults rather than teenagers. The specific factors of importance in determining the occurrence of aggressive acts are the same as those needing to be considered in assessing the risk of violence (see 📖 p. 692).

Types of violent offences

The range of recognized violent offences (excluding sexual offences) is shown in Box 17.2. The seriousness of an assault may be determined by chance factors such as the availability of medical care and the physical health of the victim. Other ways of categorizing violent offences are in terms of the victims and circumstances: domestic/spousal abuse, child abuse (see 📖 p. 663), elder abuse.

Rates of violence

Per 10 000 of the adult population there were 676 assaults and 84 robberies in England and Wales compared with 458 assaults and 54 robberies in Scotland in 1999 as estimated from the British Crime Survey 2000 (i.e. number of actual incidents, rather than number of officially recorded offences). The total numbers of officially recorded violent offences are shown in Box 17.2.

Psychiatric assessment and management

The clinical assessment of a person who has been violent or who appears to be at risk of violence involves a thorough psychiatric history and mental state examination and an assessment of risk (see 📖 p. 692). If the person is facing criminal charges then a report may have to be prepared considering the issues set out on 📖 p. 706. Management of risk is described on 📖 p. 693. The acute management of violent patients is described on 📖 p. 988.

Domestic violence

1 in 4 women experience domestic violence during their lifetimes. Women are victims of 70% of domestic violence. In over 10% of cases serious injuries occur (e.g. broken bones, loss of consciousness). May be a contributory factor in 25% of suicide attempts and in 75% of cases children witness the violence. Accounts for 25% of violent crime in Britain (which will be an underestimate).

Elder abuse

Prevalence (from US figures): 3–5% of the elderly subject to violence, neglect, or emotional abuse, particularly females. Perpetrators are usually son or daughter, perhaps under stress, with alcohol or drug problems and unable to cope with looking after victim.

Box 17.2 Recorded violent offences

The following figures are the violent offences recorded by the police in each of the jurisdictions in the British Isles in 2001 (Scotland and RoI) or 2001–2 (England and Wales and NI). Note that different jurisdictions have different ways of defining and classifying violent offences.

England and Wales (2001–2)

Homicide	886
Attempted murder	858
Threat or conspiracy to murder	13648
Child destruction	0
Causing death with vehicle	407
Wounding	16537
Endangering railway passenger or life at sea	18
Other wounding	212059
Possession of weapons	28740
Harassment	113677
Cruelty to or neglect of children	3048
Abandoning child under 2	49
Child abduction	583
Procuring illegal abortion	6
Concealment of birth	3
Assault on a constable	30010
Common assault	231625
Total violence against the person	650154
Robbery*	121375

Scotland (2001)

Serious assault (includes homicide)	7296
Handling an offensive weapon	8671
Robbery	4228
Other	3556
Total non-sexual crimes of violence	23751
Petty assault*	54870

NI (2001–2)

Homicide	55
Attempted murder	164
Threat or conspiracy to murder	740
Causing death with vehicle	23
Wounding/assault occasioning actual bodily harm	6507
Aggravated assault	941
Common assault	13971
Police assault	1563
Total violence against the person	26104
Robbery*	222

RoI (2001) Homicide

Murder	52
Murder—attempt	2
Abortion	0
Manslaughter	6
Infanticide	0
Murder—threats	14
Procuring or assisting abortion	0
Total homicide	
Assaults:	74
Assault causing harm	3114
Coercion	4
Harassment	276
Poisoning	4
Assault/obstruction/ resisting police officer	236
Endangerment	41
False imprisonment	46
Abduction	81
Total assaults	3082
Robbery*	2880

* Indicates offences not officially categorized as violent offences in the relevant jurisdiction.

1 Cordess C (1995) Crime and mental disorder I. Criminal behaviour. In Chiswick D and Cope R (eds). *Seminars in practical forensic psychiatry*. London: Gaskell.
2 Gunn J (1993) Non-psychotic violence. In Gunn J and Taylor P (eds), *Forensic psychiatry: clinical, legal and ethical issues*. Oxford: Butterworth-Heinemann.

Sexual offences 1

Offences range from prostitution and indecent exposure to rape. Other types of offences (e.g. homicide, assault, robbery, theft, and burglary) may have a sexual component. Sex offending, sexual deviation (📖 p. 480), and inappropriate sexual behaviour (a range of sexual behaviours which cause offence and/or harm to others) are overlapping but distinct concepts. A man who commits a sexual offence against a child may or may not be a paedophile and a man who exposes himself may or may not be an exhibitionist. A 17-yr-old male who has sexual intercourse with his 15-yr-old girlfriend is committing a sexual offence, but will probably not have a sexual deviation. Here the focus will be on indecent exposure and contact sexual offences against adults and children.

Types of sexual offences and offenders The range of officially recognized sexual offences is set out in Box 17.3. Legal classifications change and a legal label says little about the nature of the actual incident. Various typologies (based on the nature of the act, the motivation of the offender, the characteristics of the offender, and the characteristics of the victim) lack validity, reliability, and practical utility.

Indecent exposure The most common sexual offence. Classification:
- *Exhibitionists* Inhibited men, often previous unremarkable character, with sudden powerful urge to display genitals, who make little attempt to avoid capture and who make no further erotic or obscene gestures/attempt any contact with victim.
- *Disinhibited*—by alcohol, stress, or psychiatric disorder.
- *Aggressive, impulsive, and antisocial*—a small minority.

Most do not reoffend. A small number may progress to more serious sexual offences. Rates of further indecent exposure: first-time offenders—20%, previous sexual offences—60%, previous sexual and non-sexual offences—70%.

Rape and other sexual assaults on adults Usually perpetrated by men against women and, less often, other men. Female perpetrators uncommon. Typologies lack validity, but may be classified as: *aggressive, sexual,* or *sadistic*. Most rapists are young males from poor social and educational backgrounds who have a history of other offending. A small number of these offenders are sexual sadists. Sadistic fantasy is common in men, but sadistic sexual offending is rare—features which may be associated with acting out sadistic fantasies are social isolation, coexisting other paraphilias, lack of empathy, disinhibition (by alcohol, drugs, stress, or psychiatric disorder). 15% of rapists reoffend sexually and 20% go on to commit non-sexual violent offences.

Rape and other sexual assaults on children Female children are victimized more than males.

- *Intra-familial abuse (incest)* is usually perpetrated by fathers or step-fathers against daughters. Family pathology (dysfunctional families with generational blurring) often mixed with pathology in the perpetrator (alcohol misuse, personality disorder, paedophilia—but only in a minority).
- *Extra-familial* abuse is less common. Adolescent offending is associated with poor social skills, physical unattractiveness, and isolation from peers. Adult offenders are more likely to have paedophilic sexual fantasies than adolescent offenders and intra-familial offenders. In some cases offending against children reflects general antisocial tendencies or the expression of repressed paedophilic impulses in susceptible men disinhibited (by alcohol, stress, or psychiatric disorder). Many offenders become skilled at targeting and grooming victims to gain their trust. A very rare minority have sadistic paedophilic fantasies. Cases of sexually motivated killing of children are extremely rare.

Rates of sexual offences Rates of recorded sexual offences are shown on 📖 p. 685. Many sexual offences are not reported.

Rates of sexual reoffending Extra-familial child offenders > offenders against adults > incest offenders.

Internet offences A growing concern over the last two decades has been the role of the Internet in providing a method of distribution of obscene and/or unlawful sexual material (particularly images of children). The fast rate of technological developments and the global reach of the Internet, crossing legal jurisdictions, has left the police and legal authorities in many countries struggling to keep pace and the law in this area is still developing. The recently adopted Section 63 of the Criminal Justice and Immigration Act 2008 (in England and Wales) and Section 42 of the Criminal Justice and Licensing (Scotland) Act 2010 (in Scotland) criminalize possession of what it refers to as 'extreme pornographic images'.

Sexual offences 2

Characteristics of sex offenders A heterogeneous group—possible relevant factors: deviant sexual fantasy, sexual dysfunction, abnormal personality (impulsivity, lack of empathy, inhibition, social anxiety), relationship difficulties (poor social skills, social isolation), alcohol or drug misuse, denial and minimization of offending, cognitive distortions (regarding sex, women, or children), problems with assertiveness and control of anger, previous histories of victimization.

Mental disorder and sex offending The most common mental disorders found in sex offenders: personality disorder, paraphilias, alcohol and substance misuse; severe mental illness is rare. Sex offenders with psychosis share many of the features of other sex offenders and offending is rarely due to specific psychotic symptoms. Disinhibition due to mania or organic disorders may lead to, usually minor, sexual offences. Most sex offences committed by people with LD are associated with lack of sexual knowledge, poor social skills, and inability to express a normal sex drive appropriately. A few more serious and persistent LD offenders may share characteristics of other sex offenders.

Assessment of sex offenders Full psychiatric history and MSE—emphasis on the nature of the incident(s), psychosexual history, and previous offences, utilizing sources of information other than the accused. It may be difficult to build up a full picture of a person's sexual fantasies and activities. Some centres (mainly in North America) use penile plethysmography (measuring the extent of penile erection in response to various stimuli).

Risk assessment (📖 p. 692) Consider the following factors: sexual deviation; personality disorder; mental illness; substance misuse; relationship problems; employment problems; previous offences (sexual and non-sexual); previous supervision failure; frequency, types, and escalation in sexual offending; physical harm to victims and use of weapons; denial/minimization and cognitive distortions; future plans and attitudes towards intervention.

Management of sex offenders Some mentally disordered offenders require treatment in hospital (esp. those with mental illness or marked LD). In psychotic sex offenders it is usually important to address factors common to other sex offenders. Those with personality disorders, paraphilias, and substance misuse are normally dealt with by the criminal justice system. Within the criminal justice system, both in prison and the community, group CBT programmes have been developed. A small number of sex offenders receive psychodynamic treatment at specialist clinics. Medications such as anti-androgens, anti-gonadotrophins, and SSRIs may be used in a few offenders.

Specific legal provisions The Sex Offenders Act 1997 requires sex offenders to register their address with the police. The Crime and Disorder Act 1998 enables courts to impose Sex Offender Orders on convicted sex offenders who are not registered under the Sex Offender Act and whose behaviour gives cause for concern. The order requires the offender to register with the police and to desist from behaviour that has been identified as indicative of future risk. The same Act allows courts to impose extended sentences on sex offenders. The extended sentence comprises a custodial element with an 'extended' period of supervision post-release for up to 10yrs. Amendments to the Sexual Offences Act 2003 allow courts to apply a 'Sexual Offences Prevention Order' (SOPO) even for offences not primarily sexual in nature. Offenders issued with a SOPO are added to the sex offenders' register and are barred from specified behaviours. The 'Protection of Children and Prevention of Sexual Offences (Scotland) Act 2005 allows for the application of the similar 'Risk of Sexual Harm Order' (ROSHO) to offenders in Scotland.

Box 17.3 Recorded sexual offences

Sexual offences recorded by the police in each of the jurisdictions in the British Isles in 2001 or 2001–2. Note that different jurisdictions have different ways of defining and classifying sexual offences.

England and Wales (2001–2)

Buggery	354
Indecent assault on a male	3613
Gross indecency between males	163
Rape of a female	9008
Rape of a male	735
Indecent assault of a female	21765
Unlawful sexual intercourse with a girl	170
Unlawful sexual intercourse with a girl <16	1336
Incest	93
Procuration	130
Abduction	263
Bigamy	74
Soliciting or importuning by a man	1648
Abuse of position of trust	408
Gross indecency with a child	1665
Total offences	**41425**
Indecent exposure (recorded with other offences	8187

Scotland (2001)

Rape	589
Assault with intent to rape	164
Indecent assault	1154
Lewd and libidinous practices	1557
Indecent exposure	808
Incest	34
Homosexual acts	133
Sexual intercourse with a girl <16	179
Prostitution offences	1328
Other crimes of indecency	41
Total crimes	**5987**

NI (2001–2)

Rape	252
Attempted rape	40
Buggery	27
Indecent assault of female	286
Indecent assault of female child	308
Indecent assault of male	34
Indecent assault of male child	55
Homosexual acts	5
Indecent exposure	333
Indecent conduct towards a child	23
Other sexual offences	32
Total offences	**1431**

RoI (2001)

Sexual assault	1048
Sexual offence involving mentally impaired person	10
Gross indecency	33
Buggery	36
Unlawful carnal knowledge	78
Rape (section 4)	66
Bestiality	2
Aggravated sexual assault	18
Indecency	150
Rape of a female	335
Incest	16
Brothel keeping	5
Prostitution	142
Total offences	**1939**

Stalking

Essence A constellation of behaviours in which an individual inflicts on another repeated, unwanted intrusions and communications. Common stalking behaviours include: following, loitering nearby, maintaining surveillance, and making approaches and communications in any modality, most commonly phone calls. Stalking behaviour can arise as a result of an attempt to establish, re-establish, or impose a relationship on another who has either made clear their disinterest, or has not been consulted on the matter, or to retaliate for some perceived injustice.

History Stalking is not a new phenomenon, but the naming of this course of conduct, coupled with legal, public, and scientific interest in it is. The first state to specifically criminalize stalking was California in 1990, following a series of high-profile stalking cases. It was first made a specific criminal offence in the UK by the Protection from Harassment Act 1997. This made it an offence to pursue a course of conduct which amounts to harassment of another on two or more occasions.

Epidemiology The British Crime Survey 1998 found that 11.8% of UK adults had been subject to persistent and unwanted attention since age 16. Lifetime rates are significantly higher for females (16.1%) than males (6.8%). Perpetrators are much more likely to be male (81%). Females are usually stalked by a male (90%). Men are almost as likely to be stalked by a female (43%) as a male (57%). Most victims are stalked by someone already known to them: current or former intimate 29%; acquaintance 29%; work contact 9%; estranged friend or relative 6%. Only about of 34% victims are stalked by a stranger.

Stalker typology[1]

Rejected stalkers Pursue victims in order to reverse, correct, or avenge rejection (e.g. divorce, separation, termination of relationship).

Resentful stalkers Pursue a vendetta because of a sense of grievance against the victims. Motivated by the desire to frighten and distress.

Incompetent suitors Despite poor social or courting skills, have a fixation on, or in some cases a sense of entitlement to, an intimate relationship with those who have attracted their amorous interest.

Predatory stalkers Initially spy on victim as a precursor to a sexual assault. However, stalking can be sustained in this group due to stalker taking pleasure in voyeurism and fantasy about the coming attack.

Erotomaniac stalkers Have the delusional belief that another person, usually of higher social status, is secretly in love with them. The sufferer may also believe that the subject of their delusion secretly communicates their love through seemingly innocuous acts, or if they are a public figure through clues in the media. The object of the delusion usually has little or no contact with the sufferer, who often believes the object initiated the fictional relationship. Erotomaniac delusions are typically found as the primary symptom of a delusional disorder, and in schizophrenia or mania.

Effects of stalking on victims Stalking can have devastating conse-quences for both the victim and stalker. Victims of stalking can develop depression, PTSD-like symptoms, anxiety disorders/phobias, and substance misuse problems.

Stalking of health professionals Health professionals (especially mental health professionals) are at increased risk of being stalked compared to the general public. One study found that 53% of staff in an inpatient psychiatric unit had experienced some form of stalking harassment during their careers. Another which looked at the frequency of various diagnoses in patients who were stalking mental health staff found that 45% had a psychotic disorder, 11% had a mood disorder, and 37% had a personality disorder.

Stalking risk assessment Usually performed by a forensic psychiatrist or psychologist, a risk assessment tool such as the Stalking Assessment and Management (SAM) tool, can be used to stratify stalkers into groups depending on the level of risk of harm they pose. Various factors have been found to increase the risk of harm arising, e.g. substance misuse problems, previous criminality, persistence. The aim is to formulate a management plan to target risk factors to reduce risk.

What to do if you are being stalked

- Inform others (family, friends, neighbours, work, police) what is happening, as stalkers will use embarrassed secrecy on the part of the victim to further their stalking aims.
- Protect personal information (e.g. social networking sites, household rubbish).
- Use an answering machine (enables recording of stalker's calls).
- Retain all evidence of stalking.
- Contact the police early, and keep contacting them whenever further incidents occur, and provide them with any evidence of the stalking.
- Obtain a restraining order which, if breached, will result in the incarceration of the stalker.

⚠ Confronting the stalker is not advised due to risk of provoking an escalation to violence.

1 Mullen PE, Pathé M and Purcell R (2009) *Stalkers and their victims*, 2nd edn. Cambridge: Cambridge University Press.

Other offences

Arson

Arson (fire-setting in Scotland) is considered to be a serious offence due to its potential to threaten life and cause massive destruction. Only a small proportion (less than 20%) of arson offences lead to prosecution.

Classification As with sex offenders and other offenders, typologies are fraught with problems. The following groups have been described (but they are not mutually exclusive): insurance fraud, covering evidence of crime, politically motivated, gang activity, revenge/anger, cry for help, desire for power, desire to be hero, fascination with fire, sexual excitement, suicide, psychiatric disorder.

Psychiatric disorder Alcohol/substance misuse and personality disorder are the most frequent; less common are psychosis, organic disorders, and learning disability (a previously highlighted association due to studies of patients in secure hospitals). Pure 'pyromania' is rare—features are usually seen in individuals with personality disorders.

Assessment Full psychiatric assessment with detailed examination of current and previous offences.

Management Treatment of mental disorder if present; specific psychological interventions have been proposed but little evidence; important to take steps to prevent access to matches and lighters if ongoing risk in hospital setting.

Outcome Rates of further arson 2–20%, rates of any reoffending 10–30%. No specific indicators of risk.

Other damage to property

Acts of vandalism are common, especially in adolescence. There is little psychiatric literature on criminal damage excluding arson.

Crimes of dishonesty

Burglary, **theft**, and **fraud** are common offences which are rarely associated with psychiatric disorder. *Shoplifting* has attracted some clinical attention. About 5% of shoplifters suffer from significant mental disorder (personality disorder, substance misuse, depression, schizophrenia, dementia). Pure kleptomania is extremely rare (see 📖 p. 408).

Drug offences

Mental disorder rarely an issue (with the obvious exception of substance misuse/dependence and associated conditions).

Car crime

Impaired ability to drive may be caused by a number of disorders (see 📖 p. 902). Occasional rare cases of people disinhibited by mania or impaired by dementia who cause serious injury or death. However, mental disorder is rarely an issue in car crime.

Mental disorder and offending 1: overview

What is the relationship between mental disorder and offending?

Mental disorder is common and offending is common, so it would not be surprising to find an individual with both. But is the relationship more than coincidental? When looking at studies of this relationship one needs to consider:

- The nature of the sample studied (community vs. institutional; clinical vs. epidemiological; pre-treatment vs. post-treatment; offenders vs. non-offenders).
- The criteria used to define mental disorder (legal vs. clinical vs. operationalized) and the method used to determine its existence (case notes vs. interviews; clinically trained vs. lay interviewers).
- The criteria used to define offending (types of officially recorded offences included; inclusion of unreported or unprosecuted 'offences') and the method used to detect offences (official records vs. self-report vs. third-party report).

Most of the research has focused on violence. The following are the main conclusions to be drawn from current evidence.

- People with mental disorder as a broad group are no more or less likely to offend than the general population.
- Some specific mental disorders do increase the risk of a person acting violently, particularly alcohol- and drug-related disorders and personality disorders (especially those with predominant cluster B characteristics).
- Schizophrenia has a modest association with violence, but the overwhelming majority of people with schizophrenia are never violent, being more likely to be victims than perpetrators of violence.
- In people with mental disorders the factors most strongly associated with offending are the same as for non-mentally disordered offenders: male gender, young age, substance misuse, disturbed childhood, socioeconomic deprivation.
- When considering an offence perpetrated by a person with mental disorder, one should bear in mind that, as with any offence, there is interplay between the perpetrator, the victim, and the situational circumstances. Although mental disorder may play a part it is rarely the only factor that leads to an offence.

Mental disorder and offending 2: specific disorders and offending[1,2,3]

Schizophrenia

The lifetime risk of violence in people with schizophrenia is about 5 times that in the general population. People with schizophrenia account for less than 10% of all violent crime in Britain. The factors most commonly associated with violence in people with schizophrenia are those associated with violence in people without psychosis. Alcohol and drug misuse are particularly important. Specific symptoms may be important but clearly are not enough in themselves, otherwise virtually every person with schizophrenia would be violent. Threat control-override symptoms (delusions regarding being threatened or being controlled) have been found to be associated with violence, but again, most patients with these symptoms are never violent. The role of command auditory hallucinations is unclear. When people with psychosis are violent the victim is more likely to be known to them (particularly relatives) than when violence is committed by non-psychotic individuals.

Delusional disorders

Delusional disorders are probably over-represented among patients detained in secure psychiatric hospitals; however, the research on the association between delusional disorders and violence is difficult to interpret as the samples are usually selective and uncontrolled, and in many studies patients with delusional disorders are lumped in with patients with other psychoses, especially schizophrenia. Increased risk of violence has been reported to be associated with persecutory delusions, misidentification delusions, delusions of jealousy, delusions of love, and querulous delusions. Jealousy may be dangerous whether it is delusionally based or not. In some cases it is difficult to differentiate between premorbid personality disorder (perhaps with paranoid and/or narcissistic features) and delusional disorder. The relevant beliefs are probably no less risky if they are over-valued ideas than if they are delusional.

Affective disorders

Affective disorders have a far less strong relationship with offending and violence than schizophrenia. Mania commonly leads to minor offending due to grandiosity and disinhibition, but rarely leads to serious violence or sexual assaults. Depression is very rarely associated with violence or offending. Extended suicide (also known as altruistic homicide), in which a depressed parent (usually the father) kills members of their family before attempting and perhaps succeeding in killing themselves, is extremely rare and impossible to predict. In some cases it occurs in depressive psychosis associated with nihilistic delusions, but more commonly there is a history of marital breakdown in people who are depressed and suicidal but not psychotic. A historical association between shoplifting and depression has been highlighted, but is probably insignificant.

Alcohol- and drug-related disorders

Alcohol- and drug-related problems are more strongly linked to offending and violence than any other mental disorders. A number of aspects of alcohol and substance misuse may be relevant: direct effects of intoxication or withdrawal; funding the habit; the personal and social consequences of dependence; the neuropsychiatric sequel of prolonged misuse; the social context (peer group, socio-economic deprivation, childhood mistreatment), and personal characteristics (impulsivity and sensation seeking), which may lead to substance misuse, may also be associated with offending.

Personality disorders

Personality disorder is more strongly related to offending and violence than mental illness. Personality disordered offenders are heterogeneous: only a small number are psychopathic (see 📖 p. 496). Various aspects of personality disorder may be related to offending: impulsivity, lack of empathy, poor affect regulation, paranoid thinking, poor relationships with others, problems with anger and assertiveness.

Learning disability

Offending occurs more often in people with milder forms of learning disability than in those with severe learning disability. Offences are broadly similar to those in non-learning disabled offenders and are associated with family and social disadvantage. Evidence for increased rates of sex offending and fire-raising is based on highly selected patient samples in secure hospitals and is therefore questionable. In some learning disabled offenders poor social development, poor educational achievement, gullibility, and impaired ability to communicate may be important factors. Profound and severe learning disability may be associated with disturbed behaviour, including aggression, but would rarely come to the attention of the criminal justice system.

Organic disorders

Aggression is well recognized in dementia, but rarely leads to serious violence. Delirium and brain injury may lead to aggression. In head injury cases it may be difficult to differentiate the effects of the head injury from premorbid personality. Epilepsy is twice as common in offenders as in the general population, but this is probably due to shared environmental and biological disadvantages that predispose individuals to both. Violence resulting from epileptic activity is extremely rare.

1 Higgins J (1995) Crime and mental disorder II. Forensic aspects of psychiatric disorder. In Chiswick D and Cope R (eds), *Seminars in practical forensic psychiatry*. London: Gaskell.
2 Walsh E, Buchanan A and Fahy T (2002) Violence and schizophrenia: examining the evidence. *Br J Psychol* **180**: 490–5.
3 Chiswick D (1998) The relationship between crime and psychiatry. In: Johnstone EC, Freeman CPL and Zealley AK (eds), *Companion to psychiatric studies*. Edinburgh: Churchill Livingstone.

Assessing risk of violence[1,2,3]

Context Risk of violence to others is assessed by psychiatrists in a range of situations, (e.g. acute assessments in casualty, allowing patients leave, court reports, determining whether a patient should progress from a secure setting; see Box 17.4).

Types of violence risk assessment

- *Clinical:* Traditionally carried out in an unstructured manner, perhaps guided by the research literature. Clinical risk assessment criticized due to lack of reliability, validity, and transparency.
- *Actuarial* (e.g. violence risk appraisal guide [VRAG]): Statistical approaches based on multivariate analyses of factors in samples of forensic patients or prisoners to determine which predict further violence. Variables predictive of recidivism given weightings and combined to give score. From this score a probability of recidivism can be calculated. Criticized as factors identified invariably historical unchangeable attributes. Considered by some to be inflexible and unable to inform risk management.
- *Structured clinical* (e.g. historical, clinical and risk [HCR-20]): Intermediate approach. Combines historical factors of actuarial approach with dynamic factors in structured way. Clinically the consideration of each factor is more important than the actual scores, so act as useful aides-mémoires. The approach here is based on this method.

Information Sources of information determined by nature and context of assessment, using as many sources of information as possible: records (psychiatric, general practice, social work, prison, school, criminal), interviews (patient, relatives, staff), psychometric (e.g. PCL-R).

Factors to consider (based on HCR-20)

- **Historical** *Previous violence* (convicted and non-convicted, nature, motivation, victims, context); *relationships* (lack of relationships, unstable relationships); *employment* (poor employment record, disciplinary problems); *substance misuse*; *mental illness* (noting its relationship to previous aggression); *personality disorder* (dissocial, emotionally unstable, paranoid, psychopathy); *childhood problems* (behavioural disturbance, mistreatment); *previous difficulties with supervision* (absconding, lack of attendance, lack of compliance).
- **Current (internal)** *Symptoms* (delusions, hallucinations); *threats* (towards particular victim or group); *fantasies* (violence, sexual); *attitudes* (pro-criminal, minimization, denial); *impulsivity*; *insight* (into illness, into personality, into previous violence and precursors); *response to treatment* (pharmacological and psychosocial); *plans* (realistic).
- **Current (external)** *Weapons*; *access to victims*; *support* (formal and informal); *destabilizers* (alcohol, drugs, homelessness, victimization); *stress* (relationship problems, debt, life events).

Formulation Anchored by historical factors with current factors indicating immediate/short-term risk. Risk of what, to whom, when, under what circumstances? Acknowledge uncertainties and information gaps. Emphasize context(s) in which person may be at increased/decreased risk. If using actuarial methods: are they applicable to this person/risk? Are normative values from an appropriate sample?

Communication The assessment must be communicated in an appropriate and understandable way to others. It must also be documented. Use of scores, percentages, or terms such as low, medium, or high should be explained.

Risk management The factors identified in the risk assessment should indicate areas to be addressed in management. They may point to the need for specific treatments (pharmacological or psychological), supervision, support, or detention.

Box 17.4 Risk assessment instruments

A number of risk assessment instruments have been developed. Some are structured clinical methods, while others are actuarial. The following list indicates the type of risk assessed and whether the tool is actuarial or structured clinical in nature. Most of these tools require specific training and all require familiarity with the tool and the risk being assessed. There is no consensus as to which tools should be used and when, and some argue that risk assessment tools should not be used at all.

Historical, clinical and risk 20—(HCR-20)	Violence/structured clinical
Violence risk appraisal guide (VRAG)	Violence/actuarial
Psychopathy checklist—revised (PCL-R)	Violence/actuarial
Risk assessment, management, and audit systems (RAMAS)	Violence/structured clinical
Risk assessment guidance framework (RAGF)	Violence/structured clinical
Offender assessment system (OASys)	Violence/structured clinical
Reconviction prediction score (RPS)	Violence/actuarial
Risk of reconviction (ROR) score	Violence/actuarial
Offender Group Reconviction Scale (OGRS)	Violence/actuarial
Risk of sexual violence protocol (RSVP) (previously SVR-20)	Sex offending/structured clinical
Sexual offending risk appraisal guide (SORAG)	Sex offending/actuarial
Rapid risk assessment of sex offender recidivism (RRASOR)	Sex offending/actuarial
Static 99	Sex offending/actuarial
SONAR[1]	Sex offending/actuarial
Matrix 2000 (previously structured anchored clinical judgement [SACJ])	Sex offending/actuarial
Spousal assault risk assessment (SARA)	Spouse abuse/structured clinical

1 Sex Offender Needs Assessment Rating (SONAR)

1 Quinsey VL, Harris GT, Rice ME, *et al.* (1998) *Violent offenders: appraising and managing risk.* Washington, DC: American Psychological Association.
2 Webster CD, Douglas KS, Eaves D, *et al.* (1997) *HCR-20 Assessing risk for violence* (version 2). Vancouver: Simon Fraser University.
3 Royal College of Psychiatrists (1996) *Assessment and management of risk of harm to other people.* Council report CR53. London: Royal College of Psychiatrists.

Secure hospitals and units[1]

Within the health service there are psychiatric hospitals and units that offer varying degrees of security. The terms high, medium, and low security are used to categorize these services, and give some indication of the level of risk that can be managed within a particular unit. However, there are no clear definitions of these levels of security; different units at the same security level may operate in very different ways; there is blurring between the different levels; and rather than thinking of patients in terms of level of security required it is better to consider a particular patient's risk, how this should be managed, and how a particular unit may or may not be able to manage the risk. The network of secure services for a particular area varies considerably from region to region.

Security does not just rely on the physical barriers and monitoring, although these are important. Knowing patients well (from studying their backgrounds and interacting with them) and developing good relationships with them contribute to 'relational security'. Multidisciplinary risk assessment and management are also important.

High-security hospitals

There are five high-security hospitals in the British Isles:
- **English special hospitals**—Ashworth, Broadmoor, and Rampton Hospitals. Serve England and Wales and are each part of a local NHS Trust. Each has about 500 beds.
- **State hospital (Carstairs)**. Serves Scotland and NI. Managed by a special health board. About 250 beds.
- **Central mental hospital (Dundrum)**. Serves the RoI. Managed by the Eastern Health Board. About 80 beds.

Patients are admitted from prisons, courts, or less secure hospitals. Patients must be detained under mental health or criminal procedure legislation. Majority of patients have committed offences, but a substantial minority are transferred from other hospitals where they are unmanageable. Patients should pose a grave immediate danger to the public. Admissions are usually for several years.

Medium-security units

Medium-security units are not as virtually escape-proof as high-security hospitals but are more secure than locked wards. Vary in size from 30–100 beds. Each region in England and Wales has one or more medium-security unit, there is one in Scotland (with current plans to develop more), and one in NI. Patients are admitted from prisons, courts, and less secure units, and also from high-security hospitals. Admissions are not usually for more than 2yrs. Patients may move on to low-security units, open wards, or the community, being managed by general or forensic services depending on local service provision, patients' backgrounds, and clinical needs.

Some specialist units have developed for personality disordered patients, learning disabled patients, women, and adolescents. The State hospital, Carstairs, and the central mental hospital, Dundrum, admit many patients who would be admitted to medium-security units in England and

Wales due to the under-development of local secure forensic provision in Scotland, NI, and the RoI.

Low-security units

Low-security units and wards have locked doors but do not usually have a secure perimeter. Some regional forensic services have a combination of low- and medium-security wards; in areas of Scotland and NI there are low-security forensic wards without medium-security units. Intensive Psychiatric Care Units (IPCUs) are low-security short-stay wards primarily for the care of acutely disturbed general psychiatry patients. In a few areas they also take patients from courts, prisons, and more secure units, but they are not well-suited to providing longer-term assessment or treatment.

Referring a patient to secure forensic services

- A comprehensive assessment should be made and details of this should be sent with the referral.
- Particular attention should be given to the risk the person poses (📖 p. 692) and why this risk cannot adequately be managed in less secure services.
- Patients should meet the criteria for compulsory detention in hospital under relevant legislation.

1 Kennedy HG (2002) Therapeutic uses of security: mapping forensic mental health services by stratifying risk. *Adv Psychiat Treat* **8**: 433–43.

Police liaison 1

Prevalence of psychiatric disorder

2–5% of people held in custody by the police suffer from mental disorder. About 1–2% suffer from severe mental illness.

Liaison and diversion

- **Diversion** of people with mental disorders from the criminal justice system to health care can operate at any stage of the criminal justice process. The term is often used to refer to **early diversion**, the transfer of mentally disordered people from police custody or at their first court hearing.
- **Diversion schemes** operate in some areas whereby a specific service is provided to the police and/or courts to help identify and divert mentally disordered individuals. These schemes may also be known as police or court *liaison schemes*.
- **Police or court liaison** is the process or system by which mental health services provide assessment and/or diversion for people with mental disorder at an early stage of the criminal justice process.
- In some areas there are formal diversion schemes, but from area to area there are differences.

In many cases where a person is diverted, the police, prosecutor, or court will discontinue the criminal justice process. This will be particularly appropriate in most cases where individuals with mental disorder will have committed relatively minor offences. However, diversion does not necessitate this, and where appropriate, particularly where more serious offences have been committed, a prosecution may be pursued in parallel with diversion for care and treatment.

Powers allowing police to take a person to a place of safety (Box 17.5)

- The police have powers under mental health legislation to convey a person whom they believe is suffering from mental disorder to a place of safety. (Specific powers are set out in Box 17.5.)
- The purpose of these powers is to allow for a psychiatric assessment.
- The use by the police of these powers does not oblige mental health services to admit the person.

Arrest and detention in custody

Where an offence has been committed, a mentally disordered offender may be arrested and taken into police custody.

- **Issues to be addressed when assessing a person in police custody:**
  - Is there evidence of mental disorder?
  - Is treatment in hospital required? If so, how urgently?
  - What is the nature of the alleged offence and is there any evidence of a serious risk to others?
  - Is the person fit to remain in police custody?
  - Is the person fit to be interviewed by the police? Do they require an appropriate adult?
  - Would they be fit to plead if they appeared in court (see 🕮 p. 716)?

- Options following assessment if person appears to be mentally disordered:
  - Admission to hospital informally or under mental health legislation.
  - Treatment in the community.
  - Recommend admission on remand following first court appearance.
  - Recommend further assessment on remand in custody or on bail following first court appearance.
- **Fitness to remain in police custody** There are no legal criteria to determine whether a person is 'fit to remain in police custody'. A person may be unfit to remain in police custody due to physical illness or mental disorder. Where a person is mentally disordered such that there would be a serious immediate risk to their own health if they remained in the police cells, then they would be unfit to remain in police custody, and should usually be admitted to hospital.

Box 17.5 Powers allowing the police to take a mentally disordered person to a place of safety

England and Wales Section 136 MHA 1983 allows the police to apprehend a person who appears to be mentally disordered found in a public place, and convey them to a place of safety where they may be detained for up to 72hrs. The place of safety should be a mental health setting, but often a police station is used. The purpose of section 136 is to allow for the person to be assessed by mental health services. Following the assessment the person may be diverted to mental health services (informally or under compulsion), arrested and taken into police custody, or released.

Scotland Section 297 MH(CT)(S)A 2003 allows similar provisions in Scotland, but detention may only be for up to 24hrs.

NI Article 130 MH(NI)O 1986 allows similar provisions in NI, but detention may only be for up to 48hrs.

RoI Under section 12 MHA 2001, if a garda has reasonable grounds for believing that a person is suffering from a mental disorder and that, because of the disorder, there is a serious likelihood of the person causing harm to himself/herself or another person, the garda may take the person into custody. If necessary, the garda may use force to enter the premises where it is believed that the person is. The garda must then go through the normal application procedure for involuntary detention in an approved centre. If the garda's application is refused, the person must be released immediately. If the application is granted, the garda must remove the person to the approved centre.

Note: in England and Wales, Scotland, and NI these powers do not allow the police to enter premises if they want to remove a person who appears to be suffering from mental disorder. Under these circumstances powers are available under s135 MHA 1983, s293 MH(CT)(S)A 2003, and article 129 MH(NI)O 1986.

Police liaison 2[1,2,3]

Police interviews: fitness, false confessions, and appropriate adults

Mental disorder may affect a police interview by: impairing the ability of a person to communicate; leading to the person giving unreliable evidence; or making a person vulnerable to becoming distressed. In some cases mental disorder may be so severe that a person is unfit to be interviewed.

- There is no legal basis for *fitness to be interviewed*, but the following issues may be relevant:
  - Does the detainee understand the police caution after it has been fully explained to him or her?
  - Is the detainee fully orientated in time, place, and person and does he or she recognize the key persons present during the police interview?
  - Is the detainee likely to give answers which can be seriously misconstrued by the court?
- Where a person is mentally disordered and fit to be interviewed, an *appropriate adult* should be present during the police interview. Appropriate adult schemes operate differently in the different jurisdictions of the British Isles (see **Appropriate adults**).
- *False confessions* have been at the heart of some notorious miscarriages of justice. Three types are recognized:
  - Voluntary (the person voluntarily presents and confesses to a crime he has not committed).
  - Coerced compliant (persuasive interrogation leads to a person confessing to an offence he knows he has not committed).
  - Coerced internalized (amnesia or subtle manipulation by the interrogator leads to the person believing he has committed a crime which he has not).

Appropriate adults

- **England and Wales** The Police and Criminal Evidence Act (PACE) 1984 and its Codes of Practice provide a statutory basis for appropriate adults. Appropriate adults should be requested by the police where a detained person is under 16 or is deemed to be 'vulnerable' (perhaps due to mental disorder). The appropriate adult may be a relative or carer.
- **Scotland** No statutory basis for appropriate adult schemes. Schemes operate to provide appropriate adults, who should not be a relative or carer, and who should be requested by the police when they are interviewing any mentally disordered person. These schemes do not cover children.
- **NI** Similar statutory basis as England and Wales.
- **RoI** No specific provisions.

1 Gudjonnson GH (1993) *The psychology of interrogations, confessions and testimony.* Chichester: Wiley.
2 Birmingham L (2001) Diversion from custody. *Adv Psychiat Treat* **7**: 198–207.
3 Pearse J and Gudjonnsen G (1996) How appropriate are appropriate adults? *J Forens Psychiat* **7**: 570–80.

Court liaison

Broadly covers all aspects of psychiatric assessments for courts, but here is used narrowly to refer to psychiatric assessment at an early (usually the first) court appearance. The terms 'liaison' and 'diversion' in relation to police and courts are described on 📖 p. 696. Preparation of court reports and giving evidence in court are covered on 📖 p. 708.

Some areas have court liaison or diversion schemes, aimed at identifying people with mental disorders at an early stage of the court process and diverting them to appropriate mental health services where necessary. Some screen all detainees, but most rely on referrals from criminal justice staff when mental disorder is suspected. In many schemes the first assessment is by a CPN who then refers the person on if necessary. Back-up from psychiatrists is necessary for those cases where admission, particularly under compulsion, may be necessary.

Features of successful court liaison schemes
- 'Owned' by mainstream general or forensic services.
- Staffed by senior psychiatrists.
- Nurse-led and closely linked to local psychiatric services.
- Good working relationships with courts and prosecution.
- Good methods for obtaining health, social services, and criminal record information.
- Access to suitable interview facilities.
- Use of structured screening assessments.
- Direct access to hospital beds.
- Ready access to secure beds.
- Access to specialized community facilities.
- Integrated with police and prison liaison schemes.

In many areas there are no dedicated schemes. Under these circumstances it is important that it is clear to the police, courts, social services, and health services how an urgent assessment may be obtained if necessary.

Issues to be addressed when assessing a person at an early court appearance
- Is there evidence of mental disorder?
- Is assessment and/or treatment in hospital required?
- If so, how urgently?
- What is the nature of the alleged offence and is there any evidence of a serious risk to others?
- Is the person fit to plead (see 📖 p. 716)?

Options following assessment if person appears to be mentally disordered
- Admission to hospital informally or under mental health legislation.
- Treatment in the community.
- Recommend admission on remand (see 📖 p. 712).
- Recommend further assessment on remand in custody or on bail.

In many cases it will be appropriate for the criminal justice process to be discontinued. However, where serious offences are alleged it would usually be appropriate, if diversion is necessary, for the person to be remanded in hospital (see 📖 p. 712).

Prison psychiatry 1: overview

Introduction

The average daily population of prisons in the UK is 775 000 (7140 per 100 000 population). This places the UK 'mid-table' in a list of incarceration rates by country, but is high for Western Europe and historically high for the UK. Prisons in the UK are either local prisons (accommodating remand prisoners and prisoners serving sentences of less than 2yrs) or training prisons (taking prisoners serving sentences of more than 2yrs). In practice a number of prisons perform both functions. Security varies depending on the categories of prisoners held. All prisoners are categorized solely on security considerations: 'A' (the highest category requiring maximum security) to 'D' (the lowest category, suitable for open conditions). Most female prisoners are kept in separate prisons.

The prison remand

A person accused of committing an offence may be held on remand in prison whilst awaiting trial and/or sentence. Courts should not remand a person in custody unless there is a good reason not to grant bail. Mentally disordered offenders are more likely to be remanded in custody than other offenders perhaps because: they are more likely to be homeless; they are considered less likely to comply with bail; they are perceived as more dangerous because of their mental disorder; there are a number of statutory objections to bail for mentally disordered defendants even where the offence is not punishable by imprisonment; and even though remands in custody for reports are discouraged there is a lack of hospital or specialist bail facilities.

The prison sentence

A prison sentence is imposed on an offender by a judge. He will consider a number of factors, including any mitigating or aggravating circumstances. The sentence may serve one or more of the following functions: punishment, deterrence, reparation, incapacitation, rehabilitation. In certain circumstances there may be a mandatory prison sentence (e.g. a life sentence for murder). Most prisoners serving determinate sentences are released before the end of their sentence and subject to a period of supervision and/or recall. The exact nature of this depends on the nature of the offence and the length of the sentence imposed. Life-sentenced prisoners have a tariff (minimum time to serve as punishment) set by the judge. Following the end of the tariff period the parole board may authorize the release of the prisoner on 'life licence'. They are subject to recall to prison should they breach their parole conditions. Following legal challenge, the UK Home Secretary has lost the power to set the tariff for prisoners sentenced to life imprisonment, although the Attorney General has the power to petition the Court of Appeal to increase any prison terms which are seen as unduly lenient. The legality of 'whole-life' tariffs (i.e. where the prisoner is sentenced to die in jail) is currently being challenged in the European Court of Human Rights.

Mental disorder in prisoners

The prevalence of mental disorder in the prison population is high, especially in remand and female populations. Psychotic disorders: 2–10%; affective/neurotic disorders: 6–59%; alcohol-related disorder: 22–63%; drug-related disorder: 20–73%; personality disorder: 10–75%. It has been estimated that 23–55% of prisoners have psychiatric treatment needs, with 2–5% requiring transfer to psychiatric hospital.

Mental health services in prison

Traditionally the prison medical service has been separate from the mainstream health service. Health screening occurs on reception to prison but is cursory and ineffective. Officially prisons should give prisoners access to the same quality and range of health care services as the general public receives from the NHS. Psychiatrists from the health service provide sessions or may visit for a particular case. Prisons may have mental health nurses who provide assessment, monitoring, and support for prisoners and advice to other staff. Some prisons have multidisciplinary mental health teams. In England and Wales greater partnership between the NHS and the prison service is proposed in the provision of mental health services to prisoners.

Prison psychiatry 2: the role of the psychiatrist[1,2]

Psychiatrists may be asked to assess prisoners for the following reasons:
- To provide court reports (see 📖 p. 706).
- To provide assessment and treatment at the request of a prison medical officer.
- For statutory purposes (e.g. preparing reports for the parole board).

When arranging to see a prisoner, a psychiatrist should make an appointment which will fit in with the prison routine. There will usually be only 2–3hrs in the morning or afternoon when there is access to prisoners. The psychiatrist will have to wait to be escorted by prison staff.

Assessment of prisoners

Prisoners should be seen on their own unless prison staff or other sources indicate this would be unwise. It may be difficult to get relevant information about the prisoner's day-to-day functioning and presentation from prison staff, although attempts should be made to do this. Ask the prisoner for a relative's telephone number and permission to speak to them. The prison medical file may not contain all the necessary information, and in some cases other prison records should be examined. History-taking, MSE, and information gathering should proceed as with any other psychiatric assessment.

Options in the management of mentally disordered prisoners

If a psychiatrist assesses a prisoner and finds that they are mentally disordered he may:
- Treat the person in prison.
- Arrange for the person to be transferred to mental health services, either by arranging direct transfer from prison (see 📖 p. 712) or by recommending a mental health disposal through the courts if the prisoner has not been sentenced yet.

No prison, or prison medical centre, is recognized as a hospital under mental health legislation. Therefore compulsory treatment under the Mental Health Act cannot be given. All prisoners with severe mental illness should be transferred to hospital for treatment. Legal provisions for transferring prisoners to hospital are set out on 📖 p. 713. Similar provisions for remand prisoners are discussed on 📖 p. 712 and listed on 📖 p. 714 for each jurisdiction.

Treatment in prison

- Medication, monitoring, and modest psychological treatment (supportive psychotherapy perhaps utilizing some cognitive–behavioural or psychodynamic techniques) may be offered to prisoners with mental disorders who do not require treatment in hospital.
- Various treatment programmes to address offending behaviour have been developed in prisons. These are run by the prison service and do not involve mental health services. Programmes are available for areas

such as sexual offending, anger management, alcohol and substance misuse, problem-solving.
- Some prisons specialize in treating certain mentally disordered prisoners—e.g. HMP Grendon in England offers therapeutic community treatment for personality disordered prisoners who volunteer to be transferred there; there is a 17-bed psychiatric unit at HMP Maghaberry in NI.

Suicide in prison

Suicide is the most common mode of death in prisons. The rate is approximately 9 times that in the general population. The most common means is by hanging. Remand prisoners, young offenders, and those with histories of substance misuse and violent offences are at particular risk.

Many factors probably contribute to the increased rate of suicide in prisons, including:
- histories of psychiatric disorder;
- previous self-harm;
- alcohol and substance misuse;
- social isolation.

These are compounded by:
- uncertainty;
- powerlessness;
- bullying;
- isolation.

The task of identifying prisoners who are at risk is extremely difficult as those who kill themselves share the same vulnerabilities and stresses with many other prisoners who do not. A major factor that may reduce suicide rates is improvement in prison conditions. Isolation of prisoners at risk in strip cells still occurs, although it is becoming less frequent and is against official guidance.

1 Birmingham L (2003) The mental health of prisoners. *Adv Psychiat Treat* **9**: 191–201.
2 Chiswick D and Dooley E (1995) Psychiatry in prisons. In Chiswick D and Cope R (eds), *Seminars in practical forensic psychiatry*. London: Gaskell.

Legal provisions for transfer of prisoners to hospital

Sentenced prisoners

England and Wales

Section 47 MHA 1983 allows for the transfer of a mentally disordered sentenced prisoner to hospital. There must be reports from two registered medical practitioners addressing what category of mental disorder the person suffers from and whether this is of a nature or degree to warrant hospital detention. The reports are submitted to the Secretary of State who decides whether or not to grant a 'transfer direction'.

Section 49 MHA 1983 allows the Secretary of State to add a 'restriction direction' to a transfer direction, which has the same effect as a restriction order under section 41 and may last as long as the sentence the person was serving. In practice, section 47 is rarely made without section 49.

Scotland

Section 136 MH(CT)(S)A 2003 sets out similar provisions for Scotland. There must be reports from two medical practitioners (one approved) addressing whether the prisoner has a mental disorder, that the mental disorder is 'treatable', that the person would be at risk or pose a risk to others, and that the transfer is necessary. The reports are submitted to the Scottish Ministers who decide whether or not to grant a 'transfer for treatment direction'. All transferred prisoners are treated as restricted patients for the duration of the prison sentence that they are serving.

NI

Article 53 MH(NI)O 1986 sets out similar provisions for NI. Two medical practitioners (one appointed for the purposes of part II by the Mental Health Commission) must submit reports to the Secretary of State. The issues are similar to England and Wales, except the mental disorder must be mental illness or severe mental impairment. The order is called a 'transfer direction'. *Article 55* allows the addition of a 'restriction direction' as in England and Wales.

RoI

Section 15 Criminal Law (Insanity) Bill 2002 allows for transfer of a prisoner suffering from mental disorder to a designated centre for the purpose of receiving appropriate care and treatment. Transfer is authorized by the prison governor on the recommendation of one approved medical officer (if the prisoner agrees to the transfer) or of two approved medical officers (if the prisoner is unable or is unwilling to agree to the transfer).

Prisoners awaiting trial or sentence

England and Wales

Section 48 MHA 1983 is similar to section 47 but provides for transfer of unsentenced prisoners. Other differences from section 47: the person must have mental illness or severe mental impairment (cannot be used for psychopathic disorder or mental impairment) and there must be urgent need for treatment. This section also enables the transfer of civil prisoners and people detained under immigration legislation.

Scotland

Section 52 CP(S)A 1995 provisions ('assessment orders' and 'treatment orders'), as described on p. 714, may be used for prisoners awaiting trial or sentence. The necessary medical recommendations are made to the Scottish Ministers who then apply to a court for the person to be admitted to hospital, in the same way as for a hospital remand made at any court appearance.

NI

Article 54 sets out similar provisions for NI as section 48 MHA 1983 for England and Wales. Again, one of the two doctors must be approved under part II by the Commission. The prisoner may not be transferred to the State hospital, as it is in another jurisdiction and the court process has not been completed.

RoI

Provisions are as set out here (see p. 704) for sentenced prisoners.

Court reports and giving evidence 1

A psychiatrist may be required to provide reports and give evidence in criminal and civil proceedings: the following deals with reports in criminal proceedings. Reports may be requested by the prosecution, the court, or by a solicitor. The assessment should be objective and professional, and should not be influenced by which 'side' has made the request.

The clinical issues The clinical issues will involve those that psychiatrists usually assess: diagnosis, treatment needs, prognosis, etc. However, specific attention needs to be given to how these clinical issues interact with the legal issues in question. What is the relationship between any psychiatric disorder and past, present, and future offending? How might treatment or the natural course of the disorder impact on the likelihood of further offending? What impact might the current mental state have on the person's ability to participate in the court process?

The legal issues The request for psychiatric assessment should indicate the legal issues towards which the psychiatrist should direct the assessment. However, in many cases the instructions are not specific. The main issues to consider are usually:
- Fitness to plead (see 📖 p. 716).
- Responsibility (see 📖 p. 720).
- The presence of mental disorder and whether assessment and/or treatment under compulsion (or otherwise) is required (see 📖 p. 689)
- The risk the person poses (may be relevant in whether a restriction order is imposed, in determining if disposal should be to a secure unit or special hospital, or perhaps in determining the nature of the sentence imposed; see 📖 p. 692).

Before the interview
- Comprehensive background information should usually be provided by those requesting the report. Unfortunately this is often lacking. Ideally one should have the opportunity to examine: document specifying the charges, police summary, witness statements, records of interviews with the accused, records of previous offences, other reports. Sometimes tape recordings of interviews, photographic or video evidence may be available.
- Arrangements should be made to interview the person in prison (if they have been remanded in custody), as an outpatient (if they have been remanded on bail), or in hospital (if they have been admitted to hospital). The psychiatrist should be given reasonable time to complete the assessment and produce a considered report. If there is insufficient time then this should be stated in the report and any opinion given should be qualified.

The interview
- Check the person's correct name and details. Introduce yourself and state who has requested the report.
- Make it clear that the interview is not confidential and that the information in the report will be seen by others.

- Clarify that the person has understood this, and seek their consent to prepare the report.
- If the person refuses to be interviewed then this should be respected and reported to the person requesting the report.
- Ask the person's permission to contact a relative and/or their GP for further information.
- Follow the usual format for a psychiatric assessment.
- Enquiry about the circumstances of the offence and the person's understanding of the court process will need to be made in addition.
- More than one session may be necessary in some cases.
- Physical examination and investigations should be performed if indicated.

After the interview

Further information may be gathered from the following sources:
- Interviews with relatives or staff (health care, prison, or social services):
- Health (psychiatric or general practice), prison, social work, or educational records.
- In some cases specific psychometric testing by a psychologist may be necessary (e.g. where a person appears to be learning disabled).

Court reports and giving evidence 2

The report

- The various strands of the assessment should be brought together in the report.
- The report should be clear, concise, well structured, and jargon-free.
- Technical terms (e.g. schizophrenia, personality disorder, delusions, hallucinations, thought disorder) should be explained if they are used.
- If a number of sources of information have been used, indicate where the particular factual information in the report has come from, particularly when there are inconsistencies (e.g. 'according to…', 'he stated that…').
- The main body of the report should present the information gathered; the opinion should present the conclusions concerning the relevant issues and lead to the recommendations.
- The opinion and recommendations should confine themselves to psychiatric issues. Punitive sanctions, such as imprisonment, should never be recommended.

There are different formats for a court report, just as there are different ways of presenting history and mental state. A suggested structure is given on 📖 p. 710.

What will happen to the report?

- The report becomes the property of whoever requested it.
- Defence reports may or may not be produced in evidence in a particular case; prosecution reports must be revealed to the defence.
- Copies of the report should not be sent by the psychiatrist to others (such as the patient's GP, another psychiatrist, or a probation officer) without the consent of both the person examined and the person who commissioned the report.
- A psychiatric report may come to be included in various records (health, prison, probation), and may in the future be used for reference or in further legal proceedings.

Giving evidence

In most cases a psychiatrist will not be required to give oral evidence. However, under some circumstances this will be the case: a report requires clarification, the court finds it difficult to accept the opinion, there are conflicting reports, in specific circumstances where oral evidence is obligatory (e.g. where a restriction order is under consideration). If you are requested to attend court:

- Clarify with the court when you should attend.
- Prepare in advance by examining the papers and re-reading your report.
- Consult references and anticipate questions.
- Present in a smart, confident, professional manner and be punctual.
- Counsel may request a conference before the court sits.
- Have a brief interview with the accused in the court cells if he has not been seen for some time and particularly where fitness to plead may be an issue.

When called to give evidence you will be asked to take the oath, and then will be questioned by the barrister or solicitor who called you. You will then be cross-examined by the 'other side' before being re-examined. You may take notes with you, but ask the judge before referring to them. Speak clearly and slowly, and explain technical terms. Address the judge. If counsel's questioning is not allowing you to get the appropriate information across, then ask the judge if you may clarify your response.

A note on addressing the judge:
- **England and Wales** —High Court 'My Lord' or 'My Lady'; local judge 'Your Honour'; Magistrate's Court 'Sir' or 'Madam'.
- **Scotland**—High Court and Sheriff Court 'My Lord' or 'Sir' and 'My Lady' or 'Ma'am'.
- **NI**—as England and Wales.
- **RoI**—'Your Lordship', 'Judge', or 'Sir'.

Suggested format for criminal court report

- The following sets out a comprehensive list of the matters that may be set out in a report.
- Not all of the issues will be relevant in every case. For example:
  - Where there is little information available and the recommendation is for further assessment, then the report may be relatively brief, focusing on the issues of relevance to the making of any relevant order.
  - Where the person has been convicted, consideration of fitness to plead, insanity at the time of the offence, and diminished responsibility (in murder cases) is irrelevant.
  - Where a report is updating a previous report prepared in the same case relating to the same offence (or alleged offence) or is recommending the extension of an order, then the report may be relatively brief, as long as it addresses whether the person fulfils the criteria for that order and why extension is necessary.

Preliminary information

- At whose request the assessment was undertaken, circumstances of assessment (place, time, any constraints on assessment such as inadequate time to complete assessment due to prison routine).
- Sources of information used (interview with the person, interviews with others, documents examined).
- The person's capacity to take part or refuse to take part and understanding of the limits of confidentiality.
- If any important sources of information could not be used, there should be a statement as to why this was the case.

Background history Family history; personal history; medical history; psychiatric history; recent social circumstances; personality; forensic history.

Circumstances of offence or alleged offence
Progress since offence or alleged offence: particularly where there has been a considerable period of time since the (alleged) offence.

Current mental state

Opinion

- Fitness to plead.
- Presence of mental disorder currently and whether the criteria for the relevant order are met.
- Presence of mental disorder at the time of the offence:
  - The relationship between any mental disorder and the offence (this is still relevant even if the person has been convicted as it may affect the choice of disposal).
  - Whether the person was insane at the time of the offence.

- In murder cases, whether there are grounds for diminished responsibility.
- Assessment of risk:
  - The risk that the person might pose of reoffending.
  - The relationship between this risk and any mental disorder present.
  - Does the person require to be managed in a secure setting (medium-security unit, high-security hospital)?
- What assessment or treatment does the person require?
  - Does the person need further assessment? (Where? Does the person need a period of inpatient assessment and at what level of security? Why? What issues remain to be clarified?)
  - Does the person require treatment? (What treatment do they need and where?)
- State any matters that are currently uncertain and the reasons they remain uncertain.

Recommendation

- Should the court consider using any particular order (and if so, what arrangements have been made for the person to be received in hospital or elsewhere under this order)?
- Whose care will the person be under?

Consider whether an alternative order may be appropriate if circumstances change so that the order recommended here cannot be acted on, e.g.
- If the person is or is not found to be insane.
- If the person is or is not convicted.

Medical practitioner's details: name; current post; current employer; qualifications; whether fully registered with the GMC; approved under relevant mental health legislation; a statement that the report is given on soul and conscience (in Scotland); statements as to whether the medical practitioner is related to the person and has any pecuniary interest in the person's admission to hospital or placement on any community-based order (if a mental health disposal is being recommended); the medical practitioner should sign the report.

Overview of the pathways of mentally disordered offenders through the criminal justice and health systems

The following gives an overview of the criminal justice process, and how at each stage mental disorder may lead to certain courses of action being taken. Different procedures are available in the four main jurisdictions of the British Isles (see Table 17.3 for a summary of the legal provisions for each jurisdiction). The numbers appearing in superscript in the following bullet points give an indication as to which procedures are not applicable in all four jurisdictions: 1: England and Wales and Scotland only; 2: Not in RoI; 3: Scotland only.

Arrest and police custody

After being apprehended, an individual may be diverted to mental health services informally or under civil procedures. Police may also have specific powers allowing them to take mentally disordered individuals for assessment by psychiatric services.

Pre-trial

- At a pre-trial court appearance a mentally disordered individual may be remanded to hospital for assessment and/or treatment.[2] With more minor offences criminal proceedings may be taken no further and an individual may receive care from mental health services either informally or using compulsory measures under mental health legislation.
- If an individual is remanded in prison, but appears to be mentally disordered, procedures may allow for the transfer of that person to hospital.
- If an individual is remanded on bail, conditions may be attached so that they are required to be assessed and/or treated by psychiatric services.

Trial

- If a person's mental state is such that they cannot participate in the court process then they may be found unfit to plead and would subsequently only be liable to receive a mental health disposal.
- Mental disorder may affect a person's legal responsibility for their actions:
  - Automatic behaviour (automatism) may lead to complete acquittal or acquittal on the grounds of insanity.
  - A severe mental disorder may be such that a person is held not to be legally responsible for their actions and they are acquitted on the grounds of insanity (also known as not guilty by reason of insanity). Following such a finding they would only be liable to receive a mental health disposal.
  - In murder cases, mental disorder may lead to diminished responsibility, reducing the offence to manslaughter, thus avoiding the mandatory life sentence and allowing flexibility in disposal (which may be a penal or mental health disposal).

- Despite the presence of mental disorder at the time of trial and/or at the time of the offence, a mentally disordered offender may plead or be found guilty. Mental disorder may then be taken into account when sentence is passed.

Post-conviction/pre-sentence

- Procedures may allow a mentally disordered offender to be assessed in hospital after conviction but prior to sentencing.[2]
- Individuals remanded in prison awaiting sentence may be transferred to hospital if they appear mentally disordered, as at the pre-trial stage.[2]

Sentencing

Following conviction, a mentally disordered offender may receive a mental health disposal:[2]

- A compulsory order to hospital.
- A compulsory order to hospital with special restrictions in more serious cases.
- A compulsory order to hospital with a prison sentence running in parallel.[1]
- A compulsory order in the community.[3]
- Other community disposals.

They may alternatively, despite the presence of mental disorder, receive a penal disposal either in prison or the community. During a prison sentence if a person appears to be mentally disordered they may be transferred to hospital.

Table 17.3 Legal provisions for procedures relating to mentally disordered offenders

	England and Wales	Scotland	NI	RoI
Police				
Detention of mentally disordered person found in public place	s136 MHA 1983	s297 MH(CT)(S)A 2003	a130 MH(NI)O 1986	s12 MHA 2001
Detention of mentally disordered person in private premises	s135 MHA 1983	s293 MH(CT)(S)A 2003	a129 MH(NI)O 1986	s12 MHA 2001
Pre-trial				
Remand to hospital for assessment	s35 MHA 1983	s52B-J CP(S)A 1995	a42 MH(NI)O 1986	—
Remand to hospital for assessment	s36 MHA 1983	s52K-S CP(S)A 1995	a43 MH(NI)O 1986	—
Transfer of untried prisoner to hospital	s48 MHA 1983	s52B-J P(S)A 1995 or s52K-S CP(S)A 1995	a54 MH(NI)O 1986	*
Trial				
Criteria for fitness to plead	R v Prichard	HMA v Wilson Stewart v HMA	R v Prichard	R v Prichard (s3 CL(I)B 2002)
Procedure relating to a finding of unfitness to plead	s2–3 and sch 1–2 CP(IUP)A 1991	s54–57 CP(S)A 1995	a49 and 50A MH(NI)O 1986	Lunacy (Ireland) Act 1821, Juries Act 1976 (s3CL(I)B 2002)
Criteria for insanity at the time of the offence	M'Naghten Rules	HMA v Kidd	CJ(NI)A 1966	Doyle v Wicklow County Council
Procedure relating to a finding of insanity at the time of the offence	s1&3 and sch 1–2 CP(IUP)A 1991	s54 and 57 CP(S)A 1995	a50 and 50A CJ(NI)O 1996	Trial of Lunatics Act 1883 (s4CL(I)B 2002)
Criteria for diminished responsibility	s2 Homicide Act 1957	Galbraith v HMA	CJ(NI)O 1996	— (s5 CL(I)B 2002)
Post-conviction but pre-sentence				
Remand to hospital for assessment	s35 MHA 1983	s52B-J CP(S)A 1995 s200 CP(S)A 1995	a42 MH(NI)O 1986	—

	England and Wales	Scotland	NI	RoI
Remand to hospital for treatment	s36 MHA 1983	s52K-S CP(S)A 1995	a43 MH(NI)O 1986	—
Interim hospital/ compulsion order	s38 MHA 1983	s53 CP(S)A 1995	—	—
Transfer of untried prisoner to hospital	s48 MHA 1983	s52B-J CP(S)A 1995 s52K- S CP(S)A 1995	a54 MH(NI)O 1986	*
Sentence				
Compulsory treatment in hospital under MHA	s37 MHA 1983	s57A CP(S)A 1995	a44 MH(NI)O 1986	—
Restriction order	s41	s59 MHA 1983	a47 CP(S)A 1995	— MH(NI)O 1986
Hybrid order (hospital disposal with prison sentence)	s45A-B MHA 1983	s59A CP(S)A 1995	—	—
Compulsory treatment in community under MHA	—	s57A CP(S)A 1995	—	—
Guardianship	s37 MHA 1983	s58(1A) CP(S)A 1995	a44 MH(NI)O 1986	—
Intervention order for incapable adult	—	s60B CP(S)A 1995	—	—
Psychiatric probation order	sch2 (p5) Powers of Criminal Courts (Sentencing) Act 2000	s230 CP(S)A 1995	sch1(p4) CJ(NI)O 1996	—
Post-sentence				
Transfer of sentenced prisoners to hospital	s47 MHA 1983	s136 MH(CT)(S)A 2003	a53 MH(NI)O 1986	*
Restriction direction for transferred prisoner	s49 MHA 1983	**	a55 MH(NI)O 1986	—

Notes:

A, article; p, paragraph; s, section; sch, schedule; CJ(NI)A1 966, Criminal Justice (NI) Act 1966; CJ(NI)O 1996, Criminal Justice (NI) Order 1996; CL(I)B 2002, Criminal Law (Insanity) Bill 2002; CP(IUP)A 1991, Criminal Procedure (Insanity and Unfitness to Plead) Act 1991; CP(S) A 1995, Criminal Procedure (Scotland) Act 1995; MHA 1983, Mental Health Act 1983; MHA 2001, Mental Health Act 2001; MH(CT)(S)A 2003, Mental Health (Care and Treatment) (Scotland) Act 2003; MH(NI)O 1986, Mental Health (NI) Order 1986; –, no such procedure in this jurisdiction; (…), proposals in CL(I)B 2002 for RoI are in parentheses; *, procedure may involve various old pieces of legislation, **, all s136 MH(CT)(S)A 2003 transfer directions in Scotland are restricted.

Fitness to plead 1: assessment

Essence If a person's mental disorder is such that they cannot participate adequately in the court process, then it has long been held that it is unfair for the person to be tried. If this is the case the court finds the person unfit to plead and the trial does not proceed.

Legal criteria The details of these vary in different jurisdictions, but broadly cover the same issues (see Box 17.6).

Clinical assessment of fitness to plead

The assessment of fitness to plead is concerned with the current mental state and ability of an accused. This involves:

- Making a diagnosis of mental disorder.
- Determining the impact of this disorder on the abilities covered in the legal criteria.

Clinicians should be aware that the mental state of an individual may change and therefore if some time has elapsed between a clinical examination and the accused's appearance in court then a brief re-examination may be necessary.

Diagnoses that may be relevant:

Dementia and other chronic organic conditions, delirium, schizophrenia and related psychoses, severe affective disorders (mania and depression), LD.

Features of an individual's mental state due to their disorder to be taken into consideration:

- Ability to communicate (schizophrenic thought disorder, manic flight of ideas, depressive poverty of speech, dysphasia of dementia).
- Beliefs (e.g. the individual may have delusions that they have a divine mission and that the court process is irrelevant to them).
- Comprehension (may be impaired in dementia, acute confusion, or learning disability).
- Attention and concentration (may be impaired in any of the conditions listed here).
- Memory (as noted, amnesia for the alleged offence is irrelevant, but short-term memory failure due to organic impairment may be such as to make following proceedings in court impossible).

In some cases suggestions may be made as to how the communication and understanding of the accused may be facilitated. However, such suggestions must be practicable in court.

In most cases psychiatric evidence is unanimous and followed unquestioningly in court. A recommendation that an individual is unfit to plead should be reserved for cases where this is beyond doubt. In borderline cases certain measures (such as a hospital remand) may allow further assessment and treatment to clarify the issue. Where the index offence is relatively minor it may be appropriate for charges to be dropped and for civil detention to be initiated. In such cases prosecutors are usually keen to take this course.

Box 17.6 Fitness to plead—legal criteria for finding

England and Wales: R v Prichard (1836) 7 C&P 303

'Whether he can plead to the indictment…[and]…whether he is of sufficient intellect to comprehend the course of proceedings on trial, so as to make a proper defence—to know that he might challenge any of you [the jury] to whom he might object—and to comprehend the details of evidence…'

Scotland: Criminal Justice and Licensing (Scotland) Act 2010

This Act replaced the common law understanding of unfitness to stand trial with a new statutory definition under Section 170: *(1) A person is unfit for trial if it is established on the balance of probabilities that the person is incapable, by reason of a mental or physical condition, of participating effectively in a trial. (2) In determining whether a person is unfit for trial the court is to have regard to: (a) the ability of the person to: (i) understand the nature of the charge, (ii) understand the requirement to tender a plea to the charge and the effect of such a plea, (iii) understand the purpose of, and follow the course of, the trial, (iv) understand the evidence that may be given against the person, (v) instruct and otherwise communicate with the person's legal representative, and (b) any other factor which the court considers relevant.*

NI: As for England and Wales.

RoI: Statutory definition under s4(2) Criminal Law (Insanity) Bill 2002: *'An accused person shall be deemed unfit to be tried if he or she is unable by reason of mental disorder to understand the nature or course of the proceedings so as to: (a) plead to the charge, (b) instruct a legal representative, (c) make a proper defence, (d) in the case of a trial by jury, challenge a juror to whom he or she might wish to object, or (e) understand the evidence.'*

Fitness to plead 2: procedures

A person who is unfit to plead may not be subject to penal sanctions. Traditionally the person would be detained indefinitely in a secure hospital with special restrictions on discharge until they recovered to the extent that they could be tried (although the person would rarely go back for trial even if they recovered!). This unsatisfactory arrangement is still the case in the RoI. In England and Wales, Scotland, and NI, following a finding of unfitness to plead, there is a trial of facts where the court determines if the person did the act charged. If the facts are found the person may be subject to one of a range of mental health disposals depending on their mental state, their needs, and the risk they might pose.

Proceedings following a finding

England and Wales
- Proceedings set out in the Criminal Procedure (Insanity and Unfitness to Plead) Act 1991.
- Following a finding of unfitness to plead there is a *trial of facts* held to determine whether on the balance of probability it is likely that the person committed the offence.
- If this is not found to be the case the defendant is discharged; if it is found to be the case the person may be subject to one of the following disposals:
  - Hospital order (almost identical to s37 MHA 1983).
  - Hospital order with restriction order (almost identical to s37 and s41 MHA 1983).
  - Guardian order (almost identical to s37 MHA 1983).
  - Supervision and treatment order (similar to psychiatric probation order).
  - No order.
- If the person had been charged with murder then there is a mandatory hospital order with an unlimited restriction order.

Scotland
- Proceedings set out under s54–57 CP(S)A 1995, as amended by Criminal Justice and Licensing (Scotland) Act 2010.
- Following a finding of *unfitness for trial* there is an 'examination of facts'.
- Whilst awaiting this the person may be placed in prison, on bail, or in hospital under a temporary compulsion order.
- At the 'examination of facts' a determination is made as to whether on the balance of probability it is likely that the person committed the offence.
- If this is not found to be the case the defendant is discharged; if it is found to be the case the person may be subject to one of the following disposals:
  - Compulsion order (almost identical to s57A CP(S)A 1995) in hospital or the community.

- Compulsion order in hospital with a restriction order (almost identical to s57A and s59 CP(S)A 1995).
- Interim compulsion order (almost identical to s53 CP(S)A 1995)
- Guardianship order or intervention order (identical to such orders under the Adults with Incapacity (Scotland) Act 2000).
- Supervision and treatment order (similar to a psychiatric probation order).
- No order.
- In Scotland there is no longer a mandatory restriction order in murder cases. The interim compulsion order is to be used in all cases where the person appears to pose a considerable risk to others; following assessment, if the person is determined to pose a high risk according to the criteria set out under section 210E CP(S)A 1995, then the mandatory disposal is a compulsion order to hospital with a restriction order.

NI
- Articles 49 and 50A MH(NI)O 1986 set out almost identical procedures as for England and Wales.

RoI
Under the Criminal Law (Insanity) Bill 2002:
- If a person is found unfit to be tried, and the court is satisfied that there is a reasonable doubt that he committed the act alleged, it will acquit him and no further action under criminal proceedings will be taken.
- If that is not the case, then following a finding of unfitness to be tried the person must be examined by a doctor to determine if they meet the criteria for detention under the Mental Health Act 2001; this may occur via a 28-day period of assessment in a designated centre.
- If the person does meet such criteria then they are detained in a designated centre until they are fit to be tried or they no longer require detention in hospital. The designated centre may be a prison or hospital.

Fitness to stand trial

Fitness to stand trial is a separate issue from fitness to plead. It concerns whether a person is so unwell (either mentally or physically) that they are unable to appear in court or appearing in court would be detrimental to their health. In most circumstances an individual who was unfit to stand trial due to mental disorder would be unfit to plead.

Criminal responsibility 1

If a person was mentally disordered at the time of an offence this may affect their legal responsibility for their actions. The relevant legal issues are:

- Insanity at the time of the offence.
- Automatism.
- Diminished responsibility (📖 p. 722).
- Infanticide (📖 p. 722).

Insanity at the time of the offence

In some cases the court may find that a person's mental condition was such that they cannot be held responsible for their actions; they are then acquitted on the grounds of insanity (also known as insanity at the time of the offence, not guilty by reason of insanity, or guilty but insane [the present term in the RoI]). For legal criteria, see Box 17.7.

Automatism

- If an individual commits an offence when his body is not under the control of his mind (e.g. when asleep) he is not guilty of the offence.
- Legally this is called an *automatism*. (*Note:* this is different from the clinical concept of automatism occurring during a complex partial seizure.)
- In England and Wales two legal types of automatism are recognized: insane and sane (*automatism simpliciter*). The distinction is based on whether the behaviour is likely to recur:
  - **Insane automatism**—due to an *intrinsic* cause (e.g. sleepwalking, brain tumours, epilepsy) results in an acquittal on the grounds of insanity.
  - **Sane automatism**—due to an *extrinsic* cause (e.g. confusional states, concussion, reflex actions after bee stings, dissociative states, night terrors, and hypoglycaemia) results in a complete acquittal.

Note: the distinction is less important now that there is a flexible range of disposals available for those found insane.

- In Scotland (until recently) **sane automatism** was not recognized—it is now recognized only in cases where an *external factor* is shown to have caused the accused's dissociated state of mind.

What happens after a person is acquitted on the grounds of insanity?

- Disposal after an acquittal on the grounds of insanity is identical to that following a finding of unfitness to plead with the facts found in England and Wales, Scotland, and NI; and that following a finding of unfitness to plead in the RoI (see Box 17.7).

Box 17.7 Insanity at the time of the offence—legal criteria

England and Wales: M'Naghten Rules of 1843 (West and Walk 1977)

'Every man is presumed to be sane, until the contrary be proved and that to establish a defence on the grounds of insanity it must be clearly proved that at the time of committing the act the accused party was labouring under such a deficit of reason from disease of the mind to not know the nature and quality of the act; or that if he did know it, that he did not know that what he was doing was wrong.'

Also:

'If the accused labours under a partial delusion only [meaning an isolated delusional belief or system, rather than a partially held delusion or over-valued idea], and is not in other respects insane, he should be considered in the same situation as to responsibility as if the facts with which the delusion exists were real.'

Scotland: Criminal Justice and Licensing (Scotland) Act 2010

As for the issue of unfitness to stand trial this Act replaced the common law understanding of insanity at the time of the offence with a new statutory definition under Section 168: *'(1) A person is not criminally responsible for conduct constituting an offence, and is to be acquitted of the offence, if the person was at the time of the conduct unable by reason of mental disorder to appreciate the nature or wrongfulness of the conduct. (2) But a person does not lack criminal responsibility for such conduct if the mental disorder in question consists only of a personality disorder which is characterised solely or principally by abnormally aggressive or seriously irresponsible conduct.'*

NI: Criminal Justice (NI) Act 1966

A defendant who is found to have been 'an insane person' at the time of the alleged offence shall not be convicted. *'Insane person'* means *'a person who suffers from mental abnormality which prevents him—*
1. from appreciating what he is doing; or
2. from appreciating that what he is doing is either wrong or contrary to law; or
3. from controlling his own conduct.'
Mental abnormality is defined as *'an abnormality of mind which arises from a condition of arrested or retarded development of mind or any inherent causes or is induced by disease or injury'.*

RoI: s5 Criminal Law (Insanity) Bill 2002

'Where an accused person is tried for an offence and, in the case of the District Court or Special Criminal Court, the court or, in any other case, the jury finds that the accused person committed the act alleged against him or her and, having heard evidence relating to the mental condition of the accused given by a consultant psychiatrist, finds that—(a) the accused person was suffering at the time from a mental disorder, and (b) the mental disorder was such that the accused person ought not to be held responsible for the act alleged by reason of the fact that he or she—(i) did not know the nature and quality of the act, or (ii) did not know that what he or she was doing was wrong, or (iii) was unable to refrain from committing the act, the court or the jury, as the case may be, shall return a special verdict to the effect that the accused person is not guilty by reason of insanity.'

Criminal responsibility 2

Diminished responsibility

- In murder cases, a person's mental condition may be such that although they cannot be fully absolved of responsibility they are found to be of diminished responsibility (known as impaired mental responsibility in NI).
- A finding of diminished responsibility does not result in acquittal, but in conviction for the lesser offence of manslaughter (or culpable homicide in Scotland).

For legal criteria, see Box 17.8.

Infanticide

- In cases involving the killing of a child aged under 12mths by the mother she may be convicted of infanticide instead of murder if the court is satisfied that the balance of her mind was disturbed by reason of her not fully having recovered from the effect of giving birth to the child, or by reason of lactation consequent upon the birth (Infanticide Act 1938 for England and Wales, Infanticide Act (NI) 1939, Infanticide Act 1949 for RoI).
- These criteria set a lower threshold than those for diminished responsibility.
- Disposal in such cases is flexible, as with manslaughter.
- This defence is not available in Scotland where diminished responsibility would be used instead in such cases.

What happens following a finding of diminished responsibility?

- A person is convicted of manslaughter (or culpable homicide in Scotland) instead of murder.
- There is therefore no mandatory sentence of life imprisonment and the court may pass any sentence it sees fit: penal sanctions in the community or prison, or any of the mental health disposals available following conviction (see p. 712).

Box 17.8 Diminished responsibility—legal criteria

England and Wales: Section 2 Homicide Act 1957 states
'When a person is party to the killing of another, he shall not be convicted of murder if he was suffering from such abnormality of mind (whether arising from a condition of arrested or retarded development of mind or any inherent causes or induced by disease or injury) as substantially impaired his mental responsibility for his acts and omissions in doing or being a party to the killing.'

In **R v Byrne (1960) 44 Cr App R 246** *'abnormality of mind'* was interpreted widely:
'A state of mind so different from that of ordinary human beings that the reasonable man would term it abnormal. It appears to us to be wide enough to cover the mind's activities in all its aspects, not only the perception of physical acts and matters and the ability to form a rational judgement whether an act is right or wrong, but also the ability to exercise will-power to control physical acts in accordance with that rational judgement.'

Scotland: these were recently set out in **Galbraith v H MA Advocate 2001 SCCR 551**. The conclusions of the court were:
'In essence, the judge must decide whether there is evidence that, at the relevant time, the accused was suffering from an abnormality of mind which substantially impaired the ability of the accused, as compared with a normal person, to determine or control his acts.'
'Psychopathic personality disorder' and voluntary intoxication are excluded. The effect of a finding of diminished responsibility is that the accused is found guilty of culpable homicide rather than murder.

NI: **Criminal Justice Act (NI)** 1966 defines the defence of *'impaired mental responsibility'*:
'Where a party charged with murder has killed or was party to the killing of another, and it appears to the jury that he was suffering from mental abnormality which substantially impaired his mental responsibility for his acts and omissions in doing or being party to the killing, the jury shall find him not guilty of murder but shall find him guilty (whether as principal or accessory) of manslaughter.'

RoI: s6 Criminal Law (Insanity) Bill 2002
'Where a person is tried for murder and the jury or, as the case may be, the Special Criminal Court finds that the person—(a) committed the act alleged, (b) was at the time suffering from a mental disorder, and (c) the mental disorder was not such as to justify finding him or her not guilty by reason of insanity, but was such as to diminish substantially his or her responsibility for the act, the jury or court, as the case may be, shall find the person not guilty of that offence but guilty of manslaughter on the ground of diminished responsibility.'

Assessing 'mental state at the time of the offence'

Clinical examination

- Necessitates the reconstruction of the circumstances of the offence and in particular the mental state of the accused at that time.
- Along with interviewing the accused it is extremely helpful to peruse witness statements, police reports, and transcripts of police interviews (or if possible, to view videotaped interviews).
- Other important sources to help with 'retrospective' assessment:
  - Relatives, or other persons, who knew the defendant at the time.
  - Any psychiatric assessment carried out soon after the offence (if the police or court were sufficiently concerned about their mental state).
  - Any records of contact with psychiatric services at the time, and the views of relevant staff who were involved in these contacts.

Putting the legal criteria into clinical terms

For insanity at the time of the offence:

- The accused should have been suffering from a severe mental disorder which was the overwhelming factor in determining the occurrence of the offence.
- There should be a clear relationship between the offence and the symptoms of the mental disorder.
- However, it should be noted that the criteria for insanity at the time of the offence in Scotland, NI, and the RoI are broader than not knowing what one is doing or that it is wrong, and encompass an inability to control one's actions due to mental disorder (see criteria on 📖 p. 721).
- Diagnoses that may be relevant: dementia and other chronic organic disorders (including those secondary to alcohol or drug misuse); delirium (including delirium tremens); schizophrenia and related psychoses; severe affective disorders with psychotic symptoms; severe LD.

Note: in most successful cases the diagnosis is a psychotic disorder, and delusions or hallucinations are directly relevant to the behaviour constituting the offence.

For diminished responsibility:

- The accused should have evidently been suffering from an 'abnormality of mind' (i.e. a mental disorder not severe enough to deem them 'insane', but of sufficient degree to substantially impair their ability to determine or control their actions; see criteria on 📖 p.722).
- Diagnoses that may be relevant: any of the diagnoses listed here for insanity, as well as: non-psychotic affective disorders; acute stress reactions, adjustment disorders, and post-traumatic stress disorder; personality disorders (not primary dissocial personality disorder in Scotland); sexual deviation (not in Scotland); mild to moderate LD and pervasive developmental disorders (including autistic spectrum disorders).
- Other conditions that have been successful in gaining a diminished responsibility verdict are premenstrual syndrome and 'battered spouse syndrome'.

Learning disability

Introduction

Patients with a learning disability (LD) have unique needs, sufficiently different from those of the general population as to require specialist psychiatric services. The incidence of mental illness is approximately two to three times that of the general population and illness often presents in a different manner. It is a complex subspecialty, encompassing everything from molecular genetic diagnostic techniques to provision of adequate social supports, and which requires an enquiring mind and a truly holistic approach to medicine.

Psychiatrists in learning disability will be involved in the assessment and treatment of acute and chronic mental illness, challenging behaviour, and pervasive developmental disorders, and will require a more detailed knowledge of how physical illness, epilepsy, sensory impairments, and environmental factors affect the presentation of mental disorders (see Box 18.1). While challenging, it can be a very rewarding specialty, where appropriate management can dramatically improve quality of life for patients.

The LD psychiatrist will work with children, adolescents, adults, the elderly and families, and carers in a variety of clinical settings, usually in collaboration with a range of other professionals in a variety of disciplines:

- Paediatricians, during childhood, but particularly at the time of establishing the cause of developmental delay.
- Clinical geneticists and genetic counsellors, either in childhood or adulthood when looking both at the individual and the family for potential genetic causes.
- Social work departments when setting up and reviewing appropriate packages of care, particularly when a Mental Health Act or capacity/incapacity legislative framework is in place.
- Psychologists are often involved in both the assessment and subsequent management of patients with LD. They will often use mixed methods, drawing on behavioural, cognitive, and dynamic approaches. In some services music therapists and art therapists are involved in individual and group work.
- Speech and language therapists play an important role in the assessment and management of people with a learning disability and are vital members of the multidisciplinary health team.
- Occupational therapists, physiotherapists, and dieticians all have particular roles in the learning disability team, more so than in general adult psychiatry, and as such are often full-time members of the team.
- Family/carers are at the 'coal face' of care and it must always be remembered that they have often years of experience with their child/ward. It is essential to engage the family/carers in the assessment and management.

The LD psychiatrist will often act as a focal point in the collation and dissemination of information, being a 'fixed point' for the family/carers who may be somewhat 'at sea' with the dizzying array of professionals involved in the care of the child or adult with LD.

Box 18.1 The role of the LD psychiatrist

- Establishing the reason for developmental delay in infants and young children (📖 p. 736).
- Establishing the nature and extent of specific learning difficulties and the statement of special educational needs for children of school age.
- Assessing longer-term social care needs, particularly in advance of transitional stages (📖 p. 770).
- Assessing behavioural problems (📖 p. 766) or possible psychiatric problems (📖 p. 764) in children or adults.
- Ensuring physical problems, sensory impairments, or other disabilities are not overlooked and facilitating access to general medical services and other specialist assessments.

Historical perspective

The Mental Deficiency Act (1913) and The Elementary Education (Defective and Epileptic Children) Act (1914) were turning points in the management of those diagnosed as 'mentally defective' or 'feeble-minded' (by 'duly qualified' medical practitioners) in the UK, requiring local authorities to provide suitable care in special institutions or the guardianship of families, and educational placements in special schools or classes. These 'segregation' acts moved those with LD from home, asylum, or workhouse, to special institutions, with the aim of providing for their special needs and the hope of social treatments (through education and training).

The motivation of at least some of those who advocated institutional care may have been admirable. Unfortunately the definition of mental handicap (defined as 'idiots', 'imbeciles', and the 'feeble-minded') was related to subjective measures, such as 'ability to care for oneself', rather than objective measures, such as intelligence. This led to abuses, such as other 'deviant behaviours' (e.g. having an illegitimate child, habitual drunkenness) being used as grounds for committal to an institution. In addition the institutions became focuses for contemporary social concerns, by scapegoating the 'feeble-minded' as the cause of everything from social problems (e.g. poverty, alcoholism, unemployment, promiscuity, illegitimacy) to imperial, and even racial, decline.

Progress was gradually made in the use of more objective assessment of 'defectives', but most medical authorities believed causation was inherited (a 'neuropathic trait'). This fed directly into prevalent eugenic notions of preventing 'racial decline' by segregation, with physical stigmata (e.g. facial characteristics) seen as 'proof' that appearance (especially 'racial characteristics') and mental health were interrelated. Nowadays, such ideas seem simplistic (like the practice of phrenology at the time), but the notion that the Caucasian races were 'more civilized' had significant influence at the beginning of the twentieth century. Some doctors even advocated compulsory sterilization 'to protect social health, but permit liberty'. It would take decades, and two world wars, before social, political, and scientific pressure finally dismantled these firmly held ideas.

Impetus for change came from growing concerns about the effects of large institutions, forms of treatment, and rights of the mentally handicapped. In the 1960s, official enquiries found evidence of abuse, malpractice, and neglect. Alarm among social reformers about the conditions in institutions was fuelled by Erving Goffman's *Asylums*. Efforts were made to reduce stigma by replacing older labels with less pejorative terms (e.g. 'mental subnormality', 'mental retardation', 'mental handicap' for 'mental deficiency'; 'idiot', 'imbecile', 'trisomy 21' or 'Down's syndrome' for 'mongolism'; 'congenital hypothyroidism' for 'cretinism'). In 1968, ICD-8 (WHO) classified 'mental retardation' according to *severity* of intellectual impairment (by IQ assessment) and social factors. The 1970s and '80s saw major policy changes, emphasizing integration with mainstream resources and education, away from institutions and to the community. Many people with LD moved from hospitals to purpose-built hostels or 'group homes'.

Understanding of the aetiology of LD expanded from the 1950s onwards, with Lionel Penrose's *Biology of mental defect* in 1949, and the discovery of the genetic basis of Down's syndrome by Jérôme Lejeune in 1959. By the 1970s most standard textbooks recognized multiple aetiologies (genetic and environmental), separating pre-, peri-, and postnatal causes. Karyotyping, identifying metabolic abnormalities, and isolating infectious agents allowed for laboratory diagnoses, rather than reliance on clinical observation. Pharmacological treatments of epilepsy, behavioural disturbance, movement disorders, and psychiatric comorbidity; dietary treatments of metabolic disturbances; behavioural and cognitive approaches; improved assessment/management of social/occupational functioning, communication problems, and educational needs have allowed rational management of LD.

The last 20yrs have seen enormous changes in the way that people with learning disabilities are viewed and the way in which they are treated. The large institutions are largely gone, and indeed many of the small hospitals as well. The majority of patients live either in their own homes or in a small community placement with paid carers. Whilst this has undoubted benefits when compared to the large anonymous institutions, it has created an entirely new set of challenges and problems. Some patients miss the social aspects of the group setting and are frustrated that the only people they have contact with are paid carers/support workers. The design of care provision has come a long way but there will always be a need to keep on improving.

Classification

The clinical terms used to refer to individuals with learning disability have changed over the years as formerly neutral terms have acquired pejorative connotations and been replaced. In the UK at present the preferred term is 'learning disability', which is used interchangeably with the internationally agreed term 'mental retardation' (used in ICD-10, DSM-IV, and the American Association of Intellectual and Developmental Disabilities [AAIDD] classifications).

Both ICD-10 and DSM-IV also agree on the use of the terms mild, moderate, severe, and profound to describe the degree of mental retardation, with arbitrary cut-offs varying only slightly (see Table 18.1):

Table 18.1 Classification

IQ range for categories	ICD-10	DSM-IV
Mild	50–69	50–55 to 70
Moderate	35–49	35–40 to 50–55
Severe	20–34	20–25 to 35–40
Profound	Below 20	Below 20–25

Both the DSM-IV and AAIDD (formerly AAMR) criteria are multi-axial. In DSM-IV, mental retardation is classified in Axis II, whereas the specific learning difficulties and pervasive developmental disorders are classified in Axis I.

ICD-10 guidelines

ICD-10 defines 'mental retardation' as 'a condition of arrested or incomplete development of the mind, characterized by impairments of skills manifested in the developmental period, i.e. cognitive, language, motor and social abilities'.

Mild Delay in acquiring speech, but eventual ability to use everyday speech; generally able to independently self-care; main problems in academic settings (e.g. reading, writing); potentially capable of working; variable degree of emotional and social immaturity; problems more like the normal population. Minority with clear organic aetiology, variable associated problems (autism, developmental disorders, epilepsy, conduct disorders, neurological and physical disabilities).

Moderate Delay in acquiring speech, with ultimate deficits in use of language and comprehension; few acquire numeracy and literacy; occasionally capable of simple supervised work. Majority have an identifiable organic aetiology, a substantial minority have associated problems (autism, developmental disorders, epilepsy, conduct disorders, neurological and physical disabilities).

Severe Similar to moderate, but with lower levels of achievement of visuospatial, language, or social skills. Marked motor impairment and associated deficits.

Profound Comprehension and use of language very limited; basic skills limited at best; organic aetiology clear in most cases; severe neurological and physical disabilities affecting mobility common; associated problems (atypical autism, pervasive developmental disorders, epilepsy, visual and hearing impairment) more common.

DSM-IV additional features

- Onset before age 18 (ICD-10 only states, 'during the developmental period'). In both cases, this discriminates LD from acquired brain injury.
- Deficits/impairments in present adaptive functioning in at least 2 areas from:
  - Communication
  - Self-care
  - Home living
  - Social/interpersonal skills
  - Use of community resources
  - Self-direction
  - Functional academic skills
  - Work
  - Leisure
  - Health
  - Safety.

'Subcultural' LD

Although the concept of 'psychosocial' causation (due to physical and emotional neglect) is controversial, it is true to say that mild or border-line intellectual impairment is more common in families of lower socio-economic status. This is best viewed as a cultural norm, and individuals generally have no, or only minor, impairments in adaptive functioning (i.e. lack of disability or handicap—see 📖 p. 732). Generally the intellectual ability of family members is also in the borderline range, dysmorphic characteristics are less likely, and other impairments or disabilities are unusual. This is in contrast to biological causation where impairments are more significant, there is no difference in socio-economic status, parents and sibling are usually of normal intelligence, and dysmorphic features are more common.

Impairments, disabilities, and handicaps

The terms 'learning disability' and 'mental retardation' are sometimes inaccurately (and confusingly) used as diagnostic terms. In fact, they both describe a constellation of impairments with consequent disability and hence handicap, the aetiology of which may be known (e.g. Down's syndrome) or unknown (e.g. childhood disintegrative disorder). The WHO[1] has proposed a system of classification, which helps to define needs and to direct interventions, without making specific aetiological assumptions:

Impairment
- Any loss or abnormality of psychological, physiological, or anatomical structure or function:
  - A deviation from some norm in an individual's biomedical status.
  - Characterized by losses or abnormalities that may be temporary or permanent.
  - Includes anomalies, defects, or losses of a limb, organ, tissue, or other structure of the body, or defects in a functional system or mechanism of the body, including the systems of mental functioning.
  - Is not contingent upon aetiology.

Disability
- Any restriction or lack (resulting from impairment) of ability to perform an activity in the manner or within the range considered normal for a human being:
  - Concerned with compound or integrated activities expected of the person or of the body as a whole (e.g. tasks, skills, and behaviours).
  - Includes excesses or deficiencies of customarily expected activities and behaviour, which may be temporary or permanent, reversible or irreversible, and progressive or regressive.
  - The process through which a functional limitation expresses itself as a reality in everyday life.

Handicap
- A disadvantage for a given individual, resulting from impairment or disability that limits or prevents the fulfilment of a role that is normal for that individual:
  - Is relative to other people and represents discordance between the individual's performance, or status, and the expectations of their social/cultural group.
  - Places value on this departure from a structural, functional, or performance norm by the individual or his/her peers in their cultural context.
  - A social phenomenon, representing the social and environmental consequences for the individual stemming from his/her impairment or disability.

1 World Health Organization (1980) *International classification of impairments, disabilities, and handicaps*, 10th edn. Geneva: World Health Organization.

Aetiology

A specific cause for LD can be identified in about 80% of severe and 50% of mild cases. Modern classifications of aetiological factors are based on timing of the causative event: see Table 18.2): about 50–70% of cases will be attributable to a prenatal factor, 10–20% to a perinatal factor, and 5–10% to a postnatal factor.

The identification of aetiological factors is important because it allows for discussion of the risk of recurrence in future pregnancies. A known cause can allow for discussion of likely disabilities, possible cognitive impairments, and prognosis. This can be useful for planning supports/services, access to education, and optimizing environmental factors.

Genetic causes

- Autosomal chromosome disorders (e.g. Down's syndrome, ☐ p. 744)
- Sex chromosome disorders (see ☐ p. 755)
- Deletions and duplications (see ☐ p. 746)
- Autosomal dominant (☐ p. 748) and recessive (☐ p. 750) conditions
- X-linked recessive (☐ p. 754) and dominant (☐ p. 752) conditions
- Presumed polygenic conditions (e.g. neural tube defects, pervasive developmental disorders)
- Mitochondrial disorders, maternally inherited (e.g. myoclonic epilepsy with ragged red fibres [MERRF]).

CNS malformations of unknown aetiology About 60% of all CNS malformations do not have a known genetic or exogenous cause. The types of malformation seen indicate the timing of the causative event, but not its nature (see Table 18.2).

External prenatal factors (see ☐ p. 756) Infection; exposure to medication, alcohol, drugs, and toxins; maternal illness (diabetes, hypothyroidism, hypertension, malnutrition) and gestational disorders. These factors are particularly damaging in the early stages of foetal development during blastogenesis or organogenesis.

Perinatal factors Occurring around the time of delivery. Neonatal septicaemia; pneumonia; meningitis/encephalitis; other congenital infections; problems at delivery (asphyxia, intracranial haemorrhage, birth injury); other *newborn* complications (respiratory distress, hyperbilirubinaemia, hypoglycaemia).

Postnatal factors Occurring in the first years of life. CNS infections, vascular accidents, tumours; causes of hypoxic brain injury (e.g. submersion); head injury (e.g. RTAs, child abuse); exposure to toxic agents; psychosocial environment (i.e. deprivation).

Other disorders of unknown aetiology (see ☐ p. 757) e.g. cerebral palsies, epilepsy, autistic spectrum disorders, childhood disintegrative disorders.

Table 18.2 Types of malformation and the timing of the causative event

Timing (in gestation)	CNS event	Malformation
3–7wks	Dorsal induction	Anencephaly, encephalocoele, meningomyelocele, other neural tube closure defects
5–6wks	Ventral induction	Prosencephalies and other faciotelencephalic defects
2–4mths	Neuronal proliferation	Microcephaly or macrocephaly
3–5mths	Neuronal migration	Gyrus anomalies and heterotopias
6 mths (to 1st year of life)	Neuronal organization	Myelination. Disturbed connectivity (dendrite/synapse formation). Disturbed proliferation of oligodendrocytes and myelin sheets

Establishing the cause

This requires a comprehensive history from the parents, examination of antenatal and perinatal records, and physical examination of the child.

Factors in the history

- **Family history** Parents: ages; consanguinity; medical history; any previous pregnancies (including abortions, stillbirths). Wider family: any history of LD; specific cognitive impairments; congenital abnormalities; neurological or psychiatric disorders.
- **Gestational history** General maternal health and nutrition; maternal infections; exposure to medication, drug and alcohol use, toxins, radiation; chronic medical conditions; history of pre-eclampsia, abnormal intrauterine growth, or foetal movements.
- **Birth of child** Gestational age; whether multiple pregnancy (birth order); duration of labour; mode of delivery; any complications; any placental abnormalities. Examination of birth records (Apgar scores, weight, length, head circumference).
- **Neonatal history** Need for special care (respiratory distress, infections, hypoglycaemia, hyperbilirubinaemia), baby checks (physical examination, Guthrie test).
- **Childhood history** Weight gain, growth pattern, feeding pattern, sleeping pattern, early developmental milestones. History of childhood illnesses (esp. CNS infections or seizures, metabolic/endocrine disorders) and accidents. General systemic enquiry.

Physical examination

- Look for evidence of any dysmorphic features and note whether these are seen in close relatives (e.g. skin—pigmentation, dermatoglyphs; facial features; musculoskeletal abnormalities).
- Full physical examination of all systems including neurological examination for localizing signs.
- If suggested by the history/examination, ophthalmic and audiology examinations should be arranged.

Investigations

- Standard tests will include FBC, U&Es, LFTs, TFTs, glucose, infection screening (blood and urine), and serology (ToRCH—toxoplasmosis, rubella, cytomegalovirus, herpes simplex virus; HIV).
- Where dysmorphic features are evident, or physical signs indicate, arrange X-rays of skull, vertebrae, chest, abdomen, hands, feet, and long bones; cardiac/abdominal ultrasound.
- If metabolic disorder is suspected (e.g. progressive course), arrange screening tests of blood and urine.
- If genetic disorder suspected arrange for karyotyping (G-banding, high resolution banding, fluorescence *in situ* hybridization—FISH) or other more specific genetic tests (e.g. FraX DNA testing).
- Other more detailed investigations may include neurophysiological tests (EEG, evoked potentials), neuroimaging (cranial ultrasound, CT/MRI, functional imaging), (neuro)pathological examination (fibroblast culture; biopsies—muscle, skin, rectum).

The process of assessment

When a person with LD presents to services because of a particular problem (e.g. 'challenging behaviour' or mood disturbance), the task for the clinician is to determine the underlying *cause*, and to consider any predisposing, precipitating, and perpetuating factors. Causation will often be multifactorial, and because of this a structured assessment approach is best. Some aspects of assessment may be well documented (e.g. the aetiology of the LD), particularly when the patient is an adult. Any diagnostic formulation should always take note of previous assessments and highlight what further assessments may be helpful. It is always useful to consider any protective factors which can potentially be harnessed or used to aid improvement.

Assessment of the nature and severity of the LD

- *Intellectual impairment* Assessed using standardized tests (e.g. Wechsler scales). There are often important differences in subscale scores (e.g. verbal vs. performance IQ).
- *Severity of LD* Using ICD-10 or DSM-IV criteria (see 📖 p. 730).
- *Disabilities* Assessments of functioning (e.g. Vineland Adaptive Behaviour Scales, American Adaptive Behavior Scales, Hampshire Assessment for Living with Others [HALO]).
- *Handicap* Assessment of quality of life and life experiences (e.g. Life Experiences checklist).
- *Aetiology of LD* See **Establishing the cause** 📖 p. 736.

Assessment of the current problem

- *Full physical examination* This may identify undiagnosed problems, which the patient may be unable to communicate.
- *Mental state examination* See **Psychiatric comorbidity in LD** 📖 p. 764. Mental illness (which may go unrecognized and untreated) can be a causative or complicating factor in many presentations.
- *Environmental and social factors* In addition to assessment of the patient, attention should also be focused on the patient's living situation, relationships and current stressors, noting particularly any recent changes.

Current support network

Assessment will involve not only talking to the patient, but also gathering information from previous documentation (including previous diagnoses and current treatments), talking to the family and to any carers, and to any other support services or education services involved. The aim is to view the current problem in the light of past experiences, known problems, and current situational factors. A longitudinal approach is advised (i.e. does the current presentation reflect a recurrent problem, is it part of progressive functional decline, or does it represent a new, unidentified problem or unmet need?). It is useful to document the current supports received by the patient, and any important contacts for future reference.

Needs assessment

Should it be the case that the person's needs have changed, then there may be a statutory responsibility to undertake a formal 'needs assessment', taking into account the wishes of the person (if they have capacity to make the kinds of decisions required) and others involved in care provision. This includes social care, educational, and health care needs.

Increasingly, more joint work is being done between psychiatry of learning disability departments and social work departments. As a result, it is likely that you will be more involved in discussions and assessments of patients with a view to deciding on what their overall care needs are, in addition to their particular psychiatric needs. Naturally this will be in a multidisciplinary team but will include consideration of:

- Level of supervision by nursing/care staff, e.g. day and night staffing ratios, sleeping vs. waking night cover, same building or next door building.
- Layout of building.
- Location of building.
- Compatibility of different patients if being considered for group accommodation.

Considering management choices

The therapeutic environment

Provision of care and support should always be within an appropriate setting. Support may be: **general** (care provided by usual carers, schools, community teams) and/or **specific** (addressing particular needs, e.g. special education, parental support groups, physical or psychiatric problems, maladaptive behaviours). Although, in general, every effort will be made to sustain a 'normal' environment (remaining at home, integration into mainstream schools, use of local community resources), often more specialized environments are necessary (see **Admission to specialist environments**).

Overcoming communication difficulties

- Use of aids to overcome/improve sensory deficits (e.g. hearing aids, glasses).
- Strategies for improving communication—picture exchange communication system (PECS); symbol dictionaries; Makaton; sign language.
- Because of often unique communication styles it is important that family/carers who know the patient are available to assist/improve communication and that their expertise is shared amongst new staff.

Factors influencing management choices

- The nature of the problem (e.g. biological, psychological, social).
- The degree and aetiology of the LD.
- Comorbid physical conditions (which may restrict medication choices).
- Situational factors (e.g. practicalities of instituting various treatment options, supports, ability to monitor progress).

Admission to specialist environments

Sometimes disabilities or problems may be too severe or too complex to be managed with standard community resources because:

- The degree of LD or the specific cognitive impairments requires a well-structured, predictable environment that cannot be provided elsewhere.
- The degree of physical impairment requires more intensive specialist nursing or a safer environment where medical care is close at hand (e.g. severe treatment-resistant epilepsy).
- The severity of behavioural problems prohibits management at home (e.g. abnormally aggressive or disinhibited behaviour which constitutes a serious risk of harm to the patient or to others).
- The person requires treatment for a comorbid psychiatric disorder, which has failed to respond to initial treatment.

Other reasons for admission may include:

- Respite placements to allow individuals and their families some relief from the intensity of long-term care.
- Assessment of complex problems—to disentangle environmental from illness factors, or where treatment requires close monitoring.

- 'Crisis' admissions due to an acute breakdown of usual supports.

Cautionary notes
- Attributing treatment success to a particular intervention may miss the real reason for improvement, e.g. return of familiar carer, more structured environment (if admitted to specialist centre), or treatment effects on an undiagnosed primary condition (e.g. anticonvulsant used for aggressive behaviour may actually be treating underlying epilepsy).
- Many conditions may run *relapsing–remitting* courses, leading to mistaken conclusions about effectiveness of an intervention, which only become clear when symptoms return *despite* treatment.
- Improvement (or worsening) of symptoms may reflect *normal* maturational processes or, conversely, further pathological degeneration.
- Because of the wide variation in aetiology (genetic, environmental, psychological, social) and the complexity (and variable degree) of cognitive impairments, most trials of treatment are by nature empirical. Most management plans will inevitably be *individually* tailored and the current evidence base for many treatment modalities is limited.

Treatment methods

Behavioural treatments

May be used to help teach basic skills (e.g. feeding, dressing, toileting), establish normal behaviour patterns (e.g. sleep), or more complex skills (e.g. social skills, relaxation techniques, assertiveness training). Behavioural techniques may also be used to alter maladaptive patterns of behaviour (e.g. inappropriate sexual behaviour, pica, phobias).

Pharmacological treatments

Cautions

- Comorbid physical disorders (e.g. epilepsy, constipation, cerebral palsy) increase the need to closely monitor adverse effects.
- Atypical responses, such as increased (or reduced) sensitivity and 'paradoxical' reactions, are more common, hence low doses and gradual increases in medication are advisable.
- The evidence base for many drug treatments is lacking and many claims for efficacy are at best based on small, open, uncontrolled trials.

Antipsychotics

For the treatment of comorbid psychiatric disorders (e.g. schizophrenia and related psychosis) and acute behavioural disturbance. May also be effective in managing autistic spectrum disorders, self-injury, social withdrawal, ADHD, and tic disorders.

Antidepressants

Effective for the treatment of depression, OCD, and other anxiety disorders. They have also been used in the management of violence, self-injury, 'non-specific' distress, and other compulsive behaviours.

Anticonvulsants

There is some evidence for the use of anticonvulsants in the treatment of episodic dyscontrol (e.g. carbamazepine), but their effectiveness may be due to better control of underlying epilepsy.

Lithium

Aside from the treatment of bipolar affective disorder and augmentation of antidepressant therapy, lithium may have some utility in reducing aggressive outbursts.

β-Blockers

May be useful in conditions of heightened autonomic arousal (e.g. anxiety disorders), which may be at the root of aggressive behavioural disturbance.

Stimulants (e.g. methylphenidate)

For the treatment of ADHD, see p. 628.

Opiate antagonists (e.g. naltrexone)

May be effective in the treatment of repetitive self-injury.

Anti-libidinal drugs (e.g. cyproterone acetate and medroxyprogesterone, which reduce testosterone levels)
Used in the treatment of sexual offending (see 📖 p. 684).

Cognitive therapies and CBT

For borderline, mild, or moderate LD, cognitive approaches may be adapted to the level of intellectual impairment. These may be effective in the teaching of problem-solving skills, the management of anxiety disorders and depression, dealing with issues of self-esteem, anger management, and treatment of offending behaviours (e.g. sex offenders).

Psychodynamic therapies

May be helpful in addressing issues of emotional development, relationships, adjustment to life events (e.g. losses, disabilities, and bereavement). The range of approaches varies from basic supportive psychotherapy to more complex group and family therapies.

Down's syndrome[1]

Down's syndrome (trisomy of chromosome 21) is the most common genetic cause of LD (1:800–1:1000). It is characterized by intellectual impairment and associated characteristic facies and habitus. Although Down's syndrome is diagnosed at birth, LD only becomes evident at the end of the first year of life, with subsequent delayed developmental milestones. The IQ in adults is most often below 50 (range: low to high/ moderate LD). Those who survive into their 40s and 50s show pathological brain changes similar to Alzheimer's disease.

Aetiology

Risk factors for giving birth to a child with Down's syndrome are: maternal age over 40yrs; a previous child with the syndrome; and Down's syndrome in the mother (although pregnancy is rare). Incidence per 1000 living births is approx. 0.5 for a woman under 25, 0.7 under the age of 30, 5.0 under 35, 25 under 40, and 34.6 over the age of 45. Most children with Down's syndrome (70–80%) are born to mothers under the age of 35 (due to higher number of pregnancies in younger women).

Genetics

Full **trisomy 21** (non-disjunction) in ~95% of cases. **Robertsonian translocations** in ~5% (of which ~45% show fusion—usually 14 and 21, also 13/15/22 and 21 described). **Mosaicism** (a mixture of normal and trisomic cell lines) ~2–5%: IQ can be in the 70s and physical abnormalities may be less marked.

Clinical features

- **General** Short stature (mean 1.4–1.5m), overweight (~30%), muscular hypotonia.
- **Head and neck** Brachycephaly and reduced anterioposterior (AP) diameter, maxilla reduced more than mandible, underdeveloped bridge of nose, eyes close together, Brushfield's spots—grey or very light yellow spots of the iris, epicanthic fold, low-set ears, high-arched palate, protruding tongue, instability of atlanto-axial joint, narrowed hypopharynx (may lead to sleep apnoea).
- **Congenital heart defects** (~50%) e.g. atrial or ventricular septal defect, mitral valve disease, patent ductus arteriosus.
- **Congenital GI abnormalities** Oesophageal atresia, Hirschsprung disease, umbilical and inguinal hernia.
- **Hands** Short broad hands with a single palmar crease (simian crease), syndactyly (webbed fingers), clinodactyly (incurving of fingers), and altered dermatoglyphics.
- **Eye defects** Strabismus ~20%, myopia ~30%, blocked tear ducts, nystagmus, late-life cataracts, keratoconus.
- **Hearing defects** Structural anomalies may lead to recurrent otitis media, sensorineural deafness.
- **Immunological abnormalities** Raised IgG and IgM, lowered T-lymphocytes.
- **Endocrine abnormalities** Thyroid dysfunction (hypothyroidism ~20%), diabetes.

- **CNS abnormalities** Reduced brain weight ~10–20%, reduced gyri, cortical thinning, underdeveloped middle lobe of cerebellum, reduced neuronal numbers in cerebellum/locus coeruleus/basal forebrain, reduced cholinergic neurones, neuropathological changes similar to AD (in those over 40yrs), epilepsy (5–10%).
- **Abnormal sexual development** *Males:* normal course; delayed puberty; problems with spermatogenesis (unless mosaic). *Females:* normal onset of menstruation; fertile, but problems with ovulation and follicular growth; early menopause.

Psychiatric comorbidity In ~18% of children and ~30% of adults with Down's syndrome (usually depression ~10%; less commonly bipolar disorder, OCD, Tourette's, schizophrenia, increased risk of autism).

Dementia in Down's syndrome

A clear relationship exists between Down's syndrome and dementia. While dementia of the Alzheimer's type (DAT) is the most common in Down's syndrome, all types of dementia can occur. Unfortunately, the diagnosis is often difficult given the premorbid cognitive deficits and communication difficulties. The crucial element in diagnosis is establishing a history of change from an informant who has known the patient over a sufficient period as to be able to make a useful comparison.

Assessment

- Full history, focusing on previous abilities, presentation and behaviour.
- Exclusion of other physical/psychiatric explanations—e.g. sensory loss, delirium, hypothyroidism, depression.
- Use of a standardized cognitive assessment battery either to act as a baseline for decline or response to treatment.
- Full blood investigations including FBC, U&Es, ESR, LFTs, TFTs, glucose, folate and B12, serum drug levels if relevant.
- Consideration of CT/MRI brain or EEG if indicated.

Management

- Make diagnosis of dementia type.
- Treat all reversible additional factors
- Optimize communication: use of pictures, communication dictionary, etc. (see 📖 p. 740).
- Liaison with psychology colleagues for potential behavioural management.
- Consideration of anticholinesterase inhibitors, but titrating at a significantly slower rate than normal (e.g. donepezil 5mg nocte for 4–6wks before increasing the dose). Seek advice from local experts.
- Appropriate placement, considering client mix, age group, range of available activities.

---

1 James Langdon Down remarked in his original observations on 'mongolism' (1866) that he was surprised it had not been described earlier. In fact, the first description of this syndrome was made in 1838 by Esquirol (1772–1840), with similar observations reported by Séguin (1812–1880) in 1844. The typical phenotype has also been noted in paintings dating from the Middle Ages. In 1959 the chromosomal abnormality leading to Down's syndrome was found by the French human geneticist Jérôme Lejeune (1926–1994). In doing so, Lejeune became the first researcher to elucidate the genetic mechanism of an inherited disorder.

Deletions and duplication syndromes

Prader–Willi syndrome (PWS) Microdeletion; karyotype 15q11-q13; incidence 1:10 000–1:20 000; the complement of Angelman syndrome; 75% due to deletion of paternally derived chromosome 15, 25% due to maternal uniparental disomy (mUPD) (i.e. inheritance of 2 genes from the same parent), M:F = 4:3. *Essence* The striking feature of PWS is massive hyperphagia with associated compulsive food-seeking, and consequent marked obesity. At times, the hyperphagia may be such that questions of how to appropriately limit the person's access to food must be addressed, sometimes requiring consideration of measures under capacity/incapacity legislative frameworks. *Clinical features* Neonates: hypotonia, sleepiness, unresponsiveness, narrow bifrontal diameter, triangular mouth (feeding difficulties and swallowing problems), strabismus, acromicria (shortness of extremities). Childhood/adolescence: short stature, hypogenitalism (cryptorchidism, micropenis; amenorrhoea), behavioural disorders (overeating and obesity, self-injurious behaviour), mild–moderate LD, speech abnormalities, sleep disorders. Affective psychoses are associated particularly with the mUPD genotype. *Associated features* Small hands and feet, cleft palate, almond-shaped eyes, strabismus, incurved feet, clubfoot, congenital hip dislocation, abnormalities of the knee and ankle, scoliosis. *Other physical problems* Diabetes, GI problems (obstruction, duodenal ulcer, rectal prolapse, gallstones), heart disease, respiratory (asthma, cor pulmonale), renal calculi, hearing deficits, hypothermia.

Angelman ('happy puppet') syndrome Microdeletion (60–75% of cases); karyotype 15q11-q13; incidence 1:20 000–30 000; a contiguous gene syndrome (the complement of PWS) with 80% due to deletion of maternally derived chromosome 15, 2% paternal uniparental disomy (pUPD), the remainder due to direct mutations. *Clinical features* Ataxia (jerky limb movements, gait problems); epilepsy (86%); paroxysms of laughter; absence of speech; facial features (blond hair, blue eyes, microcephaly, flattened occiput, long face, prominent jaw, wide mouth, widely spaced teeth, thin upper lip, mid-facial hypoplasia); severe/profound LD; other behaviours (hand flapping, tongue thrusting, mouth movements); other problems (URTIs, ear infections, obesity).

β-Thalassaemia mental retardation Small deletion; karyotype 16pter-p13.3 (cryptic terminal deletion). *Clinical features* LD.

Cri du chat Partial monosomy; karyotype 5p- (varies from deletion of a small band at 5p15.2 to the entire arm of 5p); usually sporadic, occasionally inherited; incidence 1:20 000–50 000. *Clinical features* 'Cat-like' cry (possibly due to abnormal laryngeal development), microcephaly, rounded face, hypertelorism, micrognathia, dental malocclusion, epicanthic folds, low-set ears, hypotonia, severe/profound LD. Puberty occurs normally and some may survive to adulthood.

DiGeorge (velo-cardio-facial) syndrome Microdeletion; karyotype 22q11.2; incidence 1:5000. *Clinical features* ~50% have LD (mild: 2/3; moderate: 1/3), cardiac abnormalities (75%: Fallot tetralogy, VSD, interrupted aortic arch, pulmonary atresia, truncus arteriosus), facial features (microcephaly, cleft palate/submucous cleft, small mouth, long face, prominent tubular nose, hypoplasia of adenoids—nasal speech, bulbous nasal tip, narrow palpebral fissure, minor ear abnormalities, small optic discs/tortuous retinal vessel/cataracts), hypocalcaemia (60%—seizures, short stature, hearing problems, renal problems, inguinal/umbilical hernia), hypospadias (10% of males), long, thin hands (hypotonia and hyperextensible fingers), associated behavioural and psychiatric disorders (including schizophrenia, blunted/inappropriate affect).

Rubenstein–Taybi syndrome Microdeletion of the gene encoding human cAMP-regulated enhancer binding protein; karyotype 16p13.3; incidence 1:125 000. *Clinical features* LD and dysgenesis of the corpus callosum. Broad thumbs and great toes; persistence of foetal finger pads; facial features (short upper lip, pouting lower lip, maxillary hypoplasia, beaked nose, slanted palpebral fissure, long eyelashes, ptosis, epicanthic fold, strabismus, glaucoma, iris coloboma); cardiac problems (pulmonary stenosis and hypertension, mitral vale regurgitation, patent ductus arteriosus); propensity to keloid formation; genitourinary features (hypoplastic kidneys, cryptorchidism, shawl scrotum); GI problems (constipation, megacolon); collapsible larynx (leading to sleep apnoea); epilepsy (25%); behavioural problems (sleep problems, stereotypies, e.g. rocking, self-injurious behaviour).

Smith–Magenis syndrome Deletion in 17p11.2; incidence 1:50 000. *Clinical features* Moderate LD; facial features (brachycephaly, broad face, flattened mid-face, strabismus); myopia; short broad hands; upper limb deformity; insensitivity to pain. *Behavioural problems* 'Self-hugging' posturing, aggression, self-injury, hyperactivity, severe sleep problems, other autistic features.

Williams syndrome Small deletion; karyotype 7q11.23 (possibly gene for elastin or protein kinase—LIMKI); 1:55 000 live births; may also be related to excessive maternal vitamin D intake. *Clinical features* Hypercalcaemia (in ~50%) with supravalvular aortic stenosis and unusual facies. Neonates: may be irritable, have feeding problems and failure to thrive. Childhood: growth retardation, 'elfin' facial features, hoarse voice, premature wrinkling and sagging of the skin, cardiovascular anomalies (e.g. supravalvular aortic stenosis), urinary tract abnormalities (asymmetrical kidneys, nephrocalcinosis, bladder diverticuli, urethral stenosis), pulmonary artery stenosis, mild to moderate LD (verbal often better than visuospatial and motor abilities). Often there is abnormal attachment behaviour (manifest as anxiety, poor peer relationships, hypersensitivity, or conversely as social disinhibition, excessive friendliness).

Wolf–Hirschhorn syndrome Partial monosomy; karyotype 4p-. *Clinical features* Severe LD; many survive to adulthood.

Autosomal dominant syndromes

Noonan's syndrome Occuring in 1:1000–1:2000; M = F. Initial description of 9 children seen in the congenital heart disease clinic who shared a characteristic facies, anterior chest wall deformities (pectus carinatum or excavatum) and short stature. Whilst a number of genes (including PTPN11, SOS1 and KRAS) have been identified which can cause Noonan's syndrome, it remains a clinical diagnosis. *Clinical features* Varying degree of LD (from none to severe), short stature (80%), cardiac abnormalities (>80%), hepatosplenomegaly (25%), distinctive facies.

The following group of disorders is also termed the phakomatoses— a variety of conditions of ectodermal origin with neurocutaneous signs. Although Von Hippel–Lindau syndrome is not associated with LD, it is included for completeness.

Tuberous sclerosis (TSC) Occurring in 1:7000–10 000; M = F. *Clinical features* Varying degree (usually severe) of LD (50%), seizures (e.g. 'Salaam attacks' and other types, in 90%), hamartomas of the CNS (including the retina) as well as ependymomas and astrocytomas, facial angiofibroma, adenoma sebaceum, depigmented skin patches ('ash leaf spots' in 96%), shagreen patches, depigmented naevi, subcutaneous nodules, 'café-au-lait' spots, fibromas of the nails, pitted tooth enamel, hypoplasia, and occasionally tumours of the heart (rhabdomyeloma, hamartoma), kidney problems (Wilm's tumour, renal cysts), olfactory hamartomas, hypertension, and aortic aneurysm. *Subtypes* TSC1: 1:12 000; associated with a gene (for hamartin—believed to be tumour-suppressant) near the ABO blood group locus on chromosome 9 (9q34—40% of cases). TSC2: associated with a gene for tuberin (a guanosine triphosphatase-activating protein also believed to be tumour-suppressant) on chromosome 16 (16p13.3-); more psychiatric and behavioural problems. TSC3: a rare translocation of a gene on chromosome 12.

Neurofibromatosis Type 1 (NF1, von Recklinghausen's disease) Occurring in 1:2500; M = F. Autosomal dominant condition, responsible gene on chromosome 17 (approx. 50% spontaneous mutations). *Clinical features* Café-au-lait spots, freckling, dermal neurofibromas, nodular neurofibromas, Lisch nodules. Associated with mild learning disability in approx. 50%. Type 2 (NF2) Occurring in 1:35 000. Autosomal dominant condition, responsible gene on chromosome 22. *Clinical features* Bilateral vestibular schwannomas, café-au-lait spots, juvenile posterior subcapsular lenticular opacities.

Sturge–Weber syndrome Caused by spontaneous genetic mutation in unknown location. *Clinical features* 'Port-wine stain' typically covering part of the forehead and at least one eyelid, angiomas of the meninges in the temporal and occipital areas on the same side as the port-wine stain. Associated to varying degrees with LD. Epilepsy is the most common early problem, often starting before the age of one. Hemiparesis may develop, usually contralateral to the port-wine stain. Buphthalmos (bulging of the eye) and glaucoma are common in the affected eye.

Von Hippel–Lindau (VHL) syndrome A rare genetic condition caused by a mutation of the VHL tumour suppressor gene on chromosome 3p. 80% inherited, 20% new mutation. Symptoms caused by angiomas in various areas of the body. *Clinical features* Renal cysts/carcinomas, phaeochromocytomas, CNS haemangioblastomas, pancreatic cysts/tumours (can be neuroendocrine), subretinal haemorrhages 2° to retinal vessel tortuosities/aneurysms. Not associated with LD.

Autosomal recessive syndromes

These conditions include some of the lysosomal storage diseases, e.g. mucopolysaccharide storage—Hurler syndrome, Sanfilippo disease, sphingolipid storage—Tay–Sachs disease, Niemann–Pick disease (sphingomyelins), glycoprotein storage—sialidosis; phenylketonuria; and rare disorders such as Laurence–Moon syndrome and Joubert syndrome (see 📖 p. 751).

Phenylketonuria A preventable cause of severe LD, due to deficiency of phenylalanine hydroxylase (long arm of chromosome 12), leading to phenylalaninaemia and phenylketonuria; prevalence 1:15 000; diagnosed postnatally ('Guthrie test'). *Clinical features* Fair hair/skin and blue eyes (lack of pigment—tyrosine deficiency), neurological signs (stooped posture, broad-based gait, increased tone and reflexes, tremor, stereotyped movements). *Behavioural problems* Hyperactivity, temper tantrums, perseveration, echolalia. *Management* Supervised early dietary restriction of phenylalanine. *Prognosis* Even with dietary treatment, lower than average IQ.

Sanfilippo disease Due to disorders of the breakdown of heparan sulphate, of which there are 4 subtypes (types A–D). Prevalence 1:25 000–325 000. *Clinical features* Severe LD, claw hand, dwarfism, hypertrichosis, hearing loss, hepatosplenomegaly, biconvex lumbar vertebrae, joint stiffness. *Behavioural problems* Restlessness, sleep problems, challenging behaviour. *Aetiology* Type A (most severe, most common) mapped to 17q25.3 (heparan sulphate sulphatase). Type B 17q21 (N-acetyl-α-D-glucosaminidase). Type C on chromosome 14 or 21 (acetyl-CoA-α-glucosaminide-N-acetyltransferase). Type D 12q14 (N-acetyl-α-D-glucosamine-6-sulphatase). *Prognosis* Poor, many die between 10–20yrs of respiratory tract infections.

Hurler syndrome Due to deficiency in A-L-iduronidase (4p16.3); incidence 1:76 000–144 000. *Clinical features* Progressive LD (eventually severe/profound), skeletal abnormalities (short stature, kyphosis, flexion deformities, claw hand, long head, characteristic facial appearance), hearing loss, respiratory and cardiac problems, hepatosplenomegaly, umbilical/inguinal hernia. *Prognosis* Poor, some survive to 20s; may benefit from allogenic bone transplantation.

Laurence–Moon syndrome Associated with multiple loci (11q13, 11q21, 15q22, 3p13); prevalence 1:125 000–160 000 (higher in Bedouins of Kuwait and Newfoundland). Also known as *Laurence–Moon–Biedl syndrome* (incorporating Bardet–Biedl syndrome which shares clinical features, but additionally there is central obesity and polydactyly). *Clinical features* Mild–moderate LD, short stature, spastic paraparesis, hypogenitalism (most males are infertile), night blindness (due to red cone dystrophy), non-insulin dependent diabetes mellitus (NIDDM), renal problems (diabetes insipidus, renal failure).

Joubert syndrome Exceptionally rare, no loci identified, but recessively inherited. *Clinical features* Severe LD, characteristic hyperpnoea ('panting like a dog'), cerebellar dysgenesis, hypotonia, ataxia, tongue protrusion, facial spasm, abnormal eye movements, cystic kidneys, syndactyly/polydactyly. *Behavioural problems* Self-injury. *Prognosis* Poor—no specific treatments.

Gaucher's disease Most common of the lysosomal storage diseases. Caused by deficiency of glucocerebrosidase, leading to accumulation of glucosylceramide, most commonly in spleen, liver, lung, bone, and brain. Type I—brain is unaffected, onset later in adulthood. Types II and III associated with learning disability, type II being the most severe. *Prognosis* Type I—close to normal, type II—children usually die by age 2, type III—adolescence—adulthood. *Treatment* Enzyme replacement and bone marrow replacement both used in the treatment of types I and III. Unfortunately there is no treatment for the neurological effects in types II and III.

X-linked dominant syndromes

Fragile X syndrome

A common inherited cause of LD, affecting ~1:4000 males and 1:8000 females, with X-linked dominant transmission. Penetrance is low, but greater in males than females (due to the 'protective' effects of the second normal X chromosome in females). Gene sequence has been cloned[1] and designated FMR-1. The syndrome is associated with a large sequence of triplet repeats (CGG)n at a fragile site on the X chromosome (Xq27.3). In affected males n >230–1000+, in transmitting males and obligate females n = 43–200, and in the general population n = 6–54 (mean 30).

Clinical features Variable, subtle, and often cannot be detected before adulthood. May include: large testicles and ears, smooth skin, hyper-extensible fingers, flat feet, mitral valve prolapse, inguinal and hiatus hernia, facial features (long, narrow face with underdevelopment of the mid-face, macrocephaly), epilepsy (~25%), variable LD (borderline to profound); behavioural features appear to be similar to those seen in ADHD and autism: hand flapping/waving, repetitive mannerisms, shyness, gaze avoidance, poor peer relationships, communication difficulties (e.g. delayed language development, conversational rigidity, perseveration, echolalia, palilalia, cluttering, and over-detailed/circumstantial speech), psychiatric problems (e.g. prominent depression/anxiety). Many of the features of fragile X also overlap with those of autism, though debate is ongoing as to the exact nature of the relationship. *Note:* general domestic and daily living skills may be excellent. *Brain imaging* Reduced posterior cerebellar vermis, enlarged hippocampus and caudate nuclei, enlarged ventricles.

Other disorders with 'fragile' sites

Two other fragile sites have been found on the X chromosome. The original 'fragile X' site has hence been designated 'FRAX A'. FRAX E, caused by FMR-2 mutation is also associated with mild LD, with an incidence of 1:100 000, and 200–1000 triplet repeats. FRAX F has not (yet) been associated with any disorder. Another fragile site has been located on chromosome 16 (FRA 16) associated with a large GCC triplet expansion—but no specific clinical disorder.

Rett's syndrome

A pervasive developmental disorder (see 📖 p. 758) almost exclusively affecting females with an incidence of 1:10 000—20 000. Initially described by Austrian physican Andreas Rett in 1966,[2] but only fully recognized after a second paper in 1983.[3]

Clinical features Initially normal development followed by 4 stages: (1) early onset/developmental arrest, (2) rapid destructive/regressive, (3) plateau (or pseudo-stationary) and (4) late motor deterioration.
- *Stage 1* Onset usually 6–18mths. May be delays in gross motor skills. Infants may show ↓ eye contact and ↓ interest in toys. The typically described hand-wringing and ↓ rate of head growth may also be apparent.

- *Stage 2* Onset usually between 1 and 4yrs. Purposeful hand movements and spoken language are lost. Stereotypical hand movements including wringing, washing, clapping, or tapping are often seen. Emergence of some autistic symptoms and a worsening gait may be seen.
- *Stage 3* Onset usually before age 10, and can last for most of life. Seizures and motor problems more prominent. Some improvement in behaviour, with more interest in others and surroundings and some improvement in communication skills.
- *Stage 4* This stage can last for decades and is typified by gradual worsening in mobility, with scoliosis, spasticity, and muscle weakness.

Aetiology Mutations in the *MECP2* gene on the X chromosome are present in the majority of girls with Rett's syndrome. Mutations on the *CDKL5* gene have also been implicated in a variant of Rett's with notably early-onset of seizures. *Prognosis* The prognosis is poor with continued motor deterioration and usually severe learning disability.

Aicardi syndrome

Rare (only 200 reported cases—all female); dysgenesis of the corpus callosum and cerebrum, with severe LD; prognosis poor (often death in infancy). *Clinical features* Microcephaly, facial asymmetry, low-set ears, eye lesions (chorioretinal lacunae), hypotonia, scoliosis, epilepsy. *Behavioural problems* 25%—aggression, lack of communication, tiredness/sleep problems, self-injurious behaviour.

1 Verkerk AJ, Pieretti M, Sutcliffe JS, *et al.* (1991) Identification of a gene (FMR-1) containing a CGG repeat coincident with a breakpoint cluster region exhibiting length variation in fragile X syndrome. *Cell* **65**: 905–14.

2 Rett A (1966) Ueber ein eigenartiges himatrophisches Syndrom bei Hyperammoniamie in Kindesalter. *Wien Med Wschr* **116**: 723–8.

3 Hagberg B, Aicardi J, Dias K, *et al.* (1983) A progressive syndrome of autism, dementia, ataxia, and loss of purposeful hand use in girls: Rett's syndrome: report of 35 cases. *Ann Neurol* **14**: 471–9.

X-linked recessive syndromes

These include other lysosomal storage diseases, e.g. mucopolysaccharide storage—Hunter syndrome; trihexosylceramide storage—Fabry disease and other extremely rare conditions such as Lesch–Nyhan syndrome and oculocerebrorenal syndrome of Lowe.

Hunter syndrome Caused by iduronate sulphatase deficiency (mapped to Xq27-28); incidence 1:132 000–28 0000 (more common in male Ashkenazi Jews: 1:34 000). Symptoms are caused by build-up of glycosaminoglycans (GAG) in a variety of body tissues. Only 20% have complete depletion of iduronate sulphatase and two subtypes are recognized: *Type A* Progressive LD and physical disability, with death before age 15yrs. *Type B* Milder form, with minimal intellectual impairment and better prognosis. *Clinical features* Short stature, distinctive course, facies 'gargoylism', prominent forehead, enlarged tongue, flattened bridge of nose, enlarged head, degenerative hip disease, joint stiffness, claw hand, chest deformities (pes cavus or excavatum), cervical cord compression, hepatosplenomegaly, hearing loss, breathing obstruction, developmental delay, eye defects (retinitis pigmentosa, papilloedema, hypertrichosis), umbilical/inguinal hernia.

Lesch–Nyhan syndrome An extremely rare X-linked recessive condition, due to a mutation in the HPRT gene (hypoxanthine phosphoribosyl transferase) on the short arm of chromosome Xq26-27, with a nearly total loss of the enzyme leading to hyperuricaemia. Prognosis is poor and most affected individuals die in early adulthood. *Clinical features* Children appear healthy at birth, dystonias become apparent around 3–4mths with delayed developmental milestones, later there is development of spasticity, choreoform movements and transient hemiparesis (which may be misdiagnosed as cerebral palsy), variable degree of LD (usually severe), microcephaly is common, ~50% develop epilepsy. *Behavioural problems* Around age 2yrs (sometimes not until adolescence) self-mutilating behaviours may be seen (biting of lips, inside of mouth, fingers). Sometimes there is an episodic pattern, and some may show a reduction in frequency and severity after age 10yrs. May be associated with verbal and physical aggression. There is no clear cause for this behaviour— CNS findings include reduction in dopamine in the basal ganglia and at synaptic terminals (but not in the cell bodies of the substantia nigra), with other monoaminergic systems apparently intact. *Management* Even treating hyperuricaemia does not appear to reduce behavioural problems; however, there is some evidence for use of SSRIs.

Oculocerebrorenal syndrome of Lowe Very rare X-linked recessive condition (Xq24-26); incidence 1:200 000. *Clinical features* Moderate–severe LD (up to 25% have normal IQ), short stature, hypotonia, epilepsy (~30%), eye problems (e.g. congenital cataracts), renal problems (tubular dysfunction). *Behavioural problems* Temper tantrums, hand-waving movements, self-injury (~70%—esp. in early adolescence).

Sex chromosome disorders

Turner's syndrome Sex chromosome monosomy; karyotype 45XO, female phenotype; generally normal IQ with LD rare though there may be specific deficits of visuospatial learning.

Trisomy X Sex chromosome trisomy; karyotype 47, XXX; 1:1000 female births. *Clinical features* Slight increase in height, ~70% have learning disorder (usually mild), some evidence of reduced fertility (children have normal karyotypes), possibly increased incidence of schizophrenia.

Klinefelter's syndrome Sex chromosome trisomy; karyotype 47, XXY; 1:1000 male births (50% due to paternal and 50% maternal non-dysjunction). *Clinical features* Variable degree of development of secondary sexual characteristics with hypogonadism, scant facial hair (90%), gynaecomastia (50%). Taller than average (~4cm), asthenic body build, median IQ ~90 with skewed distribution—most in 60–70 range, uncertain association with psychiatric disorders.

XYY male Sex chromosome trisomy; karyotype 47, XYY; 1:1000 male births. *Clinical features* Controversial suggestion of higher incidence in prison populations, IQ may be slightly lower than average, behavioural problems commonly seen.

Non-genetic causes of learning disability

Foetal alcohol syndrome (FAS)

One of the major causes of LD, incidence 0.2–3 per 1000 live births. 10–20% of cases of mild LD may be caused by maternal alcohol use. Risk increased by: overall alcohol consumption, bingeing, other drug use (including smoking), genetic susceptibility, and low socio-economic status. May be due to the effects of alcohol on NMDA receptors, which may alter cell proliferation. *Clinical features* Postnatal signs of alcohol withdrawal (irritability, hypotonia, tremors, seizures); microcephaly; abnormal facial features—small eye fissures, epicanthic folds, short palpebral fissure, small maxillae and mandibles, underdeveloped philtrum, cleft palate, thin upper lip; growth deficits—small overall length, joint deformities; CNS features—high incidence of mild LD, associated behavioural problems (hyperactivity, sleep problems), optic nerve hypoplasia (poor visual acuity), hearing loss, receptive and expressive language deficits; other physical abnormalities—ASD, VSD, renal hypoplasia, bladder diverticuli.

Iodine deficiency disease

Worldwide the most common cause of severe intellectual impairment and largely forgotten in the West by virtue of good diet and iodized table salt. Important cause of LD, particularly because of its treatability. Mainly found in large areas of Asia, Africa, and South America.

Congenital hypothyroidism

A treatable cause of mental and growth retardation due to loss of thyroid function; incidence 1:3500–4000, but now screened for neonatally and treated early with levothyroxine. If untreated, leads to typical clinical picture of lethargy, difficulty feeding, constipation, macroglossia, and umbilical hernia.

Secondary to other toxins

E.g. cocaine, lead, bilirubin, coumarin anticoagulants, phenytoin.

Secondary to infective agents

ToRCH, syphilis (treponema pallidum), HIV, and other causes of meningitis and encephalitis.

Hypoxic damage

Secondary to placental insufficiency, pre-eclampsia, birth trauma, severe prematurity, 'small for dates' babies (foetal growth retardation), or multiple pregnancy.

CNS and skull developmental abnormalities

Micro- and macrocephalies, spina bifida, hydrocephalus, craniostenosis, callosal agenesis, lissencephalies, holoprosencephalies.

Disorders of unknown aetiology

This includes a broad range of disorders associated with LD, but for which a clear aetiology is as yet undetermined, e.g. cerebral palsies, epilepsy, autistic spectrum disorders (see 📖 p. 760), childhood disintegrative disorders, and other clearly defined syndromes with a suspected but not yet proved genetic basis (e.g. Cornelia de Lange).

Disintegrative disorder

Clinical features Characterized by normal development until the age of ~4yrs, followed by profound regression with disintegration of behaviour, loss of acquired language and other skills, impaired social relationships, and stereotypies. *Aetiology* Unknown, but may follow minor illness or viral encephalitis (e.g. measles). *Prognosis* Poor, with development of severe LD.

Cornelia de Lange syndrome (Brachmann de Lange syndrome)

Usually IQ is below 60 (range 30–86), prevalence 1:50 000–100 000, mode of inheritance unknown (possibly autosomal dominant). *Clinical features* Hypertrichosis (hirsutism, synophrys, long eyelashes), facial features (depressed nasal bridge, eye abnormalities, prominent philtrum, thin lips, downturned mouth, anteverted nostrils, bluish tinge around eyes/nose/mouth, widely spaced teeth, high-arched palate, low-set ears, micrognathia, short neck), limb deformities (esp. upper limbs), cryptorchidism/hypoplastic genitals (males), small umbilicus, low-pitched cry, small nipples. Associated with GI problems, congenital heart defects, visual and hearing problems, skin problems, epilepsy, and death in infancy.

Behavioural problems Expressive language deficits, feeding difficulties, sleep disturbance, self-injury, temper tantrums, mood disorders, and autistic features.

Pervasive developmental disorders

Pervasive developmental disorders (PDDs) are a group of lifelong developmental disorders characterized by a triad of: abnormal reciprocal social interaction; communication and language impairment; and a restricted, stereotyped, and repetitive repertoire of interests and activities. ICD-10 categorizes PDDs as follows:

* Autism and atypical autism (📖 p. 760)
* Rett's syndrome
* Childhood disintegrative disorder
* Asperger's syndrome
* Pervasive developmental disorder not otherwise specified (PDD-NOS).

Patients with PDD show either a lack of normal development of skills or the loss of already acquired skills. There is a gender bias with male > female predominance in all syndromes except Rett's syndrome (female predominance). Prevalence of PDD ranges from 10–20 cases per 10 000 individuals.

Asperger's syndrome (AS)[1]

Essence A syndrome first described by Hans Asperger in 1944, but only eponymously named in 1981 by Lorna Wing. Described by Baron-Cohen as 'The extreme male brain', with 'mind-blindness'. Characterized by severe persistent impairment in reciprocal social interactions, repetitive behaviour patterns, and restricted interests. IQ and language are normal or, in some cases, superior. Children with AS may have more striking autistic features before age 5, but later develop 'normally' in most spheres except-ing social behaviour. Social deficits commonly manifest in adolescence or early adulthood when the individual experiences difficulty with intimate relationships. Psychiatric comorbidity is high with depression most common. Bipolar affective disorder and schizophrenia are more common than in the general population.

Mild motor clumsiness (ICD-10) and a family history of autism may be present.

Epidemiology Male predominance. Prevalence may be as high as 1 in 300 as AS is almost certainly under-recognized.

'Autistic spectrum' There is some evidence that AS forms a spectrum with autism and high-functioning autism in terms of aetiology, pathology, and clinical presentation.

Rett's syndrome (RS)—see 📖 p. 752
Childhood disintegrative disorder (CDD)[2]

Rare, occurring in fewer than 5 in 10 000 children. Male predominance. There is normal development for 2–3yrs, followed by a loss of acquired motor, language, and social skills between ages 3 and 4yrs. Stereotypies and compulsions are common. Cause is unknown and prognosis is poor.

PDD-NOS

Also termed 'atypical autism', PDD-NOS is relatively common and encompasses subthreshold cases where there are impairments of social interaction, communication, and/or stereotyped behaviour patterns or interest, but where full criteria for other PDDs are not met.

1 Blasic JC (2008) *Pervasive developmental disorder: Asperger syndrome.* http://www.emedicine.com
2 Bernstein BE (2007) *Pervasive developmental disorder: childhood disintegrative disorder.* http://www.emedicine.com

Autism[1]

Autism was first described by Maudsley in 1867 and named 'infantile autism' by Leo Kanner in 1943. It is a syndrome that has engendered controversy in terms of its definition, relationship to other syndromes (e.g. schizophrenia), and aetiology. Autism is characterized by the same triad of symptoms (see 📖 p. 758) as the core symptoms of PDD: abnormal reciprocal social interaction; communication and language impairment; and a restricted, stereotyped, and repetitive repertoire of interests and activities (see Box 18.2).

Eighty per cent of patients with autism have mild to moderate LD. The remaining 20% with normal IQ are classified as either **high-functioning autism** (with language difficulties) or **Asperger's syndrome** (with normal language). *Note:* this last point is controversial and many would consider AS not to be classified as a form of autism. In general terms, 1–2% of those with autism have a 'normal' life; 5–20% have a 'borderline' prognosis (i.e. varying degrees of independence); but 70% are totally dependent upon support.

Epidemiology The onset of symptoms is typically before age 3. Male: female ratio is 3–4:1. Prevalence is 5–10 per 1000 individuals.

Aetiology The cause is unknown, but a number of hypotheses exist: genetic (in Down's syndrome and fragile X); obstetric complications; toxic agents; pre/postnatal infections (with maternal rubella); autoimmune (anecdotal MMR—not proven); association with neurological disorders (e.g. tuberous sclerosis).

Pathophysiology MRI: some have ↑ brain size; ↑ lateral and 4th ventricles; frontal lobe and cerebellar abnormalities.

Pathology: abnormal Purkinje cells in cerebellar vermis; abnormal limbic architecture.

Biochemistry: one-third have ↑ serum 5-HT; some have ↑ β-endorphin immunoreactivity.

Clinical features

- *Abnormal social relatedness:* impaired non-verbal behaviour; poor eye contact; impaired mentation; failure to develop peer relationships; reduced interest in shared enjoyment; lack of social or emotional reciprocity and empathy; attachment to unusual objects.
- *Abnormal communication or play:* delay or lack of spoken language; difficulty in initiating or sustaining conversation; stereotyped and repetitive (or idiosyncratic) language; mixing of pronouns; lack of developmentally appropriate fantasy, symbolic, or social play.
- *Restricted interests or activities:* encompassing preoccupations and interests; adherence to non-functional routines or rituals; resistance to change; stereotypies and motor mannerisms (e.g. hand or finger flapping or body rocking); preoccupation with parts of objects.
- *Neurological features:* seizures; motor tics; ↑ head circumference; abnormal gaze monitoring; ↑ ambidexterity.

- *Physiological features:* unusually intense sensory responsiveness (e.g. to bright lights, loud noise, rough textures); absence of typical response to pain or injury; abnormal temperature regulation; ↑ paediatric illnesses.
- *Behavioural problems:* irritability; temper tantrums; self-injury; hyperactivity; aggression.
- *'Savants':* a minority may have 'islands of precocity' against a background of LD (i.e. isolated abilities, e.g. incredible memory or arithmetic skills).

Differential diagnosis Other PDDs; childhood schizophrenia; LD; language disorders; neurological disorders; sensory impairment (deafness or blindness); OCD; psychosocial deprivation.

See Box 18.3 for a summary of treatment.

Box 18.2 Assessment of autism

- A multidisciplinary approach is required, involving psychiatrists, psychologists, paediatricians, neurologists, speech therapists, occupational therapists (OTs), and primary care teams
- Full clinical evaluation: including physical and mental state as well as specific developmental, psychometric, and educational assessments
- Rating scales: Autism Behaviour Checklist (ABC); Childhood Autism Rating Scales (CARS); Autism Diagnostic Interview—Revised (ADI-R); Autism Diagnostic Observation Schedule (ADOS); Diagnostic Interview for Social and Communication Disorders (DISCO)

Box 18.3 Treatment strategies for autism

- STRUCTURE, ROUTINE, PREDICTABILITY
- Aids to improve communication: symbol dictionaries, picture boards, social stories
- Educational and vocational interventions: special versus mainstream
- Behavioural interventions: includes behaviour modification, social skills training, and CBT methods
- Family interventions: education; support; advocacy
- Speech and language therapy; OT; physiotherapy; dietary advice etc.
- Pharmacotherapy: symptom management, e.g. antipsychotics for stereotypies; SSRIs for compulsive and self-harming behaviours and depression/anxiety. Risperidone now has FDA licence for autism— seek expert advice
- Treat medical conditions (e.g. epilepsy, GIT problems)

1 Brasic JR (2008) *Pervasive developmental disorder: autism.* ℘ http://www.emedicine.com.

Epilepsy and LD

Epilepsy is significantly more common in people with a learning disability than in the general population. The prevalence of epilepsy is ~40% in the hospitalized LD population and is higher in severe LD (30–50%) than in mild LD (15–20%). It may begin at any age, presentations may change over time, and multiple forms may occur in the same individual.

Diagnosis

History and examination May be difficult to obtain accurate information, often relying on third-party accounts (home video may be useful). Try to exclude other differential diagnoses (e.g. infection, trauma, hypoglycaemia, hyperventilation, withdrawal from drugs or alcohol, over-sedation, localizing signs of intracranial pathology, evidence of movement disorders). Conduct an MSE, focusing on observed behaviours. Identification of any stressors (especially if anxiety-provoking).

Investigations Baseline laboratory tests—FBC, U&Es, LFTs, glucose. Consider EEG and CT/MRI (in complex cases video-EEG monitoring may be useful), PET or SPECT (to detect areas of hypometabolism).

Co-occurrence

- Epilepsy is common in patients with LD of various causes, e.g. Down's syndrome (5–10%), fragile X (25%), Angelman syndrome (90%), Rett's syndrome (90%). This may be due to shared aetiologies such as alterations in neuronal development and function, or co-associated brain lesions (haemorrhage, ischaemia, neoplasm, vascular malformation).
- Frequent epileptic seizures may lead to (or worsen) permanent loss of intellectual functioning (e.g. 'acquired epileptic aphasia'/Landau–Kleffner syndrome, progressive partial epilepsies such as epilepsia partialis Kozhevnikov or Rasmussen syndrome type 2) emphasizing the need for early diagnosis and treatment to prevent often fatal progression.

Epilepsy syndromes in infancy and childhood

Infancy Early infantile epileptic encephalopathy due to congenital or acquired abnormal cortical development; early myoclonic epileptic encephalopathy possibly due to metabolic disorders; infantile spasms/West syndrome[1] due to intrauterine infections (toxoplasmosis, CMV, rubella), Down's syndrome, tuberous sclerosis, progressive degenerative disorders, or intracranial tumours; severe myoclonic epilepsy.

Childhood A variety of other myoclonic epilepsy syndromes are recognized: Lennox–Gastaut syndrome, myoclonic-astatic epilepsy (Doose syndrome), progressive myoclonus epilepsies (Baltic or Lafora disease), Northern epilepsy.

Treatment

Note: practice varies geographically—in some areas the lead is taken by neurologists, in other areas by LD psychiatrists and/or epilepsy specialist nurses.

Choice of treatment will depend upon a number of factors:
- Accurate classification of the type of seizures/epilepsy syndrome.
- Possible drug interactions.
- Minimizing side-effects (esp. cognitive impairment).

IASSID Guidelines[2]

Collation of evidence for different treatments of epilepsy in LD.
- Generalized seizures—sodium valproate, lamotrigine.
- Partial seizures—valproate, carbamazepine, lamotrigine.

Points to note

- Behavioural problems may be associated with anti-epileptic drugs, and may be more common in patients with brain injury or LD (e.g. phenobarbitone, primidone, BDZs, vigabatrin).
- Communication difficulties may make assessment of side-effects more difficult.
- For intractable epilepsy, neurosurgery is an option, and it should not be excluded on the basis that the person has LD.

Prognosis

There is wide variation in outcome; however, up to 70% of patients with LD can achieve good control of their epilepsy without major side-effects.

Common pitfalls

- Diagnostic overshadowing, explaining new (epileptic) symptoms as being 'only' due to the LD.
- Epilepsy may be misdiagnosed in patients with LD, particularly when there is a history of sudden unexplained aggression, self-mutilation, and other 'bizarre' behaviours, including abnormal or stereotyped movements, fixed staring, rapid eye blinking, exaggerated startle reflex, attention deficits, or unexplained intermittent lethargy. (If anti-epileptic medication has been previously prescribed for these kinds of presentations, consider careful withdrawal with close monitoring.)
- Non-epileptic (pseudo) seizure disorder can also occur in patients with epilepsy. (Cf. non-cardiac chest pain in patients with angina.)
- Epilepsy-related behaviours may also be confused for psychiatric problems, e.g. hallucinations in simple (somatosensory) partial seizures; psychosis-like episodes during complex partial seizures (esp. temporal or frontal lobe); or post-ictal confusion.

---

1 West syndrome is the triad of infantile spasms, mental retardation, and hypsarrhythmia (characteristic EEG finding of chaotic intermixed high-voltage slow waves and diffuse asynchronous spikes).
2 International Association for Scientific Study of Intellectual Impairment (2001) Clinical guidelines for the management of epilepsy in people with an intellectual disability. *Seizure* 10, 401–9.

Psychiatric comorbidity in LD

In the assessment of patients with LD it is important to always consider comorbid psychiatric illnesses as they are both common and treatable. Psychiatric illness is often missed in the LD population because of diagnostic overshadowing (symptoms of mental illness mistakenly attributed to the LD). The diagnostic criteria for people with LD (DC-LD) is published by the Royal College of Psychiatrists as an aid to the diagnosis of mental illness in the LD population.

Schizophrenia

Approximately 3 times more common than in the general population. Age of onset tends to be earlier (mean 23yrs). More commonly associated with epilepsy, negative symptoms of schizophrenia, and impairment of episodic memory.[1] In severe LD there may be unexplained aggression, bizarre behaviours, mood lability, or increased mannerisms and stereotypies.

Bipolar affective disorder

Prevalence is estimated to be greater than the general population (2–12%), with difficulty in making the diagnosis in severe LD. Symptom 'equivalents' may include: hyperactivity, wandering, mutism, temper tantrums.

Depressive disorder

Commonly missed as a quiet withdrawn person may not be a focus of clinical attention. Biological features tend to be more marked, with diurnal variations. Suicidal thoughts and acts may occur in borderline–moderate LD, but are less frequent in severe. Other causes of mood disturbance (e.g. perimenstrual disorders) should also be considered.

Other disorders

Anxiety disorders May be difficult to distinguish from depression, except where there are situational features.

OCD Reported to be more prevalent in LD. Differential diagnosis: ritualistic behaviours, tic disorders, behavioural manifestations of autism/ Asperger's disorder.

ADHD Often a prominent feature in children with LD (up to 20%). Stimulants may help in mild LD with clear symptoms, but have no clear efficacy in severe to profound LD.

Personality disorder Difficult to define in the LD population, but prevalence is estimated in ~20% of mild–moderate LD patients who are inpatients.

---

1 Doody GA, Johnstone EC, Sanderson TL, Owens DGC, and Muir WJ (1998) Pfropfschizophrenie revisited: schizophrenia in people with mild learning disability. *Br J Psychiatry* 173, 145–53.

Behavioural disorders and 'challenging' behaviour

Behavioural disorders are over-represented in LD populations, ranging from minor antisocial behaviours to seriously aggressive outbursts. Prevalence estimates are 7% of the LD population: 14% for inpatients (esp. 25–29-yr-olds), and 5% for those in the community (esp. 15–19-yr-olds).

Studies of behavioural disorders in the LD population identify 6 relatively consistent groupings of pathological behaviours,[1] which create a significant burden for parents/carers:

- Aggression-antisocial:
  - *Antisocial behaviours* Shouting, screaming, general noisiness; anal poking/faecal smearing (? 2° to constipation); self-induced vomiting/ choking; stealing.
  - *Aggressive outbursts* Against persons or property.
  - *Severe physical violence* Rare.
  - *Self-injurious behaviour* Skin picking, eye gouging, head banging, face beating (more common in severe/profound LD; prevalence 10% overall, 1–2% most severe).
- Social withdrawal.
- Stereotypic behaviours (some of which may be *self-injurious*).
- Hyperactive disruptive behaviours.
- Repetitive communication disturbance.
- Anxiety/fearfulness.

When these behaviours are particularly severe, they are often termed 'challenging' (see Box 18.4).

Associated factors

- **Cognitive functioning** Severe intellectual impairment, poor/absent language ability, poor social comprehension.
- **Temperament** Particularly high emotionality, ↑activity, poor sociability.
- **Physical problems**, e.g. epilepsy, cerebral palsy, cardiac problems, GI problems, visual/hearing impairment.
- **Medication** Psychotropic drugs may produce or mask cognitive, behavioural, or emotional problems. Sometimes a 'drug holiday' may be helpful to assess how medication contributes to the presentation.
- **Psychological factors** 1°reinforcers, e.g. food, drink, pain (often undetected). 2°reinforcers, e.g. praise, environment, aversive stimuli.
- **Communication difficulties** Frustration due to inability to utilize normal forms of communication.
- **Adverse experiences** Common to the general population, and also particular to the LD population, e.g. experience of institutions, social rejection, neglect, and emotional, physical, or sexual abuse.
- **Environmental factors** Living conditions, stability and continuity of day-to-day activities (a common precipitant is multiple short-term residential placements with multiple changes in care staff). The quality of the care environment may be directly responsible for behavioural problems and assessment should include factors such as: social

relationships, specific environmental stressors, consistency of care, and lack of stimulation.

- **Comorbidity** Psychiatric disorders may complicate the presentation of behavioural problems, e.g. *ADHD* (see 🕮 p. 726); *conduct disorder/ oppositional defiant disorder* (see 🕮 p. 625); *tic disorders* (see 🕮 p. 632); *anxiety disorders* (see 🕮 p. 639)—fears/phobias, separation anxiety (see 🕮 p. 640), PTSD (see 🕮 p. 646), OCD (see 🕮 p. 648); *depressive disorder* (see 🕮 p. 652); *bipolar disorder* (see 🕮 p. 656); *pervasive developmental disorders* (see 🕮 p. 630). Identification and appropriate treatment may significantly improve behavioural problems.

Behavioural phenotypes

Many genetic causes of LD are associated with characteristic patterns of behaviour. Recognizing these 'behavioural repertoires' may help in diagnosis and management, and forms the basis for ongoing research into the genetic basis of some behavioural problems. Examples include: *Down's syndrome* (oppositional, conduct, and ADHD); *fragile X syndrome* (autism, ADHD, stereotypies, e.g. hand flapping); *Lesch–Nyhan syndrome* (self-mutilation); *Prader–Willi syndrome* (OCD, multiple impulsive behaviour disorder, e.g. hyperphagia, aggression, skin picking); *Smith–Magenis syndrome* (severe ADHD, stereotypies—'self-hugging', severe self-injurious behaviours, insomnia); *Williams syndrome* ('pseudomature' language ability in some; initially affectionate and engaging; later anxious, hyperactive, and uncooperative).

> ### Box 18.4 Criteria for clinically significant challenging behaviour
>
> - At some time the behaviour has caused more than minor injuries to themselves or others, or destroyed their immediate living or working environment.
> - At least weekly behaviours requiring intervention by staff; placed them in physical danger; caused damage that could not be rectified; caused at least 1hr of disruption.
> - Behaviour has caused over a few minutes' disruption at least daily.
>
> Qureshi H (1994) The size of the problem.
> In Emerson E, McGill P, and Mansell J (eds),
> *Severe mental retardation and challenging behaviours:
> designing high quality services.*
> London: Chapman and Hall

1 Einfeld SL and Aman M (1995) Issues in the taxonomy of psychopathology in mental retardation. *J Autism Dev Disord* **25**: 143–67.

Management of behavioural disorders

At all stages in assessment and management, it is essential to involve parents, carers, and other allied professionals (e.g. teachers) both as sources of information and in implementing any proposed interventions.

Assessment

- Exclusion of psychiatric disorder.
- Exclusion of physical disorder and assessment of general health.
- Assessment of physical impairments (vision, hearing, etc.).
- Assessment of communication difficulties (including formal speech and language assessment).
- Assessment of specific cognitive impairments (including formal psychological testing).
- Identification of environmental and social factors.
- Use of behavioural diaries (by carers/staff): ABCs—antecedents, behaviours, consequences.

Management

Following assessment, *specific* factors should be addressed—psychiatric/physical causes, reduction of stimuli/reinforcers, modification of environmental factors.

Approaches may involve:

- **Educational interventions** Both for families/carers (to improve understanding) and for patients (to ensure educational needs are being appropriately met in a suitable setting).
- **Social interventions** To address unmet needs at home, with family/carers, or widen access to other services or facilities (to provide opportunities for social interaction and improve support networks).
- **Facilitating communication of needs** Addressing impairments of hearing, vision, and language (including use of pictures, sign language, electronic speech devices).
- **Behavioural interventions** Modification of behaviour using operant conditioning (e.g. removal of aversive stimuli, rewarding 'good' behaviour, use of appropriate attention—'neutral' response to attention-seeking behaviours), secondary reinforcers, modelling, 'positive programming'.
- **Cognitive approaches** At an appropriate level for degree of cognitive impairment and language abilities—may range from counselling on specific issues to simple imitation of relaxation/breathing techniques.
- **Pharmacotherapy** Treatment for specific comorbid conditions (e.g. ADHD—stimulants; OCD—SSRIs; antidepressant treatment; tic disorders—antipsychotics; epilepsy—anticonvulsants). Sometimes a trial of antipsychotic treatment may be useful for serious aggression, hyperactivity, or stereotypies (often depot; caution in epilepsy; increased risk of EPSEs). Other options for aggression, agitation, or self-injurious behaviours (mainly empirical evidence): anticonvulsants, lithium, β-blockers, buspirone. For self-injurious behaviours alone there is some evidence for opiate antagonists (e.g. naltrexone).

- **Physical interventions** (i.e. restraint): from splints and headgear to isolation (to protect individual and others from injury/damage to property).

Any intervention should be closely monitored to ensure compliance, acceptability, and therapeutic response. In the case of medication, side-effects should be minimized and if treatment is deemed ineffective drugs should be carefully withdrawn (to avoid secondary problems).

Transition periods

Adolescence

This may be a difficult transitional period; issues that may require attention include:

- **Engaging with adult services** Loss of the additional support provided by supported mainstream or special schools may lead to problems if there is not a smooth transition to adult services. Where appropriate (or available) this may include moving to *social educational/day centres*. Some countries have specific legislation to ensure that needs are identified early (e.g. 'transitional planning' from the age of 14 under the UK Education Act 1993).
- **Social/economic independence**
  - *Employment* Depending on the level of disability, this may be in *sheltered employment*, *workshops*, or *supported open employment*. Despite changing attitudes, there are considerable barriers to finding work in the open job market, although for some this may be worth pursuing.
  - *Living arrangements* Loss of additional social supports may actually increase the burden of care shouldered by the family. For some, the wish for independence or the lack of family support may be best met with *small group homes* where support may be tailored to individual needs.
- **Sexual relationships** Societal views may find it difficult to accept the fact that people with LD have normal sexual desires, which can be more of a problem for families/carers than the individuals themselves. Nonetheless, issues raised by appropriate sexual relationships will include consideration of contraception, understanding of the responsibilities of parenthood, issues of commitment and marriage. Many people, particularly with mild LD, are capable of being successful parents and provide a stable environment for children with appropriate support. Policy and practice guidelines will often exist on this contentious topic, for example the 'Making choices, keeping safe' policy in Lothian.

Later adulthood

- **Changing health needs** With increasing age, health needs may go unrecognized and there may be failure to access services. Patients with LD may lack capacity to consent to necessary medical treatment but this should not be allowed to prevent appropriate treatment.
- **Changing mental health needs** These may relate to changing symptomatology over time, altered tolerance of medication, and additional specific age-related cognitive impairment (e.g. due to chronic intractable epilepsy or early-onset Alzheimer's disease in Down's syndrome).
- **Ageing carers** The ability of carers to continue to provide the same level of care for their children ought to be considered *before* a crisis is reached. This requires an ongoing assessment of the patient's needs and the carer's abilities. Increasing reliance on carers may lead to social

isolation for the patient, and it is prudent to raise the issue of planning for the future at an early stage. Death of carers may produce multiple simultaneous difficulties when a patient with LD must cope with bereavement, loss of a familiar home setting, and adjustment to new carers and living with other individuals in a group setting.

Family issues

Having a child with LD is a major and often unexpected blow to any family. Individual responses vary, but the majority of parents adapt well to the situation and show remarkable resilience and resourcefulness. Depression is quite common in parents and should not be overlooked. Important positive factors include having a good relationship with their partner and the support of relatives and friends. Needs and priorities will vary over time and should be identified early and addressed collaboratively with the involvement of parents and other carers in any key decisions (see **Needs and priorities** 📖 p. 773).

Early impact

Prenatal diagnostic screening can place parents in the unexpected position of having to make difficult choices even *before* the birth of their child. Advice and counselling are a necessary and important part of the screening process, and should not be ignored even when testing is regarded as 'routine'. The mistaken assumption that screening 'guarantees' a healthy child may lead to even greater feelings of disappointment and anger, magnified further by anxious times after the birth, with a baby in a special care unit. Although some conditions can be diagnosed at birth, often parents only realize there is a problem when their child fails to reach developmental milestones, or develops seizures after an apparently 'normal' infancy. Often the response is one of bereavement (see 📖 p. 388) or guilt, and parents may need support to 'work through' their feelings.

The importance of diagnosis

Clear diagnosis is essential and may greatly relieve the anxieties of many parents who may blame themselves for their child's problems. It may allow access to specific supports including parent groups and support organizations. These can provide valuable support and education and help answer the many questions which parents have (e.g. usual course, associated problems, prognosis). For inherited conditions, the issue of further genetic counselling/testing of family members needs to be addressed. Provision of clear information allows individuals to make informed decisions about being tested and to weigh the risks of having other affected children.

The effect on other family members

Although it was previously thought that having a child with LD impacted adversely on other unaffected siblings (often leading to the removal of the child from the family), there is little evidence that this is the case and worries about long-term damage appear unfounded. In fact, brothers and sisters of individuals with LD often appear to be drawn to the caring professions and many end up working as doctors, nurses, teachers, or providing support for children with special needs. Grandparents may be a useful supportive resource for parents, but may also need to come to terms with their own feelings of having a disabled grandchild.

The 'burden of care'

For carers, informal support may actually be more valuable than formal (professional) support. Frequent appointments or regular home visits may be more disruptive than helpful. Developmental delay brings with it associated problems (e.g. longer time until the child can walk, achieve continence, acquire language/communication skills, establish a normal sleep pattern). The social, financial, and psychological impact on carers should be acknowledged and appropriate help and support provided. For infants and children, schooling may be both a benefit (in terms of learning social skills, support/respite for parents, and close contact with teachers/other parents) and a burden (particularly if necessary specialist schooling is not locally available). Transitional periods (e.g. adolescence/early adulthood) are accompanied by parental anxieties as well as changes in how needs are met (see **Transition periods** 📖 p. 770). Advance planning will go some way to alleviate increased carer stress. Carers may also be concerned about what will happen to their child when they are no longer able to care for them and the open discussion of these issues, with provisional planning, may help avert crises.

Needs and priorities

- Early, accurate diagnosis.
- Informative genetic advice to parents and other family members.
- Access to high-quality primary (and secondary) health care.
- Advice and access to appropriate help and support (practical help, financial assistance, social and educational needs).
- Help and advice with any communication problems (communication aids, learning of sign language).
- Consideration of the needs of carers (education, support groups, respite care).
- Provision of specialist and domiciliary help with specific behavioural problems.
- 'Safety net' of open access to increased support when necessary.
- Acknowledgement that needs will change over time (and planning for this—see 📖 p. 770).

Liaison psychiatry

Introduction

Liaison psychiatry[1] is concerned with the assessment and management of psychiatric and psychological illnesses in general medical populations. The subspecialty is a relatively recent innovation and has expanded considerably in both role and practitioner numbers over the last 25yrs. It offers an opportunity for interesting and varied clinical practice and research at the interface between psychiatry and medicine.

History The development of a distinct subspecialty of liaison psychiatry arose in large part due to the physical separation of psychiatric specialists from their medical and surgical colleagues with the establishment of asylums separate from the general hospitals in the nineteenth century. Following this separation, a number of practitioners remained within the general hospitals with a special interest in 'nervous disorders', working at the boundary between neurology and psychiatry. At that time the distinction between the two specialties was not as clear as it later became.

As neurological practice became more scientific, the role of psychological factors became less an object of clinical attention for neurologists. At the same time, psychoanalytic theories were pre-eminent within psychiatry, and interest in, and involvement with, organic illnesses declined. However, by the early twentieth century there was increasing attention to psychosomatic factors in the aetiology and maintenance of disease and their role in recovery. With the onset of 'biological psychiatry' in the mid-twentieth century, a number of pioneering individuals began psychiatric practice within the general hospitals. They advocated the need for recognition and treatment of psychological factors in physical illness and began the process of establishing links with medical colleagues, identifying appropriate cases for intervention and gaining funding for service development and research.

The development of the subspecialty was motivated by the low rate of outside referral in proportion to prevalence of the disorders in the medical population and increasing medical specialization leading to lack of confidence and competence with psychiatric/psychological problems in physicians and surgeons. By the 1970s a distinct subspeciality was recognized in both the UK and the US. It was staffed mainly by sole practitioners who were generally confined to the larger hospitals. They developed services and established models and ways of working and in particular developed links with individual departments with particular needs. In the last quarter-century there has been growth in both role and practitioner numbers. This growth has often been service-led, with demand and hence funding from individual clinical services who see the need for regular psychiatric input.

Roles and responsibilities The role of the liaison psychiatrist and the types of referral seen will vary by the hospital type, the population served, and the specialty mix within the hospital.
- *Direct consultation on the general wards* Requests for advice on diagnosis, prognosis, and management of psychiatric disorder.
- *Direct liaison with specialist units* A closer relationship with a specialist unit, with involvement in unit planning, staff support, policy

development, and training as well as involvement in individual clinical cases.

- *Emergency department* Assessment of patients presenting with symptoms suggestive of mental disorder, following deliberate self-harm, and of patients brought in by the police to a 'place of safety'.
- *Outpatient referrals* Outpatients referred from general medical, surgical, or obstetric clinics. Some services also take GP referrals, particularly of cases with somatization or medically unexplained symptoms.
- *Teaching and training* Formal teaching of undergraduate and postgraduate medical trainees and training of paramedical and nursing staff.
- *Research and audit* Particularly research into the psychological and psychiatric effects of medical illness and into deliberate self-harm.

Presentations

The range of psychiatric presentations and disorders seen in the general hospital is very wide and liaison psychiatrists can expect to see conditions described in all of the chapters of this handbook. In our clinical practice we have found the following 12 referral types to be the most common.

- Patients presenting after deliberate self-harm or with suicidal thoughts or plans (📖 p. 784).
- Assessment of mood or anxiety symptoms (📖 p. 780).
- Issues of consent, capacity, or detainability (📖 p. 794).
- Assessment of confusion or cognitive impairment (📖 p. 790).
- Assessment of psychotic symptoms (📖 p. 782).
- Request for advice in a patient with pre-existing psychiatric problems.
- Patients referred during pregnancy or in the puerperium (📖 p. 470).
- Medically unexplained symptoms (📖 p. 796).
- Alcohol or drug problems (📖 p. 552, p. 592).
- Assessment prior to listing for organ transplantation (📖 p. 816).
- Psychiatric symptoms secondary to organic illness (Chapter 5).
- Eating disorders (Chapter 10).

---

1 The subspecialty is generally known as 'liaison psychiatry' within the UK, but is also referred to as 'psychosomatic medicine', 'consultation–liaison psychiatry', and 'psychological medicine'.

Working in the general hospital

While working as a psychiatrist in a medical setting you are in a sense acting as an ambassador for psychiatry[1] in general. You may well be the only psychiatrist whom colleagues in other specialties will regularly meet. You should therefore aim to be available, approachable, considerate, practical, and strive to be a 'problem-solver'. In this role as 'ambassador for psychiatry' you will have the opportunity to meet and encourage medical students and doctors in training, some of whom may not have previously thought of psychiatry as a career. You will also have the opportunity to teach staff in multiple professions and grades, both on a case by case basis, and during formal teaching sessions.

When you first come to work in the general hospital you may feel overwhelmed. There are many new disorders, altered presentations of familiar disorders, a new tempo of working, and patients suffering medical conditions about which you may know very little. Additionally, general hospital doctors in the various specialties will have their own ideas about psychiatry, as well as about the indicated treatment in each case (which may differ from yours). Nonetheless it is well to remember that you have a range of skills and knowledge that will be useful and are not shared by other members of staff. You should rely on these and your own judgement, backed up by senior colleagues, in difficult situations.

Taking referrals The person receiving the referral should take details of the patient, their GP, their treating team, and the nature of the problem, including its urgency. It is important to clarify what questions the treating team wants addressed. It is vital to clarify that the patient understands that psychiatric referral has been made and agrees to this.

Gathering information Where the situation is not an emergency, it is useful to review any departmental or other psychiatric records for previous contacts, prior to assessing the patient. A discussion with the GP may also be helpful. On arrival on the ward, review the medical record of this and previous admissions and speak to a senior member of the treating team. Clarify the patient's diagnosis and any investigations or treatments planned. Discuss the patient with the nursing staff—they may have useful information regarding the patient's symptoms around the clock and their mood day to day.

Approach to the patient Arrange a private room for the interview if at all possible. Introduce yourself to the patient as a psychiatrist or a psychological medicine specialist. Explain your role, which may be misunderstood by the patient, who may feel you are there to 'see if I'm crazy'. Stating that the medical team is concerned about some of the patient's symptoms and they want a specialist in these symptoms to give them some advice is often an acceptable phrasing for patients.

Assessing psychiatric symptoms on the general wards The assessment of psychiatric symptoms in the general hospital is broadly similar to their assessment in psychiatric settings. There are, however, a number of important differences:

- The patient's medical condition, the clinical urgency of the situation or the setting (e.g. A&E, ITU) may make full or normal assessment impossible.
- The patient's medical symptoms may confuse the issue: symptoms of psychiatric disorders overlap with those of many medical conditions.
- The differential diagnosis and relative likelihood of various psychiatric diagnoses is different between the general medical and psychiatric populations.

The assessment of depressive, anxiety, and psychotic symptoms and of confusion on the general wards is described on 📖 pp. 780–91, as well as the differential diagnosis for these symptoms in the general setting.

Management of psychiatric illness on the general wards The pharmacology and psychology of particular psychiatric disorders is broadly similar in the psychiatric and the general hospital setting. The differences relate to factors imposed by the patient's medical condition and the environment. When considering medication, consult 📖 pp. 968–79 which describe the prescribing of psychotropics in specific medical conditions.

Documenting your findings When documenting your findings in the medical notes remember that the written record has a dual purpose—it acts both to document the clinical contact and to communicate information about your findings and opinion. In general, the medical team will be more interested in the opinion and any associated management advice than in detailed history or psychiatric formulation. You should avoid any jargon or acronyms which are specific to psychiatry.

Stating your opinion Aim to specifically answer any questions you have been asked. If a definitive psychiatric diagnosis is possible, write this clearly in the notes, along with a provisional management plan and any treatment recommendations. Clarify in the notes if further psychiatric review is planned and when, and which symptoms should cause them to seek an earlier review. If at all possible, discuss your findings with the medical team face to face. Remember that general hospital doctors will have less experience than you in psychiatric issues and it will be necessary to 'spell out' some things—e.g. what is the implication of detention? What side-effects should they look out for after antipsychotic prescription?

1 Masterton G (2003) Liaison psychiatry and general hospital management. *Br J Psychiat* **183**: 366.

Assessment of depressive and anxiety symptoms

Depressive symptoms

One of the most common referrals in liaison psychiatry is of patients with low mood. Apparent low mood is a common presentation of hypoactive delirium (📖 p. 790) and so assessment of orientation and basic cognitive testing is an important part of the assessment of mood symptoms in the general setting. If delirium is ruled out, the next step is to assess the nature and severity of the mood disorder and, if depressive illness is present, to make suggestions as to appropriate management.

Differential diagnosis

Depressive illness (📖 p. 788 and p. 248), hypoactive delirium (📖 p. 790), normal emotional response to illness or loss, adjustment reactions (📖 p. 386), drug or alcohol misuse, depression secondary to organic cause.

Organic causes of depressive symptoms

- Neurological (CVA, epilepsy, Parkinson's disease, brain tumour, dementia, multiple sclerosis, Huntington's disease, head injury)
- Infectious (HIV and related opportunistic infections, EBV/CMV, infectious mononucleosis, Lyme disease)
- Endocrine and metabolic (hypothyroidism, hyperprolactinaemia, Cushing's disease, Addison's disease, parathyroid disease)
- Cardiac disease (MI, cardiac bypass surgery, heart failure)
- Systemic disease (systemic lupus erythematosus [SLE], rheumatoid arthritis, cancer)
- Medications (analgesics, antihypertensives, levodopa (L-dopa), anticonvulsants, benzodiazepines, antibiotics, steroids, combined oral contraceptive, cytotoxics, cimetidine)
- Substance misuse (alcohol, BDZs, cannabis, cocaine, opioids).

Key points in assessment

- *Is there evidence of confusion?* Examine for orientation and perform a basic test of cognitive function (e.g. abbreviated mental test [AMT], MMSE). Acute onset of confusion (or acute deterioration of existing impairment) together with an apathetic, 'depressed' presentation, is seen in patients with hypoactive delirium (📖 p. 790).
- *How does the patient describe their mood?* It is vital to gain an understanding of the patient's subjective mood. Often referrals are made without this information because patients 'look depressed'.
- *Explore cognitive depressive symptoms* Biological depressive features may be less useful as diagnostic features in physically ill patients—impairment of sleep, appetite, energy levels, concentration, and libido may be due to depression or may be due to the medical condition itself. For this reason cognitive symptoms are more important diagnostically:
  - *Do they describe hopelessness?* How do they view their situation? What do they think the future holds for them? Do they think things will ever improve? Patients with depressive illnesses tend to maintain

a gloomy and pessimistic view of the future, while non-depressed patients will often remain optimistic about improvements in their condition and look forward to rehab or discharge.
* *Anhedonia* Are they still doing things they enjoy doing (if they are physically able to)? If not, do they still wish they could do those things or have they lost interest altogether? Do they seem to retain pleasure in family visits?
* *Lack of reactivity* Are they flat in affect? Emotionless? These are more indicative of a clinical depression.
* *Collateral information* Obtain information from close family or others who know the patient well. This can add insight into the severity, duration, and temporal relationship of the symptom course.

Anxiety symptoms

Anxiety is a common phenomenon in medically ill patients and may often be viewed as appropriate to their current situation. Where it is severe, prolonged, out of keeping with the current situation, or is interfering with appropriate medical management it may become a focus of clinical attention. Often medical patients don't meet full diagnostic criteria for diagnosis of an anxiety disorder—it is important to make an individual assessment and make a decision based on symptom severity and impairment whether treatment would help the anxiety.

Differential diagnosis

Realistic worry over medical condition, primary medical condition, alcohol withdrawal, prescribed or illicit drug withdrawal (esp. benzodiazepine or opiate), drug intoxication (esp. stimulants), generalized anxiety disorder or panic disorder (new or exacerbation of pre-existing disorder), anxiety as part of a depressive illness, specific phobia (esp. needle phobia).

Organic causes of anxiety symptoms

* Neurological (epilepsy, dementia, head injury, CVA, brain tumour, MS, Parkinson's disease).
* Pulmonary (COPD, asthma, airway-assisted patients on weaning trials).
* Cardiac (arrhythmias, heart failure [CHF], angina, mitral valve prolapse).
* Hyperthyroidism, hypoglycaemia, metabolic acidosis/alkalosis, phaeochromocytoma.
* Medications (antidepressants, antihypertensives, antiarrhythmics).
* Drugs of abuse (alcohol, BDZs, caffeine, cannabis, cocaine, LSD, ecstasy, amfetamines).

Key points in assessment

* *Medical work-up* Assess for medical causes for symptoms first. Has the patient had a complete medical evaluation for the physical complaints?
* *Consider substance abuse/ingestion* Always take a drug/alcohol history, and selected patients should have urine drug screen.
* *Past psychiatric history* Does the patient have an underlying anxiety disorder that is being made worse by a new medical stressor?
* *Are there psychological anxiety symptoms?* Do the subjective match the objective findings? Does the patient feel like or fear they are going to die? Have a sense of doom? Fear they are going crazy?

Assessment of psychotic symptoms and confusion

Psychotic symptoms

While referrals for assessment of apparent psychotic symptoms are common in the general setting, presentations with functional psychoses are rare in comparison with psychiatric hospitals. They *are* seen in the emergency department, in patients brought in by police to a 'place of safety' and after self-harm (especially in those using violent or bizarre methods). However, in the majority of cases in the general hospital psychotic features represent organic illnesses—commonly delirium, or are part of a withdrawal syndrome.

Differential diagnosis

Delirium (📖 p. 790), drug intoxication or withdrawal, alcohol withdrawal, epileptic phenomena (📖 p. 156), dementia (📖 p. 132), schizophrenia (📖 p. 178), acute/transient psychotic disorders (📖 p. 226).

Organic causes of psychosis

- Neurological (epilepsy, head injury, brain tumour, dementia, encephalitis, e.g. HSV, HIV, neurosyphilis, brain abscess, CVA).
- Endocrine (hyper/hypothyroidism, Cushing's, hyperparathyroidism, Addison's disease).
- Metabolic (uraemia, electrolyte disturbance, porphyria).
- SLE ('lupus psychosis').
- Medications (steroids, levodopa (L-dopa), interferon, anticholinergics, antihypertensives, anticonvulsants, stimulants).
- Drugs of abuse (cocaine, LSD, cannabis, PCP, amfetamines, opioids).

Key points in assessment

- *The nature of any hallucinations* Auditory hallucinations are characteristic of functional psychoses, while visual hallucinations (and visual illusions and misperceptions) are seen in organic conditions.
- *Presence of fluctuations* Note whether symptoms are fluctuating in nature or associated with confusion and/or behavioural disturbance. A waxing and waning picture with alterations in attention and alertness suggest delirium as opposed to a primary psychotic disorder.
- *Previous history* Note any previous history of psychotic illness or previous or current history of drug or alcohol use.
- *Time course of illness* How long have psychotic symptoms been present? Was there a gradual or sudden onset? Have previous similar episodes occurred before?
- *Vital signs* Withdrawal syndromes can present with psychotic symptoms. It is helpful to look for any autonomic instability, vital sign changes, sweating, and tremor which may suggest an underlying withdrawal from alcohol or other sedatives. Such changes would be less likely in a primary psychotic disorder.

Confusion

A common referral is the request to assess for the severity and possible cause of confusion. A wide range of disorders and insults to the brain produce three common clinical presentations: (1) acute confusional state or delirium, (2) dementia (progressive or non-progressive), and (3) acute or chronic confusion. A common question is the extent to which a confusion reflects acute or chronic deficit—often linked to requests for opinion about capacity/consent and placement issues. Another key question is whether there is a reversible component to the condition.

Differential diagnosis

Delirium (📖 p. 790), dementia (📖 p. 132), alcohol withdrawal, drug intoxication or withdrawal, Wernicke–Korsakoff syndrome, epileptic phenomena, functional psychoses.

Key points in assessment

- *Bedside cognitive testing* Assess conscious level (via GCS— 📖 p. 69), orientation in time, place, and person, and make an objective measurement of confusion (e.g. AMT, MMSE, ACE— 📖 p. 70).
- *Previous history* For an accurate account of the previous history in a confused patient it is *vital* to have corroboration of the patient's account—this should ideally be by a live-in or close relative or friend, but in their absence a neighbour or GP may provide useful information. Note any previous history of cognitive impairment or functional decline; any history of alcohol of drug use; and any history of previous similar episodes.
- *Previous functional level* It is important to consider the degree of cognitive deficit now, and the level of cognitive function over the lifespan, reflected in the educational achievement of the patient and their work status, and their recent cognitive function as reflected in their self-care, etc.
- *Medical status* Note current medical condition as recorded in the case records and nursing notes/observations. Note recent investigation findings, noting particularly any abnormal results or recent changes. Examine drug kardex for any medications associated with confusion—have any medications recently been started or stopped?
- *Consideration of specialist testing* In selected cases specialist neurocognitive assessment may be helpful.
- *Consideration of imaging* In consultation with medical and radiology colleagues, consider whether cerebral imaging (e.g. CT, MRI) is indicated.

Parasuicide assessment

Parasuicide is a deliberately undertaken act which mimics the act of suicide but does not result in death. Psychiatric assessment of such patients is mandatory once their medical condition allows. The involvement of mental health professionals in the assessment of patients following parasuicide relates to the following observations:

- In this population of patients, roughly 1% will die by completed suicide in the 24mths after the initial parasuicidal act, with the risk highest in the weeks following the original act. This represents a mortality by suicide 50–100 times that of the general population.
- The rates of completed suicide are significantly raised in all mental disorders excepting mental handicap and dementia. Studies examining completed suicides in patients with mental illness show inadequate doses of therapeutic drug treatment, increased dropout rate from follow-up and increased presence of untreated comorbidity.
- Clear risk factors exist for completed suicide (see Box 19.1) and the closer the parasuicidal patient approximates to these demographics, the greater the relative risk. However, the absolute risk is low and estimate of the risk in a particular case relies on assessment of the individual act and the mental state.

Assessment The initial management of the patient following overdose or other deliberate self-harm will be by specialist toxicologists or general medical/surgical specialists. Early psychiatric assessment may be required for advice regarding detainability, behavioural disturbance, drug/alcohol withdrawal, or delirium, but assessment of the parasuicide itself should be deferred until conscious level is full. The history should focus on the act itself, the patient's mental state and recent life events, and past medical/psychiatric history. It may be easier to assess these in reverse order, moving from the factual history towards the emotive descriptions of the parasuicidal act itself after building rapport.

Features of act

- **Method** ~90% of parasuicides are by self-poisoning with self-cutting making up most of the remainder. Use of method likely to be fatal (e.g. jumping, hanging) is indicative of clear intent to die.
- **Patient's belief in the lethality of the method** Did the patient believe that that combination of tablets was likely to be fatal? Serious suicidal intent is associated with medically trivial overdoses—and vice versa.
- **Length of planning** Was the act impulsive—'on the spur of the moment', or planned in advance—and for how long?
- **Triggers** Was there a clear precipitant (e.g. row with partner)? Were they intoxicated at the time? Was there any direct 'gain' (e.g. patient in custody at the time of act)?
- **Final acts** Was there a suicide note? Did they make any other 'acts of closure' (e.g. setting affairs in order, arranging for the care of children)?
- **Precautions to avoid discovery** Where did the act take place? Would they have anticipated being found? Did they signal or tell their intentions to another? Was anyone else actually present at the time?

- **Previous similar acts** Is this act a repeat of a previous non-fatal act? Are there any different features?
- **Actions after act** What did they do after the act? How did they end up coming to hospital?

Mental state
- **Attitude now to survival** Are they relieved or disappointed to be alive? Do they have ongoing wish to die? How do they feel about the future and what plans (if any) do they have?
- **Affective symptoms** Current affective symptoms. Recent symptoms of low mood, anhedonia, and hopelessness. Biological depressive features.
- **Substance misuse problems** Evidence for current drug or alcohol misuse or dependence.
- **Other mental disorder** Enquire directly about other symptoms of mental disorder as directed by the history.
- **Risk to others** Is there any evidence of intent to harm anyone else? Did the parasuicidal act put anyone else at risk?

Personal and past medical/psychiatric history
- **Recent life events** Describe recent events involving loss or change (e.g. bereavements, job loss, relationship break-up).
- **Current life situation** State of current significant relationships. Type and security of job and accommodation. Presence of legal/criminal problems.
- **Previous or current psychiatric diagnoses** Clarify with hospital records if further details required or if significant history.
- **Physical health problems** Again clarify with records or GP if required.

Box 19.1 Risk factors for completed suicide

Sociodemographic factors
- Male sex.
- Elderly.
- Single, divorced, or widowed.
- Living alone, poor social support.
- Unemployed or low socio-economic class.

Personal/mental health factors
- Previous parasuicide or DSH.
- Any mental disorder (greatest risk in major depression and anorexia nervosa, then functional psychosis, then neurotic and personality disorders).
- Dependence on alcohol or drugs.
- Recent inpatient psychiatric treatment.
- Concurrent physical disorder.
- Recent bereavement.

Management after parasuicide

Reasons for act Only a minority of patients presenting after parasuicide have evidence of clear intent to die. Assessment will reveal a mixture of the following types of case:

- Those whose intent was unequivocally to die but were prevented by discovery, chance, or overestimation of the lethality of the method.
- Those who were ambivalent whether they lived or died, 'letting the chips fall as they may'.
- Those whose act was impulsive and 'in the heat of the moment' in response to an immediate stressor.
- Those whose actions were designed to communicate distress—the classical 'cry for help'.
- Those whose actions were manipulative in nature and designed to provoke changed behaviour from others.
- Those attempting to escape from intolerable symptoms or an intolerable situation.
- Those whose intent is later unclear even to themselves.

There may initially be diagnostic confusion with the following groups: (1) deliberate overdoses of drugs taken for intoxicating effect; (2) deliberate self-harm (e.g. wrist cutting) which is a repetitive, ritualistic action whose intent is to relieve tension, not to kill or seriously injure; (3) accidental overdoses of prescribed or OTC medication. (1) and (2) may merit psychiatric evaluation in their own right and (3) should be examined carefully for evidence of post hoc rationalization of a parasuicide.

Assessment aims By the end of assessment you should aim to answer the following questions:

- **Is there ongoing suicidal intent?** Evidenced by: continuing stated wish to die; ambivalence about survival; sense of hopelessness towards future; clear intent to die at time of act.
- **Is there evidence of mental illness?** Diagnosed in the normal way. Most common diagnoses are depressive illness and alcohol misuse. Be alert to comorbid substance misuse and to the combination of an acute stressor on the background of a chronic condition.
- **Are there non-mental health issues which can be addressed?** Many patients will reveal stressors such as: family or relationship difficulties; emotional problems (particularly relating to previous abuse; school or employment problems; debt; legal problems; problems related to immigration). They can be usefully directed to appropriate local services.

Management

- **Ongoing suicidal intent** In many cases this will be managed by admission to a psychiatric ward, on a compulsory basis if necessary.
- **Mental illness**
  - *Patients already known to mental health services* Here close liaison with the usual team is required to agree a joint management plan.
  - *New diagnoses* Here the focus should be on integrating with an appropriate service for follow-up, rather than necessarily starting

new treatments. The type of appropriate follow-up depends on the type of disorder (e.g. GP review for moderate depressive illness, referral to alcohol services for alcohol abuse). Short-term community outreach from liaison psychiatry can 'bridge' the patient to the general services. Try to ensure follow-up is as soon as possible, even if non-urgent, as otherwise non-attendance is very high.

- *Admission required* For both new and established mental illnesses, admission will sometimes be indicated after parasuicide even where there is no ongoing suicidal intent. This may be due to seriousness of condition (e.g. new psychotic illness) or to allow for a period of inpatient assessment of mental state. It should not simply be in order to defer or devolve the decision about discharge—ask yourself what will have changed to mean discharge in a few days will be safer than now.

- **Other issues** With the patient's permission discuss the case with an appropriate agency (e.g. abuse counselling service, school counsellor). Clarify the appropriateness of the referral and referral method and feed these back to the patient.

- **In all cases** Discuss and agree management plan with patient. In most cases discuss with GP (mandatory if GP input is required). Consider provision of emergency crisis card giving details of emergency psychiatric service and telephone contact for emergency counselling/ support services.

Frequent attenders A small minority of patients attend emergency services repeatedly with parasuicidal acts or deliberate self-harm without suicidal intent. A management plan for such patients should be agreed on a case-by-case basis. The aim should be to avoid 'rewarding' maladaptive behaviours (e.g. by repeated admissions providing 'time-out' from stressful situations), while providing appropriate support and treatment.

Depression in physical illness

Depressive illness is more common in those with physical illness than in the healthy population. In primary care the prevalence of depressive illness is ~5%, while in medical outpatients it is 5–10% and in medical inpatients it is 10–20%, with higher rates reported in some studies. The frequency of depressive illness is raised in those with more severe illnesses, and some conditions (e.g. cardiac and neurological disorders) show very high rates.

Occurrence of depression in physically ill patients adds to their morbidity, both due to the depressive symptoms themselves, and by hampering the treatment of the underlying medical condition (e.g. by impairing compliance or by diminishing interest in rehabilitation). Additionally there is increased risk of cardiac mortality in depressed patients, which is directly correlated with the severity of the depression.

Depression is poorly recognized and undertreated in general patients. In some medical settings there is a lack of focus on psychiatric symptoms—'not willing to ask the question'. There is also often a reluctance to prescribe antidepressants in context of medical illness. More often the possibility of treatment is simply overlooked with the patient assuming that the symptoms are due to their underlying disorder and the treating physician making assumptions (e.g. 'I'd be depressed in his situation') and not thinking of offering treatment.

Reasons for the association of depression and physical illness

- The physical illness causes the depression:
  - Biological cause—e.g. hypothyroidism, Cushing's disease, Parkinson's disease.
  - Psychological cause—related to loss or change, life events secondary to illness, e.g. amputation, loss of sexual function. Particularly potent are fatal or potentially fatal, disfiguring, or disabling diseases.
- The depression is a side-effect of the treatment for the physical illness:
  - Drug treatments, e.g. steroids, β-blockers, digoxin, calcium channel blockers, aminophylline, theophylline, NSAIDs, cimetidine, metoclopramide, levodopa, methyldopa, isotretinoin, α interferon.
  - Disfiguring, painful, or prolonged treatments.
- The physical illness is a result of the depression—e.g. liver failure after paracetamol overdose in context of depressive relapse.
- The physical illness and the depression have a common cause—e.g. stressful life events acting as precipitants to both MI and depression.
- Their co-occurrence may be coincidental—depressive illness is common and its co-occurrence with other common illnesses can be expected by chance.

Presentations of depression in physical illness

Low mood, tearfulness, hopelessness regarding recovery, biological depressive features (poor sleep, appetite, energy, and concentration)—which may be misinterpreted as symptoms of the physical disorder, poor compliance, increase in somatic complaints or complaints of pain severity, apparent cognitive impairment (pseudodementia).

Diagnosis

Nursing staff are often more proficient than medical colleagues at identifying medical inpatients with depressive disorders. While operational diagnostic criteria are the same in physically ill as in physically well patients, biological features may be less useful in making the diagnosis. Features:

* Depression of mood (is it pervasive or do some activities—e.g. family visits—still provide pleasure?)
* Hopelessness (is the patient's attitude that although things are bad now they can still look forward—e.g. to going home, to moving to the rehab ward, or are they hopeless about any prospects for recovery?)
* Morning depression (do the nurses note a diurnal variation in mood, or in other marker symptoms, e.g. interest in rehab, talkativeness?)

Screening tools are available (e.g. Geriatric Depression Scale) and are used in some centres. They do not replace individual clinical assessment.

Treatment (see also pp. 256–9)

Effective treatment offers the possibility of improvement in mood (which is of course valuable in itself) but also improved rehabilitation, better compliance, decreased hospital stay, and an overall reduction in morbidity, mortality, and eventual disability.

* *Practical interventions*: e.g. attention to specific worries (e.g. clarification of prognosis, about which the patient may be unduly pessimistic); attempt to improve social contacts; aim to optimize medical condition, mobility, and pain control.
* *Psychological support*: often the liaison psychiatrist will have a key role here, but you should also attempt to engage the nursing and paramedical staff in supportive psychotherapeutic interventions—often these staff members are enthusiastic about constructive involvement but fearful of 'doing the wrong thing', and will appreciate your guidance.
* *Consideration of drug treatment:* treatment strategies are similar to those in patients without medical illness while taking note of the advice given for treatment in specific medical conditions (pp. 968–79).
* *Specific psychological treatments:* individual psychotherapy is often unavailable in or unsuited to the general setting, but some therapies, e.g. CBT, are now incorporated into rehabilitation and pain management programmes.

Acute confusional state (delirium)

Essence

Stereotyped response of the brain to a variety of insults, very commonly seen in hospital inpatients. Syndrome characterized by **acute** onset of fluctuating cognitive impairment (or deterioration in pre-existing cognitive impairment) associated with behavioural abnormalities. Like other acute organ failures it is commoner in those with chronic impairment of that organ (e.g. dementia, may be undiagnosed).

Epidemiology

Extremely common in medical and surgical inpatients (10–20%). Particularly vulnerable include: elderly; pre-existing dementia; blind or deaf; very young; post-operative (especially cardiac); burn victims; alcohol- and benzodiazepine-dependent; serious illness, particularly multiple. Carries significant mortality, as well as morbidity to patient and others. Common cause of delayed discharge.

Clinical features

- Impaired ability to direct, sustain, and shift attention.
- Global impairment of cognition with disorientation, and impairment of recent memory and abstract thinking.
- Disturbance in sleep–wake cycle with nocturnal worsening.
- Psychomotor agitation.
- Emotional lability.
- Perceptual distortions, illusions, and hallucinations—characteristically visual.
- Speech may be rambling, incoherent, and thought disordered.
- There may be poorly developed paranoid delusions.
- Onset of clinical features is rapid with fluctuations in severity over minutes and hours (even back to apparent normality).

Three clinical presentations are commonly seen, distinguished by differing combinations of symptoms: *hyperactive or agitated delirium* (psychomotor agitation, increased arousal, inappropriate behaviour, delusions, and hallucinations); *hypoactive delirium* (psychomotor retardation, lethargy, excess somnolence); and *mixed delirium* (combination of these features with varying presentation over time).

Differential diagnosis

Mood disorder; psychotic illness (new major mental disorder very much less likely than delirium in a hospitalized patient, particularly if elderly); post-ictal; dementia (characteristically has insidious onset with stable course and clear consciousness).

Aetiology

The cause is frequently multifactorial and the most likely cause varies with the clinical setting in which the patient presents:

- **Infective** UTI; chest infection; wound abscess; cellulitis; subacute bacterial endocarditis (SBE).

- **Metabolic** Anaemia; electrolyte disturbance; hepatic encephalopathy; uraemia; cardiac failure; hypothermia.
- **Intracranial** CVA; head injury; encephalitis; primary or metastatic tumour; raised ICP.
- **Endocrine** Pituitary, thyroid, parathyroid, or adrenal diseases; hypoglycaemia; diabetes mellitus; vitamin deficiencies.
- **Substance intoxication or withdrawal** Alcohol; BDZs; anticholinergics; psychotropics; lithium; antihypertensives; diuretics; anticonvulsants; digoxin; steroids; NSAIDs.
- **Hypoxia** Secondary to any cause.

Course and prognosis

Delirium usually has a sudden onset with a fluctuating clinical course thereafter. There is gradual resolution of symptoms with effective treatment of the underlying cause. Symptom resolution may be much slower in the elderly. There is often patchy amnesia for the period of delirium following recovery. Mortality is high (~20% of patients will die during that hospital admission, up to 50% at 1yr). May be a marker for the subsequent development of dementia.

Assessment (see also 📖 p. 782)

- Attend promptly (situation only tends to deteriorate and behaviourally disturbed patients cause considerable anxiety on medical wards).
- Review time course of condition via notes and staff report—note recent investigation findings, particularly any abnormal results or recent changes. Examine kardex for any drugs associated with confusion—have any medications recently been started or stopped?
- Establish premorbid functional level (e.g. from relatives or GP).

Management

Four main principles of management:

- Identify and treat precipitating cause and exacerbating factors.
  - Likely primary cause varies according to setting and examination finding—remember cause may be multifactorial.
  - Optimize patient's condition—attention to hydration, nutrition, elimination, pain control.
- Provide environmental and supportive measures.
  - Education of those who interact with the patient.
  - Make environment safe.
  - Create an environment which optimizes stimulation—e.g. adequate lighting, reduce unnecessary noise, mobilize patient whenever possible, and correct any sensory impairment (e.g. hearing aids, glasses).
  - Reality orientation techniques. Firm clear communication, preferably by same staff member (or small group of staff). Use of clocks and calendars.
- Avoid sedation unless severely agitated or necessary to minimize risk to patient or to facilitate investigation/treatment.
  - Use single medication, start at a low dose and titrate to effects.
  - Give dose and reassess in 2–4hrs before prescribing regularly.

- Consider oral haloperidol 0.5–1mg up to max of 6mg daily, oral lorazepam 0.5–1mg up to max of 4mg daily, or oral risperidone 1–4mg up to max of 6mg daily—consider giving preference to antipsychotic management in the first instance, benzodiazepines tend to worsen delirium with the exception of alcohol withdrawal and gammabutyrolactone (GBL) withdrawal.
- For delirium related to alcohol withdrawal, BDZs are the drugs of choice—see 📖 p. 560.
- Review dose regularly and aim to stop as soon as possible.
- Regular clinical review and follow-up (MMSE useful in monitoring cognitive improvement at follow-up).

Capacity and consent[1]

A fundamental principle of medical practice is that treatment of a patient should be with their valid consent. Valid consent is that which is informed freely given, and obtained from a patient with *capacity*. The medical team will often ask for a psychiatric opinion as to a patient's capacity to make treatment decisions. While all doctors should be familiar with assessment of capacity and be prepared to make decisions regarding consent, liaison psychiatrists are often consulted on such matters due to their experience in assessing mental disorder and abnormal mental states and their (usually) greater knowledge of applicable law.

Incapacity legislation Specific incapacity legislation exists in England and Wales (the Mental Capacity Act 2005—📖 p. 876), and Scotland (the Adults with Incapacity Act 2000—📖 p. 878). These Acts and their accompanying codes of practice should direct and guide clinical practice relating to incapacity for doctors working in these jurisdictions.

Referral types Occasionally, these referrals will take the form of a specific question, e.g. does this patient with dementia have capacity to give consent to a hip operation? More often they reflect a number of worries about a patient's capacity, ability to care for themselves, and decisions which balance a patient's autonomy against best exercising their duty of care. The two most common referrals ask the following questions:
- Does this patient have the capacity to consent to or refuse consent for a procedure or treatment?
- Does this patient have the capacity to make personal welfare decisions (e.g. to choose to go home rather than accept residential care)?

Occasionally a referral is phrased as a capacity assessment when the patient is seeking to leave hospital against medical advice and what is actually required is a decision as to the patient's detainability under the Mental Health Act. In these cases the patient should be assessed for the presence of mental disorder justifying detention in the normal way. In these cases remember that detention under the Mental Health Act does not allow for the compulsory treatment of medical conditions.

Assessment of incapacity

1. Identify the question
The question—'does this patient have capacity?' is essentially meaningless. Incapacity law and common law in the UK presume capacity in adults, and incapacity law explicitly encourages the exercise of residual capacity. Incapacity must therefore be assessed in relation to the particular decision required of the patient and the nature of this decision should be established prior to the interview. Additionally you should clarify with the medical team what treatment is proposed, and what information has already been discussed with the patient.

2. Consider whether the patient has capacity to make the decision
Incapacity cannot be presumed on the basis of any individual patient factors (e.g. diagnosis of dementia, learning disability, brain injury, mental disorder)

but must be assessed specifically for each decision. The questions to ask are—*for the decision required*, does the patient have the ability to:
- Make a decision?
- Understand the information relevant to the decision?
- Use or weigh that information in making the decision?
- Retain memory of the decision?
- Communicate the decision?

For example, in considering whether a patient can refuse an amputation in the setting of osteomyelitis and early gangrene, we need to establish whether the patient is aware of the nature of their illness, the treatment being offered to them, the risks and potential benefits associated with that treatment, and any alternative treatment options, as well as the consequences of refusing treatment.

3. Evaluate the presence of psychiatric illness and determine whether it is influencing the patient's decision

Even if the patient's decision reflects a fair grasp of the elements of consent, it is necessary to determine whether their judgement is being influenced by mental illness. For example, if the patient with gangrene understands the nature of their infection and the risks of surgery versus delaying treatment, we would not support their making a decision to avoid surgery if the decision was based on auditory hallucinations telling them that they don't deserve to live. Therefore, a comprehensive psychiatric assessment, screening for the presence of mental disorder, and including an evaluation of how they have made their decision, is essential.

The psychiatric evaluation for a capacity assessment needs to be comprehensive, particularly focusing on cognitive functions, reasoning and judgement; however, it is otherwise similar to any thorough psychiatric examination. The primary difference lies in the additional examination of how the patient has made similar choices in the past and what role psychiatric symptoms are playing in their current decision.

4. Gather additional information

If the opinion is that the patient lacks capacity, then it will be important to establish: (1) what were the patient's views on the matter when greater capacity existed (e.g. did they discuss treatment outcomes with relatives?, is there an advance directive?), (2) what are the views of the patient's relatives or carers?, is there a relative with surrogate decision-making powers (e.g. attorney, court-appointed deputy in England and Wales, or guardian in Scotland)?

5. Report and document opinion

You should formally document your opinion and the reasons for it, as well as speaking to the treating team directly if at all possible.

---

1 This page should be read in conjunction with those pages in the **Legal issues** chapter describing consent (□ p. 870), treatment without consent (□ p. 872), common law (□ p. 874), and incapacity legislation (□ pp. 876–9).

Medically unexplained symptoms 1: introduction

A substantial proportion of patients presenting to primary care, or to an individual hospital specialty, will have symptoms for which, after adequate investigation, no cause can be found. Non-specific symptoms without underlying organic pathology are very common and usually transient. Where they become prolonged enough to merit medical attention they may present to any specialty, with presentations such as pain, loss/disturbance of function, and altered sensation.

Symptom 'meaning' The 'problem' of medically unexplained symptoms (MUS) arises, in part, from the different meanings symptoms hold for patient and doctor. Patients present to doctors with illness (symptoms and behaviours); doctors diagnose and treat disease (pathology and other recognized syndromes). The patient wants explanation and treatment for their symptoms and the route to this is generally through being given a diagnosis. If there is no recognized diagnosis available the doctor may respond with 'there's nothing wrong', expecting to be met with pleasure. The patient, however, is baffled—there is 'something wrong' and the symptoms are still there. The doctor may then undertake a number of courses of action: continue to investigate in the hope of finding something; treat the patient anyway as a therapeutic trial; refer to another specialty; or dismiss the patient.

Psychiatric role The role of psychiatry in the assessment and management of these patients has changed substantially over recent years (hopefully for the better). Formerly patients were referred 'at the end of the line', often after prolonged, inconclusive tests and unsuccessful interventions. Patients often misinterpreted (and resented) the referral as suggesting that symptoms were 'all in your mind', or were feigned. Psychiatrists sometimes took an overly narrow view of their role and responsibility unhelpfully dismissing patients as having 'no psychotic or depressive illness', or colluding with the patient's desire for a 'clean bill of mental health' in order to return to treatment-seeking behaviour. We are currently at an early stage of our understanding of medically unexplained illnesses. While no specialty has all the answers in the management of this patient group, psychiatry can offer: experience of the presentation of MUS across the hospital specialties; ability to assess and treat the frequently comorbid depressive/anxiety symptoms; and a tolerance for diagnostic uncertainty and ability to take a long-term view of improvements.

Misdiagnosis A frequently expressed concern doctors hold about this group of patients is the risk of 'getting it wrong' (often associated with poorly formed worries about litigation). A long-held belief was that, despite repeated negative findings, all such patients (or a majority) would eventually be found to suffer from an organic disease which would, in retrospect, account for their symptoms. This concern was largely based on older, poorly conducted studies with significant methodological flaws. Recent follow-up studies suggest that the misdiagnosis rate for functional illness is ~5% (e.g. comparable to other medical and psychiatric diagnoses).

such as idiopathic epilepsy and schizophrenia). This improvement has followed both the development of modern imaging and investigatory techniques, and the use of operational diagnostic criteria for psychiatric diagnosis.

Iatrogenic harm A problem common to all members of this group of disorders is the potential for iatrogenic harm. These patients often accrue considerable morbidity and even mortality due to excess negative investigations, irradiation, operative procedures, etc. Those disorders associated with chronic pain carry the risk of iatrogenic opiate dependency. Often at the later stages of the patient's illness this secondary morbidity is more problematic than the original symptoms. A major positive intervention in these patients is therefore the avoidance of iatrogenic harm.

Classification Patients presenting with somatic symptoms for which no adequate physical cause can be found make up a large and heterogeneous group in all clinical settings, from primary to tertiary care. Our lack of full understanding of this group of disorders is reflected in the confusing and disputed classification system adopted. Our modern concepts arose from the concept of 'hysteria'—of repressed emotions being expressed as physical symptoms. There are differences between ICD-10 and DSM-IV in the classification of this group of disorders and each classification contains a number of disputed and unsatisfactory categories. One difficulty has been the residual old labels still in use; another has been the confusion of names indicating symptom and disorder; a third has been the substantial overlap between the syndromes described.

Differential diagnosis The differential diagnosis for relatively acute, isolated, medically unexplained symptoms includes:
- Symptoms directly related to psychiatric disorders, such as depression, anxiety disorders, or psychosis.
- Functional somatic illness (📖 p. 798).
- Conversion and dissociative disorders (📖 p. 806).
- Pain disorders (📖 p. 804).
- Somatization disorder (📖 p. 802).
- Factitious disorder (📖 p. 814).
- Malingering.
- Uncommon medical syndromes which have not yet been diagnosed.

Causative mechanisms These are currently unclear, but the following may play a part: patient psychological factors; patient's health beliefs; affective state; underlying personality; degree of autonomic arousal; increased muscle tension; effects of hyperventilation; effects of disturbed sleep; effects of prolonged inactivity; impaired ability to filter afferent stimuli.

Medically unexplained symptoms 2: clinical presentations

Somatization This is the experience of physical symptoms with no—or no sufficient—physical cause, with presumed psychological causation. Somatization is a symptom of various disorders commonly seen in liaison psychiatry and may occur: (1) as a normal accompaniment of physical illnesses; (2) as a common presentation of depressive illness; (3) as a core component of illness ('functional somatic syndromes'); (4) as part of a long-standing pattern of behaviour ('somatization disorder').

1. As a normal accompaniment of physical illnesses

Complaint of symptoms and help-seeking behaviour is adaptive. All illnesses have emotional components which deserve attention. Both doctor and patient may be more comfortable dealing with specialty-appropriate symptoms (e.g. a patient presenting with pain post-radiotherapy may be articulating a desire for reassurance that the tumour has not recurred). While some doctors may be reluctant to deal with the emotional context of illness, patients may have worries and express these as somatic complaints. These should often be understood as part of the emotional reaction to illness, not dismissed as 'functional overlay'. Their appropriate treatment is via consultation with the responsible clinician. Psychological factors may (positively or negatively) influence outcome in treatment of physical illnesses by their effects on advice-seeking, treatment compliance, and perceived quality of life.

2. As a common presentation of depressive illness

A frequent cause of medically unexplained symptoms is somatized depression and anxiety. Somatic complaints (e.g. pain, GI complaints, weakness, loss of appetite) are common presentations of depression, with prevalence increased in certain subgroups (e.g. elderly, children, certain immigrant populations). Anxiety disorders (e.g. atypical panic attacks) can be the cause of unexplained cases of chest pain and shortness of breath. Conversely, anxiety and depressive symptoms are a common finding in both the physically ill and those with somatization.

3. As a core component of illness ('functional somatic syndromes')

These conditions are usually reported as individual clinical syndromes; however, several factors are common to them all. There is presentation by the patient with symptoms which are suggestive of an underlying organic illness; these symptoms cause distress; there is no identifiable organic illness which is sufficient to explain the symptoms; and the causation is attributed to psychological factors which may be more or less apparent. A variety of presentations are seen across the medical and surgical specialties:

- Cardiology—atypical chest pain.
- Respiratory medicine—hyperventilation syndrome (see 📖 p. 356).
- GI medicine—irritable bowel syndrome.
- Infectious diseases—chronic fatigue syndrome.
- Rheumatology—fibromyalgia.

- Neurology—tension headache.
- ENT—globus syndrome.
- General surgery—unexplained abdominal pain.
- Gynaecology—chronic pelvic pain.
- Dentistry—atypical facial pain.

4. As part of a long-standing pattern of behaviour
Somatization disorder (📖 p. 802).

Hypochondriasis (📖 p. 808) This is the belief that one has a particular illness, despite evidence to the contrary—usually takes the form of an over-valued idea, although is more rarely frankly psychotic in nature. A particular form of hypochondriasis is dysmorphophobia (📖 p. 810): the belief that one has a significant deformity.

Conversion/dissociation (📖 p. 806) 'Conversion' or 'dissociation' is the theorized process by which thoughts or memories unacceptable to the conscious mind are repressed from consciousness, and either 'converted' into physical symptoms, sometimes with symbolic meaning to the patient, or result in disruption to the normal integrated functioning of the mind—as evidenced in symptoms such as amnesia, fugue, or stupor.

Factitious symptoms Factitious symptoms are those which are intentionally produced or elaborated, with the aim of receiving a medical diagnosis. Where there is secondary gain (e.g. obtaining opiate prescription, obtaining legal compensation), this is referred to as *malingering*.

Medically unexplained symptoms 3: management principles

Accepting cases for assessment Psychiatrists should be reluctant to accept patients for assessment of MUS where significant doubt still exists in the treating doctor's mind as to the diagnosis (e.g. where significant further investigations are planned). They should also be reluctant to be put in the position of 'last hurdle' before an otherwise planned intervention (e.g. 'I'll perform your operation if the psychiatrist gives the go-ahead').

Management principles Definitive treatments validated by RCT evidence are not currently available for MUS. In addition, these patients present a heterogeneous group, in terms of presentation, 'psychological mindedness', and severity. Nonetheless, the following principles may be helpful. Management should include: (1) thorough assessment; (2) confident diagnosis; (3) clear explanation; (4) minimization of iatrogenic harm; (5) empirical use of potentially beneficial treatments; and (6) consideration of involvement in treatment trials.

Assessment

- Prior to the consultation, obtain the full hospital case records for all specialties. Discuss the case with the GP and obtain copies of GP records if available. Clarify whether the patient is seen in other hospitals or health care services and aim to obtain these records. Establish whether there are any pending investigations and what the patient has been told about their presumed diagnosis.
- At the interview: establish full details of current symptoms; circumstances of symptom onset; and 'life context' of symptom development.
- Explore their illness beliefs: specific worries about cause and possible prognosis; ask the patient to describe their understanding of their symptoms and what they feel they may represent.
- Full details of past medical history (may be reticent—'no problems before current symptoms' or overly dramatic); what were they told at the time by the doctors treating them?
- Remember to explore possible psychiatric differential diagnoses— full mental state as normal, even if no symptoms spontaneously mentioned.
- Observe patient in waiting room/onward/entering and leaving room—be alert to inconsistencies in symptoms.

Diagnosis

- A positive and confident diagnosis is crucial.
- Be willing to make organic and non-organic diagnosis (e.g. where there is undoubted organic disease but also significant MUS morbidity).
- Acknowledge the patient's distress and disability; a diagnosis of MUS should not mean to the patient that you believe that there is 'nothing wrong with them'.

Explanation

- Terminology in this field is variable, imprecise, and potentially offensive (e.g. supratentorial, hysterical). The terms 'functional illness' or 'medically unexplained illness' are generally acceptable to patients.
- Begin with a clear explanation of what is (and what is not) wrong: 'You are suffering from a functional, not structural, problem of your nervous system. This is a common problem which we have seen in other patients.' Various analogies may be used as appropriate (e.g. computer hardware vs. software problem; piano working, but out of tune).
- Emphasize what can and cannot be done: 'We can help train the body to function normally again', 'We might not be able to pinpoint the exact cause'.
- Allow the patient to query what you have said (you should have allowed sufficient time at the end of the interview). Allow carers/relatives to become involved in this exploration of your explanation.
- Copy your clinic letter to the GP and the hospital professionals caring for patient. Consider, in certain situations, copying the letter to patient.

Minimize iatrogenic harm

- In all MUS patients, be aware of the risk of iatrogenic harm and justify any risks taken by benefit to the patient, over and above the gratification of seeming to give the patient 'what they want'.
- Accept that there may be a chronic illness which can be managed, but not 'cured'.
- Appropriately investigate *genuinely new* symptoms.
- In planning further investigations in patients with MUS, greater weight should be placed on objective rather than subjective change.
- Clear verbal, written (and in some cases, face-to-face) communication between all involved professionals is especially crucial in this group of patients: everyone should 'know what's going on'.
- Accept that there will be a proportion of severe cases who are unable to leave the sick role and who must be managed by changing how the system responds to them.

Empirical use of potentially beneficial treatments

- Often there is improvement in patient perception of symptoms following confident diagnosis and explanation.
- All patients with prominent depressive/anxiety symptoms should have these treated in the normal way.
- Consider empirical trial of antidepressant medication even where affective features are not prominent.
- Consider use of physiotherapy to aid regaining of functional loss.
- Consider referral for assessment for formal psychotherapy.
- Consider referral to other resource (e.g. pain management).

Involvement in treatment trials

- Little is known about the course of these disorders over time and less about appropriate treatments: consider patients for involvement in research.

Somatization disorder

Somatization disorder is a disorder in which there is repeated presentation with medically unexplained symptoms, affecting multiple organ systems, first presenting before the age of 40. It is usually chronic in adults. In children, it usually involves one or a few organ systems, often for shorter periods of time. At all ages, it is associated with significant psychological distress, functional impairment, and risk of iatrogenic harm. Full-blown somatization disorder or 'Briquet's syndrome' probably represents the severe end of a continuum of abnormal illness behaviour.

Clinical features Somatization disorder patients have long, complex medical histories ('fat-file' patients), although at interview they may minimize all but the most recent symptomatology. Symptoms may occur in any system and are to some extent suggestible. The most frequent symptoms are non-specific and atypical. There may be discrepancy between the subjective and objective findings (e.g. reports of intractable pain in a patient observed by nursing staff to be joking with relatives). Symptoms are usually concentrated in one system at a time but may move to another system after exhausting diagnostic possibilities in the previous one. The patient's life revolves around the illness as does their family life. There is excessive use of both medical services and alternative therapies.

Diagnosis is usually only suspected after negative findings begin to emerge because normal medical practice is to take a patient's complaints at face value. The key diagnostic feature is multiple, atypical, and inconsistent medically unexplained symptoms in a patient under the age of 40. Chronic cases will have had large numbers of diagnostic procedures and surgical or medical treatments. There is high risk of both iatrogenic harm and iatrogenic substance dependence. Hostility and frustration can be felt on both sides of the doctor–patient relationship with splitting (⌨ p. 830) between members of the treating team. Psychological approaches to treatment are hampered by ongoing investigations to ever rarer diagnostic possibilities and by the attribution of symptoms to fictitious but 'named' medical entities.

Two-thirds of patients will meet criteria for another psychiatric disorder, most commonly major depressive or anxiety disorders. There is also association with personality disorder and substance abuse. Patients characteristically deny emotional symptoms or attribute them directly to physical handicaps—'the only reason I'm depressed is this constant pain'.

Aetiology Observable clinical association with childhood illnesses in the patient and a history of parental anxiety towards illness. Increased frequency of somatization disorder in first-degree relatives. Possible neuropsychiatric basis to the disorder with faulty assessment of normal somatic sensory input. Association with childhood sexual abuse.

Epidemiology Lifetime prevalence of ~0.2%. Markedly higher rate in particular populations. ♀:♂ ratio 5:1. Age of onset is childhood to early 30s.

Differential diagnosis *Undiagnosed physical disorder:* particularly those with variable, multi-system presentations (e.g. SLE, AIDS, porphyria, tuberculosis, multiple sclerosis). Onset of multiple symptoms for the first time in patients over 40 should be presumed to be due to unexposed physical disease. *Psychiatric disorder:* major affective and psychotic illnesses may initially present with predominately somatic complaints. Diagnosis is by examination of other psychopathology, however over half of somatization disorder patients exhibit psychiatric comorbidity. *Other somatoform disorders:* distinguish from: hypochondriasis (presence of firm belief in particular disorder), somatoform pain disorder (pain rather than other symptoms is prominent), conversion disorder (functional loss without multi-system complaints), factitious disorder (intentional production or feigning of physical symptoms to assume sick role), and malingering (intentional production of false or grossly exaggerated physical symptoms with external motivation). In practice the main distinction is between the full and severe somatization disorder and somatization as a symptom in other disorders.

Assessment (see 📖 p. 800). Establish reasons for referral, experience of illness, attitudes to symptoms, personal and psychiatric history, and family perspective.

Initial management (see **management principles**, 📖 p. 800) Make, document, and communicate the diagnosis. Acknowledge symptom severity and experience of distress as real but emphasize negative investigations and lack of structural abnormality. Reassure patient of continuing care. Attempt to reframe symptoms as emotional. Assess for and treat psychiatric comorbidity as appropriate. Reduce and stop unnecessary drugs. Consider case conference involving GP and treating physicians. Educate parents/family.

Ongoing management

• Regular review by single, named doctor.
• Reviews should be at planned and agreed frequency, avoiding emergency consultations.
• Symptoms should be examined and explored with a view to their emotional 'meaning'.
• Avoid tests 'to rule out disease': investigate objective signs only.
• All secondary referrals made through one individual.
• Disseminate management plan.
• These patients can exhaust a doctor's resources—plan to share the burden over time.

Some evidence for the effectiveness of patient education in symptom re-attribution, brief contact psychotherapy, group therapy, or CBT if the patient can be engaged in this.

Prognosis Poor in the full disorder; tendency is for chronic morbidity with periods of relative remission. Treatment of psychiatric comorbidity and reduction of iatrogenic harm will reduce overall morbidity. Key for recovery in children and adolescents is rehabilitation and return to usual activities as soon as possible.

Somatoform pain disorder

In somatoform pain disorder there is a complaint of persistent severe and distressing pain which is not explained or not adequately explained by organic pathology. The causation of the symptom is attributed to psychological factors. This disorder is diagnosed where the disorder is not better explained by somatization disorder, another psychiatric diagnosis, or psychological factors in a general medical condition.

All pain is a subjective sensation and its severity and quality as experienced in an individual are dependent on a complex mix of factors including the situation, the degree of arousal, the affective state, the beliefs about the source, and 'meaning' of the pain. The experience of pain is modified by its chronicity and associations and there is a 'two-way' relationship with affective state, with chronic pain predisposing to depressive illness, while depressive illness tends to worsen the subjective experience of pain.

Comorbidity In common with the other somatoform disorders there is substantial overlap with major depression (~40% in pain clinic patients) and anxiety disorders. Substance abuse (including iatrogenic opiate dependency) and personality disorder patients are over-represented.

Epidemiology No population data are available. The prevalence of patients with medically unexplained pain varies by clinical setting; higher in inpatient settings, particularly surgery, and highest in pain clinic patients.

Differential diagnosis Elaboration of organic pain, malingering (e.g. patient with opiate dependency seeking opiate prescription), genuine organic cause with absence of other manifestations (e.g. sickle cell crisis, angina).

Assessment History from patient and informants, length of history (may be minimized), relationship to life events, general somatization, experience of illness, family attitude to illness, periods of employment, treatments, beliefs about cause, comorbid psychiatric symptoms.

Management (see **management principles**, 📖 p. 800). It is important to recognize and treat occult comorbid depression. It is often helpful to adopt an atheoretical approach: 'let's see what works', and to resist pressure for 'all or nothing' cure or a move to investigation by another specialty. Opiates are not generally effective in chronic pain of this type and add the risk of dependence. *Psychological treatments*: these are directed towards enabling the patient to manage and 'live with' the pain, rather than aspiring to eliminate it completely; can include relaxation training, biofeedback, hypnosis, group work, CBT. *Pain clinics*: these are generally anaesthetist-led with variable psychiatric provision. They offer a range of physical treatments such as: antidepressants, transcutaneous electrical nerve stimulation (TENS), anticonvulsants, and local or regional nerve-blocks.

Conversion (dissociative) disorders

In conversion or dissociative disorders there is a loss or disturbance of normal motor or sensory function which initially appears to have a neurological or other physical cause but is later attributed to a psychological cause. These disorders were initially explained by psychodynamic mechanisms—repression of unacceptable conscious impulses and their 'conversion' to physical symptoms, sometimes with symbolic meaning. In ICD and DSM, the presumed psychodynamic mechanisms are not part of the diagnosis, although the initiation or worsening of the symptom or deficit is often preceded by conflicts or other stressors. Symptoms are not produced intentionally and the presence of 'secondary gain' is not part of the diagnosis.

Classification ICD-10 and DSM-IV classify these disorders differently. In ICD-10 dissociation and conversion are used synonymously, with dissociation preferred as it does not imply a definite psychological explanation. All expressions of such disorders are classified together under the heading 'F44, dissociative (conversion) disorders'. In DSM-IV 'conversion' refers to motor or sensory deficit, while 'dissociation' refers to disturbance in function of consciousness. Conversion disorders are classified with the somatoform disorders, while dissociative disorders are classified separately.

Clinical features These vary depending on the area affected but the following are commonly seen:

- **Paralysis** One or more limbs or one side of the face or body may be affected. Flaccid paralysis is common initially but severe, established cases may develop contractures. Often active movement of the limb is impossible during examination but synergistic movement is observed (e.g. Hoover's test: the patient is unable to raise the affected limb from the couch but is able to raise the unaffected limb against resistance with demonstrable pressing down of the heel on the 'affected' side).
- **Loss of speech (aphonia)** There may be complete loss of speech, or loss of all but whispered speech. There is no defect in comprehension and writing is unimpaired (and becomes the main method of communication). Laryngeal examination is normal and the patient's vocal cords can be fully opposed while coughing.
- **Sensory loss** The area of loss will cover the patient's beliefs about anatomical structure rather than reality (e.g. 'glove' distribution, marked 'midline splitting').
- **Seizures** Non-epileptic seizures are found most commonly in those with genuine epilepsy. The non-epileptic attacks generally occur only in the presence of an audience, no injury is sustained on falling to the ground, tongue biting and incontinence are rare, the 'seizure' consists of generalized shaking, rather than regular clonic contractions, and there is no post-ictal confusion or prolactin rise.
- **Amnesia** Memory loss, most often for recent events, not attributable to organic mental disorder, and too severe to attribute to ordinary forgetfulness. Usually patchy and selective amnesia—true global amnesia is rare. There is expectation of recovery and usually a history of recent traumatic event gradually emerges.

- **Fugue** Here there is dissociative amnesia plus a history of travel outside the patient's normal environs. The patient may 'come to' far from home, without memory of how they came to be there, and with a variable amnesia for other personal information. Although there is amnesia for the period of fugue, the patient has apparently functioned normally during this time (e.g. able to buy travel tickets, etc.). Again recovery can be expected in time, and a history of recent traumatic events is commonly found.

Diagnosis The diagnosis will usually be suspected due to the non-anatomical or clinically inconsistent nature of the signs. It is established by (1) excluding underlying organic disease, or demonstrating minor disorder insufficient to account for the symptoms; (2) finding of 'positive signs' (i.e. demonstration of function thought to be absent); (3) a convincing psychological explanation for the deficit. Additionally helpful though non-specific is a prior history of conversion symptoms or recurrent somatic complaints or disorder, family or individual stress and psychopathology (recent stress, grief, sexual abuse) or the presence of a symptom model.

Treatment Clear presentation of diagnosis in collaboration with the treating medical team. Aim to present the diagnosis as positive (emphasizing the likelihood of recovery) rather than negative ('we couldn't find anything; it's all in your head'). In general, avoid interventions which could maintain the sick role or prolong abnormal function (e.g. provision of crutches to those with dissociative gait disturbance) and instead consider interventions directed towards graceful resumption of normal function (e.g. physiotherapy). Treat psychiatric comorbidity if present. Controlled treatment studies are absent, CBT, IPT, supportive psychotherapy, family therapy, biofeedback are all potentially helpful.

Prognosis For acute conversion symptoms, especially those with a clear precipitant, the prognosis is good, with expectation of complete resolution of symptoms (70–90% resolution at follow-up). Poorer outcomes for longer-lasting and well-established symptoms.

Hypochondriasis

Hypochondriasis is the preoccupation with the fear of having a serious disease which persists despite negative medical investigations and appropriate reassurance with subsequent distress and impaired function.

Clinical features The central and diagnostic clinical feature is the preoccupation with the idea of having a serious medical condition, usually one which would lead to death or serious disability. The patient repeatedly ruminates on this possibility and insignificant bodily abnormalities, normal variants, normal functions, and minor ailments will be interpreted as signs of serious disease. The patient consequently seeks medical advice and investigation but is unable to be reassured in a sustained fashion by negative investigations.

The *form* of the belief is that of an over-valued idea; the patient may be able to accept that their worries are groundless but nonetheless be unable to stop dwelling and acting on them. Where the belief in illness is of delusional intensity, the patient should be treated as for delusional disorder (📖 p. 220).

Aetiology As in somatization disorder there may be a history of childhood illness, parental illness, or excess medical attention-seeking in the parents. Childhood sexual abuse and other emotional abuse or neglect are associated. In one aetiological model, individuals with a combination of anxiety symptoms and predisposition to misattribute psychical symptoms, seek medical advice. The resulting medical reassurance provides temporary relief of anxiety which acts as a 'reward' and makes further medical attention-seeking more likely.

Epidemiology Equal sex incidence. Very variable prevalence depending on group studied (0.8%–10.3%), higher in secondary care.

Differential diagnosis The main differentiation is from the feared physical disease. In most cases this is straightforward, but the possibility of an early, insidious disease with vague physical signs and normal baseline investigations should be considered.

Comorbidity High (>50%) incidence of generalized anxiety disorder. Hypochondriasis may also coexist with major depressive illness, OCD, and panic disorder. Examination of the time course of symptom development and most prominent clinical features helps to distinguish primary hypochondriasis from a secondary clinical feature of these disorders.

Management

• *Initial* Allow patient time to ventilate their illness anxiet-ies. Clarify that symptoms with no structural basis are real and severe. Aim to plan continuing relationship and review, not contingent upon new symptoms. Explain negative tests and resist the temptation to be drawn into further exploration. Patients will in the early stages often change or expand symptomatology. Emphasize aim to improve function. Break cycle of reassurance and repeat presentation—family education may help in this.

- *Pharmacological* Uncontrolled trials demonstrate antidepressant benefit, even in the absence of depressive symptoms. Try fluoxetine 20mg, increasing to 60mg, or imipramine up to 150mg.
- *Psychotherapy* Behavioural therapy (response prevention and exposure to illness cues); CBT (identify and challenge misinterpretations, substitution of realistic interpretation, graded exposure to illness-related situations, and modification of core illness-beliefs), 75% symptom reduction in one controlled trial.[1]

1 Warwick HM, Clark DM, Cobb AM, et al. (1996) A controlled trial of cognitive–behavioural treatment of hypochondriasis. *Br J Psychiat* **169**: 189–95.

Body dysmorphic disorder

The core clinical feature of body dysmorphic disorder is preoccupation with the belief that some aspect of physical appearance is markedly abnormal, unattractive, or pathological. This preoccupation causes distress and has the characteristics of an over-valued idea; it is not amenable to reassurance. The bodily part is found to be normal, or if abnormal is only trivially so compared with the degree of distress.

It is an unusual condition which has only relatively recently come prominently to clinical attention. It rarely presents directly, but such individuals may present requesting plastic surgery or mutilating surgical procedures, and hence come to psychiatric attention. There are many similarities to OCD in terms of clinical features and treatment response.

Clinical features There is preoccupation with the idea that some specified aspect of their appearance is grossly abnormal, markedly unattractive, or diseased. Any part of the body may be affected, most usually the face, head, and secondary sexual characteristics. Patients believe that the supposed deficit is noticeable to others and attempt to hide or minimize it. These beliefs may develop delusional intensity. There is associated functional impairment, agoraphobia, and risk of suicide. Comorbid behaviours such as skin picking, rubbing, topical applications may cause worse secondary problems. Clinically significant disorder causes severe functional impairment, restriction of relationships and employment opportunities, and the risk of iatrogenic morbidity by unwarranted surgical procedures.

Aetiology Begins in late childhood or early adolescence, overlap with normal worries at this age.

Epidemiology Equal sex incidence. Less than 1% prevalence but markedly over-represented in some groups (e.g. plastic surgery [10%] and dermatology). 10% incidence in first-degree family members.

Comorbidity 60% risk of major depression.

Differential diagnosis There is a significant overlap in terms of symptom profile with social phobia, hypochondriasis, OCD, somatic delusions in schizophrenia, and anorexia nervosa. Where the concerns are persistently delusional, ICD-10 reclassifies as delusional disorder, while DSM-IV allows diagnosis of a delusional form.

Treatment
- **Operative** Plastic surgery to the affected part is generally not indicated, even successful surgery risks being followed by a new preoccupation or a focus on surgical scarring.
- **Pharmacological** Evidence for clinical effectiveness of SSRI, try fluoxetine 20mg increasing to 60mg. If ineffective try clomipramine up to 250mg. If delusional features, add antipsychotic.
- **Psychological** Evidence for CBT, treatment focused on response prevention, challenging cognitive errors, and behavioural tasks.

Prognosis Chronic course with fluctuating symptom severity. Partial rather than full remission.

Chronic fatigue syndrome

Chronic fatigue syndrome (CFS) is a clinical syndrome whose central feature is severe fatigue, unrelated to exertion or triggered by only minimal activity, and unrelieved by rest. The fatigue is experienced as a subjective feeling of lethargy, lack of energy, exhaustion, and a feeling of 'increased effort to do anything'. Patients also often complain of aching muscles, sleep disturbance, aching joints, headaches, and difficulties with concentration. They may date the onset of symptoms very precisely to an episode of viral infection with sore throat, fever, and tender lymph nodes. The syndrome is also referred to as myalgic encephalomyelitis (ME), post-viral fatigue syndrome, and previously as neurasthenia. The term CFS is currently preferred as it does not imply knowledge of underlying pathology or aetiology.

It should be understood that CFS is not a disorder in the conventionally accepted sense, but a characteristic clinical syndrome. It shows diagnostic overlap with major depression, somatization disorder, and hypochondriasis but cannot be subsumed into these diagnoses because of substantial areas of lack of fit. Any operational diagnostic criteria for CFS will be contentious and will include people with chronic organic illnesses. Patients with this syndrome will often have passionately held beliefs about the cause of their symptoms and the appropriate management. A practical and pragmatic approach is advised from treating clinicians.

Aetiology Currently the aetiology of CFS is unknown, with immunological, genetic, viral, neuroendocrine, and psychological causes suggested. While a minority of cases have a confirmed onset with viral illness, ongoing viral replication or chronic infection is not the cause. The condition is likely to be heterogeneous, without a single or simple aetiology. At the moment it may be best regarded as a spectrum of illness that is triggered by an acute reaction to stress or minor illness in a vulnerable individual with a persisting clinical syndrome caused by deconditioning and other secondary phenomena. Vulnerable individuals are those with abnormal symptom attribution, increased awareness of normal bodily processes, cognitive errors, and perfectionist personality types.

Epidemiology Population prevalence of 0.2–0.4% with women affected at four times the rate of men. Most common in people in their 40s and 50s. Occasionally occurs in children, particularly during adolescence.

Diagnosis CFS should be considered where there is complaint of fatigue which: (1) is persistent and/or recurrent; (2) is unexplained by organic conditions or other psychiatric diagnoses; (3) results in substantial reduction in previous activity level; and (4) is characterized by post-exertion malaise and slow recovery after effort, AND one or more of the following symptoms:

- sleep disturbance (e.g. insomnia, hypersomnia, unrefreshing sleep, disturbed sleep–wake cycle)
- muscles and/or joint pain without evidence of inflammation
- headache
- painful lymph nodes

- sore throat
- minor cognitive dysfunction (e.g. impaired concentration, impairment of STM, word-finding difficulty)
- worsening of symptoms following mental or physical exertion
- recurrent flu-like symptoms
- dizziness, nausea and palpitations.

Comorbidity Many patients with CFS will meet the criteria for another psychiatric diagnosis, most commonly major depression. Many patients resist a 'psychiatric' diagnosis and attribute any mood disturbance to the restriction on activities caused by their illness. Nonetheless, treatment of comorbid depressive or anxiety symptoms can produce clinical improvement.

Investigation findings Non-specific subjective cognitive impairment similar to that found in depression. Normal muscle function with poor performance on tolerance testing related to deconditioning. No characteristic blood abnormalities or immune system abnormalities. There are no definite and replicable abnormal findings. Do minimum indicated tests.

Assessment Establish the diagnosis and identify comorbid psychiatric disorders. Avoid confrontation with the patient and attempt to agree a common understanding of the disorder. Acknowledge the severity of the symptoms and the consequent disability. Aim to take the focus of the interview towards potentially beneficial interventions and away from unwarranted investigations.

Management

There is no specific pharmacological treatment. The best evidence base exists for graded exercise therapy and cognitive behaviour therapy.

- **Graded exercise therapy (GET)** Establish via diary record the patient's daily activity level, establish with them their maximal tolerable level even on their worst day, and encourage them to perform this level of activity every day, no more and no less, with gradual negotiated increase over time. The aim is to break the cycle of inactivity, brief excess activity, and consequent exhaustion.
- **Cognitive behavioural therapy (CBT)** (see 📖 p. 850).
- **Psychotropic medication** Consider antidepressant treatment trial even where no clear-cut evidence of affective symptoms. Try SSRI first (e.g. paroxetine 20mg) as this patient group is intolerant of side-effects.
- **Symptomatic medication** Patients may experience greater intolerance and more severe side-effects from drug treatment. Where appropriate, drugs used for symptom control should be initiated at a lower dose than in usual clinical practice, and should be increased gradually.

Prognosis Outcome is difficult to predict but the severely affected cases and those with very chronic symptoms appear to do worse. Many patients with mild to moderate symptoms do show some degree of improvement over time. A proportion of cases show a fluctuating course with periods of relative remission followed by relapse. Of the severe cases, a proportion will remain significantly disabled.

Factitious disorder (Munchausen's syndrome)

In factitious disorder, patients intentionally falsify their symptoms and past history and fabricate signs of physical or mental disorder with the primary aim of obtaining medical attention and treatment. The diagnostic features are the intentional and conscious production of signs, falsification, or exaggeration of the history and the lack of gain beyond medical attention and treatment. Three distinct subgroups are seen.

* **Wandering**: mostly males who move from hospital to hospital, job to job, place to place, producing dramatic and fantastic stories. There may be aggressive personality or dissocial PD and comorbid alcohol or drug problems.
* **Non-wandering**: mostly females; more stable lifestyles and less dramatic presentations. Often in paramedical professions; overlap with chronic somatization disorder. Association with borderline PD.
* **By proxy**: mostly female. Mothers, carers, or paramedical and nursing staff who simulate or prolong illness in their dependants—here the clinical focus must be on the prevention of further harm to the dependant.

The behaviours can mimic any psychical and psychiatric illness. Behaviours include: self-induced infections, simulated illnesses, interference with existing lesions, self-medication, altering records, reporting false physical or psychiatric symptomatology. Early diagnosis reduces iatrogenic morbidity and is facilitated by: awareness of the possibility; a neutral interviewing style using open rather than closed questions; alertness to insistencies and abnormalities in presentation; use of other available information sources; and careful medical record keeping.

Differential diagnosis Any genuine medical or psychiatric disorder. Somatization disorder (no conscious production of symptoms and no fabrication of history), malingering (secondary gain for the patient, e.g. compensation, avoiding army service), substance misuse (also gain, i.e. the prescription of the drug), hypochondriasis, psychotic and depressive illness (associated features of the primary mental illness).

Aetiology Unknown, there may be a background of childhood sexual abuse or childhood emotional neglect. Probably more common in men and those with a nursing or paramedical background. Association with personality disorder. Production of psychiatric symptoms associated with borderline PD, CSA, or emotional abuse.

Management

There are no validated treatments. Patients are often reluctant to consider psychiatric assessment and may leave once their story is questioned. Management in these cases is directed towards reducing iatrogenic harm caused by inappropriate treatments and medications.

* **Direct challenge** Easier if there is direct evidence of feigned illness; the patient is informed that staff is aware of the intent to feign illness

and the evidence is produced. This should be in a non-punitive manner with offer of ongoing support.

- **Indirect challenge** Here the aim is to allow the patient a face-saving 'way out', while preventing further inappropriate investigation and intervention. One example is the 'double bind' 'if this doesn't work then the illness is factitious'.
- **Systemic change** Here the understanding is that there is no possibility of change in the individual and the focus is on changing the approach of the health care system to assessing them in order to minimize harm. These strategies can include dissemination of the patient's usual presentation and distinguishing marks to regional hospitals, 'blacklisting', 'Munchausen's registers', etc. As these strategies potentially break confidentiality and can decrease the risk of detecting genuine illness, they should be drawn up in a multidisciplinary fashion involving senior staff.

Assessment prior to organ transplantation

For patients with end-stage organ disease (e.g. kidney, liver, heart, lung, bowel, or pancreas), a transplant offers the prospect of significant improvement in their mortality and quality of life. Unfortunately, the supply of donor organs is less than the number of potential recipients. Because of this, patients requiring transplantation will suffer declining health while on the waiting list, and a proportion of listed patients will die while awaiting transplant. This places a responsibility on the assessing team to consider carefully each potential candidate for listing for transplantation in order to ensure the best use of the donor organs. Psychiatric assessment of patients prior to listing for organ transplantation may be requested in the following situations:

- In some patients being considered for liver transplantation:
  - Fulminant liver failure following overdose (usually paracetamol)
  - Liver disease secondary to alcoholic liver disease (ALD)
- Patients with history of mental illness
- Patients with previous or current drug misuse
- Patients with history of non-compliance
- Living related donors

The involvement of the psychiatrist in the assessment prior to listing for transplantation should in no sense be a moral judgement as to the patient's suitability. The issues are whether there are psychiatric factors which would jeopardize the survival of the donor organ. The psychiatric opinion may have the most profound implications for the patient and so assessment should be as thorough as time allows. In addition to taking psychiatric history and MSE, family members, GP, and hospital case records should be consulted.

Fulminant liver failure This will often follow on from a late presenting paracetamol overdose. At the point patients are seen it is often unclear whether they are going to recover or to deteriorate to the point of requiring transplant. They should be seen as soon as possible after presentation as encephalopathy may develop as their condition worsens. The issue is whether there is: ongoing intent to die or refusal of transplant (which would normally preclude transplantation); or whether there is a history of repeated overdoses in the past, significant psychiatric disorder, or ongoing drug or alcohol misuse (which would be relative contraindications).

Liver disease secondary to ALD Suitably selected patients transplanted for ALD have similar outcomes in terms of survival and quality of life to patients transplanted for other indications. Units will have individual policies regarding these patients which should be consulted if available. The issue is whether the patient, who has already damaged one liver, will damage a second. There is a wider issue of maintaining the public confidence in the appropriate use of donated organs. Consider:

- How long have they been abstinent (is there independent verification of this)?
- Do they accept alcohol as the cause of liver failure?

- Do they undertake to remain abstinent post-transplant?
- Do they have a history of dependence or harmful use?
- What is their history of involvement in alcohol treatment services and, in the past, how have they responded to relapse?
- When were they told that their drinking was causing liver damage, and what was their response?

Given these findings and your routine psychiatric assessment, the transplant team will seek your opinion as to:
- The patient's psychiatric diagnosis
- Their risk of relapse
- Their risk of re-establishing harmful/dependent drinking
- The potential for successful intervention should this occur

History of mental illness/drug misuse Generally speaking, a diagnosis of mental disorder (other than progressive dementia) will not preclude transplant. The important issues are whether the mental disorder will affect compliance or longer-term mortality in its own right. Close liaison with the patient's normal psychiatrist is clearly crucial here. Ongoing substance dependence is generally a contraindication to transplantation and should be addressed before listing.

History of non-compliance with treatment Non-compliance with treatment may be the reason for a patient's need for transplant, or place the patient at risk for future morbidity or mortality and the loss of a donated organ if not recognized early in assessment. Past medical records and discussions with past treatment teams will provide information regarding this area of risk for a given patient or family. In addition, pre-transplant evaluation by multiple team members, including behavioural health, should identify psychosocial factors that place a patient or family at risk for non-adherence, and provide the team an opportunity to be proactive to increase the likelihood of future adherence and transplant success.

Living related donors This type of transplant uses organs or tissues from a matched and usually biologically related donor. Examples include bone marrow, single kidney or portion of liver. In this case, the donor is an additional focus of evaluation, with the goal of establishing that there is valid consent and the absence of coercion.

Psychotherapy

Introduction

The psychotherapies are a collection of treatments for mental disorder which employ language and communication, and the relationship with a skilled therapist, as their means of producing change. Psychotherapeutic methods are used both to conceptualize abnormal mental states (to understand why symptoms have developed in this patient at this particular time), and to treat symptoms and disorders.

Generally the aim of therapy is to enable patients to improve their relationships with themselves and others as well as to manage and treat symptoms. The core components of psychotherapy, regardless of the underlying theoretical basis, are an **empathetic and non-judgemental** stance towards the patient, an awareness of the importance of the **setting** in which therapy takes place and the use of the **therapeutic relationship** between the therapist and patient as both a diagnostic and therapeutic agent.

Types of psychotherapy

Supportive psychotherapy

This form of psychotherapy aims to offer practical and emotional support, opportunity for ventilation of emotions, and guided, problem-solving discussion. There is no explicit attempt to alter underlying cognitions or to dismantle adaptive defence mechanisms. Supportive psychotherapy is sometimes preferred where fundamental behavioural change is not aimed for, or where patient factors (e.g. learning difficulty, psychotic illness) preclude exploratory therapies. Examples include counselling and general psychiatric follow-up.

Psychodynamic psychotherapy

This form of therapy aims to produce changes in individuals' thinking and behaviour by exploring childhood experience, the unconscious mind including **transference** (see 📖 p. 828), and the quality and nature of relationships both in the past, the present, and in the here-and-now with the therapist. The latter receives particularly close analysis as it allows for understandings to come directly rather than via third party report by the patient. Ideally patients should be highly motivated, able to tolerate frustration and anxiety, have good impulse control, be able to form meaningful relationships and be capable of insight and abstract thought. These traits however could be regarded as being the markers of health rather than the sign that somebody needs treatment and as such a balance needs to be struck between a triad of factors—does the patient *want* therapy, do they *need* therapy, and can they *use* therapy?

Cognitive and/or behavioural therapies

These are based on learning and cognitive theories with the rationale that a patient's thoughts, feelings, and actions are interdependent on one another. Attention in these therapies is directed towards the patient's *current* thoughts and behaviours which are closely examined and challenged, with a view to modification to improve symptoms. Unconscious processes, childhood experience, and the specific nature of the therapist–patient relationship receive less attention. Cognitive and behavioural therapy sessions are generally more structured than in other psychotherapies and often take place over a relatively brief and predetermined period of time. These therapies are useful in a wide range of disorders including depression, anxiety disorders (including OCD), eating disorders and, more recently they have been applied to psychotic disorders.

Psychotherapeutic training

As a psychiatric trainee, you are required to gain competency in five areas of psychotherapy—supportive psychotherapy, psychodynamic psychotherapy, brief psychotherapies, cognitive behavioural therapy, and combined psychopharmacology/psychotherapy. Training generally consists of formal teaching, experience working with a range of patients, and regular supervision with experienced therapists. It is only through the process of conducting therapy under supervision that you will really understand psychotherapeutic techniques. These notes on general concepts and specific psychotherapies aim to familiarize you with theories, guide your referrals, and assist you in explaining the process to patients.

Recommended further reading

Dewan M, Steenbarger B, and Greenburg R (2004)*The art and science of brief psychotherapies.* Arlington: American Psychiatric Publishing, Inc.

Gabbard GO (2000) *Psychodynamic psychiatry in clinical practice,* 3rd edn. Washington, DC: American Psychiatric Press, Inc.

Malan D (1995) *Individual psychotherapy and the science of psychodynamics.* London: Hodder Arnold Publications.

Padesky CA and Greenberger D (1995) *Mind over mood: change how you feel by changing the way you think:* New York: Guilford Publications.

Winston A, Rosenthal R, and Pinsker H (2004) *Introduction to supportive psychotherapy.* Arlington: American Psychiatric Publishing, Inc.

Assessment for psychotherapy

Indications and contraindications

- Psychotherapeutic methods can be useful in the treatment of many psychiatric illnesses, including mild to moderate depressive illness, neurotic illnesses, eating disorders, and personality disorders.
- Specific therapies also have a place in the management of patients with learning disabilities, those with psychosexual problems, substance misuse disorders, and chronic psychotic symptoms.
- They are generally *contraindicated* in:
  - **acute psychosis** (due to increasing expressed emotion and the inherent neuropsychological deficits associated with this mental state);
  - **severe depressive illness** (because of psychomotor retardation);
  - **dementia/delirium** (where treatment of organic pathology is first-line);
  - some individuals where there is **acute suicide risk**.

Goals of assessment

The assessment of a patient for psychotherapy has three major goals:
- What does the patient expect (or **want** from therapy)?
- Obtaining a careful history/narrative of the problem from the patient (do they **need** therapy?)
- Establishing whether the patient can form a therapeutic relationship and make **use** of the type of therapy being potentially offered.

Different therapies will have a varying focus in the initial assessment, e.g. psychodynamic assessments will often focus more on relational aspects of the patient's life whereas cognitive behavioural therapists may concentrate more on the (A)ntecedents, (B)ehaviours/(B)eliefs, and (C)onsequences of the patient's behaviours or beliefs.

Psychological factors in assessment for psychotherapy

'Psychological-mindedness'

Refers to the capacity for insight and to understand problems in psychological terms: 'can the patient think about their thoughts?'. If this is lacking, a supportive method may be preferred over a cognitive or exploratory method.

Motivation for insight and change

Many patients (and trainees!) do not want to 'get better' or change. Often we are more comfortable playing by the rules of the game we know, even if this means we find ourselves caught in difficult situations, rather than learning a new game. An important part of assessment is to establish whether the potential patient is willing to take responsibility for their situation and use therapy as a means of changing it.

Adequate ego strength and reality testing

Important when considering exploratory psychotherapies, especially those based on exploring **transference** dynamics. Includes the ability to sustain feelings and fantasies without impulsively acting upon them, being over-whelmed by anxiety, losing the capacity to continue the dialogue, or treating 'as if' situations as though they 'actually are' real.

Ability to form and sustain relationships

Where there is inability to enter into trusting relationships (e.g. in paranoid personality disorder) or where there is inability to maintain relationship boundaries (e.g. in borderline personality disorder), this may preclude exploratory methods.

Able to tolerate change and frustration

As with any potentially powerful treatment, psychotherapy has the potential to exacerbate symptoms, particularly when maladaptive coping mechanisms are examined and changed.

Selection of psychotherapeutic method

Local availability

In practice, often the main determinant of therapy choice is local availability and the practical availability determined by the length of the waiting list. The waiting times associated with most forms of therapy should encourage all practitioners to exercise care in patient referral.

Practitioner experience and view of modality

Where the treating psychiatrist also provides the psychotherapy, his or her area of expertise may determine choice of psychotherapeutic method.

Illness factors

Varying illnesses and states of mind have been shown, within the evidence base, to respond differentially to different treatments.

Patient choice

Patients may express a preference for a particular therapeutic model because of previous positive experience or having read or been told about the approach. A method which 'makes sense' to the patient given their understanding of their symptoms is often preferred.

A brief history of Sigmund Freud

Freud remains far and away the world's best-known psychiatrist and his image, of a scholarly, bearded man sitting behind a distressed patient lying on a couch, is many lay-people's archetype for our profession. He made a huge contribution to our understanding of the mind, but many of his ideas are now so much a part of our general view of the world that it is easy to overlook the breakthroughs they originally were.

He was born in 1856 in Moravia (now part of the Czech Republic, but then part of the Austro-Hungarian Empire). He moved to Vienna when he was a child and lived there until his last year. On entering medical training he was influenced by scientific empiricism—the belief that through careful observation the un-understandable could be understood. On qualification he began laboratory work on the physiology of the nervous system under Brücke, later entering clinical medical practice after his marriage in 1882. He chose neurology as his specialty and received a grant to study at the Salpêtrière in Paris, where he was exposed to the ideas of Charcot, who interested Freud in the study of hysteria and the use of hypnosis. In Paris with Charcot, and later in Nancy with Liébault, he studied the behaviour of hysterical patients under hypnosis and developed his ideas of the unconscious mind and its role in normal and disordered behaviour.

Returning to Vienna, Freud began collaboration with Josef Breuer on the study of hysteria. The subsequent development of psychoanalysis was prompted by the case of Anna O., treated by Breuer between 1880 and 1882. This patient, a 21-yr-old woman (real name Bertha Pappenheim), presented with a range of hysterical symptoms including paralysis, visual loss, cough, and abrupt personality change. These symptoms had developed while her father was terminally ill. Breuer observed that her symptoms resolved during hypnotic trances. Breuer also noted that not only did the symptoms recur after the sessions ended, but that after he terminated the treatment relationship she suffered a full-blown relapse. Breuer wrote up the case after discussing it with his younger colleague. Later they published *Studies in hysteria*, detailing their ideas on the aetiology and treatment of hysterical symptoms. This book postulated that trauma is unacceptable to the patient and hence repressed from conscious memory. This repression produces an increase in 'nervous excitation'—which is expressed eventually as hysteria—with a conscious remnant, often in a disguised form, which can be accessed and resolved during hypnosis.

Freud explored these ideas during his clinical practice in the 1890s, using a variety of methods to uncover the repressed memories. Later he developed the technique of *free association*, where the patient is encouraged to say whatever comes to mind. Experience in the 1890s led Freud to develop the ideas of *repression* of unacceptable memories and their expression as hysterical symptoms. The initial memory was generally of a sexual nature. At first Freud thought this was a real, remembered assault, but later realized that in the majority of cases the patients were describing a sexualized fantasy towards parental figures. Freud described these ideas in his most famous book, *The interpretation of dreams*, published in 1900. It described the basis of his psychoanalytic technique including analysis of the content of dreams, descriptions of defence mechanisms, and his *topographical model* of the mind. Freud's early insights tended to come directly from clinical experience, particularly from patients with hysteria. His later ideas were more theoretical and aimed to develop a model of the normal and abnormal development of mind through psychoanalytical ideas. His drive theory postulated the existence of basic drives, which included the *libido*, the sexual drive, and the *eros* and *thanatos* (the drives towards life and death). He described the *pleasure principle*, the drive to avoid pain and experience pleasure, and its modification through the *reality principle*.

In 1905 he published *Three essays on the theory of sexuality*, describing his theories regarding childhood development including the ideas of developmental phases and the Oedipal and Electra complexes and their relationship with the development of adult neuroses. *The ego and the id*, published in 1923, saw the replacement of the topographical with the structural model of the mind. He described his theories of ego psychology and the production of anxiety symptoms in *Inhibitions, symptoms and anxiety* in 1926. Although he recognized the importance of unconscious defences in response to anxiety, the first systematic account of these mechanisms was written by Freud's daughter Anna in *The ego and the mechanisms of defence* in 1936. Freud's repeated revision of his own theories was mirrored by repeated disagreements and splits in the psychotherapeutic movement and the formation of separate psychotherapeutic 'schools', usually strongly associated with one charismatic individual. Freud died from cancer in England in 1939 after fleeing Vienna following the rise to power of the Nazis. His daughter Anna continued to refine and publicize her father's work, which has recently been retranslated and reprinted in full.

Other pioneers of psychoanalysis

Anna Freud (1895–1982) Although Freud recognized the importance of unconscious defences, the first systematic account of these mechanisms was written by his daughter Anna in *The ego and the mechanisms of defence* in 1936. She also helped to develop child psychoanalysis and play therapy.

Carl Jung (1865–1961) Associated with Freud until their views over the sexual aetiology of the causes of neuroses differed and he founded his own school of analytic psychology. Key concepts include the 'collective unconscious' in which humanity's shared mythological and symbolic past is represented in the unconscious mind of an individual by symbols called 'archetypes'. He also described 16 personality types, including differentiation between 'introverted' and 'extroverted' types.

Erik Erikson (1902–1994) Expanded Freud's developmental theory by explaining that there were not only sexual conflicts at each phase but also a conflict related to how individuals adapt to their social environment. Described eight stages of psychosocial development of the identity throughout the lifespan, characterized by the following conflicts: trust vs. mistrust (infancy), autonomy vs. shame and doubt (early childhood), initiative vs. guilt (play age), industry vs. inferiority (school age), identity vs. role confusion (adolescence), intimacy vs. isolation (early adulthood), generativity vs. stagnation (middle adulthood), integrity vs. despair (old age).

Alfred Adler (1870–1937) Theorized that all people are born with an 'inferiority complex', an unconscious sense of inadequacy, which may lead them to over-compensate. Disagreed with Freud's emphasis on sexuality in the development of both normal personality and the neuroses.

Melanie Klein (1882–1960) A controversial figure and one of the founders of the object relations school. She demonstrated that a child's unconscious development can be understood by observing the child at play—felt to be analogous to free association. While her resulting developmental theories are not widely accepted by contemporary psychologists, play therapy is still commonly practised. She emphasized primitive defence mechanisms such as projection/projective identification, introjection, and splitting as well as the emotions of love, hate, anger, and envy.

Donald W. Winnicott (1897–1971) Another object relations theorist who studied the infant's growth of a sense of self. He described the 'transitional object', which was an item such as a teddy or blanket that aided the infant's transition to independence by standing in for the mother–infant object relationship. He described the 'good-enough mother' to refer to the environment needed for normal psychological development. He also developed the concept of true and false selves—the true self responds instinctively and spontaneously, but when parenting is not 'good enough' a false self-persona may develop to maintain relatedness with the parents while protecting the more vulnerable true self.

Wilfred R. Bion (1897–1979) A pioneer in thinking about groups whose 'basic assumptions' describe three ways in which groups may function:

dependency, fight–flight or pairing. He moved away from emphasizing the content of patients' narratives to thinking about how we structure the world around us through our thinking, and how this in turn allows our internal worlds to develop.

Carl Rogers (1902–1987) Worked on therapeutic technique. He conceived 'client-centred therapy'. He felt that the therapeutic attributes of genuineness, unconditional positive regard, and accurate empathy could help patients achieve what he called 'self-actualization', a complete sense of self, which was beneficial to their recovery.

John Bowlby (1907–1990) Worked on *attachment theory*, which has been developed from ethological studies and empirical research in humans such as observing infants' behaviours when separated from and then reunited with their mothers. Attachment theory stresses the importance of the feelings of closeness and security an infant develops with the caregiver as well as the role the caregiver plays in helping the infant to form these feelings. The child can, if such feelings have developed, then use the mother as a 'secure base' from which to explore and then return to when their anxiety increases. Bowlby delineated four different attachment styles which have been found to be transmitted from parent to child with reasonable reliability: secure, ambivalent, avoidant, and disorganized.

Basic psychoanalytical theory

Topographical model of the mind In *The interpretation of dreams* Freud theorized that the mind consisted of the unconscious, the preconscious, and the conscious. Only those ideas and memories in the conscious mind are within awareness. The preconscious contains those ideas and memories capable of entering the conscious mind. The preconscious performs a 'censorship' function by examining these ideas and memories and sending those which are unacceptable back to the unconscious ('repression'). The unconscious mind acts according to the 'pleasure principle'—the avoidance of pain and the seeking of gratification. This is modified by the 'reality principle' of the conscious mind: that gratification often must be postponed in order to obtain other forms of pleasure. Freud's psychoanalytic techniques would attempt to interpret unconscious content based on access to preconscious content, such as free associations, the content of dreams, transference, jokes, and 'parapraxes' (📖 p. 837).

Structural model of the mind Freud reconfigured the *topographical model* in light of his clinical experience. In the *structural model* an infant's mind was comprised of id ('the it', which wishes to pursue its own desires regardless of the constraints of morality or external reality) which is entirely unconscious. As time goes on and development occurs the mind further differentiates into the ego and then the superego. The ego ('the me') is mostly conscious, emerges during infancy, and is the part of the personality which negotiates between the 'three harsh masters': the desires of the id; the hold of reality; and the superego. The superego (the 'conscience') is the conscious and unconscious internalization of the morals and strictures of parents and society, which provides judgements on which behaviours are acceptable and which are not. When the ego is unable to successfully moderate between the id and superego it may defend the individual's sense of self by repressing the impulse to the unconscious, where its presence may produce disturbance. Alternatively, the ego may be tormented by an over-harsh superego.

Drive theory Freud postulated the existence of basic drives, which included 'libido', the sexual drive (📖 p. 832), which made up part of 'eros', the life drive, in opposition to 'thanatos', the drive towards death. He described the pleasure principle, the drive to avoid pain (or unpleasure) and experience pleasure as well as its modification through the reality principle. Additionally he described the *repetition compulsion*—the tendency of people to compulsively repeat their early experiences throughout their lives.

Transference reactions

Transference The unconscious development, in the patient, of feelings, thoughts, attitudes, and patterns of behaviour towards the therapist which recapitulate earlier life relationships, most usually the patient's relationships with their parents. Transference is viewed as a defence against the reality of relationships with others. The analysis of the transference is a prime feature of psychoanalysis.

Countertransference Describes the equivalent reaction in the therapist towards the patient, though this concept has now been extended by some schools to encompass all thoughts, feelings, imagery, etc. that patients evoke and engender in therapists. The examination of transference and countertransference is a central part of dynamic psychotherapies and guides diagnostic formulation and the exploration of the patient's pathology.

Thought processes

Dreams were felt by Freud to be the product of the unconscious mind as they occur when the internal censor is relaxed by sleep. They allow insight into unconscious thought process which is described as *primary process thinking*. In this form of thought there is no negation (yes and no can mean the same thing), there is no sense of time, ideas can be condensed into single symbols, and it is primarily symbolic and non-linear. *Secondary process thinking*, in contrast, is found within preconscious and conscious parts of the mind and is orientated to time, operates in a linear fashion, is predominantly word-orientated, and negation applies (i.e. yes is not no).

Psychoanalytical techniques

Free association The *fundamental rule* within psychoanalysis is for the patient to say whatever comes into his mind and then associate from this.

Resistance Blocks to free association, e.g. forgetting or changing the subject, demonstrate where resistance and hence psychological problems are present, i.e. the mind says 'don't even go there!'. These points of resistance are to be analysed, thus making the unconscious conscious, or more famously 'where it is, let ego be'.

Evenly suspended attention As a corollary to the patient's free association the analyst is asked to maintain themselves in a state of 'evenly suspended' attention to allow themselves to hear both what the patient is saying and what they are not.

Defence mechanisms

Freud conceived the idea of *repression* acting as a *defence* to prevent unacceptable thoughts from reaching conscious awareness. Subsequently other *defence mechanisms* were described, viewed as developing to prevent conflict between the conscious mind and unconscious desires and developing in the course of normal maturation. Mental disorder can be characterized by the persistence of primitive defence mechanisms, with immature defences seen in early childhood, mental illness and personality disturbances and neurotic defences seen in older children or adults experiencing stress or anxiety. Mature defences are seen in functioning adults. A full list of defence mechanisms is given on 📖 p. 830.

Defence mechanisms

Primitive defence mechanisms

Denial Remaining unaware of difficult events or subjective truths which are too hard to accept by pushing them into the unconscious.

Introjection Our perceptions of significant figures in our lives are internalized where they form the part of the structure of the personality (e.g. someone who was raised by a hostile and critical father may themselves feel persecuted by the introjection of this object but also may 'become like' this object at other times). Freud's theory on depression suggests that it is caused by introjection of the aspects of others that make the depressed patient feel anger, leading to 'anger turned inwards'.

Projection Attributing one's own internal unacceptable ideas and impulses to an external target, such as another individual, and reacting accordingly to them (e.g. an angry child looks at his dog and accuses it of being angry).

Projective identification Behaving toward another in a manner that causes them to take on one's own internal unacceptable ideas and impulses. Not to be confused with projection. Whereas during projection an individual with a certain emotion might perceive someone else as feeling the same way, in projective identification, the individual causes the other to feel that emotion (e.g. an angry child behaves in such a way that his mother becomes angry with him).

Idealization and denigration Perceiving others as ideal in order to avoid conflicting feelings about them. Humans find it less anxiety-provoking to avoid ambivalence and grey areas within people. The converse of idealization is denigration where only bad is seen within others.

Splitting Separating polarized and contradicting perceptions of self or others in order to disregard awareness of both simultaneously (e.g. a patient believing that a doctor is 'the best doctor they have ever had' at one point, and 'the worst doctor they have ever had' at another). This utilizes both idealization and denigration. Splitting can also happen intrasubjectively where patients split off parts of themselves that they find unacceptable and project these parts onto another person.

Acting out Literally acting out in ways that may reveal unconscious desires (e.g. a patient self-harming to express disgust at themselves).

Regression Responding to stress by reverting to a level of functioning of a previous maturational point (e.g. a teenager sucking their thumb around exam time).

Neurotic defence mechanisms

Repression Preventing unacceptable aspects of internal reality from coming to conscious attention. (A victim of childhood abuse may not have conscious awareness of the abuse as an adult.) The associated emotional reaction may remain in the conscious mind but divorced from its accompanying memory.

Identification Taking on the characteristics, feelings, and/or behaviours of someone else as one's own. Differs from introjection in a similar manner to the way projective identification differs from projection. Whereas in introjection, one may perceive themselves as being like someone else, in identification one may actually feel the way someone else does, and become more like the other person. An extension of this is found in the defence of identification with the aggressor wherein those who have been victims of aggression become aggressive themselves as this feels to the person like a less vulnerable position (e.g. a young man who was physically abused may grow up to be violent to others rather than remain in the vulnerable position of victim).

Intellectualization Focusing on abstract concepts, logic, and other forms of intellectual reasoning to avoid facing painful emotions (e.g. a victim of a traumatic abuse experience may discuss the statistics of abuse instead of talking about the particular experience).

Isolation of affect Separating an experience from the painful emotions associated with it (e.g. a victim describing a traumatic abuse experience without displaying any of the affect the experience has evoked).

Rationalization Justifying feelings or behaviours with a more acceptable explanation, rather than examining the unacceptable explanation known to the unconscious mind (e.g. a mourner stating that the deceased person is 'in a better place now' in order to ease feelings of guilt associated with the death).

Reaction formation Externally expressing attitudes and behaviours which are the opposite of the unacceptable internal impulses (e.g. being extra polite to a person to avoid expressing anger towards them).

Undoing and magical thinking The former is found when performing an action which has the effect of unconsciously 'cancelling out' an unacceptable internal impulse or previous experience. The action symbolizes the opposite outcome of the impulse or experience. Magical thinking is found when one attributes magical properties to thoughts or behaviours, e.g. 'if I throw this piece of paper in the bin five times in a row then I'll pass my exams'. Both these defences are associated with OCD.

Displacement Transferring the emotional response to a person to someone else that in some way resembles the original but is not associated with as much conflict or risk (e.g. a boy feeling anger towards a man who reminds him of his father, rather than towards his father).

Mature defence mechanisms

Humour Finding aspects of an unpleasant experience funny or ironic in order to manage the experience without the associated painful emotions.

Altruism Attending to the needs of others above one's own needs.

Compensation Developing abilities in one area in response to a deficit in another.

Sublimation Expressing unacceptable internal impulses in socially acceptable ways.

Theory of psychosexual development

Freud theorized that everyone is born with an instinctive sex drive called the libido, a primary source of tension if unsatisfied. He developed a theory that attempted to explain the development of the personality during infancy and childhood. He visualized five phases, characterized by particular satisfactions and conflicts. Infants progressed from a state of primary narcissism, in which they find gratification in their own body processes, to 'object love', in which they can more clearly separate themselves from other 'objects', or people. Inability to resolve the conflicts of a particular stage could lead to a lack of psychosexual development, while regression to an earlier state could result in the development of neurotic symptoms (Table 20.1).

Table 20.1 Phases of psychosexual develpoment

Phase	Source of pleasure	Conflicts
Oral phase Birth to 15–18 mths	Suckling and investigation of objects by placing them in the mouth.	Love for breast of nursing mother vs. 'aggressive' urge to bite or spit.
Anal phase 15–18 to 30–36 mths	Anal sensations, the production of faeces and, later, the ability to withhold faeces.	Need to control sphincter enough to avoid shame of making a mess (related to pleasing authority and keeping orderly), but not so much that there is faecal retention.
Phallic phase 30–48 mths to around the end of the fifth year	Manipulation of the penis.	Boys: Move through the Oedipal phase (Box 20.1). Girls: 'Penis envy' leading to feelings of inferiority (*Note*: this theory has been rejected or modified by many modern dynamic theorists) and pass through the Electra complex (the inverse of the Oedipal complex).
Oedipal phase 48 mths–6 yrs	Fantasies of sexual intercourse with opposite sex parent with a corresponding wish to kill the same sex parent.	Boys: Love for mother vs. fear of castration by father, leading to 'castration anxiety'. Boy's unconscious desires were characterized by the 'Oedipus complex'. Girls: Desire for a baby leads to attachment to father as someone who potentially can give her one. Called the 'Electra complex'.
Latency phase 6 yrs until puberty	Period of relative quiescence of sexual thoughts	The anxieties from the previous phase are repressed. The sexual drive remains latent through this period.
Genital phase Adult sexuality, beginning at puberty	The sexual drive returns with greater strength than before.	Improper resolution of previous phases may be manifest in symbolic ways.

Box 20.1 The story of Oedipus (Sophocles ~430 BC)

King Laius of Thebes is told by the oracle at Delphi that his son will kill him and marry his wife. When his wife Jocasta gives birth to a boy, Oedipus, he orders a slave to abandon the child on a mountain. The slave takes pity on the child and, instead of leaving him to die, gives him to a shepherd, who brings him to the King of Corinth who is childless. Oedipus grows up thinking that Polibus, King of Corinth, is his father.

As a youth, Oedipus visits the oracle at Delphi and is told that he will grow up to kill his father and marry his mother. At this, Oedipus vows never to return to Corinth and sets out for Thebes instead. On a narrow part of the road he meets an old man in a chariot who angrily orders him aside and strikes him with a spear. Oedipus seizes the spear to defend himself and strikes the old man on the head, killing him. The man is Laius, King of Thebes, his real father.

Approaching Thebes, Oedipus meets the Sphinx which is terrorizing the city. The monster is stopping all passers-by and challenging them with its riddle; those who fail to answer the riddle are devoured. Oedipus solves the riddle of the Sphinx and the monster jumps to its death. He enters the city as a hero. He is told that the king has been murdered and is offered the throne, together with the hand of Jocasta in marriage.

Oedipus is a wise and successful king and Jocasta bears him two sons and two daughters. Many years later Thebes is afflicted by a terrible plague. The people appeal to Oedipus to save them and he sends his brother-in-law to the oracle at Delphi for advice. The oracle states that the plague will abate when the murderer of Laius is banished. Oedipus promises to bring the murderer to justice and forbids the people of Thebes from offering him any shelter.

Oedipus asks the prophet Teiresias to help him discover the killer's identity. Teiresias tries to dissuade him from pursuing the matter but the king persists, eventually accusing the prophet of being a fraud. Teiresias them angrily tells him that before nightfall he will find himself 'both a brother and a father to his children'. The king is bewildered and Jocasta tries to comfort him by telling him about the prophecy given to Laius—it was prophesied that he would be killed by his son, when in fact his son had died as an infant and he had been killed by bandits—hence prophecies could not be trusted. This story only increases Oedipus's worry and he suspects that he murdered Laius but does not yet realize that Laius was his father.

A messenger arrives to inform him of the death of the King of Corinth. The messenger also reveals that Oedipus was adopted. He begins to suspect that he is the son of Laius and continues to investigate, ignoring the pleas of Jocasta who has already realized the whole truth. Eventually he finds the shepherd who took him to the household of the King of Corinth and the full truth is revealed. At this point he hears anguished cries coming from the palace and rushes to his apartments. Oedipus breaks down the door of the royal bedchamber to find the queen, his wife and mother, has hanged herself. He seizes her dress pin and gouges out his eyes so as not to have to look at the atrocity he has unwittingly committed. He enters into exile, having failed to avoid the fate laid out for him.

Object relations theory

In the mid-twentieth century Winnicott, Klein, Fairbairn, and others developed object relations theory which emphasized the importance of relationships, rather than drives such as sexuality and aggression, in affecting the mind. This theory describes a model of infant psychological development, links abnormal early experiences to symptoms in later life, and uses this as a basis for interpretation in therapy. Object relations theory remains significant in modern psychoanalytical practice.

Essence Our 'sense of self' and our adult personality are developed as a result of the relationships we form in our lives. The earliest, and hence the most important, relationship is that between mother and child. Our early relationships form a template for future relationships, with abnormal early experiences being associated with psychological symptoms and abnormal relationships later in life.

Theory The mind is viewed as blank at birth with the newborn unable to distinguish between 'myself' and 'everything else'. Then the infant begins to view the external world as a series of (initially unconnected) 'objects'. These objects may be things (e.g. a toy, a blanket), people (e.g. mother, father), or parts of people or things (e.g. the mother's breast, the mother's face). The infant creates an internal representation of each object and has relationships with, and feelings towards, the internal as well as the external objects.

There are three primitive emotions (or 'affects') which an infant can display towards each object—attachment, frustration, and rejection. There is a tendency for a single affect to become associated with one object. Inevitably even a caring mother will create some feelings of frustration and rejection: mothers comfort their children and provide food and love, but also scold, punish and are sometimes simply unable to meet their child's needs. Consequently the child will view the mother as comprising a number of objects, some of which he views positively and some with hostility.

The child will initially deal with this by keeping the 'good objects' (associated with attachment) separate from the 'bad objects' (those causing frustration and rejection)—a phenomenon known as 'splitting'. This is the initial primitive defence mechanism—the 'paranoid–schizoid position'. As the child develops, this defence becomes increasingly untenable and, in normal development the child will unify the good and bad maternal objects to a single 'mother object' containing both good and bad—the so-called 'depressive position'.

The relationships we form later in life have a strong tendency to echo relationships from earlier in our development. Interestingly, we can take on either role in these recapitulated relationships. Hence a child, one of whose parental relationships was with an aggressive/abusive father, can take on a 'victim' posture in some later relationships but may instead take on the role of the aggressor in others.

In therapy The therapist's neutral stance provides an ideal environment for the recapitulation of previous relationships. Most relationships are moulded by both parties, but in therapy the therapist aims to allow the relationship model to be developed by the patient. The subsequent examination of the role and relationship forced onto the therapist (the transference) is a key part of therapy. Most therapies incorporating object relations theory help the patient resolve the pathological qualities of the transference through the experience of the real relationship between the therapist and the patient. Once these relationships are identified they can begin to explore with the patient how the relationship in the consulting room reflects the patient's experience growing up as well as their current life-situations.

Psychoanalysis 1

Dynamic therapies, including psychoanalysis or psychodynamic psychotherapy and group analysis are derived from the psychoanalytic principles and practice of Sigmund Freud and those who have subsequently developed his ideas. Most therapies which conceptualize an unconscious mind affecting our perceptions and actions can be considered part of the school of the dynamic psychotherapies.

Rationale

Traumatic experiences, particularly those in early life, give rise to psychological conflict. The greater part of mental activity is unconscious and the conscious mind is protected from the experience of this conflict by inbuilt defences, designed to decrease 'unpleasure' and to diminish anxiety. These defences are developmentally appropriate but their continuation into adult life results in either psychological symptoms or in a diminished ability for personal growth and fulfilment. Conflict can be examined with regard to the anxiety itself, the defence, or the underlying wish or memory. The individual's previous family and personal relationships will have symbolic meaning and be charged with powerful emotions. Representations of these relationships will emerge during therapy and provide a route towards understanding and change.

How illness is viewed

Both mental illness and normal psychological development can be understood using psychoanalytic theories. In psychoanalysis overt symptoms are viewed as merely the external expression of underlying psychic abnormality. Symptoms continue, despite the suffering they cause to the individual because of what Freud called primary gain. This is the benefit to the individual of not having unacceptable ideas in the conscious mind. While a typical descriptive assessment of a patient by a psychiatrist may categorize patients into groups using diagnostic criteria, a dynamic assessment of a patient uses psychoanalytic theory to explore the unique layout of the individual patient's conscious and unconscious mind.

Techniques

Psychoanalysis is an intense therapy that usually involves one to five, 50-min sessions per week possibly for a number of years. Psychoanalysis typically features traditional techniques to attempt to interpret unconscious content, including the 'fundamental rule' of free association, analysis of the transference/countertransference, the interpretation of dreams, 'parapraxes', and the symbolism of neurotic symptoms. Therapists of different schools will utilize these techniques in slightly different ways, e.g. by choosing what to interpret and why. The three mainstays of analyst–analysand interaction are enquiry, clarification, and interpretation.

Free association The patient agrees to reveal everything which comes to mind, no matter how embarrassing or socially unacceptable (i.e. 'speaking without self-censorship'). Traditionally the patient is speaking in a reclining position with minimal eye contact with the therapist, i.e. 'on the couch'.

The therapist assumes a position of neutrality, in which reassurance and directive advice are withheld. Areas where free association 'breaks down' and areas of resistance to pursue associative thought may represent difficulties which are important to explore.

Exploration of transference/countertransference

(See **Transference reactions** 📖 p. 828.) The intense and frequent nature of psychoanalysis often results in a patient forming powerful feelings towards a therapist, who adopts a stance of neutrality—a blank screen on which the patient can project their internal world. Important repressed aspects of past relationships and defence mechanisms used by the patient in current relationships find expression in the transference relationship. Through adopting a mindset called 'reverie' (similar to evenly suspended attention), psychoanalysts, through monitoring their own countertransference, attempt to avoid fulfilling the patient's unconscious expectations that they will act like the people from their past as well as using thoughts that enter consciousness as information about the patient's inner world.

Examination of dreams

Dreams are traditionally viewed as being formed by a mix of daytime memories, nocturnal stimuli, and representations of unconscious desires, which are then distorted by the ego to protect us from conscious knowledge of the content. The actual or 'latent' dream is eventually reconstructed from the 'manifest' dream, the portions of the dream that patients remember in therapy, by a process of symbolization and elaboration which can potentially expose the hidden unconscious meanings.

Examination of parapraxes

A parapraxis is a slip of the tongue, which today is often referred to as a 'Freudian slip'. They may reveal unconscious desires, thoughts and feelings.

Examination of symbolism

In individual patients, neurotic symptoms may have symbolic meaning which can be usefully explored. Symbolism may also be analysed in child psychotherapy when observing play and drawings.

Interpretation

Expression of the therapist's understanding of the meaning of what is occurring in therapy. Interpretations commonly include descriptions of defence mechanisms, explanations for current anxiety in the context of underlying desires and making links between what is happening in the here-and-now of the transference relationship between patient and therapist and how that connects to their earlier experiences.

Psychoanalysis 2

Phases of treatment

Assessment and early sessions

The analyst will typically explain methods of therapy, establish boundaries (e.g. about times of sessions), and begin to produce a psychodynamic formulation of the case. The therapist will assess patient suitability and motivation while exploring potential risk factors.

Middle sessions

As the patient progresses in psychoanalysis, the therapist, who will typically work with a supervisor (providing a valuable third position view of the case outwith the close relationship between analyst and analysand), identifies unconscious defence mechanisms, key conflicts, personality structure, patterns of object relations and transference/countertransference.

Later sessions

The therapist may use more interpretive techniques, which may increase anxiety. Towards the end of therapy, which is in the main mutually negotiated, increasing focus will be placed on the patient's thoughts, feelings, and attitudes to termination of therapy as loss and abandonment are often key areas in patients' pathology.

Indications and contraindications

(See also **Assessment for psychotherapy** 📖 p. 822.)

- Commonly chosen by the patient rather than prescribed though this may be due to its lack of availability through the public sector.
- Not reserved only for specific mental illnesses—those with relatively sound mental health may find it improves the quality of their lives.
- Commonly sought by patients where there are anxious or emotional symptoms, such as mild to moderate depressive symptoms, somatic symptoms, dissociative or other neurotic symptoms
- Patients with substantial personality difficulties are increasingly seen.
- May be a good choice for patients who are looking for change, motivated to explore past experiences, and are emotionally stable and willing to re-experience some emotional challenges in doing so.
- Psychoanalysis is not absolutely contraindicated for drug or alcohol dependence, suicidal thoughts or harmful/violent behaviours, psychotic illness, severe depressive features, limited cognitive ability, but most practitioners would be aware of the potential pitfalls present in each of these classes of patient.

Efficacy and limitations of dynamic therapies

Evidence base?

Studies have demonstrated benefits in decreased symptoms, decreased need for medication, as well as long-term and enduring improvements in personality-disordered individuals. The volume, validity, and reliability of the evidence, however, is limited. Some clinicians criticize all dynamic therapies because they have arisen primarily from theory and clinical observations instead of evidence-based medicine. This may not reflect on the inefficacy of psychodynamic therapies as much as it reflects the inherent difficulties in designing research studies. There is a lack of standardization in diagnosis, in method of therapy delivery (as by its very nature it is delivered by individuals to other individuals, both of whom are bewilderingly complex), problems with gaining sufficient numbers of patients and controls for statistical analyses to be viable, and determining how improvement is measured as even Freud regarded the task as converting 'neurotic misery into ordinary unhappiness'. Psychodynamic researchers also stress the point that much of psychoanalysis is process- and not outcome-orientated. Nonetheless, the future may bring more of an evidence base to support dynamic therapies, both alone and in combination with psychotropic medications. Studies may also show more support for the theories behind psychodynamic therapies. There is already experimental psychological research to support that mental activity can be unconscious, such as studies that show initiation of action by pre-frontal cortex begins before 'consciousness' in the frontal areas is involved.

Possible harm?

While dynamic therapies do not have the biological side-effects of psychiatric medications, they are not free of risk. These therapies aid in increasing the insight of the patient, which may involve the removal of defence mechanisms that play a protective role, and therefore must be done with caution, especially with patients whose 'psychic scaffolding' is integral to their managing day to day life. The risks and benefits of such phenomena are a subject of study and controversy, although most dynamic therapists would agree that patient readiness determines when to explore painful experiences in therapy.

Training

Involves education in psychoanalytic history, theory and practice, extensive supervised case work, and personal psychoanalysis for the therapists themselves. Many major British and Irish cities have a local psychoanalytic institute that may offer formal psychoanalytic training to those with doctoral or master's degrees in mental health and 2yrs of clinical experience. Training usually consists of a 5yr postgraduate curriculum specifically in psychoanalysis. For doctors, this training would typically be completed after completion of a basic specialist psychiatric training. Most institutes also offer supervision and classes for therapists who are interested in dynamic psychotherapy, but have not chosen the 5yr psychoanalytic programme.

Psychodynamic psychotherapy

Psychodynamic psychotherapy is an intervention where the concepts of symptom development are based on those of psychoanalysis, but the methods of therapy are adjusted for a reduced frequency of sessions and decreased number of total sessions. Supporters of this type of therapy state that some of the insights and opportunity for change and growth available from long-term psychoanalysis can be achieved in a shorter time and that introducing directive elements and focus on particular topics does not reduce overall effectiveness.

Rationale and **How illness is viewed** As for psychoanalysis (📖 p. 836).

Techniques

- Psychodynamic psychotherapy is modified from psychoanalysis in that it often involves active therapy, where the therapist may say more in an attempt to allow therapy to be more structured. It can vary in length depending on both the therapist and the needs of the patient. It may be significantly more brief than psychoanalysis, often lasting 6mths or 1yr with the termination date decided at the outset. Shorter treatments (of around 16 sessions) may be placed under the heading of 'brief psychodynamic psychotherapy'. The frequency may be 1–2 sessions a week.
- The therapist usually develops a working psychodynamic formulation early on which is then referred to throughout the therapy.
- Methods employed are similar to those of psychoanalysis (📖 p. 836), but with therapist–patient eye contact (i.e. both sitting on chairs rather than the patient lying on a couch) and more verbal interaction from the therapist.
- Both transference and countertransference give the therapist valuable information about the nature of past relationships (📖 p. 837).
- The therapist will help the patient to explore symptom precipitants and associated early trauma and avoidance.
- The therapist may guide therapy by use of interpretation at an earlier point than in psychoanalysis.
- In the case of patients with more severe mental illness, such as psychosis, or in acute crisis or decompensation, these techniques are sometimes further modified to be less focused on improving insight, and instead, the emphasis is more supportive, particularly focusing on encouraging the expression of emotions. This can be combined with drug treatment.

Phases of treatment

Initial assessment

Diagnosis, including consideration of appropriateness of this method of therapy in this patient. Consideration of appropriate use of medication.

Early sessions

Identification of main problems, goals, and issues. Limited comments from therapist. Usually there is positive transference due to expectation of 'magical' change. Identification of main defences, coping styles, and ability to accept and work with interpretations.

Middle sessions
Exploring present emotions and emotions evoked by past experiences. Exploration of transference, countertransference, and resistance in discussion with supervisor.

Closing sessions
Exploring anticipation of termination. Arrangements for aftercare.

Indications and contraindications
See **Assessment for psychotherapy** 📖 p. 822 and **Efficacy and limitations of dynamic therapies** 📖 p. 838.
- Indications and contraindications are similar to those of psychoanalysis 📖 p. 838.
- Particular emphasis on the ability and motivation to form a collaborative relationship with a therapist.

Training
Similar to training for psychoanalysis, including education in psychoanalytic history, theory and practice, supervised case work, and personal psychoanalysis. Local psychoanalytic institutes may offer courses varying in length and required time commitment.

Group psychotherapy

Group psychotherapy is a form of treatment in which selected individuals are brought together under the guidance of a therapist with the goals of reducing distress and symptoms, increasing coping, or improving relationships. Group methods were first developed in the early twentieth century following observations of beneficial group effects with TB patients. Like individual psychotherapy, the term group psychotherapy encompasses a range of modalities, settings, and techniques.

Groups may be homogeneous or heterogeneous (e.g. in terms of diagnosis, age, gender), and may vary as to the frequency and duration of meetings, the degree of therapist involvement, and whether they are time-limited or ongoing. The basic tasks of the therapist include making decisions about these factors, preparing and assessing patients for the therapy, formulating goals for therapy, and building and maintaining a therapeutic environment that promotes group interaction.

Yalom[1] described a set of therapeutic factors common to many types of group: instillation of hope, universality, imparting information, altruism, corrective recapitulation of the primary family group, development of socializing techniques, imitation of adaptive behaviour, interpersonal learning, group cohesion, catharsis, and existential factors.

Indications and contraindications

Group therapy generally requires that members:

- Are able to tolerate the task of interacting in a group.
- Have problem areas that are compatible with the goals of the group.
- Are consciously motivated for change.

While most patients may benefit from some form of group therapy, exclusion criteria include:

- Inability to comply with the group norms for acceptable behaviour (e.g. assaults on other patients or therapist).
- Inability to tolerate the group setting (e.g. paranoid ideas).
- Severe incompatibility with one or more group members (which may only be discernible after members have joined the group).

Types of group therapy

Supportive groups

Features

- Focus on promoting and strengthening adaptive defences, giving advice, providing encouragement.
- Goals include re-establishing and/or maintaining function, improving coping.

Indications May be useful in psychotic disorders, anxiety disorders, and in a self-help context.

Problem-focused cognitive–behavioural groups
Features
- Useful where the goal is modification of dysfunctional thoughts, feelings, and behaviours, such as in anxiety, depressive, and eating disorders.
- Focus is on psychoeducation, mutual support, and group examination of strategies for change within a CBT framework, rather than on the nature of interpersonal interactions between members.
- Therapist takes an active and central role.
- Peers may be experts at identifying resistance and rationalization for avoiding change in other group members.

Indications Can include anxiety or anger management, assertiveness training, acute or chronic depression, alcohol or drug dependence.

Psychodynamic groups, including group analysis
Features
- The individual is viewed as embedded in a social network or 'matrix'.
- Members' interactions with each other and the therapist reflect their interactions with others outside the group (i.e. the interpersonal difficulties which have brought them to therapy). An individual's range of relationship styles derives from early experience (e.g. the position they tended to take up within the family, at school, etc.). Examination of interactions between group members and with the therapist aims to increase patients' understanding of this repeating repertoire of contact with people, and to change dysfunctional patterns.
- Techniques include close examination of transference, counter-transference, resistance, and unconscious conflict.
- Goal is lasting change through modification of personality factors.

Indications See **Psychoanalysis** p. 838.

Activity groups
Generally helpful for patients with intellectual impairment, or severe and persistent mental illness. Examples include art, music, computing, exercise, and social activity groups. Can foster social skills and adaptive behaviours. Helpful for psychosocial and vocational rehabilitation.

Self-help groups
Strictly speaking, not a form of group therapy, though may have beneficial therapeutic effects. Groups tend to be organized around a specific problem, have strong peer support and group cohesion, and be led from within the group. Examples include Alcoholics Anonymous, Narcotics Anonymous, Gamblers Anonymous, Overeaters Anonymous.

1 Yalom ID (1995) *The theory and practice of group psychotherapy*, 4th edn. New York: Basic Books.

Basic learning theory

Behavioural psychology is a method for understanding the development of knowledge and behaviours in organisms. In an individual organism these are shaped by environmental influences and can change as a result of experience. Learning theory concerns the testing of methods to produce behavioural adaptation through changing environmental influences. The two basic learning processes are *classical (Pavlovian) conditioning*—involuntary behaviours which become associated with stimuli, and *operant (Skinnerian) conditioning*—learning to obtain reward and avoid punishment related to voluntary behaviours. Although most abnormal mental processes and mental illnesses are not amenable to understanding purely in terms of conditioning, understanding of learning theory is helpful in conceptualizing the development and maintenance of abnormal mental processes and provides a rationale for behavioural and cognitive behavioural treatment approaches.

Classical conditioning

In his initial experiment, Pavlov presented a dog with food which produced the response of salivation. Here the food is the unconditioned stimulus (US) and the salivation is the unconditioned response (UR). A neutral stimulus such as a bell ringing is not associated with any unconditioned response. However, if a bell is rung immediately before the food is presented, after a number of repetitions the dog will salivate in response to the bell alone. Now the bell is a conditioned stimulus (CS) producing a conditioned response (CR), the salivation.

Acquisition
The development of the association between the UR and the US producing a CR. In animal experiments this can take between 3 and 15 pairings. Where there is sufficient emotional involvement, acquisition can occur with as few as one pairing.

Extinction The loss of the association between the CR and the CS. Occurs when the CS is repeatedly *not* followed by the US.

Generalization The phenomenon where similar stimuli to the initial CS produce the response. The subject then demonstrates the conditioned response (CR) to these similar stimuli (e.g. to a buzzer as well as a bell).

Higher-order conditioning
Process in which conditioned trials cause the subject to demonstrate the CR to new stimuli by pairing them with the CS (e.g. where the dog has been conditioned to salivate to a bell, pairing the bell with a light stimulus so the dog becomes conditioned to salivate to the light).

Spontaneous recovery During extinction trials, following a rest period, the conditioned response (CR) often briefly reappears.

Habituation The subject becomes accustomed to and less responsive to a stimulus after repeated exposure.

Note: for emotional disorders the response is usually an emotion rather than a behaviour. For example, an initial encounter with a large, barking dog which bites the individual can produce the CR of fear to the generalized CS of seeing a dog. The affected individual may then avoid all contact with dogs and so avoid the unpleasant CR. However, because there is no occasion when the CS of seeing a dog is not paired with the CR of fear, there is no opportunity for extinction to take place.

Techniques based on classical conditioning concepts

- *Systematic desensitization* (📖 p. 848): presentation of situations more similar to the CS are paired with relaxation techniques, in order to eventually break the association between the CS and the CR. Frequently used in the treatment of phobic anxiety disorders.
- *Flooding* (📖 p. 848): presentation of full CS without the possibility of withdrawal from the situation. The initial unpleasant experience of the CR gradually diminishes, and the patient learns that they can survive exposure to the feared situation without coming to harm.

Operant conditioning

The experimental techniques and rules of operant conditioning were developed by Thorndike and Skinner. The basic principles of operant conditioning are that if a response to a stimulus produces positive consequences for the individual it will tend to be repeated, while if it is followed by negative consequences it will tend not to be repeated. In the original experiments rats were placed in a box containing a lever which, when pressed, delivered a pellet of food. Eventually the rat would press the lever and be rewarded. The rat would then press the lever with increasing frequency. (Note that operant conditioning doesn't rely on insight on the part of the rat.)

Acquisition The linkage of the response (pressing the lever) with the reinforcer (receiving the food).

Reinforcement

Can be *positive* (behaviour is followed by a desirable outcome) or *negative* (behaviour is followed by removal of an aversive stimulus). Can occur after every response (continuous reinforcement) or only after some responses (partial reinforcement). Behaviours conditioned by partial reinforcement extinguish at a much slower rate than those conditioned by continuous reinforcement.

Punishment

In *positive* punishment an operant response is followed by the presentation of an aversive stimulus in an attempt to decrease the likelihood of a behaviour occurring in the future. In *negative* punishment an operant response is followed by the removal of an aversive stimulus.

Shaping

Used to produce a complex behaviour which is not in the organism's initial repertoire. Initially, component parts of the desired behaviour are rewarded, then reward is limited to behaviour which approximates the desired result. As appropriate behaviour appears it is only rewarded if it is 'in the right direction' and further reward is contingent upon continued advancement until the organism is only rewarded once the entire behavior is performed.

Extinction

Occurs over time when the response is no longer followed by the reinforcer.

Techniques based on operant conditioning concepts (📖 p. 848)

- Behaviour modification.
- Aversion therapy.

Behaviour therapy

Techniques based on learning theory are used in order to extinguish maladaptive behaviours and substitute more adaptive ones.

Systematic desensitization

Holds as a central tenet the principle of reciprocal inhibition (i.e. anxiety and relaxation cannot coexist). Systematic graded exposure to the source of anxiety is coupled with the use of relaxation techniques (the 'desensitization' component). Effective for simple phobias, but less so for other phobic/anxiety disorders (e.g. agoraphobia). Process in a typical case is as follows:

- Patient identifies the specific fear (e.g. cats).
- Patient and therapist develop a hierarchy of situations listing the most anxiety-provoking situation at the top (e.g. stroking a cat on one's knee > touching a cat > having a cat in the room > looking at pictures of cats > thinking about cats).
- Patient is instructed in relaxation technique.
- Patient experiences the lowest item on the hierarchy while practising the relaxation technique and remains exposed to the item until the anxiety has diminished.
- The process is repeated until the item no longer produces anxiety.
- The next item in the hierarchy is tackled in similar fashion.

Flooding/implosive therapy

High levels of anxiety cannot be maintained for long periods, and a process of 'exhaustion' occurs. By exposing the patient to the phobic object and preventing the usual escape or avoidance, there is extinction of the usual (maladaptive) anxiety response. This may be done *in vivo* (flooding) or in imagination (implosion).

Behaviour modification

Based on operant conditioning. Behaviour may be shaped towards the desired final modification through the rewarding of small, achievable intermediate steps. This can be utilized in behavioural disturbance in children and patients with learning disability. Other forms of behavioural modification include the more explicit use of secondary reinforcement, such as 'token economy', in which socially desirable/acceptable behaviours are rewarded with tokens that can be exchanged for other material items or privileges, or 'star charts' where children's good behaviour is rewarded when a certain level is achieved. May also be used for less voluntary actions such as childhood nocturnal enuresis.

Aversion therapy and covert sensitization

The use of negative reinforcement (the unpleasant consequence of a particular behaviour) to inhibit the usual maladaptive behavioural response (extinction). True 'aversion' therapy (e.g. previously used to treat sexual deviancy) is not used today; however, covert techniques (e.g. the use of antabuse in alcohol dependency) can be (at least partially) effective.

Cognitive behavioural therapy 1

The theory and method of cognitive behaviour therapy (CBT) were developed by Aaron Beck and outlined in a series of papers published in the 1960s.[1] CBT development was prompted by the observation that patients referred for psychotherapy often held ingrained, negatively skewed assumptions of themselves, their future, and their environment. Treatment is based on the idea that disorder is caused not by life events, but by the view the patient takes of events. It is a short-term, collaborative therapy, focused on current problems, whose goals are symptom relief and the development of new skills to sustain recovery.

Rationale

A person's emotions, thoughts, behaviours, physiological sensations and their external environment all exist together in equilibrium. Altering any component of this system will bring about change in the others. While pathological emotions may not be directly amenable to change, the unhelpful cognitions and behaviours associated with these emotions may be examined and modified, leading to change in the underlying emotion. CBT aims to 'change how you feel by changing the way you think'.[2] The cognitive model is a guide for therapy, not a comprehensive model of illness causation, and precludes neither neurochemical or other factors as important in symptom development, nor the use of pharmacological treatments.

How illness is viewed

In some personality types and in mental illness there are errors in the evaluation and processing of information (i.e. cognitive distortions). These distortions relate to the self, the world, and the future (Beck's cognitive triad) and originate from the child's early learning and experience of the world around him. Cognitive errors are associated with unpleasant emotions and maladaptive behaviour.

An example of this vicious circle is: an event (friend doesn't call when she said she would) → negative automatic thought ('friend doesn't like me because she thinks I'm a loser') → emotional response (sadness) → maladaptive behaviour → (avoiding friend → self-isolation → worsening of low mood) = pathology (depression). In CBT with this patient, the therapist would facilitate their recognition of the faulty cognitive appraisal (cognitive error) and then teach skills to address it—see Box 20.2 and Box 20.3.

Modes of delivery

CBT can be delivered on an individual basis, in groups, or as self-help via books or computer programs (including online). As such it is a cost-effective treatment with evidence of good efficacy. It is worth stressing that CBT is at its most effective when delivered 'by the book', following established protocols. Sessions by trainees are therefore often taped to ensure adherence to a standard regimen.

Box 20.2 Cognitions

Cognitions are appraisals of events. They may be elicited by asking the patient about thoughts, ideas, or images in their head. CBT describes three types of thoughts or beliefs:

- *Automatic thoughts* are the most superficial and accessible. They are involuntary and appear plausible, but may be distorted, e.g. 'my friend phoned to cancel meeting me tomorrow—she must not like me any more.'
- *Underlying assumptions* are a person's 'rules' for behaving, based on fundamental beliefs and shaped by experience, e.g. 'I can't enjoy myself unless I'm with other people.'
- *Schemas or core beliefs* are a person's most fundamental beliefs about themselves and the world around them, e.g. a neglected child believing 'I am unlovable.'

Box 20.3 Common types of cognitive error

- Selective abstraction—drawing a conclusion based only on part of the information, e.g. 'My whole dinner party was a failure because my dessert didn't turn out as I'd hoped.'
- Arbitrary inference—drawing an unjustified conclusion, e.g. 'My partner appears stressed, s/he must be about to leave me.'
- All or nothing thinking—seeing things only as extremes of black or white with no shades of grey, e.g. 'I must win or else I'm a failure.'
- Magnification/minimization—emphasizing negatives and playing down positives, e.g. 'My career hasn't been successful, even my few achievements weren't all that impressive.'
- Disqualifying the positive—e.g. 'I only came first by chance.'
- Personalization—assuming responsibility for all negative events, e.g. 'My sister is in a bad mood, she must be angry with me.'
- Catastrophic thinking—e.g. 'I embarrassed myself in front of my colleagues—I'll never be able to face them again.'
- Over-generalization—viewing a single negative event as the norm, e.g. 'I made a mistake, therefore I'm incompetent to do my job.'
- Emotional reasoning—using emotions as evidence, e.g. 'I feel very anxious, therefore that spider must be really dangerous.'
- Jumping to conclusions—mindreading or fortune-telling, e.g. 'I know the exam will ask about topics I haven't had time to study.'

1 Wright JH (2006) Cognitive behaviour therapy: basic principles and recent advances. *Focus* **4**(2): 173–8.
2 Padesky CA and Greenberger D (1995) *Mind over mood*. New York: Guilford.

Cognitive behavioural therapy 2

Techniques

The CBT therapist works together with the patient in a spirit of scientific inquiry to explore the problem and possible solutions. Through a process of psychoeducation and guided discovery, the therapist assists the patient in monitoring cognitions and their associated emotions and behaviours; identifying and challenging cognitive distortions; and exploring alternative strategies for approaching distressing situations. Progress is measured against objective rating scales (e.g. the Beck Depression Inventory[1]), as well as the patient's own goals for therapy.

Phases of treatment

Initial assessment is usually followed by 6–20 hour-long sessions. There may be a review after 6 sessions to share a formulation, take stock of progress so far and refocus goals if therapy is to continue. Attention is primarily focused on events in the 'here and now'. Each session generally proceeds as follows: deal with emergencies; jointly set agenda; review homework task; focus on specific items guided by current problems; suggestion of cognitive or behavioural techniques (see Box 20.4); jointly agree on homework task.

Indications and contraindications

CBT is an active treatment requiring patient understanding and collaboration (see Box 20.4). Patients should be motivated and be able to recognize, articulate, and link their thoughts and emotions (i.e. be psychologically minded). The general contraindications to psychotherapy (📖 p. 822) apply. It is indicated for:
- Mild to moderate depressive illness.
- Eating disorders.
- Anxiety disorders.
- Bipolar disorder (reduce risk of relapse).
- Substance abuse disorders.
- Schizophrenia and other chronic psychotic disorders as an adjunct to pharmacotherapy, for both positive and negative symptoms.
- Chronic medical conditions such as fibromyalgia, chronic fatigue, or chronic pain, where there may be a psychological component and misinterpretation of physiological phenomena.

Efficacy

There is good evidence for effectiveness in depressive illness, eating disorders and anxiety disorders. CBT is at least as effective as pharmacotherapy in mild to moderate depression and may be more effective in long-term follow-up (e.g. in preventing relapse).

Box 20.4 CBT techniques for depression and anxiety

Depression
- Psychoeducation, including straightforward reading material about depression and introducing the cognitive model—a useful first homework assignment.
- Activity diary: over a week, ask the patient to record what they did in the morning, afternoon and evening of each day. The patient may rate the sense of pleasure associated on a scale of 0–10, and assign a score of 0–10 for their mood each day.
- Activity and pleasant event scheduling: make plans for the week in advance to increase general physical activity and enjoyable events, both of which are often reduced and contribute to the vicious cycle of depression. Goals should be small and achievable.
- Thoughts diary: ask the patient to make a record at the times when they feel particularly distressed, noting the trigger situation, their mood rating, and the thoughts which they experience.
- Teach the patient to identify cognitive errors in their automatic thoughts.
- Socratic questioning to elicit further thoughts ('If that were true, what would it mean?…and what would that mean?…etc.').
- Examine the evidence for and against the patient's faulty beliefs and generate rational alternatives.
- Behavioural experiments: designed collaboratively to test the hypothesis that the patient's beliefs are true, e.g. inviting a friend to meet for coffee to test the thought 'my friends don't want to know me any more'

Anxiety
- Psychoeducation, introducing the cognitive model of anxiety.
- Diary keeping: to record and monitor episodes of anxiety, their triggers, the intensity of anxiety on a scale of 0–10, and the associated thoughts and physical symptoms.
- Relaxation techniques: e.g. through breathing or progressive muscular relaxation.
- Distraction to divert the cognitive focus elsewhere.
- Challenge negative thoughts by examining the evidence for and against them, generating rational alternatives, and identifying cognitive errors.
- Construct a hierarchy of the patient's most anxiety-provoking situations, consisting of many small steps.
- Graded exposure: starting with the least threatening step of the hierarchy, coupled with relaxation techniques. Role play/rehearsal or attempting an activity together with the therapist (e.g. going into a shop) may be helpful.
- Behavioural experiments: e.g. recording anxiety repeatedly during exposure to a stressful situation, to challenge patient's assumption that, unless they escape, their anxiety will continue to rise.

1 Beck AT, Ward C, and Mendelson M (1961). The Beck Depression Inventory (BDI). *Arch Gen Psychiat* **4**: 561–71.

Interpersonal psychotherapy

Interpersonal psychotherapy (IPT) was developed in the 1970s by Klerman and Weissman as a treatment for depressive illness and later developed for use in other disorders. Its development followed the observation that depression is frequently associated with impaired interpersonal functioning. IPT aims, by improving interpersonal functioning, to improve emotional symptoms. It is a practical, short-term psychotherapy which may be offered in conjunction with medication and is suitable for delivery by a variety of health care professionals. It is described in a manual for practitioners[1] and a guide for patients.[2]

Rationale

Emotional disturbance (e.g. depression) tends to be associated with 'here and now' deficits in interpersonal functioning. Emotional problems are best understood by studying the interpersonal context in which they arise. Life events related to illness development include: grief, interpersonal disputes, change of role, and interpersonal deficits. These events are not viewed as directly causing the episode of illness, but helping the patient to understand their role in the evolution of illness and resolving the interpersonal problem is seen as a route to recovery.

How illness is viewed

Illnesses are viewed as medical disorders and are diagnosed according to standard criteria (e.g. ICD-10) and rated in severity by rating scales (e.g. BDI). IPT makes no attempt to differentiate whether the cause of depression is biological or psychosocial. In fact, psychoeducation about both is key, and the use of antidepressant medication is encouraged when indicated. Depressive symptoms, regardless of aetiology, are viewed as modifiable through the application of IPT techniques.

Techniques

After a thorough assessment, patient and therapist contract to meet weekly for 12–16 hour-long individual sessions. A key feature of IPT involves 'giving the sick role' to the patient: this entails educating them about the depressive illness, ascribing their symptoms to the current episode of depression, offering appropriate treatment, and giving the patient responsibility for change. Depending on the focus, specific techniques are applied as outlined in the IPT manual. The relationship between symptoms, interpersonal functioning, and personality factors are common to all four foci. Depressive symptom reduction is reviewed weekly and linked to changes in attitude or behaviour in the interpersonal arena.

A focus in one of the following four areas is mutually agreed upon:
- Role transitions (difficulty with life changes, e.g. graduating from school, marriage, job change, childbearing or retirement).
- Interpersonal disputes (differing opinions and expectations about relationship roles between the patient and another person, e.g. a partner, family member or in the workplace).
- Grief (abnormal reactions to bereavement).
- Interpersonal deficits (long-standing difficulties with impoverished social environment and unfulfilling relationships).

The IPT therapist is an active advocate and facilitator to encourage the patient to see their problems from different perspectives, to make attempts at change, and to return to discuss their successes or failures at subsequent weekly sessions. Transference interpretations are avoided in order to keep the patient focused on how to negotiate better with people in their current life outside of therapy.

Phases of treatment

- *Phase I* (sessions 1–2): Standard psychiatric history; risk assessment; communication of diagnosis to patient; assessment of need for psychotropic medication; establishment of the 'sick role'; completion of interpersonal inventory (description of current relationships); setting of the patient's depression within their interpersonal context; identification of focus for therapy; explanation of rationale for treatment and its aims and processes; agreement of therapeutic contract.
- *Phase II* (sessions 3–12): Commence work on the focus utilizing specific techniques outlined in the IPT manual. These include: facilitation of the grieving process; mourning the loss of the old role and learning to embrace the challenges of the new role in the role transition focus; teaching of specific communication, problem-solving or conflict resolution skills; and role play. Review progress in depressive symptom reduction weekly. Review overall progress at the 'halfway point' which encourages sustained effort before 'time runs out'.
- *Phase III* (final 3–4 sessions): Anticipate termination as scheduled from the outset in the contract with encouragement to continue to apply what the patient has learned from therapy in their real-life interpersonal sphere. The IPT therapist points out that progress toward better coping (leading to reduced depressive symptoms) has been 'earned' by the patient who did the work of changing. The therapist also reminds the patient that the therapist's own role was merely to facilitate that which the patient now knows they can do for themselves.

Indications

Non-psychotic depressive disorders. Adaptations of IPT have been applied to various subgroups such as adolescents, geriatric patients, primary care clinic patients, and patients with HIV, bulimia, panic disorder, bipolar disorder, dysthymic disorder, bereavement, post-partum depression, social phobia, and insomnia. Modifications of IPT for groups, couples therapy, maintenance therapy, and via telephone have been developed. IPT is not indicated for treating substance abuse or personality disorders.

Efficacy

Several randomized controlled trials in adults, adolescents, elders, and primary care patients have demonstrated efficacy for IPT either alone or in combination with antidepressant medication.

1 Klerman GL, Weissman MM, Rounsaville BJ, *et al.* (1984) *Interpersonal psychotherapy of depression.* New York: Basic Books Inc.
2 Weissman MM (1995) *Mastering depression: a patient guide to interpersonal psychotherapy.* Albany: Graywind Publications.

Dialectical behaviour therapy

Dialectical[1] behaviour therapy (DBT) was introduced in 1991 by Linehan[2,3] and colleagues as a treatment for borderline personality disorder (BPD). Patients with BPD are supported in understanding their own emotional experiences and are taught new skills for dealing with their distress through a combination of group and individual therapy sessions. By learning more adaptive responses to distress and more effective problem-solving techniques, patients' quality of life and functioning may be improved, and their morbidity and mortality reduced.

Rationale

Patients with borderline personality disorder suffer from significant psychiatric morbidity and mortality related to completed suicide. They are a difficult group of patients to treat as their characteristic patterns of behaviour tend to challenge therapeutic progress and exhaust therapist resources ('burnout'). Such individuals can however learn more adaptive responses later in life, with subsequent improvement in functioning and quality of life and reduction in morbidity and mortality.

How illness is viewed

BPD occurs as a product of emotional vulnerability (which may have a biological basis) and a childhood experience of an 'invalidating environment'. Here, the child's experiences and emotions are repeatedly disqualified or invalidated by others, and their difficulties with self-control or problem-solving are not acknowledged. As a consequence, the child grows up with difficulty in recognizing, understanding and trusting their emotions, and in order to have feelings acknowledged and needs for care met, may display extremes of emotion and behaviour. As certain skills (e.g. tolerating emotional distress, problem-solving) have not been taught, the individual tends to set unrealistic goals and then respond with shame and self-loathing when they cannot be met. These patterns are reinforced as the child grows and develops, with self-harming behaviour frequently emerging as a way to cope with the intense extremes of emotion experienced.

Techniques

DBT is a complex treatment which combines cognitive–behavioural interventions with Eastern meditative practice, notably mindfulness (in which a person intentionally becomes aware of their thoughts and actions in the 'here-and-now').

- *Individual therapy*, where the therapist validates the patient's responses (recognizing their distress and behaviours as legitimate and understandable but ultimately harmful), reinforces adaptive behaviours, and facilitates analysis of maladaptive behaviours and their triggers.
- *Group skills training* where the following modules are taught in a group context:
  - Mindfulness skills.
  - Interpersonal effectiveness skills (e.g. problem-solving, assertiveness training, communication skills).
  - Emotion modulation skills (to change distressing emotional states).
  - Distress tolerance skills (e.g. distraction, self-soothing strategies).

- *Telephone contact* according to the contract agreed between patient and therapist, to support the patient in applying DBT skills in real life situations between sessions and find alternatives to self-harming.
- *Therapist consultation groups* where therapists support each other, according to the DBT model, to prevent 'burnout'.

Phases of treatment

Each stage of treatment has specific targets, arranged hierarchically by importance. Within each session, targets should also be attended to in this order, e.g. addressing episodes of self-harm first. Each stage of therapy must be completed, with the targeted behaviours for that stage modified, before progressing to the next stage. DBT takes a hierarchical view of treatment aspirations, with the focus first on reducing behaviours which cause self-harm, then on reducing those behaviours which interfere with therapy and finally aiming to reduce behaviours which diminish quality of life and personal relationships.

- *Pre-treatment:* Assessment, orientation to therapy, commitment to therapeutic contract.
- *Stage 1:* Focuses on reducing life-threatening behaviour (episodes of deliberate self-harm with or without suicidal intent), behaviour which may interfere with the progress of therapy (e.g. inappropriate use of telephone contact, unreliable attendance for therapy), and behaviour which interferes with quality of life (e.g. substance misuse, interpersonal conflicts). In individual therapy sessions, exploration of internal and external antecedents to these behaviours, and generation of possible solutions. Weekly DBT skills group introduces basic skills.
- *Stage 2:* Focuses on emotional processing of previous traumatic experiences, to target post-traumatic stress-related symptoms such as flashbacks. Examines underlying historical causes of dysfunction, including exposure to memories of abuse or trauma, in combination with distress tolerance techniques.
- *Stage 3:* Aims to develop self-esteem and establish future goals— individual targets negotiated with the patient.

Indications and contraindications

DBT methods are described specifically for patients with borderline personality disorder.

Efficacy

The original DBT group produced RCT evidence of reduced rates of deliberate self-harm and admission to hospital, and improved retention in therapy compared with 'treatment as usual'. Subsequent RCTs have supported the efficacy of DBT, including studies in other patient populations (e.g. substance abusers) for whom it has been adapted.

---

1 Dialectic refers to a means of arriving at the truth by examination of the argument (the 'thesis' and the contradictory argument the 'antithesis') in order to resolve them into a coherent 'synthesis'.
2 Linehan MM (1993) *Cognitive-behavioral treatment of borderline personality disorder.* New York: Guilford Press.
3 Linehan MM (1993) *Skills training manual for treating borderline personality disorder.* New York: Guilford Press.

Cognitive analytic therapy

Cognitive analytic therapy (CAT) is a therapy method introduced by Anthony Ryle in 1990. It aims to bring together ideas from dynamic cognitive and behavioural therapies by attempting to explain psychoanalytic ideas in cognitive terms.

Rationale

Problems such as depression, anxiety disorders, and interpersonal difficulties cause emotional suffering and also hinder the ability of the individual to make positive change. These problems can often be understood in the context of an individual's history and early experiences and can be prolonged by habitual coping mechanisms. Through collaborative therapy these mechanisms can be identified, understood, and changed.

How illness is viewed

Traumatic childhood and adolescent experiences can give rise to coping mechanisms to protect the individual from conscious distress. These maladaptive mechanisms can be inappropriately maintained into adult life when they give rise to emotional symptoms such as anxiety and depression and destructive behaviours such as self-harm. Although harmful these behaviours are maintained by 'neurotic repetition'. Neurotic repetition has three essential patterns:

- *'Traps'*: negative assumptions generate acts that produce consequences, which in turn reinforce assumptions.
- *'Dilemmas'*: a person acts as if available actions or possible roles are limited and polarized (called 'false dichotomy') and so resists change.
- *'Snags'*: appropriate goals or roles are abandoned either because others would oppose them or they are thought to be 'forbidden' or 'dangerous' in light of personal beliefs.

Techniques

The 'three Rs' of CAT are **recognition** of maladaptive behaviour and beliefs, **reformulation** of these (the main 'work' of therapy), and **revision**. The reformulation is agreed between therapist and patient and documented in a 'psychotherapy file'. This reformulation is expressed in narrative and diagrammatic form and considers both past history and current problems. It is used throughout therapy to guide the active focus, to set homework, and to enable recognition of transference/countertransference.

Phases of treatment

Therapy involves active participation from both parties.

- *Assessment* Explanation of rationale of method of therapy. Planning of number and timing of sessions (8–24 sessions, normally 12).
- *Early sessions (1–3)* Patient asked to begin 'psychotherapy file' exploring common traps, dilemmas, and snags. Diary keeping to monitor moods and behaviours. Recapitulation of early experiences and narrative of current relationships.
- *Middle sessions (4–8)* Agreement on reformulation of problems with written and diagrammatic description of 'target problem procedures'.

Exploration of methods of change, (called 'exits') via work in sessions and in homework.

- *Ending sessions (9–12)* Identification and recapitulation of key themes which emerged during therapy. Both therapist and patient write 'goodbye' letters summarizing progress and formally closing the relationship. There may be a planned 3-mth review appointment.

Indications and contraindications

As for other cognitive therapies.

Efficacy

Ongoing RCTs examining effectiveness in personality disorders and comparing CAT with other methods.

Solution-focused therapy

This therapy, developed by de Shazer,[1] aims to empower patients to recognize and make use of their own strengths. It is a brief intervention which may be delivered in a single session.

Rationale

The patient is more than the sum of their problems and already has a range of skills for coping with adversity. The best way for the patient to achieve their goals is for them to discover and harness those capabilities and resources which are already helpful and to make even better use of them. The solution-focused therapist facilitates this process.

How illness is viewed

Solution focused therapy avoids viewing problems or symptoms as goals for therapy. Rather, it prompts the patient to visualize a future without the problem and to plan the stages necessary to achieve this. In-depth consideration of the development of current difficulties is avoided, as this may imply that the problems are inevitable and unchangeable.

Techniques (Box 20.5)

- *Problem-free talk* Discussion of other areas of the patient's life—this helps the therapist to understand the 'patient behind the problems' and may elicit areas of strength or competence. If the patient discusses their problems, the therapist listens actively, reflects on the coping strategies described by the patient, and highlights the possibility of change.
- *Preferred future* The patient identifies future goals, shifting focus away from the current complaints.
- *Exception finding* The patient identifies situations when the preferred future seemed more attainable. Rather than seeing them as 'the exception which proves the rule', these situations are examined to determine which skills the patient used to help bring about a favourable outcome.
- *Scales* Rating their preferred future as 10, the patient rates their current position numerically between 0 and 10. They are invited to discuss the difference between 0 and where they are now, the resources responsible for this, and to identify the steps or signs of progress between points on the scale.

Phases of treatment

First session Establishes the patient's goals or best hopes from therapy, recognizes what the patient already does or has done which helps them to cope or moves them towards this preferred future, and identifies what the next signs of progress may be.

Subsequent sessions Explore what the patient has done since the previous session which has been helpful, place this in the context of the patient's goals for therapy, and identify what may be further evidence of progress.

Indications Depression, substance misuse, interpersonal relationship difficulties, presentation in crisis or after self-harm. May be used with children and adolescents and people with learning disability.

Efficacy Few controlled trials but some evidence of effectiveness for adults with depression and for children and adolescents with emotional and behavioural problems.

Box 20.5 Solution-focused questions[2]

Problem-free talk
How do you spend your time? What do you enjoy? What are you good at? How would your friends describe you?

Preferred future (the miracle question)
Imagine that tonight, while you are asleep, a miracle happens and your hopes from coming here are realized (or the problems that bring you here are resolved), but because you are asleep you don't realize this miracle has happened. What are you going to notice different about your life when you wake up that begins to tell you that this miracle has happened?

Exceptions
When doesn't the problem happen? When doesn't it last as long? When does it feel less intense? When do you feel less upset by it? When do you manage to resist the urge to…? What are the signs that the miracle has already started to happen?

Scales
On a scale of 0–10, where 0 is the worst things have ever been and 10 represents your best hopes, where are you today? Where on that scale would be good enough, the point that you would settle for? What are you doing that means you are at 2 and not at 0? If you are at 2 now, what will you be doing that will tell us that you have reached 3?

Locating resources
It sounds as if things are very stressful; how do you cope? What helps you to keep going? How did you manage to get here? What have you been doing that has stopped things from getting even worse? When you've faced this sort of problem before, how did you resolve it?

1 De Shazer S (1985) *Keys to solution in brief therapy.* New York: Norton.
2 BRIEF (2007) *BRIEFER: A solution-focused manual.* London: BRIEF.

Counselling methods

Counselling may be thought of as a method of relieving distress under-taken by means of a dialogue between two people. The aim is to help the client or patient find their own solutions to problems, while being supported to do so and being guided by appropriate advice. In Western countries over the last fifty years, counselling has emerged as a profession in its own right and individual forms of specific counselling have been developed. In its more general sense—helping others by the provision of advice, non-judgemental reflection, and emotional support—counselling takes place all over the world in the guise of family members, priests, tutors, teachers, etc.

Counselling skills are integral to the practice of medicine, particularly in primary care and psychiatry, where counselling techniques are useful in history-taking, assessing and ensuring compliance, etc. Counselling should not be thought of as 'cut-down' or 'half-price' psychotherapy. There is clearly overlap in the methods and skills of a psychotherapist and a counsellor. However, the decision to use counselling as a specific treatment (e.g. for postnatal depression) should be made after considering both the disorder and the patient. There are a variety of counselling services in the voluntary and private sectors, some directed towards specific problems and some more general.

Rationale Behaviour and emotional life are shaped by previous experience, current environment, and the relationships the individual has. Many life problems can be viewed as arising from resolvable difficulties in one of these three areas, rather than as an 'illness'. People have a tendency towards positive change and fulfilment which can be retarded by 'life problems'. A collaborative relationship with a counsellor (however defined) is one method of addressing these issues. This relationship will proceed according to agreed rules, towards a goal, and will be based on developing the client's strengths.

Techniques
- *Information giving* Key to all psychiatric treatment and psychotherapeutic work. Information should be provided in a form the patient can understand and information giving should not be a 'one-off' but should continue throughout counselling.
- *Client-focused discussion* The client should 'lead' the sessions, particularly beyond the early information gathering sessions. Time constraints may hinder this.
- *Problem solving* A variety of techniques, particularly those borrowed from cognitive behavioural therapy, are employed here. The basic goal is to use the session time to explore current and potential future problems and to help the client consider the optimum solution.

Different types of counselling
- *Information sharing/discussion* In some contexts is also called psychoeducation. Aim is to properly inform a client prior to them making their own decision. Techniques of guided learning, providing verbal and written information, collaborative enquiry (cf. CBT).

- ***Crisis management*** Views crisis as stressor providing both risk and opportunity to change/learn/develop. Short-term, immediately follows trauma (first few weeks). Facilitates adaptive and normal emotional responses, discourages maladaptive responses. Focus on end point of intervention. Alternative to hospital admission in some cases. Should have access to alternative treatments if necessary.
- ***Problem-based counselling*** Directed towards a specific primary problem (e.g. drug misuse, CSA). Counsellor may or may not have had similar experiences themselves.
- ***Risk counselling*** Used to guide an informed decision (e.g. prenatal interventions, genetic counselling). Differentiated from other forms of counselling by the fact that the counsellor is clearly 'the expert' and has access to specialist information. Nonetheless, the basic goal, of enabling the patient to come to their own decision, with appropriate information and support, remains the same.

Indications

Absolute advice limited by lack of comparative trials and tendency for local availability of services to be the main factor in the decision to use counselling methods. Clinical usefulness in:

- Adjustment disorder.
- Mild depressive illness.
- Normal and pathological grief.
- Sequelae of childhood sexual abuse.
- After other forms of trauma (e.g. rape, accidents).
- Postnatal depression.
- Pregnancy loss and stillbirth.
- Drug and alcohol problems.
- Reaction to chronic medical conditions.
- Prior to decision such as undergoing genetic testing or HIV testing.

Legal issues

Introduction

Practising psychiatrists must be familiar with the laws in their country relating to mental health. There are five broad areas of law of interest to psychiatrists: (1) the common law as it relates to medical treatment decisions; (2) the law relating to incapable adults; (3) the law regulating the treatment of patients with mental disorder; (4) laws and regulations relating to confidentiality; and (5) the criminal law in relation to mentally disordered offenders.

In this book the subjects of criminal law and mentally disordered offenders are dealt with in Chapter 17, Forensic psychiatry. The remaining topics are covered within this chapter. As has been noted in the chapter on forensic issues, law is both parochial and dynamic. The last decade has seen significant changes in the laws relating to psychiatric practice, and further changes are likely over the decade to come. The current mental health and incapacity legislation covering the four legal jurisdictions within the British Isles is summarized is Box 21.1.

Although it is useful to have access to the relevant statute law, it is impossible to get a good understanding of how the law works in practice through reading the text of the legislation. This develops through training, experience, and discussion with colleagues. The trainee psychiatrist should be aware of the current laws in their jurisdiction which affect their current area of practice. They should aim to have a detailed knowledge of the parts of the legislation used day to day, and particularly in emergency situations.

Alongside the Acts themselves, codes of practice and guidance notes are available that give practical advice on the use of the Acts. Beyond these the trainee should know where to go for further information and advice (e.g. senior colleagues, hospital legal office, commissions). They should be wary of mental health 'lore'. Much misinformation about legislation is promulgated without reference to what is actually correct. For example, some believe that UK legislation does not permit the detention of someone who is drunk, even if they are also depressed or acutely psychotic.

It is important to remember that the law often cannot resolve clinical dilemmas. For example, if a detained patient takes an overdose, mental health legislation cannot be used to impose physical treatment. This does not mean that you can do nothing knowing that you are acting (or not acting) legally. In this situation common law may allow, and medical ethics may dictate, that physical treatment be imposed.

Box 21.1 Legislation across the British Isles

England and Wales
Care and treatment of patients with mental disorder is regulated by
the Mental Health Act 1983. Following failed attempts to produce a
completely updated Act, the Westminster parliament passed the Mental
Health Act 2007 in July 2007. This amends the 1983 Act in several
important areas. The majority of its provisions will be enacted between
October 2007 and October 2008. The Mental Capacity Act 2005, which
regulates decision-making on behalf of incapable adults, was implemented in 2007.

Scotland
The Mental Health (Care and Treatment) (Scotland) Act 2003 replaced
the previous Mental Health (Scotland) Act 1984 in October 2005. The
Adults with Incapacity Act 2000 consolidated and clarified the law relating to incapable adults, replacing a number of outdated legal instruments
which had previously been used for the role. This act received Royal
Assent in May 2000 and its provisions came into force between April
2001 and October 2003.

Northern Ireland
Care and treatment of patients with mental disorder is regulated by the
Mental Health (Northern Ireland) Order 1986, amended by the Mental
Health (Amendment) (Northern Ireland) Order 2004. There is no specific incapacity legislation. An independent and wide-ranging review
of mental health law was initiated in 2002 under the chairmanship of
Professor David Bamford. The resulting report was published in August
2007 and proposed comprehensive reform of mental health legislation
and the introduction of incapacity legislation.

Republic of Ireland
The Mental Health Act 2001 replaced the Mental Treatment Act 1945
and various modifying Acts passed in 1953, 1961, and 1981. There is no
specific incapacity legislation.

The development of mental health law

Mental health legislation in the UK has its origins in the eighteenth century, which saw the passing of both the Vagrancy Law, allowing local magistrates to order the confinement of the 'furiously mad and dangerous', and the Act for the Regulation of Private Madhouses which allowed for licensing and inspection of private asylums and required a medical certificate of insanity before the confinement of 'non-pauper' patients. The former law primarily arose out of concerns about the risk posed to the general public by the mentally ill; the latter from concern to protect the interests of vulnerable patients.

The Lunacy Act of 1890 gave magistrates authority to detain 'lunatics, idiots and persons of unsound mind' within private asylums. The Mental Deficiency Act 1913 expanded and clarified these powers, but also expanded the role of the state in the regulation and supervision of the care of the mentally disordered by reorganizing the Victorian Lunacy Commission as the Board of Control for Asylums. This was established as a department of central government with powers to inspect asylums, to review compulsory detention, to investigate complaints about treatment of patients, and to monitor the working of the compulsory measures.

In 1926 the Royal Commission on Lunacy and Mental Disorders produced a report which led to the Mental Treatment Act 1930. This Act was based on a view of mental disorders as similar to medical illness and envisaged treatment and rehabilitation, rather than preventative detention, as the goal of admission to hospital. It allowed for outpatient work by medical staff in mental hospitals, and for the first time provided for voluntary treatment in hospital.

In 1957 the report of the Royal Commission on the Law Relating to Mental Illness and Mental Deficiency (the Percy Report) was published. The Commission recommended that: 'the law should be altered so that whenever possible suitable care may be provided for mentally disordered patients with no more restriction of liberty or legal formality than is applied to people who need care because of other types of illness', and noted that: 'the majority of mentally ill patients do not need to be admitted to hospital as inpatients'. The subsequent Mental Health Act (1959) allowed most psychiatric admissions to occur voluntarily and changed the procedure for compulsory detention in hospital from a judicial to an administrative process. The Percy Report marked the turning point in official policy from hospital-based to community-based systems of care.

The 1983 Mental Health Act narrowed the definitions of categories of mental disorder, excluding certain categories of patient from compulsory treatment. It also established regulations and safeguards governing treatment without consent. Similar Acts were passed for Scotland in 1984 and for Northern Ireland in 1986.

At the end of the twentieth century the UK government established the Richardson Committee to again review mental health legislation in England and Wales, and a draft bill followed in 2002. This attracted widespread criticism for a perceived over-emphasis on public protection and under-emphasis on the rights of individuals with mental disorder, seeming to reverse progress made over the previous century. An Act amending rather than replacing the 1983 Act was finally passed in 2007.

The most recent innovation in mental health law has been the passage of Acts specifically covering the care and treatment of incapable patients—in Scotland in 2000, and in England and Wales in 2005. A future challenge for lawmakers across the British Isles is the implementation of the rights specified in the European Convention of Human Rights into UK and Irish mental health law.

Consent to treatment

A fundamental principle of medical care is that treatment of a patient should be with their consent. A patient has a right to decide for themself which treatments to undergo and which treatments to refuse. This right is retained even where refusal of treatment could result in death or significant deterioration in health. In the majority of cases doctors should treat their patients according to this principle; treatment without consent (📖 p. 872) is possible only in certain circumstances, constrained by appropriate laws.

Validity of consent

For consent to be valid the patient must have *capacity* to make medical treatment decisions, the consent must be *informed* (i.e. the patient has fully understood the details and implications of what is proposed), and it must be *freely given* (i.e. not given under duress).

Capacity to make treatment decisions

Capacity is a legal concept meaning the ability to enter into valid contracts. It is gained on adulthood and is presumed to be present throughout the lifespan unless permanently or temporarily lost. Under common law there is a presumption of capacity in adults—i.e. it is to be assumed that an adult retains full capacity unless there is evidence that it has been lost. Assessments of capacity are made on the balance of probabilities.

Capacity is not an 'all-or-nothing' quality—i.e. one may have capacity for some decisions but not others. Within incapacity law (📖 pp. 876–9), capacity is divided into two broad categories—capacity for financial decisions and capacity for personal welfare decisions. A patient's capacity or incapacity should be judged in relation to the required decision rather than being inferred from the presence of any mental illness or disability.

In order to have capacity to make medical treatment decisions the patient must understand the decision, understand the alternative possible courses of action, assess the merits and risks of these choices, retain memory of the decisions and the reasons for them, and be able to communicate their intent.

Informing consent

Doctors have a duty to provide to the patient sufficient information about any proposed treatment to enable them to make an *informed* treatment decision. The amount and type of information provided will depend on the nature of the condition, the complexity and risks of the proposed treatment, the clinical situation, and the patient's own wishes. The aim should be to provide the patient with a balanced and accurate view of their diagnosis and prognosis, the nature and purpose of the proposed treatment, any alternative treatment options, and the likely risks and side-effects, answering any questions honestly and only withholding information if its disclosure would cause the patient serious harm.

Forms of consent

Consent may be *implied* (i.e. the patient does not object to, and cooperates with, the procedure) or may be *express* (i.e. oral or written permission is explicitly asked for and recorded, often on a detailed consent form). Generally, express consent is obtained for non-trivial or invasive procedures, and for some interventions (e.g. operations) it is mandatory.

Advance statements

Sometimes, in cases where a patient has a progressive disease, although they currently lack capacity to consent or refuse treatment, they may, when greater capacity existed, have indicated their treatment preferences in an advance statement ('advance directive' or 'living will'). These wishes should be given due regard provided:

• The decision in the advance statement is clearly applicable to the present circumstances.

• There is no reason to believe that the patient has changed their mind.

If you act against an advance statement, then you should be able to justify this. Where such a statement is not available, the patient's known wishes should be taken into account using the common law principle of 'best interests' (☐ p. 874).

You must be satisfied that you have consent or other valid authority before you undertake any examination or investigation, provide treatment or involve patients in teaching or research. Usually this will involve providing information to patients in a way they can understand, before asking for their consent. You must follow the guidance in 'Seeking patients' consent: The ethical considerations', which includes advice on children and patients who are not able to give consent.

General Medical Council (2006) *Good medical practice*, paragraph 36

Treatment without consent

In general, treatment of a patient can and should only proceed with their valid consent. There are, however, situations where treatment can take place without consent, and these situations (appropriately) have legal safeguards. There are four broad areas where treatment may take place despite lack of consent: (1) treatment undertaken under common law; (2) treatment under the provisions of an incapacity act; (3) treatment under the provisions of a mental health act; and (4) treatment authorized by a court.

For psychiatrists, the majority of treatment decisions involving consideration of non-consensual treatment will relate to psychiatric patients. However, in other fields of medicine, situations may arise where decisions must be made regarding treatment without consent. Often a psychiatrist's opinion will be sought because, by the nature of their work, most psychiatrists will have greater knowledge of, and familiarity with, legal issues than their medical counterparts. Also, a patient's reasons for withholding consent may be thought to be due to a (possibly undiagnosed) mental disorder. Where this is the case, other professionals may not feel they have the clinical skills to make this diagnosis.

Treatment undertaken under common law

As noted on 📖 p. 874, *common law* 'necessity' may provide a doctor with a defence against assault where non-consensual treatment is given. There may be situations, for example the use of sedation in a patient with acute behavioural disturbance where there is a suspected physical or psychiatric cause, when the doctor has to act against a patient's wishes, in order to adequately carry out their *duty of care*. Treatment in these situations is given under *common law* even if the patient fulfils the criteria for emergency detention under mental health legislation.

Treatment under the provisions of an incapacity act

The Mental Capacity Act 2005 and the Adults with Incapacity (Scotland) Act 2000 provide the legal framework guiding the care of incapable adults in England and Wales, and in Scotland respectively. These Acts define incapacity and establish processes and safeguards regulating decision-making on behalf of incapable adults.

Treatment under the provisions of a mental health act

The majority of patients with mental disorder receive treatment informally and with their consent. For a proportion, however, treatment is authorized by a mental health act. Four mental health acts cover the four legal jurisdictions within the British Isles. These vary, but all allow for detention in hospital and for compulsory treatment of mental disorder. They all specify restrictions on the use of certain treatments (psychosurgery, ECT, and compulsory prescription of medication beyond a certain period) and describe processes of appeal and oversight of the treatment of detained patients. In general, treatment of unrelated medical disorders cannot be authorized by a mental health act.

Treatment authorized by a court

In a small number of cases doctors will ask for a court's decision regarding a decision to treat a patient without their consent. In general these will be non-urgent but potentially controversial cases where statute law has no clear role and where there does not appear to be any relevant legal precedent. Often the judgements in these test cases become important subsequently in guiding the approach to similar cases.

Common law

Common law is that body of law which is derived from previous decisions of the courts, in contrast with statute law—which is law created by legislative bodies (e.g. regional, national, and supranational parliaments). Common law can arise from:

- Long established custom and practice.
- Clarification of the meaning and extent of statute by the courts.
- Statements of law by judges ruling on cases where no applicable law exists or fits precisely.

The common law is dynamic and changes and expands as cases are heard and judgements are handed down. For this reason it is impossible to be aware of all potentially applicable judgements. Doctors should make every effort to be up to date with current debates and decisions within their own specialty. They should also seek clarification from senior colleagues, their hospital legal advisors or their professional bodies in potentially contentious cases.

Common law principles for medical treatment decisions

- *Act in accordance with the patient's wishes:* a fundamental principle of the doctor–patient relationship. Doctors should, in general, respect the patient's autonomy in decision-making, only acting against the patient's wishes in very limited circumstances.
- *Presume capacity in adults:* a patient over the age of 16 is presumed to have capacity to make treatment decisions unless there is evidence to the contrary (assessed on the balance of probabilities).
- *Apply 'reasonableness' test:* a frequently used consideration in law is the test of what a hypothetical 'reasonable man' would do in the circumstances. For medical treatment decisions the test is what the 'reasonable doctor' would have done in those circumstances.
- *Act in the patient's 'best interests':* in emergency situations, it may not be possible to obtain consent (e.g. in an unconscious RTA victim requiring drainage of an extradural haematoma); here, it is accepted that the doctor's overriding duty is to preserve life.
- *Doctrine of necessity:* 'necessity' provides a defence against a potential criminal charge that you have assaulted a patient by giving non-consensual treatment. A doctor may therefore give emergency treatment to preserve life and prevent significant deterioration in health.
- *Act in accordance with a recognized body of opinion:* it is accepted in law that medicine is not an exact science—that in any situation, multiple courses of action may be potentially reasonable. However, there is an expectation that any treatment decision is considered suitable by a body of professional opinion (the 'Bolam test').
- *Act in logically defensible manner:* the Bolitho case (see Box 21.2) added a consideration to the Bolam test by stating that medical decisions made must, in addition to being in accordance with a recognized body of opinion, be logically defensible in the circumstances.

- *Consider use of applicable law:* the treating doctor should consider whether the provisions of any statute law provide guidance and addition protections for the patient. However, they should not delay urgent treatment to enact the provisions of statute law.
- *Consider request for court judgement:* in difficult situations consult more experienced colleagues; where appropriate, seek legal advice on whether it is appropriate to apply to the court for a ruling.

Box 21.2 Significant rulings

The Gillick case[1] *Victoria Gillick, a mother of five daughters, challenged the right of her local health authority to advise doctors that contraceptives could be prescribed for under-16s without parental consent. The House of Lords ruled that, in relation to medical treatment, 'the parental right to determine whether or not their minor child below the age of 16 will have medical treatment terminates if and when the child achieves sufficient understanding and intelligence to understand fully what is proposed'. This ruling established the concept of 'Gillick competence' which applies to treatment decisions made by minors in England and Wales. Section 2(4) of the Age of Legal Capacity (Scotland) Act 1991 established the same principle within Scottish statute law.*

The Bolitho case[2] Prior to this case, the standard of care expected in medical negligence cases had been judged according to the 'Bolam test'.[3] This established the principle that a doctor is not guilty of negligence if he has acted in accordance with a responsible body of professional opinion. This case centred on an individual who, as a child, had suffered brain damage as a result of a cardiac arrest induced by respiratory failure. The court's finding was that, even if a body of professional opinion existed which held that the action was reasonable, the defendant could still be judged negligent if the judge held the opinion that no logical basis for the opinion had been shown to the court.

The Ms B case[4] As a result of a serious illness a Ms B had been rendered paralysed and dependent on artificial ventilation for survival. She refused consent for continued ventilation but, in view of the inevitable fatal outcome, the hospital refused to accept her refusal. She was assessed by several consultant psychiatrists whose opinion was that she retained full capacity. She applied for a court decision where the ruling was that, once her capacity had been established, any further treatment without consent was unlawful. The court also gave the opinion that, should doctors treating her feel unable to treat her in accordance with her wishes, they had a duty to transfer her care to other doctors. Ms B was subsequently transferred to another hospital where, following withdrawal of artificial ventilation, she died.

1 Gillick v West Norfolk and Wisbech AHA ALL ER [1985], 3 ALL ER 402.
2 Bolitho v City and Hackney HA [1997] 3 WLR.
3 Bolam v Friern Hospital Management Committee [1957] 2 All ER 118.
4 Re B (Adult: Refusal of Treatment) [2002] 2 FCR1; [2002] 2 All E R. 449.

Mental Capacity Act: England and Wales

The Mental Capacity Act 2005 provides the legal framework guiding decision-making on behalf of those who lack capacity to make decisions for themselves. The Act applies to individuals over the age of 16 in England and Wales. The Act introduces a new criminal offence of ill treatment or neglect of a person who lacks capacity.

Principles

The Act is underpinned by a set of five key principles set out in Section 1.

- *Presumption of capacity* A person is assumed to have capacity unless it is established that they lack capacity.
- *All practical steps taken to allow autonomy* A person is not to be treated as unable to make a decision unless all practicable steps to help him to do so have been taken without success.
- *Allow unwise decisions* A person is not incapable merely because they make an unwise decision.
- *Best interests* An intervention under the Act on behalf of a person who lacks capacity must be in their best interests.
- *Least restrictive option* Any intervention under the Act on behalf of a person who lacks capacity should restrict as little as possible their basic rights and freedoms.

Assessment of incapacity

Sections 2 and 3 of the Act set out a two-stage test for assessing incapacity:

- A person lacks capacity if he is unable to make a decision for himself in relation to any matter because of a permanent or temporary impairment in the functioning of the mind.
- A person is unable to make a decision for himself if he is unable:
  - to understand the information relevant to the decision;
  - to retain that information for a sufficient period to make a decision;
  - to use or weigh that information as part of the process of making the decision;
  - to communicate his decision.

Judgements about incapacity are to be made on the balance of probabilities. Lack of capacity is not to be presumed based on a person's age or appearance, on any aspect of his behaviour, on any condition or disorder from which he suffers. The Act specifies certain decisions that cannot be made by one person on behalf of another. These are: agreeing to marriage, civil partnership or divorce, consent to a sexual relationship, and casting a ballot in an election.

Techniques covered by the Act

Lasting Powers of Attorney (LPA) A person may appoint an attorney to act on his behalf if he should lose capacity in the future. This is like the current Enduring Power of Attorney (EPA) in relation to property and affairs, but the Act also allows people to empower an attorney to make health and welfare decisions. Before it can be used an LPA must be registered with the Office of the Public Guardian.

Court appointed deputies The Act provides for a system of court appointed deputies to replace the current system of receivership in the existing Court of Protection. Deputies will be able to be appointed to take decisions on welfare, health care, and financial matters as authorized by the new Court of Protection, but will not be able to refuse consent to life-sustaining treatment. They will only be appointed if the Court cannot make a one-off decision to resolve the issues.

Advance decisions The Act allows patients to make an advance decision to refuse treatment if they should lack capacity in the future. The Act sets out safeguards of validity and applicability in relation to advance decisions. Where an advance decision concerns treatment that would be necessary to sustain life the decision must be in writing, signed and witnessed, and there must be an express statement that the decision stands 'even if life is at risk'.

Protection from liability when providing care and treatment to an incapable adult Section 5 of the Act authorizes health care staff to carry out personal care, health care, and medical treatment in an incapable adult without fear of liability. The care provider must establish that the patient lacks capacity, and that the proposed treatment is in their best interest. If this is the case then the care provider does not incur any liability in relation to the Act that they would not have incurred if the adult had had capacity to consent in relation to the matter, and had consented to the treatment.

Where the proposed treatment involves physical restraint, the care provider must additionally ensure that it is necessary in order to prevent harm and that it is a proportionate response to the likelihood of the patient suffering harm, and the seriousness of that harm. Section 5 does not authorize acting in a way which conflicts with decisions made by a lasting power of attorney or court-appointed deputy; however, life-sustaining treatment or treatment necessary to prevent serious deterioration is acceptable while a decision is sought from the court.

Bodies with powers under the Act

Court of Protection This Court has jurisdiction relating to the whole Act. It will have its own procedures and nominated judges. It will be able to make declarations, decisions, and orders affecting people who lack capacity and make decisions for or appoint deputies to make decisions on behalf of people lacking capacity. It will deal with decisions concerning both property and affairs, as well as health and welfare decisions.

The Public Guardian has several duties under the Act and will be supported in carrying these out by an Office of the Public Guardian (OPG). The Public Guardian and his staff will be the registering authority for LPAs and deputies. They will supervise deputies appointed by the Court and provide information to help the Court make decisions.

Incapacity Act: Scotland

The Adults with Incapacity (Scotland) Act 2000 provides the legal framework regulating those who make decisions on behalf of adults with impaired capacity in Scotland. It covers financial and personal welfare decisions (which includes decisions about medical treatment). The Act applies to individuals over the age of 16yrs.

Principles

Those making decisions on behalf of another are required to take account of the following fundamental principles, as in Section 1:

- *Benefit* Any intervention in the affairs of an incapable adult must benefit the adult concerned and this benefit must not be reasonably achievable without the intervention.
- *Least restrictive option* Any intervention must restrict the freedom of the adult as little as possible.
- *Consider the adult's wishes* Decisions made on behalf of an incapable adult must take account of their currently expressed and previously expressed wishes on the subject.
- *Consultation with relevant others* Anyone making decisions on behalf of an incapable adult must take account of the views of the adult's nearest relative or primary carer, and of the adult's guardian, welfare attorney, or continuing attorney (if they exist).
- *Encourage residual capacity* The adult should be encouraged to exercise whatever capacity is still present.

Assessment of capacity

Under the Act, incapacity means to be incapable of:

- acting; or
- making decisions; or
- communicating decisions; or
- understanding decisions; or
- retaining the memory of decisions.

Capacity is task-specific and must be judged in relation to the decision under consideration. In assessing capacity under the Act the practitioner should consider *for this particular decision* whether the individual:

- understands what is being asked and why;
- understands that the information is personally relevant to them;
- is aware of the alternative choices available;
- can weigh up the risks and benefits associated with the alternative choices;
- has sufficient memory ability to retain the relevant information.

Additionally the practitioner should consider whether the decision is consistent with the patient's background, beliefs, and previously expressed wishes when greater capacity existed. It is important to note that a person is *not* incapable simply because they have a mental or physical illness or a learning disability.

Techniques covered by the Act

Powers of attorney A capable adult can provide for eventual incapacity by granting power of attorney to another person. A continuing power of attorney relates to financial decisions; a welfare power of attorney relates to personal welfare decisions. The latter becomes active only when the adult loses capacity in relation to the welfare decision in question.

Intromission with funds An individual can apply to the Public Guardian for authority to gain access to the adult's finances, in order to fund the adult's living expenses.

Management of residents' finances Following review by a medical practitioner certifying incapacity in relation to financial affairs, registered establishments (e.g. nursing homes) can manage the financial affairs of residents with impaired capacity up to a prescribed limit.

Guardianship and intervention orders Following application, supported by at least two medical recommendations, the Sheriff Court can grant an individual ongoing authority to make financial or personal welfare decisions on behalf of an adult. The former is financial guardianship, the latter is welfare guardianship. For decisions which require a 'one-off' intervention the Sheriff can grant a financial or welfare intervention order covering the proposed intervention.

Medical treatment Under part 5 of the Act, if a medical practitioner responsible for the medical treatment of an adult is of the opinion that the adult is incapable in relation to a decision about the medical treatment in question, he may issue a *certificate of incapacity* authorizing the treatment. The certificate must state the nature and likely duration of the incapacity and the proposed treatment.

Bodies with powers under the Act

The Office of the Public Guardian This body supervises those individuals authorized under the Act to make decisions on behalf of another. It maintains a register of continuing and welfare powers of attorney, guardianships and intervention orders, authorizes access to funds, and has powers to investigate complaints on matters related to the financial affairs of an incapable adult.

The Mental Welfare Commission for Scotland In addition to its duties under the Mental Health Act, the MWC has duties to guide and supervise the actions of those appointed to make welfare decisions on behalf of an incapable adult.

The Sheriff Court Applications for guardianships or intervention orders are made to the Sheriff Court. This court is also the forum for appeals against medical treatment decisions.

Local authorities The local authority has a duty to investigate circumstances where the personal welfare of an adult in the community may be at risk due to incapacity, to supervise appointed attorneys and guardians, and to investigate complaints in relation to those exercising welfare powers. Additionally they have a duty to apply for intervention or guardianship orders and to subsequently act as welfare guardian where necessary and no-one else is applying to do so.

Mental Health Act: England and Wales 1

Introduction

The Mental Health Act 1983 governs the care and treatment of patients with mental disorder within England and Wales. The Act was amended in several significant areas by the Mental Health Act 2007 (see Box 21.3 for changes).

Principles

The 1983 Act did not contain a statement of principles. In the 2007 Act, section 8 directs the Secretary of State to include a statement of principles in a future revision of the code of practice. At the time of writing this amended code of practice was in draft form. The draft principles are:

- Decisions under the Act should be taken with a view to minimizing the harm done by mental disorder, by maximizing the safety and health of patients and protecting the public from harm.
- Any intervention without the patient's consent must be the least restrictive alternative intervention.
- Decision-makers must recognize and respect the diverse needs, values, and circumstances of each patient. They should consider the patient's wishes and feelings and respect those wishes wherever that is practicable and consistent with the purpose of the decision.
- Patients, their carers and family members should be involved, as far as is practicable, in planning and developing their care.
- Decision-makers must seek to use the resources available to them and to patients in the most effective, efficient, and equitable way.

Definition of mental disorder

The 2007 Act defines mental disorder as 'any disorder or disability of the mind', replacing the four subdivisions of mental disorder described in the 1983 Act. The draft code of practice states that conditions which could fall within this definition include: organic mental disorders; disorders due to substance use; schizophrenia and other delusional disorders; affective disorders; neurotic disorders; eating disorders, non-organic sleep disorders and non-organic sexual disorders; personality disorders; learning disabilities; autistic spectrum disorders; and behavioural and emotional disorders of children and adolescents.

Other definitions

Approved doctor Under section 12(2) the Secretary of State may approve a registered medical practitioner as having special experience in the diagnosis and treatment of mental disorder. This is done in practice through the regional health authority.

Responsible clinician The practitioner in charge of the patient's treatment, usually a consultant psychiatrist. (Previously referred to as RMO.)

Approved Mental Health Professional (AMHP) A professional (usually a social worker) who has undergone specific training and assessment and is appointed for the purposes of the Act as having competence in dealing with individuals with mental disorder (previously referred to as ASW).

Nearest relative Determined by who is first on the following list: spouse or civil partner, child, parent, sibling, grandparent, grandchild, uncle or aunt, nephew or niece. If two relatives are of equal standing then the elder prevails. If a patient lives with a relative, or has lived with a non-relative as a spouse for 6mths, then that person is the nearest relative.

Mental Health Review Tribunal (MHRT) Legal forum to which a patient or a nearest relative can appeal against detention. The MHRT has three members: a legally qualified chair, a medical practitioner, and a lay member. It must discharge a patient if criteria for detention no longer apply.

Mental Health Act Commission (MHAC) The MHAC monitors the use of the MHA and the care of patients subject to it. It also investigates certain complaints, appoints second opinion doctors, and maintains the Code of Practice. It produces a biennial report.

Second Opinion Appointed Doctor (SOAD) An independent doctor appointed by the Secretary of State (in practice by the Mental Health Act Commission), who gives a second opinion regarding treatment which can be given without the patient's consent under section 57 or section 58.

Box 21.3 Changes to the 1983 Act made by the 2007 Act

- *Definition of mental disorder* A single definition of mental disorder applies throughout the Act, which abolishes the previous four sub-categories of disorder.
- *Criteria for detention* The previous 'treatability' and 'care' tests are abolished and replaced by a new 'appropriate medical treatment' test applying to the longer-term powers of detention. This does not allow continued compulsory detention unless medical treatment which is appropriate to the patient's mental disorder and all other circumstances of the case is available to that patient.
- *Broadened professional roles* Approved Social Workers (ASWs) are replaced by Approved Mental Health Professionals (AMHPs), and non-social workers can enter this role, subject to appropriate training. The responsible medical officer (RMO) role is replaced by that of the responsible clinician, allowing non-medical staff such as psychologists, social workers, and nurses to undertake this role.
- *Nearest relative (NR)* Patients are given the right to make an application to change their NR and courts are enabled to displace an NR where there are reasonable grounds for doing so. The list of nearest relatives is amended to include civil partners.
- *Supervised community treatment* The 2007 Act introduces supervised community treatment (SCT) which is described on 📖 p. 885.
- *Mental Health Review Tribunal (MHRT)* The Act introduces a single Tribunal for England alongside one in Wales and introduces an order-making power to reduce the time before a case has to be referred to the MHRT by the hospital managers.
- *Age-appropriate services* Hospital managers must ensure that patients aged under 18 admitted to hospital for mental disorder are accommodated in an environment that is suitable for their age.
- *Advocacy* There is a right to independent mental health advocacy (IMHA).
- *Use of ECT* New safeguards are introduced.

Mental Health Act: England and Wales 2

Compulsory measures

The main procedures allowing compulsory detention in hospital are section 2 (admission for assessment), section 3 (admission for treatment), section 4 (emergency admission), and section 5(2) (emergency detention of informal inpatient). Compulsory admission should usually be under section 2 or 3; section 4 is only used rarely, in a genuine emergency where an approved doctor is not available soon enough.

Emergency detention Section 4 allows the emergency detention of patients who have not yet been admitted to hospital (this includes those in A&E, outpatient departments, and day hospitals); section 5(2) is similar but applies to patients who have already been admitted to hospital (whether in a psychiatric or non-psychiatric ward).
- For section 4 the application is made by the nearest relative or AMHP and requires a recommendation from one registered medical practitioner.
- For section 5(2) the medical recommendation must be by the responsible clinician or his nominated deputy; this will usually be the duty psychiatrist, but the nomination should be made before the relevant period of duty. Involvement of the nearest relative or AMHP is not required for section 5(2).
- The duration of detention is 72hrs, during which an assessment must be undertaken to determine if detention under section 2 or 3 is warranted.
- Section 5(4) allows nurses (of the prescribed class) to hold an informal inpatient in hospital for up to 6hrs to allow for a medical assessment.

Admission for assessment An application for detention under section 2 may be made by the nearest relative or AMHP and requires two medical recommendations, one of which must be by an approved doctor. Duration of detention is 28 days. Following the section 2 an application may be made for detention under section 3. Alternatively the patient may remain in hospital informally or be discharged.

Admission for treatment An application for detention under section 3 is made in a similar manner to section 2. Duration of detention is initially 6mths, which may be renewed for a further 6mths, and then 12-monthly thereafter.

Treatment of patients subject to compulsion

- A patient detained in hospital (except under emergency provisions) may be given *medication* for mental disorder for up to 3mths, whether they consent and/or have capacity or not.
- Under section 58, *medication* for over 3mths or ECT requires the patient's consent (the responsible clinician completes form 38) or, if the person refuses or is incapable of consenting, agreement of a SOAD (who issues a form 39).
- Under section 62, *treatment that is urgently necessary* may be authorized by the responsible clinician without consent or a second

opinion; this is usually used for giving ECT to severely ill and at-risk patients while awaiting a second opinion.
- Under section 57, the patient's consent and agreement of a SOAD are required if any patient (whether detained or informal) is to receive neurosurgery for mental disorder or surgical implantation of hormones to reduce male sex drive.

Leave, absconding, and transfer

Procedures allow for patients to be granted leave of absence with the authorization of the responsible clinician (section 17); for patients to be taken into custody and returned to hospital if they abscond (section 18); and for patients to be transferred between hospitals (section 19).

Review

Patients subject to emergency detention have no right of appeal. Patients detained under section 2 or 3, or subject to guardianship under section 7, may appeal to an MHRT. The nearest relative may also appeal against section 3 or 7. One appeal is allowed during each period of compulsion. The responsible clinician may terminate a patient's detention at any point.

Mental Health Act: England and Wales 3

Aftercare following detention

Care programme approach and section 117 aftercare

Section 117 places a statutory duty on health and social services to provide aftercare for patients who have been discharged from detention under sections 3, 37, 47, or 48 (the last 3 are sections used for mentally disordered offenders, see ☐ Chapter 17). The framework within which this aftercare is planned and implemented is the Care Programme Approach (CPA), which was introduced in 1991, but has since been significantly modified. The CPA should be used for all patients where appropriate, even if they have not been detained in hospital. For patients in hospital the CPA process should start well before discharge.

The key aspects of CPA are:
- A co-ordinated assessment of the patient's health and social care needs.
- The development of a care plan addressing the identified needs, which will be agreed by the patient and any carers who are involved.
- An identified care coordinator (e.g. CPN, social worker, psychiatrist) who will be the main contact and will monitor the care plan.
- Regular reviews of the care plan with changes as necessary (at a minimum there must be an annual review).

The CPA should be integrated with care management (the process of care coordination used by social services).

There are two levels of CPA: *standard and enhanced*:
- *Standard CPA* may be appropriate for patients who: require the support or intervention of one agency or discipline; require only low-key support from more than one agency or discipline; are more able to self-manage their mental health problems; have an active informal support network; pose little danger to themselves or others; are more likely to maintain appropriate contact with services.
- *Enhanced CPA* may be appropriate for patients who: have multiple care needs requiring inter-agency coordination; are only willing to cooperate with one professional or agency but have multiple care needs; may be in contact with a number of agencies (including the criminal justice system); are likely to require more frequent and intensive interventions; are more likely to have mental health problems coexisting with other problems such as substance misuse; are more likely to be at risk of harming themselves or others; are more likely to disengage with services.

Supervision registers, which identify patients particularly at risk to themselves or others, have been abolished with the introduction of enhanced CPA.

A patient may not be compelled to accept or participate in any aspect of aftercare under section 117. When the aftercare services are no longer required, the section 117 duty ends.

Supervised community treatment

The 2007 Act introduces supervised community treatment (SCT) as an option for patients following a period of detention in hospital. The stated aim is to address the mental health needs of that group of patients who recover following a period of compulsory hospital treatment but repeatedly leave hospital, discontinue treatment, and relapse, requiring further compulsory treatment (so-called 'revolving door' patients).

Community Treatment Order Section 32 of the 2007 Act introduces the Community Treatment Order (CTO), a new power to discharge a patient detained under section 3 from hospital subject to his being liable to recall. A CTO is authorized by the Responsible Clinician with the agreement of an AMHP. To be valid a CTO must be in writing and the relevant criteria must be met:

- The patient is suffering from mental disorder of a nature or degree which makes it appropriate for him to receive medical treatment.
- It is necessary for his health or safety or for the protection of other persons that he should receive such treatment.
- Subject to his being liable to be recalled, such treatment can be provided without his continuing to be detained in a hospital.
- It is necessary that the responsible clinician should be able to exercise the power under section 17E(1) to recall the patient to hospital.
- Appropriate medical treatment is available for the patient.

A CTO may specify conditions to which the patient is subject and a patient can be recalled to hospital if the conditions are not met or if there is a risk of harm to the patient or to other persons if the patient were not recalled. The conditions must be for the purpose of ensuring that the patient receives medical treatment, or to prevent risk of harm to the patient or to other people, and should be kept to a minimum number consistent with achieving their purpose. The responsible clinician can vary and suspend conditions. A CTO lasts for 6mths and can be renewed for a further 6-mth period and yearly thereafter.

Mental Health Act: Scotland 1

Introduction

The Mental Health (Care and Treatment) (Scotland) Act 2003 replaced the Mental Health (Scotland) Act 1984 in 2005. The 2003 Act emphasizes the protection of the rights of mentally disordered patients and shifts the emphasis from detention in hospital to treatment for mental disorder, whether in hospital or the community.

Principles

Anyone using the Act must take account of the ten guiding principles:

- *Non-discrimination* Patients with mental disorder should retain wherever possible the same rights as those with other health needs.
- *Equality* Powers should be exercised without any direct or non-direct discrimination on any grounds.
- *Respect for diversity* Patients should receive care and treatment sensitive to their individual backgrounds and needs.
- *Reciprocity* Where an obligation is placed on a patient through the Act there is a parallel obligation on the health service to provide an appropriate service for the patient, including ongoing care following discharge from detention.
- *Informal care* Wherever possible, care and treatment should be provided without use of compulsory powers.
- *Participation* Patients should, as far as they are able, be involved in planning all aspects of their care and support.
- *Respect for carers* Those who provide informal support to patients should receive appropriate support and advice and have their views taken into account.
- *Least restrictive alternative* Patients should receive care in the least restrictive manner which is compatible with safe and effective care, taking appropriate account of the safety of others.
- *Benefit* Any intervention under the Act should be likely to produce a benefit for the patient, not achievable without use of the Act.
- *Child welfare* The welfare of any child with mental disorder is paramount in any interventions imposed on a child by the Act.

Definition of mental disorder

Section 328 defines '*mental disorder*' as 'any mental illness, personality disorder or learning disability' however caused or manifest. None of these terms is further defined.

A person is *not* mentally disordered solely by reason of sexual orientation, sexual deviancy, transsexualism or transvestism, dependence on or use of alcohol or drugs, 'exhibiting behaviour that causes or is likely to cause, harassment, alarm, or distress to any other person', or 'acting as no prudent person would act'.

Other definitions

Approved medical practitioner (AMP) Under section 22 these are doctors with the necessary qualifications and experience, who have undertaken training, and are approved by a Health Board as having special experience in the diagnosis and treatment of mental disorder.

Responsible medical officer (RMO) The registered medical practitioner in charge of the patient's treatment, usually the consultant.

Mental health officer (MHO) A social worker, with the necessary registration, experience, education, training, and competence in dealing with individuals with mental disorder; appointed under section 32 of the Act.

Designated medical practitioner (DMP) Medical practitioners appointed by the MWC to give second opinions regarding the medical treatment of patients subject to compulsion.

Care plan A document that sets out the care, treatment, and services that it is proposed that a patient subject to compulsion should receive. It will include compulsory and non-compulsory measures.

Named person Someone nominated by a person under section 250 to support them and protect their interests. Entitled to be informed about certain decisions and to act on the patient's behalf in certain circumstances. If one has not been nominated then it is the primary carer or nearest relative. For a child under 16 it is a parent.

Advance statement May be made under sections 275 and 276. When making this the person must have capacity and must make it in writing with a witness. Those carrying out duties under the Act must 'have regard to the wishes specified in the advance statement'. If acting against these wishes this must be recorded in writing with reasons, and a copy of this record must be sent to patient, named person, welfare attorney, guardian, MWC.

Advocacy Under section 259 every person with mental disorder has right of access to independent advocacy, and it is the duty of local authority and health board to ensure availability of this.

Mental Health Tribunal for Scotland (MHTS) The legal forum for making decisions regarding applications for certain compulsory orders, proposals to amend compulsory orders, and appeals against compulsory orders. Consists of three members: one legal, one medical and one lay.

Mental Welfare Commission (MWC) Similar to the MHAC for England and Wales but has wider remit and powers.

Criteria for compulsory intervention

Less stringent for emergency and shorter-term measures (i.e. parts 5 and 6) than they are for longer-term measures (i.e. part 7). The criteria for compulsion under a part 7 compulsory treatment order (CTO) are:

- The person has a mental disorder.
- Medical treatment is available which would be likely to prevent that disorder worsening or be likely to alleviate the effects of the disorder.
- There would be a significant risk to the patient's health, safety, or welfare, or to the safety of another person if such treatment were not provided.
- The patient's ability to make decisions about the provision of medical treatment is significantly impaired because of their mental disorder.
- The making of the order is necessary.

For short-term (part 6) or emergency (part 5) detention it only has to be likely that the criteria apply, and the second criterion above regarding treatability does not need to be considered.

Mental Health Act: Scotland 2

Compulsory measures

The main compulsory orders are set out under part 5 (emergency detention), part 6 (short-term detention), and part 7 (compulsory treatment order).

Emergency detention Under part 5, section 36, any fully registered medical practitioner may grant an *emergency detention certificate* (EDC) authorizing the detention of a person in hospital for 72 hrs. Consent from an MHO is necessary (unless impracticable), the situation must be urgent and such that making arrangements for short-term detention under part 6 would involve 'undesirable delay'. There are no separate procedures for inpatients and outpatients. As soon as practicable the patient should be assessed by an AMP to determine if detention under part 6 should be applied or if the patient should be dealt with informally.

Nurses' holding powers (section 299) may be used for up to 2hrs and continue for 1hr after the doctor has arrived.

Short-term detention Under part 6, section 44, any AMP may grant a Short Term Detention Order (STDO) authorizing the detention of a person in hospital for 28 days. Consent from an MHO is necessary in all cases. At the end of the order the patient may be discharged, remain as an informal patient, or may be placed on a CTO.

Compulsory treatment order (CTO) Under part 7 an application may be made to the MHTS for a patient to be made subject to a CTO authorizing compulsory treatment in hospital or in the community for 6mths. The application is made by an MHO and has three components: two medical reports (one by an AMP and the other by the patient's GP or another AMP), a report prepared by the MHO, and a proposed care plan (prepared by the MHO in consultation with the RMO and others who will be involved in the care and treatment of the patient).

The MHT must be satisfied that the criteria for a CTO are met; if there are issues that require clarification the MHT may grant an interim compulsory treatment order instead. A CTO in the community may make requirements as to residence, attendance for treatment and other services, access of staff to the patient's residence, and acceptance of medication for mental disorder. A CTO may be renewed for 6mths, then annually thereafter, without further application to the MHTS unless some variation to the order is proposed.

If a patient on a community-based CTO refuses medication then they may be taken to hospital and detained there for up to 6hrs to receive this. If the patient is non-compliant with other aspects of the order, then detention in hospital for up to 72hrs can be authorized by the RMO; this may be extended by a further 28 days with the approval of the RMO and MHO to allow an assessment as to whether an application should be made for the CTO to be varied.

Treatment of patients subject to compulsion (part 16)

- A patient subject to compulsion (except under emergency provisions) may be given *medication* for mental disorder for up to 8wks, whether they consent and/or have capacity or not. Patients in the community cannot be given medication using physical force.
- Medication for over 2mths requires the patient's consent or, if the person refuses or is incapable of consenting, authorization by a DMP.
- ECT may only be given if a patient can and does consent, or—if incapable of consenting—with the authorization of a DMP. ECT cannot be given, even in an emergency, to a patient with capacity who refuses.
- Treatment that is *urgently necessary* may be authorized by the RMO without consent or a second opinion; this may be used for giving ECT to severely ill and at-risk patients lacking capacity while awaiting a second opinion and for giving medication to acutely disturbed patients on emergency detention.
- To receive *neurosurgery for mental disorder* there must be an independent opinion from a DMP that the treatment will be beneficial, two opinions from lay people appointed by the MWC that the person has capacity and consents, or if they do not have capacity, that they do not object. If the person is incapable but is not objecting, the treatment must be authorized by the Court of Session.

Leave, absconding, and transfer

Procedures allow for 'suspension of detention' of patients detained in hospital so that they may leave hospital; the taking into custody and return of patients who abscond either from hospital or the residence specified in a community-based CTO; and for patients to be transferred to other hospitals.

Review

A patient or their named person may appeal to the MHTS against being subject to a CTO or short-term detention (but not emergency detention), against transfer to another hospital, and against being held in conditions of excessive security. This may happen once during each renewed period of compulsion for CTOs. An RMO must refer a case to the MHTS if a variation is proposed in an order (e.g. from a community-based to hospital-based order). The MWC may also refer cases to the MHTS. If the MHTS has not reviewed a case for 2yrs then it must do so without a specific referral being made. The MHTS must cancel an order if the criteria for compulsion are no longer met. The RMO and MWC also have the power to cancel an order at any point if these criteria are no longer met.

Mental Welfare Commission

The MWC has a statutory duty to protect individuals with mental disorder whether they are liable to detention or not. It also has the power to discharge patients subject to compulsion. It has a responsibility to visit and inspect services and the power to conduct enquiries into deficiencies in care. It has new duties to monitor the operation of the Act and promote best practice.

Mental Health Act: Northern Ireland 1

Introduction

The Mental Health (Northern Ireland) Order 1986 sets out the mental health provisions for Northern Ireland. The Bamford review of Mental Health and Learning Disability reported in August 2007 and proposed comprehensive reform of mental health legislation and the introduction of incapacity legislation.

Definition of mental disorder

Article 3 defines 'mental disorder' as meaning 'mental illness, mental handicap and any other disorder or disability of mind'. There are further definitions of types of mental disorder:

- *Mental illness* defined as 'a state of mind which affects a person's thinking, perceiving, emotion or judgement to the extent that he requires care or medical treatment in his own interests or the interests of other persons'.
- *Mental handicap* defined as a state of arrested or incomplete development of mind which includes significant impairment of intelligence and social functioning'.
- *Severe mental handicap* defined as 'a state of arrested or incomplete development of mind which includes severe impairment of intelligence and social functioning'.
- *Severe mental impairment* defined as 'a state of arrested or incomplete development of mind which includes severe impairment of intelligence and social functioning and is associated with abnormally aggressive or seriously irresponsible conduct on the part of the person concerned'.

The following are *excluded* if they are the *only* 'conditions' present: personality disorder, promiscuity or other immoral conduct, sexual deviancy, or dependence on alcohol or drugs.

Other definitions

Mental Health Review Tribunal for Northern Ireland (MHRTNI) Legal forum to which a patient or a nearest relative can appeal against detention. The MHRTNI has 3 members: a legally qualified chairperson, a medical practitioner, and a lay member. It must discharge a patient if the criteria for detention no longer apply.

Mental Health Commission for Northern Ireland (MHCNI) Like the MWC in Scotland, has broader remit than the MHAC in England and Wales.

Appointed doctor The MHCNI appoints medical practitioners for the purposes of Part II (compulsory admission to hospital and guardianship). These doctors are analogous to approved doctors in England and Wales. Doctors may also be appointed for the purposes of Part IV (consent to treatment). The term 'appointed doctor' on these pages is used to refer to Part II.

Responsible medical officer (RMO) The registered medical practitioner in charge of the patient's treatment, usually the consultant.

Approved social worker (ASW) A social worker who has undergone specific training and assessment and is appointed for the purposes of the Order as having competence in dealing with individuals with mental disorder.

Nearest relative The person caring for the patient who is first on the following list (article 32): spouse, child, parent, brother or sister, grandparent, grandchild, uncle or aunt, nephew or niece. If there was no carer, then the first person on the list is the nearest relative. If two relatives are of equal standing then the elder prevails.

Criteria for compulsory intervention

The criteria for compulsory intervention are less stringent for emergency and shorter-term measures (i.e. articles 4 and 7(2)) than they are for longer-term measures (i.e. article 12). The criteria for compulsion under article 12 are:

- The patient is suffering from mental illness or severe mental impairment of a nature or degree which warrants his detention in hospital for medical treatment.
- Failure to so detain the patient would create a substantial likelihood of serious physical harm to himself or to other persons.
- Consideration has been given to whether other methods of dealing with the patient are available and to why they are not appropriate.

For article 4 the type of mental disorder does not need to be specified, and for article 7(1) it must appear that the article 4 criteria are met.

Mental Health Act: Northern Ireland 2

Compulsory measures

Article 4 allows detention in hospital for assessment which may be followed by detention for treatment under article 12. Article 7(2) allows for the detention of a patient already in hospital.

Admission for assessment An application for detention under article 4 may be made by the nearest relative or ASW and requires one medical recommendation. This should be by the patient's GP or a doctor who knows the patient, if this is practicable, and should not, except in urgent cases, be by a doctor on the staff of the admitting hospital. Immediately on admission to hospital the patient must be examined by the RMO, an appointed doctor, or another doctor, who must submit a report to the responsible authority. They may then be detained for 7 days from the point of admission (this is limited to 2 days where the examination is not by the RMO or an appointed doctor, during which the RMO should examine the patient). Detention may be extended by a further 7 days on one occasion following a further report from the RMO. Following detention under article 4 a patient may be detained under article 12, remain informally, or be discharged.

Assessment of patient already in hospital Under article 7(2), where a person is a voluntary inpatient, if it appears to a doctor on the staff of the hospital that an application for assessment ought to be made, then a report may be furnished to the responsible authority, allowing detention for 48hrs. This may be followed by detention under article 4.

Detention for treatment Where a patient has been detained under article 4, they may be further detained for 6mths under article 12. This requires a recommendation from an appointed doctor (not the doctor who made the assessment recommendation). This may be renewed for a further 6mths and annually thereafter.

Guardianship Article 18 allows for guardianship. The application is made by the nearest relative or ASW, and there must be two medical recommendations and an ASW recommendation. The patient must be suffering from mental illness or mental handicap, and guardianship should be necessary in the interest of the patient's welfare. Renewal is as for article 12.

Nurses' holding powers Article 7(3) allows nurses (of the prescribed class) to detain an inpatient in hospital for up to 6hrs to allow for a medical assessment regarding detention. Detention under article 7(3) ends when the doctor arrives.

Treatment of patients subject to compulsion

Articles 62–69 set out very similar provisions regarding consent to treatment as set out for England and Wales by the 1983 Act (📖 p. 880).

Leave, absconding, and transfer

Procedures allow for patients to be granted leave of absence with the authorization of the RMO (article 15); for patients to be taken into custody and returned to hospital if they abscond (article 29); and for patients to be transferred between hospitals (article 28).

Review

The MHRTNI operates in a very similar way to England and Wales, but must review a detained patient if they have not been reviewed for 2 yrs. After reviewing a case the MHCNI may refer a patient to the MHRTNI or may recommend that the patient be discharged. The RMO may discharge a patient at any point. The nearest relative may also discharge a patient if not opposed by the RMO.

Mental Health Commission for Northern Ireland

The functions of the MHCNI are very similar to those of the MWC in Scotland: the duty to protect individuals with mental disorder whether they are liable to detention or not; the power to recommend discharge of patients subject to compulsion; the responsibility to visit and inspect services; and the power to conduct enquiries into deficiencies in care.

Mental Health Act: Republic of Ireland 1

Introduction

The Mental Health Act 2001 replaced the Mental Treatment Act 1945 and various modifying Acts passed in 1953, 1961, and 1981. The new Act was implemented in November 2006.

Principles

Section 4 sets out some principles to be considered in operating the Act. The best interests of the person should be the principal consideration with due regard being given to the interests of others who may be at risk of serious harm; the person should be notified of proposals and should be allowed to make representations regarding these which should be given due consideration; any decision should give due regard to the right of a person to dignity, bodily integrity, privacy, and autonomy.

Definition of mental disorder and criteria for compulsion

Section 3 sets out the definition of mental disorder, which also includes the criteria for compulsory detention.

'Mental disorder' is defined as 'mental illness, severe dementia, or significant intellectual impairment where:

(a) because of the illness, disability or dementia, there is a serious likelihood of the person concerned causing immediate and serious harm to himself or herself or to other persons, or

(b) (i) because of the severity of the illness, disability or dementia, the judgement of the person concerned is so impaired that failure to admit the person to an approved centre would be likely to lead to a serious deterioration in his or her condition or would prevent the administration of appropriate treatment that could be given only by such admission, and

(ii) the reception, detention and treatment of the person concerned in an approved centre would be likely to benefit or alleviate the condition of that person to a material extent.'

- 'Mental illness' means a state of mind of a person which affects the person's thinking, perceiving, emotion, or judgement and which seriously impairs the mental function of the person to the extent that he or she requires care or medical treatment in his or her own interest or in the interest of other persons.
- 'Severe dementia' means a deterioration of the brain of a person which significantly impairs the intellectual function of the person thereby affecting thought, comprehension, and memory and which includes severe psychiatric or behavioural symptoms such as physical aggression.
- 'Significant intellectual disability' means a state of arrested or incomplete development of mind of a person which includes significant impairment of intelligence and social functioning and abnormally aggressive or seriously irresponsible conduct on the part of the person.

Under section 8 the following are excluded if they are the only conditions present: personality disorder, being 'socially deviant', and being addicted to drugs or intoxicants.

Other definitions

Approved centre Hospitals or other inpatient facilities for the care and treatment of people suffering from mental illness or mental disorder. Must be registered with the MHC.

Review tribunal The legal forum which reviews the making of every admission and renewal order. Has three members: a legally qualified chairperson, a consultant psychiatrist, and another member.

Mental Health Commission (MHC) The body responsible for monitoring the standards of mental health services and protecting detained patients. Has a more direct role in the latter than similar bodies in the UK.

Inspector of Mental Health Services Consultant psychiatrist appointed by the MHC to visit and inspect approved centres and to review mental health services. Will also review individual cases when visiting centres.

Mental Health Commission (MHC)

The MHC was established in April 2002. Its main purpose is to promote, encourage, and foster the establishment and maintenance of high standards and good practices in the delivery of mental health services, and to protect the interests of detained patients. It is notified of every episode of detention and renewal, appoints tribunals, maintains a panel of consultants to undertake independent examinations, appoints an Inspector of Mental Health Services, maintains a register of approved centres, makes regulations as to the use of seclusion and restraint, and prepares codes of practice and other documents.

Mental Health Act: Republic of Ireland 2

Compulsory measures

Application for involuntary admission (section 9)

An application for admission may be made under section 9 by a spouse or relative, an authorized officer (of the health board), a garda, or any other person (with certain exclusions applying). The applicant must have seen the person within the last 48hrs.

Medical assessment (section 10)

Within 24hrs of the application being made, a medical practitioner (who does not work at the approved centre where the person may be admitted) should examine the person. The doctor should inform the person about the purpose of the examination, unless this would be detrimental to the person. If the doctor considers the person to be mentally disordered then a recommendation may be made allowing involuntary admission to an approved centre. This remains in force for 7 days.

Power of the garda to detain and apply for involuntary admission (section 12)

The garda may take a person into custody if they have reasonable grounds to believe that the person is mentally disordered and because of this there is a serious likelihood of the person harming themselves or others. They may forcibly enter premises if necessary. The garda would then follow the usual application for an involuntary admission procedure (section 9). If this application is granted the garda must take the person to the approved centre.

Removal to an approved centre (section 13)

The applicant is responsible for getting the person to the approved centre. If not possible then the doctor making the recommendation may request that staff from the centre do this. The garda may be asked for assistance.

Admission to approved centre (sections 14 and 15)

When the person is admitted to the approved centre, a consultant psychiatrist must examine them as soon as is practicable (section 14). They may be held for 24hrs to allow this examination. If this psychiatrist is satisfied that the person is suffering from mental disorder then an 'admission order' is made.

Under section 15 an admission order authorizes the detention and treatment of the patient in the centre for 21 days. This may be renewed (as a 'renewal order') for 3mths initially, then 6mths, and then annually thereafter. The consultant responsible for the patient must make the renewal following an examination in the week before making the renewal order. When an order (admission or renewal) is made, the consultant must send a copy to the MHC and a written notice to the patient (section 16).

Voluntary patients wishing to leave an approved centre

Previously a voluntary patient had to give 3 days' notice of intention to leave. Under section 23 a voluntary patient may leave hospital at any point unless a consultant psychiatrist or doctor or nurse on the staff considers that they suffer from mental disorder. If this is the case they may be detained for up to 24hrs. During this period the responsible consultant must either discharge the patient or arrange an examination by another consultant. If this consultant is of the opinion that the patient is mentally disordered then they issue a certificate and the patient is detained as they would be under an admission order (section 14).

Treatment of patients subject to compulsion (Part 4)

The consent of a patient to treatment is required except where the consultant psychiatrist considers that the treatment is necessary to safeguard the life of the patient, to restore his or her health, to alleviate his or her condition, or to relieve his or her suffering, and the patient is incapable of giving such consent because of mental disorder.

- Neurosurgery for mental disorder may not be performed unless the patient consents and it is authorized by a tribunal.
- ECT may not be given unless the patient gives consent in writing, or where the patient is unable or unwilling to give consent, the therapy is authorized by the responsible consultant psychiatrist and another consultant psychiatrist.
- Medication for the amelioration of the mental disorder for more than 3mths cannot be given unless the patient consents in writing, or, where the patient is unable or unwilling to give consent, the continued medication is authorized by the consultant psychiatrist responsible for the patient and by another consultant psychiatrist. This must be renewed every 3mths.

Review

When the MHC receives a copy of an order it must refer the case to a tribunal, assign a legal representative to the patient if they do not have one, and direct that a member of the panel of consultant psychiatrists appointed by the MHC reviews the case (section 17).

Within 21 days of the making of the order the tribunal must review the detention. The tribunal may affirm or revoke the order depending on whether the criteria for detention are met (section 18). An appeal against a tribunal's decision may be made to the Circuit Court (section 19).

Leave, absconding, and transfers

Procedures allow for patients to be allowed to be absent from the approved centre with the authorization of the consultant responsible for their care (section 26); for patients to be taken into custody and returned to an approved centre if they abscond (section 27); and for patients to be transferred to other approved centres and hospitals (sections 20, 21, and 22).

Issues of confidentiality

Whatever…I may see or hear in the lives of men which ought not to be spoken abroad I will not divulge, as reckoning that all such should be kept secret.

Hippocratic Oath

Patients' right to confidentiality

Patients have a right to expect that information about them will be held in confidence by their doctors. Confidentiality is central to trust between doctors and patients. Without assurances about confidentiality, patients may be reluctant to give doctors the information they need in order to provide good care. If you are asked to provide information about patients you should:

- Seek patients' consent to disclosure of information wherever possible, whether or not you judge that patients can be identified from the disclosure.
- Anonymize data where this will serve the intended purpose.
- Keep disclosures to the minimum necessary.
- Always document and be prepared to justify your decisions.

Protecting information

- Doctors have a professional responsibility to ensure patient information is effectively protected against improper disclosure at all times.
- Many improper disclosures are unintentional—do not discuss patients where you can be overheard or leave patients' records, either on paper or on screen, where they can be seen by other patients, unauthorized health care staff, or the public (see Table 21.1).
- Allowing for issues of personal safety, ensure that as far as possible your consultations with patients are private.

Sharing information with others providing care

- Make sure that patients are aware that personal information about them will be shared within the health care team, and of the reasons for this.
- Respect the wishes of any patient who does not wish specific information to be shared in this way, unless to do so would put others at risk of death or serious harm.
- Where patients have consented to treatment, express consent is not usually needed before relevant personal information is shared, to enable the treatment to be provided safely and ensure continuity of care (e.g. medical secretaries typing letters to GPs, referrals for further investigations, referrals to other specialists).

Medical reports

This includes both specific requests for a particular report on *current* medical problems and disclosure of information from existing medical records for a third party (e.g. court report, insurance claim, benefits claim). In these circumstances:

- Satisfy yourself that the patient has been told about the purpose of the examination and/or disclosure, the extent of the information to be disclosed, and the fact that relevant information cannot be concealed or withheld. (Showing the form or letter of request to the patient may assist in ensuring the patient understands the scope of the information requested.)
- Obtain evidence of written consent to the disclosure from the patient or a person properly authorized to act on the patient's behalf.
- Disclose only information relevant to the request made.
- Include only factual information you can substantiate, presented in an unbiased manner.
- Always check whether the patient wishes to see their report (the Access to Medical Reports Act 1988 entitles patients to see reports written about them before they are disclosed, in most circumstances).
- Disclosures without consent to employers, insurance companies, or any other third party, can be justified only in exceptional circumstances (e.g. to protect others from risk of death or serious harm—see **Breaking confidentiality** ☐ p. 900).

Recent developments

In its report in 1997 the Caldicott Committee made a number of recommendations aimed at improving the way the NHS handles and protects patient information. A key recommendation was the establishment of organizational guardians to oversee access to patient-identifiable information. These 'Caldicott Guardians' have been established and are responsible for internal protocols and policies on the use of such information, and on its disclosure. A key principle is that of 'the need to know'.

Confidentiality expectations: the reality

Despite confidentiality being one of the main foundations of the 'privileged' doctor–patient relationship, expectations about where personal information may be reasonably disclosed varies amongst patients and medical professionals at different stages of their training.

Table 21.1 Confidentiality expectations

Where information revealed	Patients (%)	House staff (%)	Medical students (%)
Large professional meeting	69	94	81
To office nursing staff	50	69	83
Identified by name to other physicians	23	60	55
Told as a story at a party:			
To other physicians	18	60	57
To non-physicians	9	36	45
Told to spouse or 'friend'	17	51	70

Weiss B (1982) Confidentiality expectations of patients, physicians, and medical students. *JAMA* **247**: 2695.

Breaking confidentiality

Personal information should not be disclosed to a third party (e.g. relative, partner, solicitor, police officer, or officer of a court) without the patient's express consent, except in the circumstances described here (p. 900). If you decide to disclose confidential information against a patient's wishes, you must document this decision in the patient's notes and be prepared to explain/justify your decision (and communicate this decision to the patient).

Disclosures to protect the patient or others

In this case, the risk to third parties is so serious that it outweighs the patient's privacy interest, and the appropriate person or authority should be informed without undue delay. Examples of such circumstances include:

- Where a colleague, who is also a patient, is placing patients at risk as a result of illness or other medical condition. (If you are in doubt about whether disclosure is justified, consult an experienced colleague, or seek advice from a professional organization. The safety of patients must come first.)
- Where a patient continues to drive, against medical advice, when unfit to do so. In such circumstances you should disclose relevant information to the medical adviser of the Driver and Vehicle Licensing Agency without delay. Fuller guidance is given on 🕮 p. 902.
- To assist in the prevention or detection of a serious crime (i.e. where someone may be at risk of death or serious harm) (e.g. threats of violence—see the Box 21.4) or suspected child abuse (🕮 p. 662).

Disclosure in connection with judicial or other statutory proceedings

Under certain circumstances disclosure of information is required by law:
- Notification of a known or suspected communicable disease.
- If ordered to do so by a judge or presiding officer of a court (unless the information appears to be irrelevant, e.g. details of relatives or partners of the patient not party to the proceedings).
- To assist a Coroner, Procurator Fiscal, or other similar officer in connection with an inquest or fatal accident inquiry (only *relevant* information should be provided).
- An official request from a statutory regulatory body for any of the health care professions, where disclosure is necessary in the interests of justice and for the safety of other patients.

Difficult situations

- Children and other patients who may lack competence to give consent (see 🕮 p. 870).
  - Always try to persuade them to allow an appropriate person (e.g. individual with parental responsibility) to be involved in the consultation.
  - Always inform the patient (and their relative or carer) prior to passing on information to another responsible person or statutory agency (e.g. social services).

- Document in the patient's record the steps you have taken to obtain consent and the reasons for deciding to disclose information.
- Where a person lacks capacity, disclosure should be in that person's best interests and follow the other basic principles regarding confidentiality.
- Situations of dual responsibilities (i.e. contractual obligations to third parties, such as companies or organizations) (e.g. occupational health services, insurance companies, benefits agencies, police forensic medical advisors, armed forces, prison services), as well as obligations to patients. Always ensure patients are aware of the purpose of the consultation, and to whom you are contractually obliged to release information.
- If in doubt, consult (in UK):
  - General Medical Council (GMC): guidance may be found in the document: *Confidentiality: Protecting and Providing Information*.
  - Royal College of Psychiatrists (RCP): guidance may be found at ✍ http://www.rcpsych.ac.uk/files/pdfversion/cr133.pdf
  - Consider seeking the advice of your Medical Defence body.

Box 21.4 The Tarasoff case

On 27 October 1969, Prosenjit Poddar killed his ex-girlfriend, Tatiana Tarasoff. Two months earlier, Poddar had declared his intentions during an outpatient appointment with his psychotherapist, Dr Lawrence Moore, at the University of California at Berkeley's Cowell Memorial Hospital. Dr Moore tried to have Poddar confined to a mental institution for observation (including asking the university police for assistance). When law enforcement agents decided that Poddar was harmless and released him, Moore's director, Dr Harvey Powelson, requested that all evidence of contact between Moore and the police department be destroyed. No one, including Dr Moore, pursued the case further.

After the murder, Tatiana's parents became aware of this prior knowledge and sued the university regents, hospital, and police department, claiming that, at least, a warning should have been issued to her. On 1 July 1976 (more than six-and-a-half years after the murder), the Supreme Court of California found that the defendants had breached their duty to exercise reasonable care. In other words, physicians and therapists have a duty to warn third parties of threatened danger arising from a patient's violent intentions. As a final statement, the Court stated that 'protective privilege ends where public peril begins'.

Note: although often quoted when discussing issues of confidentiality, this case has no legal bearing in the UK. Even in the USA the impact of the Tarasoff case has been less dramatic and intrusive than one might expect.

Fitness to drive

Principles and legal definitions

- The Driver and Vehicle Licensing Agency (DVLA) in the UK sets out minimum medical standards of fitness to drive and the requirements for mental health in broad terms.
- A clear distinction is made between the standards needed for Group 1 (cars and motorcycles) and Group 2 (lorries and buses) licences, the latter being more stringent due to the size of vehicle and the greater time spent at the wheel.
- 'Severe mental disorder' is defined by section 92 of the Road Traffic Act 1988 as 'mental illness, arrested or incomplete development of the mind, psychopathic disorder or severe impairment of intelligence or social functioning'.
- The standards set reflect not only the need for an improvement in the mental state but also a period of stability, such that the risk of relapse can be assessed should the patient fail to recognize any deterioration.
- The standards for patients with misuse of or dependency on alcohol or drugs are detailed on 📖 p. 606.

Notes on medication

- Section 4 of the Road Traffic Act 1988 states that 'any person who is driving or attempting to drive on the public highway, or other public place whilst unfit due to any drug, is liable to prosecution'.
- All drugs acting on the central nervous system can impair alertness, concentration, and driving performance. This is particularly so at initiation of treatment or soon after and when dosage is being increased. **Driving must cease if adversely affected**.
- When planning the treatment of any patient (particularly professional drivers, e.g. of taxis, lorries, buses, or construction vehicles), always consider adverse side-effect profiles which may impair driving ability:
  - Antidepressants—anticholinergic/antihistaminic effects (sedation).
  - Antipsychotics—both sedation and EPSEs (assess regularly).
  - BDZs—the most likely psychotropic medication to impair driving performance; avoid long-acting compounds.
  - For all psychotropics—consider the epileptogenic potential.

Duties and other considerations

- **Duty of care** Doctors have a duty to advise their patients of the potential dangers of adverse effects from medication and interactions with other substances, especially alcohol.
- **Confidentiality** When a patient has a condition which makes driving unsafe and the patient is either unable to appreciate this or refuses to cease driving, GMC guidelines advise breaking confidentiality and informing the DVLA (see Box 21.5).
- **Patients detained under the MHA** Similar rules as for *informal* patients (i.e. drivers must be able to satisfy the standards of fitness for their respective conditions and be free from any effects of medication which will affect driving adversely).

Further advice on fitness to drive

- Doctors may write to the DVLA or may speak to one of the medical advisors during office hours to seek advice about a particular driver (identified by an M number), or about fitness to drive in general.
- All of the DVLA advice is available online at: http://www.dvla.gov.uk (including an email facility for use by medical professionals only).

Box 21.5 GMC guidelines for informing the DVLA

- The DVLA is legally responsible for deciding if a person is medically unfit to drive. They need to know when driving licence holders have a condition which may, now or in the future, affect their safety as a driver.
- Therefore, where patients have such conditions, you should:
  - Make sure that the patients understand that the condition may impair their ability to drive. If a patient is incapable of understanding this advice (e.g. because of dementia), you should inform the DVLA immediately.
  - Explain to patients that they have a legal duty to inform the DVLA about the condition.
- If the patient refuses to accept the diagnosis or the effect of the condition on their ability to drive, you can suggest that the patient seeks a second opinion, and make appropriate arrangements for the patient to do so. You should advise patients not to drive until the second opinion has been obtained.
- If patients continue to drive when they are not fit to do so, you should make every reasonable effort to persuade them to stop. This may include telling their next of kin.
- If you do not manage to persuade patients to stop driving, or you are given or find evidence that a patient is continuing to drive contrary to advice, you should disclose relevant medical information immediately, in confidence, to the medical advisor at the DVLA.
- Before giving information to the DVLA you should inform the patient of your decision to do so. Once the DVLA has been informed, you should also write to the patient, to confirm that a disclosure has been made.

DVLA requirements for specific psychiatric conditions

Anxiety or depression without significant memory or concentration problems, agitation, behavioural disturbance, or suicidal thoughts.
Group 1 drivers: DVLA need not be notified and driving may continue.
Group 2 drivers: Very minor short-lived illnesses need not be notified.

Severe anxiety or depression with significant memory or concentration problems, agitation, behavioural disturbance or suicidal thoughts.
Group 1 drivers: *Driving should cease* pending the outcome of medical enquiry. A period of stability depending upon the circumstances will be required before driving can be resumed. Particularly dangerous are those who may attempt suicide at the wheel.
Group 2 drivers: *Driving may be permitted* when the person is well and stable for a period of 6mths. Medication must not cause side-effects which would interfere with alertness or concentration. Driving is usually permitted if the anxiety or depression is long-standing, but maintained symptom-free on doses of psychotropic medication which do not impair. DVLA may require psychiatric reports.

Acute psychosis (any cause)

Group 1 drivers: *Driving must cease* during the acute illness. Re-licensing can be considered when all of the following conditions can be satisfied:
• Has remained well and stable for at least 3mths.
• Is compliant with treatment.
• Is free from adverse effects of medication which would impair driving.
• Subject to a favourable specialist report.

Note: drivers who have a history of instability and/or poor compliance will require a longer period off driving.

Group 2 drivers: *Driving should cease* pending the outcome of medical enquiry. The person must be well and stable for a minimum of 3yrs with insight into their condition before driving can be resumed. At that time, the DVLA will usually require a consultant examination. Any psychotropic medication should be of minimum effective dosage and not interfere with alertness, concentration, or in any other way impair driving performance. There should be no significant likelihood of recurrence.

Hypomania/mania

Group 1 drivers: *Driving must cease* during the acute illness. Following an *isolated episode*, re-licensing can be reconsidered when *all* the following conditions can be satisfied:
• Well and stable for at least 3mths.
• Compliant with treatment.
• Insight has been regained.
• Free from adverse effects of medication which would impair driving.
• Subject to a favourable specialist report.

Note: hypomania or mania are particularly dangerous to driving when there are repeated changes of mood. Therefore, when there have been 4 or more episodes of mood swing within the previous 12mths, at least 6mths' stability will be required, with evidence of treatment compliance and a favourable specialist report.

Group 2 drivers: *Driving must cease* pending the outcome of medical enquiry. The person must be well and stable for a minimum of 3yrs with insight into their condition before driving can be resumed. At that time, the DVLA will usually require a consultant examination. Any psychotropic medication should be of minimum effective dosage and not interfere with alertness, concentration, or in any other way impair driving performance. There should be no significant likelihood of recurrence.

Schizophrenia or other chronic psychoses

Group 1 drivers: The driver must satisfy *all* the following conditions:
- Stable behaviour for at least 3mths.
- Adequately compliant with treatment.
- Free from adverse effects of medication which would impair driving.
- Subject to a favourable specialist report.

Note: for patients with *continuing symptoms*, even with limited insight, these do not necessarily preclude licensing. Symptoms should be unlikely to cause significant concentration problems, memory impairment, or distraction whilst driving. Particularly dangerous are those drivers whose psychotic symptoms relate to other road users.

Group 2 drivers: *Driving must cease* pending the outcome of medical enquiry. The person must be well and stable for a minimum of 3yrs with insight into their condition before driving can be resumed. At that time, the DVLA will usually require a consultant examination. Any psychotropic medication should be of minimum effective dosage and not interfere with alertness, concentration, or in any other way impair driving performance. There should be no significant likelihood of recurrence.

Dementia or any organic brain syndrome

It is extremely difficult to assess driving ability in those with dementia. Those who have poor short-term memory, disorientation, lack of insight and judgement are almost certainly not fit to drive. The variable presentations and rates of progression are acknowledged. Disorders of attention will also cause impairment. A decision regarding fitness to drive is usually based on medical reports.

Group 1 drivers: In early dementia when sufficient skills are retained and progression is slow, a licence may be issued subject to annual review. A formal driving assessment may be necessary.

Group 2 drivers: *Refuse* or *revoke* licence.

Learning disability

Group 1 drivers: Severe learning disability is not compatible with driving and the licence application must be refused. In milder forms, provided there are no other relevant problems, it may be possible to hold a licence, but it will be necessary to demonstrate adequate functional ability at the wheel.

Group 2 drivers: Recommended permanent refusal or revocation if severe. Minor degrees of learning disability when the condition is stable with no medical or psychiatric complications may be compatible with the holding of a licence.

Persistent behaviour disorder

Includes post-head injury syndrome, psychopathic disorders, and non-epileptic seizure disorder.

Group 1 drivers: If seriously disturbed (e.g. violent behaviour or alcohol abuse) and likely to be a source of danger at the wheel, licence should be revoked or the application refused. Licence will be issued after medical reports confirm that behavioural disturbances have been satisfactorily controlled.

Group 2 drivers: Recommended refusal or revocation if associated with serious behaviour disturbance likely to make the individual a source of danger at the wheel. If the person matures and psychiatric reports confirm stability a consideration would be given to restoration of the licence but a consultant psychiatrist report would be required.

Chapter 22

Transcultural psychiatry

Introduction

Psychiatry is undeniably a branch of Western medicine and our conception of psychiatric illness (and how best to treat it) is undoubtedly heavily influenced by Western social and cultural factors. However, the scientific validity of these concepts can be readily tested if they can be shown to cross cultural boundaries.

Emil Kraepelin recognized this argument when he visited Java in 1896, and found that the clinical symptoms of dementia praecox could be seen in patients he met there, just as they were manifest in his own patients in Germany. It was not until the WHO International Pilot Study of Schizophrenia in 1973 that the incidence of schizophrenia (defined by narrow criteria) was found to be 0.7–1.4 per 10 000 aged 15–54 across all nine countries studied worldwide. Despite variations in the *content* of delusions and hallucinations (which were culturally derived), the *form* was found to be the same. These conclusions have been supported by a large number of epidemiological studies and similar results have been found for bipolar affective disorder.

The manifestations of depressive, stress-related, and anxiety disorders show the greatest cultural variations (see 📖 p. 910). The myth that these are predominantly Western diseases held sway for a long time (based on views of Western civilization articulated most eloquently by Freud in *Civilization and its discontents* in 1930).

Certain manifestations of emotional distress, termed 'culture-bound syndromes' by P.M. Yap, a former professor of psychiatry in Hong Kong, are particular to different cultures. These present as mixed disorders of behaviour, emotions, and beliefs and many have local names (see 📖 p. 916). Some are clear symptom-correlates of disorders found in ICD-10 and DSM-IV; others have no Western equivalent but appear to be variations of somatoform, conversion, or dissociative disorders. Some Western disorders (e.g. anorexia nervosa, deliberate self-harm) are rarely seen in non-Western countries. However, as we move towards a more global society, 'Western influences' appear to be making these types of disorder increasingly frequent in non-Western societies.

Debate continues as to whether Western diagnostic categories are universally valid. Understanding the biological underpinnings of the common disease entities (e.g. schizophrenia, bipolar affective disorder, depression, anxiety) and the development of treatments based upon our understanding of neurophysiological and neuropharmacological mechanisms will inform this debate. However, awareness of cultural issues as they impact upon an individual, their illness (and illness beliefs), and the relationship between psychiatrist and patient, is critical if we are to provide appropriate interventions successfully.

Cultural context and the presentation of psychiatric disorders

Schizophrenia Some apparently psychotic experiences may be normal when viewed within a cultural context. This applies to delusions (e.g. belief in magic, spirits, or demons) and hallucinations (e.g. seeing 'auras', the appearance of divine entities, hearing God's voice). Other evidence of apparent psychosis, such as disorganized speech, may actually reflect local variations in language syntax, or the fact that the person is not completely fluent in the language used by the interviewer. Differences in non-verbal communication (e.g. eye contact, facial expression, body language) may also be misinterpreted. Historically there has been a tendency in the UK and US to diagnose schizophrenia more readily in certain cultural groups (e.g. Afro-Caribbeans). This probably does not reflect differences in the incidence of schizophrenia, but rather a lack of understanding of cultural differences. Some symptoms of schizophrenia (e.g. catatonia) are more common in non-Western countries, and even between Western countries the diagnosis of brief psychoses (e.g. bouffée deliriante) varies. Interestingly the course of schizophrenia appears to be more acute and have better long-term outcome in some developing countries.

Mania Often used colloquially to mean 'changes in normal behaviour', rather than its strict definition. It may be difficult to distinguish periods of frenzied activity (e.g. in *amok*—see 🕮 p. 916) from increased activity, energy, and reduced need for sleep in a manic episode. This may be particularly difficult when such episodes are preceded by apparent depressive symptoms.

Depression Cultural expressions of depressive symptoms vary across populations. In some cultures there is greater emphasis on somatic terms, e.g. 'nerves' or 'headaches' (Mediterranean cultures); 'problems of the heart' (Middle East); 'imbalance', 'weakness', or 'tiredness' (China and Asia). This often makes the use of Western diagnostic classifications difficult, as symptoms may cross diagnostic boundaries (e.g. mood, anxiety, somatoform disorders). Equally difficult may be the interpretation of culturally normal explanations for symptom causation—which may appear delusional (e.g. spirit possession), or associated somatic symptoms (see 🕮 p. 802)—that need to be distinguished from actual hallucinations.

Anxiety and stress-related disorders

Agoraphobia Social sanctions against members of certain populations (e.g. women) appearing in public may sometimes be confused with agoraphobic symptoms.

Panic attacks In some cultures these may be interpreted as evidence of magic or witchcraft (particularly when they come 'out of the blue').

OCD Religious and cultural beliefs strongly influence the content of obsessions and nature of compulsions. It may often be difficult to assess the significance of ritualistic behaviours unless the clinician has a knowledge of local customs.

PTSD Immigrants may have emigrated to escape military conflict or particularly harsh regimes. They may have had experience of significant traumatic events, but may be unwilling (or unable) to discuss them because of language problems or fears of being sent back.

Somatization disorder Common types of somatic symptoms vary across cultures (and genders within cultures). These reflect the principal concerns of the population (or individual), e.g. worms/insects in the scalp/under the skin—seen in South East Asia and Africa; concern about semen loss—seen in India (see *Dhat* 📖 p. 917) and China (see *Shenk-k'ui* 📖 p. 920).

Conversion and dissociative disorders More common in rural populations, in 'less educated' societies, and may be culturally normal. Certain religious rituals involve alteration in consciousness (including trance states), beliefs in spirit possession, and varieties of socially sanctioned behaviours that could be viewed as conversion or dissociative disorders (e.g. *falling out* 📖 p. 917, *spell* 📖 p. 920, *zar* 📖 p. 921). 'Running' subtypes of culture-bound syndromes have symptoms that would meet criteria for dissociative fugue (📖 p. 806).

Anorexia nervosa More prevalent in Western societies, with an abundance of food, and where there are strong cultural influences promoting thinness as the ideal of body shape. Immigrants from other cultural backgrounds may assimilate this ideal, or may present with primary symptoms other than disturbed body image and fear of weight gain (e.g. stomach pains, lack of enjoyment of food).

Alcohol and substance misuse Cultural factors heavily influence the availability, patterns of use, attitudes about, and even the physiological or behavioural effects of alcohol and other substances.

Alcohol Social, family, and religious attitudes towards the use of alcohol may all influence patterns of use and the likelihood of developing alcohol-related problems. Although it is difficult to separate cause from effect, low levels of education, unemployment, and low social status are all associated with increased misuse of alcohol. In some populations (e.g. Japanese and Chinese) up to 50% may have a deficiency of aldehyde dehydrogenase (complete absence in 10%), with low rates of alcohol problems in these populations because the physiological effects of consuming alcohol may be extremely unpleasant (e.g. flushing and palpitations due to accumulation of acetylaldehyde). How individuals behave when intoxicated may also be culturally determined, with aggressive and antisocial behaviour (typified by 'football hooligans') not seen to the same extent in cultures where alcohol is more of a 'social lubricant', despite levels of alcohol consumption being similar.

Other substances Use of hallucinogens and other drugs may be culturally acceptable when part of religious rituals (e.g. peyote in the Native American Church, cannabis in Rastafarianism). Equally, secular movements, typified by the hippie movements of the 1960s and '70s, or more recently the 'dance culture', provide a context in which psychedelic experiences (e.g. induced by LSD or MDMA) may be experienced without any adverse social sanctions.

Cultural formulation of psychiatric disorders

When there are clear cultural issues impacting upon the presentation of a psychiatric disorder it is important to have a systematic way of describing the nature and form these take. This may help by engaging the patient more directly in the assessment process; identifying other predisposing, precipitating, or perpetuating factors; and allowing any proposed management plans to be more tailored to the individual patient.

Issues that ought to be considered include:

- Cultural identity—how the person regards themselves; affiliations with ethnic or religious subgroups.
- Preferred language.
- If an immigrant—integration into host society and culture.
- Specific psychosocial factors that may be culturally determined.
- Particular social stressors.
- Support within the community (including the role of religious institutions) and from family and friends.
- Availability and access to appropriate services.
- Culturally determined illness beliefs and behaviour.
- What the patient believes to be wrong with them (the particular illness model used to explain perceived causation and nature of the condition).
- How the patient expresses their symptoms (language used, local idioms, behavioural manifestations).
- How the local community and family view their problems.
- The doctor–patient relationship—differences in culture, perceived social status, communication difficulties (due to language) and how they impact on:
  - Eliciting symptoms and understanding their significance.
  - Forming a 'therapeutic alliance'.
  - Discussing the possible treatment options (when 'disease models' may be at odds with each other).
- The attitude of their culture towards mental illness and the implications of a psychiatric diagnosis (e.g. will preclude marriage in some cultures).

Culture-bound syndromes

Culture-bound or culture-specific syndromes comprise a wide range of disorders occurring in particular localities or ethnic groups. The behavioural manifestations or subjective experiences particular to these disorders may or may not correspond to diagnostic categories in DSM-IV or ICD-10. They are usually considered to be illnesses and generally have local names. They also include culturally accepted idioms or explanatory mechanisms of illness that differ from Western idioms and outside of their cultural setting may be mistaken for psychosis. Awareness of culture-bound syndromes is important to allow psychiatrists and physicians to make culturally appropriate diagnoses.

According to Littlewood and Lipsedge (1987),[1] these disorders share a number of common general characteristics:

- Occur in young men or women who are 'powerless' and socially neglected.
- Usually dramatic with the individual unaware or not responsible.
- The disorder has symbolic cultural significance ('mystical sanction') and show a typical triphasic pattern:
  - Dislocation of an individual as representative of a particular group.
  - Emergence of symptoms as exaggerated form of this extrusion.
  - Restitution into normal relationships.

In fact, these features could also be applied to many of the Western neuroses (where 'mystical sanction' is provided by the medical model). Although controversial, some commentators regard the neuroses (including dissociative states, somatoform, and conversion disorders) as examples of Western culture-specific syndromes.[2] This would include a range of specific syndromes such as neurasthenia, fugue, and trance states, as well as the more modern neuroses: multiple personality disorder, anorexia nervosa, chronic fatigue syndrome, alien abduction syndrome, recovered memory syndrome, ritual or satanic abuse, Gulf War syndrome, and even shoplifting and overdosing(!).

If culture-bound syndromes are categorized according to primary phenomenology, a number of common subtypes emerge (see Box 22.1). Descriptions of specific syndromes are outlined in the following glossary (📖 p. 916), illustrating the vast range of manifestations.[3]

Box 22.1 Subtypes of culture-bound syndromes

- **Startle reaction** e.g. latah, amurakh, irkunii, ikota, olan miryachit, menkeiti, bah-tschi, bah-tsi, baah-ji, imu, mali-mali, silok.
- **Genital retraction** e.g. koro, suo yang, jinjinia bemar, rok-joo.
- **Sudden assault** e.g. amok, cafard/cathard, mal de pelea, fighting sickness, juramentado, Puerto Rican syndrome, iich 'aa, going postal.
- **Running** e.g. pibloktoq/arctic hysteria, grisi siknis.
- **Semen loss** e.g. dhat, jiryan, sukra prameha, shenkui.
- **Food restriction** e.g. anorexia nervosa, bulimia nervosa, anorexia mirabilis/holy anorexia.
- **Spirit possession** e.g. bebainan, spell, zar.
- **Obsession with the deceased** e.g. ghost sickness, hsieh-ping, shin-byung.
- **Exhaustion** e.g. neuraesthenia, chronic fatigue syndrome/ME, brain fag/brain fog, shenjian shuairuo, nervios.
- **Suppressed rage** e.g. hwa-byung/wool-hwa-bung, bilis, colera.

1 Littlewood R and Lipsedge M (1987) The butterfly and the serpent: culture, psychopathology and biomedicine. *Cult Med Psychiat* **11**: 289–335.
2 Showalter E (1998) *Hystories.* London: Picador Press.
3 For further reading see: Simons RC and Hughes CC (eds) (1985) *The culture-bound syndromes: folk illnesses of psychiatric and anthropological interest.* Dordrecht: D. Reidel Publishing Company.

Glossary of culture-bound syndromes

Amok, Amuck (Malayan males) Literally 'battling furiously': sudden, unprovoked, random acts of violence, for which the subject is amnesic, and after which they may commit suicide. May be preceded by a period of depression or brooding, anxiety, or feelings of hostility following perceived loss of face or being insulted. Also called **Matal/Mata Elap** ('darkened eye'). Similar syndromes are reported in other countries of South East Asia, the Philippines, Polynesia (**cafard** or **cathard**), New Guinea (**ahade idzi be**), Puerto Rico (**mal de pelea; fighting sickness; Puerto Rican syndrome**), the Andes of Bolivia, Columbia, Ecuador, and Peru (**colerina**), and the US (**going postal; iich'aa** in Navajo Native Americans).

Amurakh (Siberian women) 'Copying mania' characterized by echopraxia. (See **Lata**.)

Arctic hysteria (See **Piblokco**.)

Ashanti (West African women, e.g. Ghana) Consists of two subtypes: **frenzied guilt and fear** (FGF) where, sometimes following physical illness and fever, the person believes they are being punished for some offence, becomes frightened, and then frenzied, followed by a period of withdrawal, hallucinations, hebephrenic behaviour, dancing, singing, tearing off clothes, and eating faeces; and **depressive** (DP) where those affected accuse themselves of being witches and harming someone else without conscious intent. In younger women this often follows a difficult childbirth and subsequent illness, or the death of an infant.

Ataque de nervios (Puerto Ricans and other Hispanics) Dissociative trance disorder, usually following an acute stressful event (e.g. death or conflict) with brief symptoms including: a trance-like state (with narrowing of awareness, perceptual distortions, depersonalization, loss of consciousness, and partial or global amnesia), anxiety, somatic complaints, impulsive behaviour, and depression.

Bangungut (young male Filipinos) 'Oriental nightmare-death syndrome' where a series of terrifying dreams culminate in death from presumed cardiac arrhythmia. (See also **Hmong sudden death syndrome**.)

Bebainan (Indonesia) Possession state, believed to be caused by a spirit power, deity, or other person, in which the subject assumes a new identity, associated with stereotyped involuntary movements and amnesia.

Beserk, Berserk, Beserkergang (Northern Europe) 'Fighting fever', very similar to amok.

Bilis and colera (Latin America) An idiom of distress in which physical or mental illness is explained as due to extreme emotion (anger) that upsets the humours (described in terms of hot and cold).

Brain fag, brain fog syndrome (West African students) 'Brain fatigue', an idiom of distress with symptoms attributed to over-work, tiredness, and 'too much thinking'. The subject complains of reduced concentration, poor memory, blurred vision, and head/neck pain (often described as tightness, pressure, heat, or burning). Symptoms closely resemble anxiety, depressive, or somatoform disorders.

Cathard, cafard (See **Amok**.)

Colerina (See **Amok**.)

Curanderismo (Mexican Americans and other Spanish-speaking people) Folk medicine in which the healers (curanderos [male] or cunderas [female]) use a combination of herbal infusions, dramatic healing rituals, and prayers to treat a variety of physical and psychological symptoms including: **embrujo** (witchcraft), **empacho** (intestinal distress), **mal ojo** (evil eye), **mal puesto** (hexing), and **susto** (soul loss).

Delahara (Philippine women) A syndrome similar to **amok**.

Dhat (India, rural areas of Nepal, Sri Lanka, and Bangladesh) Semen-loss syndrome—a belief in the passage of semen in the urine following the breaking of taboos concerning masturbation or sexual intercourse. Associated with somatic symptoms (weakness, exhaustion), severe anxiety, hypochondriasis, whitish discolouration of the urine, and sexual dysfunction. Traditional remedies consist of herbal tonics to restore semen/humoral balance. Similar to **jiryan** (India), **sukra prameha** (Sri Lanka), and **shenkui** (China).

Echul (Native Americans of South California) Sexual anxiety and convulsions following severe stress (e.g. the death of a child).

Evil eye, mal Ojo (See **Curanderismo**.)

Falling out, blacking out (African Americans and Afro-Caribbeans) Collapse, without loss of consciousness, sometimes preceded by dizziness. The subject feels paralysed, but can hear and understand, and may claim to be blind. A type of dissociative/conversion disorder, usually following a traumatic event.

Fighting sickness (See **Amok**.)

Frenzied anxiety state (Kenya) Another syndrome similar to amok.

Frigidophobia (See **Wind illness**.)

Ghost sickness (Native Americans) Preoccupation with death or the deceased. Subjects may say they have been 'bewitched' and complain of nightmares, weakness, dizziness, episodes of collapse, anxiety, poor appetite, hallucinations, confusion, feelings of futility or apprehension, and sometimes a sense of suffocation.

Grisi siknis (Miskito Indians, Nicaragua) Headache, anxiety, anger, and aimless running. Similar to **pibloko**.

Gururumba episode ('wild man behaviour') (New Guinea) Subject (usually male) breaks into houses to steal small items (they believe to be valuable) and then runs off into the forest for some days, later returning (without the items) to their normal life. There is associated amnesia and during the episode they may appear vague, agitated, behave in a clumsy way, and have disturbance of normal hearing and speech.

Hi-wa itck (Mohave American Indians) Insomnia, depression, loss of appetite, and sometimes suicide associated with unwanted separation from a loved one.

Hmong sudden death syndrome (Laos) The death of a person whilst sleeping, attributed to being attacked by spirits in a dream, and often following a traumatic event. (See **Bangungut**.)

Hsieh-ping (Taiwan) A brief trance state during which the subject is believed to be possessed by an ancestral ghost, who often attempts to communicate to other family members. Symptoms include tremor, disorientation, delirium, and (visual/auditory) hallucinations.

Hwa-byung, wool-hwa-bung, 'anger syndrome' (Korea) Epigastric pain attributed to a mass in the upper abdomen that the patient fears will lead to death. The belief is related to ideas of bodily imbalances caused by anger (cf. **bilis and colera**.) Other symptoms may include tiredness, muscular aches and pains, breathlessness, palpitations, insomnia, dysphoria, panic, loss of appetite, and other GI problems (indigestion, anorexia).

Imu (See **Lata**.)

Juramentado (Malays and Moros) Marked agitation, indiscriminate assault or stabbing, followed by stupor, and subsequent amnesia on awakening. (Similar to **amok**.)

Kimilue (Native Americans of Southern California) Apathy, anhedonia, loss of appetite, and vivid sexual dreams.

Koro (Malaysia) Literally 'to shrink' or referring to a 'tortoise' (a popular word for penis). 'Genital retraction syndrome'—the fear or delusion that the genitals are retracting into the abdomen, and that death will occur once this has happened. Prodromal depersonalization usually occurs and elaborate measures may be taken to prevent the penis from retracting (e.g. grasping of the genitals, splints or other devices, herbal remedies, or fellatio). Occurs more frequently in predominantly young, single males, in Asia and the Middle East (epidemics have been described in the Malay Archipelago, Thailand, China, India, Singapore, and Israel). Sporadic cases have been reported in Africa, Europe, and North America. The female equivalent (fear or delusion that the labia or nipples are retracting) occurs rarely and most reported cases have been during epidemics. There are no specific associations with other psychiatric disorders, although phobic anxiety disorders, depression, schizophrenia, and depersonalization syndromes are described. Other names for this syndrome include: **suk-yeong/suo yang** (Chinese: 'shrunken penis'), **kattao** (Indian: 'cut off'), **jinjinia bemar** (Assam), and **rok-joo** (Thailand).

Lata, latah, lattah (Malay population) Exaggerated startle reaction seen predominantly in young girls. Following sudden fright/trauma, there is a behavioural response consisting of echopraxia, automatic obedience, coprolalia, and dissociative or trance-like behaviour. May be a symptom of disease (e.g. acute psychosis, conversion/dissociative state) or be an isolated behavioural abnormality. Related syndromes include: **amurakh, irkunii, ikota, miryachit, menkeiti**, and **olan/olonism** (Siberia), **imu** (Ainu of Japan), **bah-tschi, bah-tsi,** and **baah-ji** (Thailand), **mali-mali** and **silok** (Philippines), **Lapp panic** (Lapps), the **Jumpers of New England** (a nineteenth-century Shaker sect), and **jumping Frenchman** (Canada).

Locura (Latin America) Severe form of chronic psychosis, attributed to an inherited vulnerability and/or adverse life events, characterized by incoherent speech, agitation, auditory/visual hallucinations, impaired social interactions, and unpredictable (possibly violent) behaviour.

'Lost hunter' sequence (New Guinea) After period of social withdrawal (following perceived criticism of actions) the person (typically male) goes hunting alone in the bush and describes five episodes of tracking a large game animal, which suddenly disappears, before he is rescued by a search party. He feels he has been led astray by supernatural beings.

Mal de pelea (See **Amok.**)

Miryachit, mirachat (Russian: 'to fool' or 'play the fool') (See **Lata.**)

Nerfiza, nerves, nervios (Latino populations in United States, Latin America, Egypt, Northern Europe) Chronic somatic, emotional, and behavioural symptoms (e.g. headache, sleep problems, reduced appetite, nausea, fatigue, dizziness, paraesthesia, anxiety, concentration difficulties, and emotional lability/distress). More common in women; associated with anger, emotional distress, and low self-esteem. Usually treated with traditional herbal teas, 'nerve pills', rest, isolation, and increased family support. (Similar to nevra in Greece.)

Olonism (See **Lata.**)

Pibloko, pibloktoq (Polar Eskimo women) 'Arctic hysteria'—an acute dissociative state (lasting about 30 min) following the actual (or symbolic) loss of someone or something important to the individual. Usually mild irritability or withdrawal precedes impulsive or dangerous acts (e.g. screaming, tearing off clothes, breaking furniture, shouting obscenities, eating faeces, or rushing out into the snow). May be followed by convulsions and coma (lasting up to 12 hrs) with associated amnesia. Although some researchers have suggested it may be due to hypocalcaemic tetany, it is most probably an anxiety state.

Puerto Rican syndrome (See **Amok.**)

Qi-gong psychotic reaction (China) 'Excess of vital energy'—an acute episode characterized by dissociative, paranoid, or other symptoms after participation in the health-enhancing practice of qi-gong.

Rootwork (Haiti and Sub-Saharan Africa) A variety of complaints attributed to hexing, witchcraft, sorcery, voodoo, or the evil influence of another person. Symptoms include anxiety, GI complaints, and fear of being poisoned or killed. Can result in death. Associated syndromes: **voodoo death** (Haiti), **mal puesto** or **brujeira** (Latin America), and **hex.**

Sangue dormido, 'sleeping blood' (Cape Verde Islanders) Somatic symptoms including pain, numbness, tremor, paralysis, convulsions, blindness, and increased risk of heart attack, infection, and miscarriage.

Sar (Somalian women) A possession state attributed to Sar spirits that are said to hate men. The syndrome may legitimize behavioural disturbance in women who feel neglected by their husbands. (See also **Zar**.)

Shenjian shuairuo (China) Similar to **neurasthenia**—symptoms include: fatigue, irritability, poor concentration/memory, sleep disturbance, and other somatic symptoms (dizziness, headaches, pain, GI upset, sexual dysfunction, and other signs of autonomic dysfunction). Most cases would meet criteria for depressive or anxiety disorders.

Shenk-k'uei (Taiwan), **shenkui** (China) Anxiety and panic with somatic complaints, especially sexual dysfunction (premature ejaculation and impotence). Symptoms are attributed to excessive semen loss from sexual activity or 'white turbid urine', which reduces 'vital energy'. It is viewed as a life-threatening condition and described in areas with a Chinese ethnic population. Similar to **dhat** and **jiryan** (India), and **sukra prameha** (Sri Lanka.)

Shin-byung (Korea) Possession (dissociative) state attributed to ancestral spirits with associated anxiety/fear and somatic complaints (generalized weakness, dizziness, insomnia, loss of appetite, and GI problems).

Shinkeishitsu (Japan) Syndrome marked by obsessions, perfectionism, ambivalence, social withdrawal, fatigue, and hypochondriasis.

Spell (Southern United States) A trance state in which individuals 'communicate' with deceased relatives or with spirits, often accompanied by brief periods of personality change. In context, 'spells' are culturally normal and do not indicate psychiatric illness.

Susto, espanto, 'magic fright', 'fallen fontanel syndrome' (Peru) An acute anxiety state, seen in children and adolescents, usually following an acute stressor or violent (often supernatural) fright. Characterized by anxiety, agitation, dejection/apathy, sleep disturbance, significant weight loss, other somatic symptoms, and a belief that the soul has been, or will be, stolen from the body. (See **Curanderismo**.) It is also seen in Latinos of the United States, Mexico, and other Central/South American countries. Related syndromes: **lanti** (Philippines), **malgri** (Aborigines of Australia), **mogo laya** (New Guinea), **narahati** (Iran), and **saladera** (in regions around the Amazon).

Tabanka (Trinidad) Depression associated with a high rate of suicide that is seen in men abandoned by their wives.

Taijin kyofusho (Japan) Fear and guilt about embarrassing others with one's appearance or behaviour, prominent in younger people and similar to the Western concept of social phobia.

Ufufuyane, saka (Kenya, Southern Africa; Bantu, Zulu; and affiliated groups) Anxiety state attributed to the effects of magical potions (given to them by rejected lovers) or spirit possession, with characteristic sobbing, repeated neologisms, paralysis, trance-like states, or loss of consciousness. Usually seen in young, unmarried women, who may also experience nightmares with sexual themes, and rarely episodes of temporary blindness.

May be related to **aluro** (Nigeria), **phii pob** (Thailand), and **zar** (Egypt, Ethiopia, Sudan).

Uquamairineq (Inuits of the Arctic Circle) Syndrome akin to a sleep-state transition disorder or dissociative disorder in which sudden paralysis is associated with a sleep state, marked anxiety/agitation, and hallucinations. Usually lasts minutes and may be preceded by a transient sound or smell. Traditionally viewed as the result of soul loss, soul wandering, or spirit possession.

Vimbuza (Northern Malawi and Zambia) A culturally specific response to sickness involving herbal medicines and 'vimbuza dancing' that is performed late at night. Often others will dance on behalf of the patient, keeping the rhythm with metal belts, and inducing a trace state from which the 'healed' patient emerges. If the illness is considered severe, the family of the patient may sponsor a 'chilopa'—an entire night of dancing followed by an animal sacrifice at dawn. The patient drinks some of the animal's blood and then begins to dance again. The larger the animal (usually either a chicken, a goat, or a cow), the more effective the expected cure.

Voodoo death (See **Hmong sudden death syndrome** and **Rootwork**.)

Wacinko (Native American groups—Oglala Sioux—of North America) Anger, withdrawal, mutism, and immobility frequently leading to suicide. Often related to disappointment or interpersonal problems.

Wihtigo, whitigo, witiko, windigo, wendigo (Native American groups, e.g. Cree, Algonkian Indians of central and northeastern Canada) The fear or delusion of being transformed into a **wihtigo**, or giant monster that eats human flesh. There is a prodrome of anxiety about physical symptoms (e.g. reduced appetite, nausea and vomiting) and the person may commit suicide or be the target of violence. The existence of this syndrome is questioned as no single case has been described in the psychiatric or anthropological literature.

Wind illness, p'a leng, frigidophobia (China, South East Asia) Anxiety/fear of being cold or of the wind; associated with a loss of yang and upset of natural balance in the body (believed to produce fatigue, impotence, and death), leading a person to do everything they can to stay warm. Described in areas with Chinese ethnic populations. May be related to **agua frio**, **aire frio**, **frio** of Mexico, Central and South America.

Wild man behaviour (See **Gururumba episode**.)

Zar (East and North Africa, the Middle East, e.g. Ethiopia, Somalia, Sudan, Egypt, and Iran) Dissociative symptoms including shouting, laughing, head banging, singing, weeping, and other demonstrative behaviours. The person believes they are possessed by a spirit, and may develop a long-term relationship with the spirit. Other symptoms may include apathy, withdrawal, refusal to eat, and refusal to carry out tasks of daily living. Such behaviour may be regarded as culturally normal (see **Sar**).

Therapeutic issues

Medication adherence

Is adherence important?

- It has been estimated that only one-third of patients prescribed medication actually adhere to the treatment plan (this applies to *all* medical specialties, not just psychiatry) and that ~80% of psychiatric admissions relate to medication non-adherence. Adherence is a particular problem when the illness runs a chronic course and requires the patient to be on medication *for life* (e.g. diabetes, IHD, pulmonary disease, schizophrenia).
- Patients with schizophrenia who comply with a sufficient dosage of antipsychotic medication have only about one-fifth the risk of relapse compared to patients who do not take their medication.
- There is good evidence that prophylactic lithium treatment of bipolar disorder reduces the likelihood of relapse (particularly manic relapse), as well as the risk of suicide.
- Continuation of antidepressant treatment for *at least* 6mths after symptom resolution significantly reduces the risk of further depressive episodes.

Reasons for non-adherence

It is important to realize that the patient may have understandable reasons for being reluctant to take prescribed medication. Uncovering these reasons may help in negotiation and developing strategies to improve the situation.

- Continued symptoms of the underlying disorder (e.g. delusions, lack of motivation, impaired insight, and disorganization) or comorbid disorders (e.g. substance misuse, personality disorder).
- Negative attitude towards medication in general (versus other forms of treatment) or stigma associated with being 'on medication', particularly where there are external stigmata of treatment such as Parkinsonism ('looking like a zombie').
- Unacceptable (or unexpected) side-effects (e.g. weight gain—📖 p. 930, sedation, EPSEs— 📖 p. 944, sexual dysfunction— 📖 p. 938, perceived loss of 'good' symptoms, e.g. hypomania).
- Forgetting (genuine oversight, disorganization, cognitive impairment).
- Lack of communication (reasons for medication not fully explained or understood).
- Failure to obtain (or renew) prescription (through non-attendance, poor communication or poor relationship with responsible prescriber, e.g. GP).
- Belief that the medication is 'not working'.
- Feeling well and no longer seeing the need for medication. The 'reward' of freedom from side-effects may be immediate, while the 'punishment' of relapse may be more distant, not taken seriously, or not directly associated with stopping treatment.

Strategies to improve adherence

Education
- Promote insight and understanding about the illness and the benefits of treatment.
- Provide information about the medication, how to take it, possible side-effects, the length of time needed to see benefits, and the potential problems of suddenly stopping.
- Discuss the reasons for prophylactic or continued treatment, especially when patient feels well (e.g. to reduce risk of relapse and improve long-term outcome).
- Encourage discussion of pros and cons of suggested treatment plan.
- Encourage openness about potentially embarrassing issues that may lead to non-adherence (e.g. sexual side-effects).
- Regularly ask about and document side-effects at each review.

Sensible prescribing
- Simplify drug regime—use single dose where possible (most psychotropic medications have long half-lives and can be given once daily or are available in slow-release preparations).
- Minimize side-effects through choice of a medication with lowest potential for side-effects, and using lowest therapeutic dose.
- If side-effects are problematic, consider a change to an alternative preparation or (where an alternative would be less effective) co-prescribing agents to counter significant problems.
- Rational medication choice based on individual acceptability of side-effects (e.g. *any* weight gain may be unacceptable to a young female patient).
- Clear communication of any changes in regime both to patient and primary care team (including written instructions for patient and direct communication with GP) especially if the primary care physician is main prescriber.
- Consider use of depot antipsychotic preparations—this may sometimes be requested by the patient, but is more often necessary when the patient lacks insight, or has had significant serious relapses related to non-adherence.
- Regularly review the need for continued medication.

Practical/behavioural measures
- Written information to patient, particularly where regime is complex or where change of dose/medication is planned.
- Establish a regular daily routine for taking medication.
- Use of a multicompartment compliance aid (e.g. Dosette® box).
- Supervised administration (e.g. by relative/carer, at pharmacy, in day hospital, by CPN).
- Active monitoring (e.g. tablet count, blood levels—p. 928).

Off-label prescribing[1]

Essence

In the UK, licensed medicines are granted a Marketing Authorization (previously called a product licence) by the Medicines and Healthcare products Regulatory Agency under the Medicines Act 1968. For each drug, the *British National Formulary* (BNF) specifies the doses, indications, cautions, and adverse effects, which reflect those in the manufacturer's data sheet. However, in spite of various licensed treatments, patients will often remain symptomatic and psychiatrists will consider prescribing medications outside the narrow terms of their licence. Unlicensed prescribing does not imply lack of evidence in support of the proposed intervention and can still be safe and beneficial to the patient. In fact, it has also been argued that the product licence for a drug does not necessarily represent the best use of that compound.

General points

- The real extent of unlicensed prescribing in the UK is largely unknown; however, cross-sectional surveys in general adult inpatient settings have shown the rate of off-label prescribing can be as high as 40% of all prescriptions.
- Drug companies do not usually test their medicines on children; hence they cannot apply to license their medicines for use in the treatment of children. Nonetheless, the British Association for Psychopharmacology[2] has stated that it seems reasonable to extrapolate what is known about drug treatment responses in adults to children and adolescents with schizophrenia and OCD, but caution is required with mood and anxiety disorders.
- No psychotropic medication is currently licensed for use in pregnancy or in breastfeeding mothers.
- It has been argued that the final prescribing decision should rest with the clinician, based on the availability of other therapeutic options and a careful assessment of the potential risks and benefits (see Box 23.1 for legal considerations).

Types of unlicensed prescribing

- The prescription of a medication for an indication that is not covered within the terms of the Market Authorization.
- The prescription of a medication to a patient who lies outside the age range specified within the Summary of Product Characteristics.
- The prescription of a medication at doses above the maximum recommended dosage.
- The use of a licensed medication for longer periods than those specified within the Marketing Authorization.

Recommendations for unlicensed prescribing

- Unlicensed prescribing should only occur when licensed treatments have been used or considered but excluded on clinical grounds (e.g. contraindications, risk of interactions).

- The prescriber should be familiar with any possible benefits and risks of the proposed treatment (ask specialist pharmacist for further guidance).
- Particular consideration is needed with children, older patients, and patients lacking capacity (see 📖 p. 870).
- Whenever possible a full explanation of the treatment should be given to the patient (and/or his/her relative, when relevant) and documented in the notes.
- Whenever possible the agreement of the patient (and/or his/her relative, when relevant) should be obtained, but if not possible, this should be noted.
- Prescription should be started cautiously and patient's progress monitored closely with full documentation of treatment effectiveness and tolerance.
- If unsuccessful, treatment should be withdrawn carefully.

Box 23.1 Legal principles applying to unlicensed prescribing

- Legally unlicensed prescribing would not be held as a breach of the duty of care, if that treatment was supported by a respected body of medical opinion, as the Bolam test (Bolam v. Friern Hospital Management Committee, 1957) in medical negligence claims asks for proof that a body of doctors would act similarly to the doctor in question.
- According to the case of Bolitho v. City and Hackney Health Authority (1997), medical opinion should also be capable of withstanding logical analysis. In unlicensed prescribing this implies that doctors consider the risks and benefits of varying treatment options, with due regard to the available evidence.

1 Royal College of Psychiatrists: CR142 (Jan 2007) Use of licensed medicines for unlicensed applications in psychiatric practice. 🔗 http://www.rcpsych.ac.uk/files/pdfversion/cr142.pdf
2 British Association for Psychopharmacology (BAP) Consensus Statement (1997) Child and learning disability psychopharmacology. *J Psychopathol* **11**: 291–4. 🔗 http://jop.sagepub.com/content/11/4/291.full.pdf+html

Plasma level monitoring

There are a limited number of drugs with well-established plasma levels that equate with efficacy. Plasma monitoring is a regular procedure only for lithium therapy. However, there may be a number of other reasons for requesting plasma levels (bear in mind that assays for *specific* drugs may not be locally available and may need special arrangements). Many psychiatric drugs have marked variations in metabolism, or large numbers of active metabolites, making plasma levels difficult to interpret.

Reasons for monitoring

- Established therapeutic plasma levels (see Table 23.1).
- Monitoring of any changes in plasma level that might affect efficacy (e.g. due to drug interactions, intercurrent illness, pregnancy, or altered pharmacokinetics over time).
- Clinical evidence of toxicity (e.g. lithium, anticonvulsants).
- Where there is doubt about patient compliance (e.g. lack of effect despite adequate or even high-dose treatment).
- In cases where the patient may be unable to report adverse effects (e.g. children, severe LD, dementia).
- After overdose, to confirm it is safe to restart medication.

Plasma level monitoring of other psychotropics (aripiprazole [and dehydroaripiprazole], olanzapine, risperidone [and 9-hydroxy-risperidone], quetiapine, amisulpiride, lamotrigine, sulpiride) is available in the UK[1] and could be used in assessing adherence, dose optimization, and if acute poisoning is suspected. However, it is not advised in routine practice and other ways of establishing treatment adherence are preferred (e.g. measurement of serum prolactin if patient is on risperidone—see 📖 p. 936).

Table 23.1 Reference ranges for selected drugs

Lithium (see 📖 p. 336)	0.6–1mmol/L (0.6–0.8mmol/L—as an augmentative agent)
Valproate (see 📖 p. 342)	50–100mg/L
Carbamazepine (see 📖 p. 346)	4–12mg/L (>7mg/L may be more efficacious in bipolar disorder)
Clozapine (see 📖 p. 210)	350–500mcg/L (0.35–0.5mg/L)

1 Toxicology Unit, KingsPath Laboratory, King's College Hospital, London. 🖰 www.kingspath. co.uk/tests/toxicology/

Paradoxical reactions to benzodiazepines[1]

Essence

Paradoxical or 'disinhibitory' reactions to BDZs occur in a minority of patients (less than 1% of general population) and are characterized by acute excitement and altered mental state:

- Increased anxiety.
- Vivid dreams.
- Hyperactivity.
- Sexual disinhibition.
- Hostility and rage ('aggressive dyscontrol').

Recognition is important as behavioural disturbance may be exacerbated by inappropriate use of higher doses of BDZs. *Note:* similar types of reaction are described for most CNS depressants (e.g. alcohol, barbiturates).

Aetiology Incompletely understood; theories include: 'release behaviour' due to loss of frontal lobe inhibition through $GABA_A$ mechanism; BDZ related reduction in 5-HT neurotransmission; BDZ related reduction in ACh neurotransmission.

Risk factors

Children, learning disability, history of brain injury, dementia, borderline PD, antisocial PD, history of aggression/poor impulse control, family/personal history of paradoxical reaction, use of high-dose/high-potency BDZs (e.g. alprazolam, clonazepam, flunitrazepam, triazolam), IV/intra-nasal administration.

Management

- Nurse in safe environment, with constant supervision.
- Use sedative antipsychotic to treat acute behavioural disturbance if necessary.
- In extreme cases consider use of IV flumazenil (may require repeated doses).
- Clearly record occurrence of paradoxical reaction so future episodes of acute behavioural disturbance can be managed appropriately.

1 Paton C (2002) Benzodiazepines and disinhibition: a review. *Psychiat Bull* **26**: 460–2.

Weight gain with psychiatric medication

General points

Weight gain is a significant cause of non-compliance with psychiatric medication, and patients often complain about increases in weight, even when clinicians may regard it as 'clinically insignificant'. Effects on general health, self-esteem, and social embarrassment should not be overlooked.

Antipsychotics

Proposed mechanisms

Sedation (reduced activity), thirst (anticholinergic side-effects), reduced metabolism, fluid retention, endocrine effects (increased prolactin, altered cortisol, altered insulin secretion), increases in leptin levels (changes in 'set-point' weight), and altered neurotransmitters ($5-HT_{2C}$ blockade, histamine affinity, D2 blockade, CCK changes) have all been proposed.

Increased risk Female, previous pattern of overeating, narcissistic traits, family or personal history of obesity.

Effects of specific agents (see Table 23.2).

Management[1]

- Routine measurement of baseline weight.
- Warn patient of possibility.
- Encourage 'healthy diet' (involve dietician if necessary), moderate physical exercise, avoid high-calorie fluids.
- Use lowest therapeutic dose, introduce medication increases slowly, consider intermittent dosing.
- Consider adjunctive prescribing (e.g. clozapine *plus* quetiapine, to allow lowering of clozapine dose).

Antidepressants

Proposed mechanisms Reduced metabolism, carbohydrate craving (*Note:* may be a symptom of depression itself), central serotonin mechanisms in regulating food intake (appetite/satiety).

Effects of specific agents (see Box 23.2).

Management

- General advice about diet and exercise.
- Use lowest therapeutic dose.
- Consider switching to alternative antidepressant.
- Adjunctive prescribing (e.g. naltrexone, ranitidine at night: may reduce 'midnight snacks').

Table 23.2 Weight gain with antipsychotics[1]

Antipsychotic	Average weight gain (kg)
Pimozide	−2.7
Aripiprazole	−1.3
Placebo	−1.0
Trifluoperazine	0.3
Ziprasidone	0.3
Haloperidol	0.5
Polypharmacy	0.5
Loxapine	0.7
Non-drug controls	0.8
Fluphenazine	1.1
Risperidone	1.7
Quetiapine	2.5
Thioridazine	2.8
Sertindole	2.9
Olanzapine	4.2
Chlorpromazine	4.2
Clozapine	5.7
Perphenazine	5.8

1 Adapted from Fenton WS (2000) Review: most antipsychotic drugs are associated with weight gain. *Evidence Based Ment Hlth* **3**: 58.

Box 23.2 Weight changes with antidepressants

- *SSRIs:* fluoxetine, weight loss; paroxetine, fluvoxamine: slight weight loss; sertraline: limited weight gain; citalopram: no change.
- *TCAs:* weight gain (amitriptyline > imipramine > clomipramine).
- *MAOIs/RIMAs:* weight loss (tranylcypromine)—rarely weight gain; weight gain (phenelzine > moclobemide).
- *Others:* mianserin, mirtazapine; weight gain; reboxetine, trazodone: no change; venlafaxine: weight loss.

Lithium[2]

Proposed mechanisms Increased intake of high calorie drinks, hypothyroidism, increased insulin secretion.

Management Counselling and advice about diet and exercise, use of low-calorie drinks, avoidance of salty foods (or adding salt to foods).

Other mood stabilizers

Carbamazepine Weight gain due to increased appetite.

Valproate Weight gain which may be due to increased serum leptin and insulin.

Gabapentin Marked weight gain in some cases (up to 10% above baseline weight).

Lamotrigine Not associated with weight gain—making it the 'drug of choice' for those who have experienced marked weight gain with other mood stabilizers.

1 Baptista T (1999) Body weight gain induced by antipsychotic drugs: mechanisms and management. *Acta Psych Scand* **101**: 3–16.
2 Baptista T (1995) Lithium and body weight gain. *Pharmacopsychiat* **28**: 35–44.

Antipsychotics and diabetes

There have been recent concerns about the potential of SGAs to cause abnormalities in insulin sensitivity and diabetes (type II), yet the evidence that they are associated with increased risk for diabetes compared with FGAs is tentative. It is worth noting:

- The aetiology of diabetes in a patient receiving antipsychotics may not be wholly attributable to the drug—many risk factors are shared with metabolic syndrome (see Box 23.3).
- For as yet unknown reasons, schizophrenic patients have a 2–3-fold higher risk of developing diabetes than the general population even when drug use is controlled.
- Psychiatrists ought not to initiate treatment of diabetes themselves without consulting the patient's primary care physician and/or considering referral to a diabetes specialist.
- Younger patients treated with antipsychotics may be at higher risk of developing diabetes than older adults.

Pathophysiology

Not fully understood. Proposed mechanisms are: increased visceral adiposity through histaminergic H_1 antagonism, leptin resistance, $\uparrow$ TNF-α levels; inhibition of insulin secretion in pancreatic β-cells through antagonism of muscarinic M3 receptors; $\downarrow$ glucose sensitivity through antagonism of serotonergic 5-HT_{1A} receptors; $\uparrow$ insulin release through antagonism of adrenergic $\alpha 2$ receptors; inhibition of GLUT glucose transporter.

Management

- *Prior to initiating antipsychotic treatment* determine baseline measures, ideally oral glucose tolerance test (OGTT) or fasting plasma glucose (FPG); otherwise random plasma glucose (RPG) or urine glucose (UG) will suffice.
- *When a patient gains 5% or more of their initial weight* at any time during therapy, consideration should be given to switching to an antipsychotic with less weight gain liability (see 🔲 p. 930).
- *A general rank ordering of the SGAs* that have the greatest to the least risk of metabolic effects is: clozapine > olanzapine > quetiapine > risperidone > aripiprazole. *Note:* weight gain can occur with all of these drugs and considerable variability exists among patients receiving the same drug regarding the risk of metabolic effects.
- *For patients at risk of diabetes* changing to an antipsychotic less likely to cause metabolic effects should be balanced against the risks and benefits from continuing treatment with the same drug. Adjunctive treatments include: oral hypoglycaemics (e.g. metformin) or insulin; rosiglitazone and orlistat have been used with olanzapine and clozapine respectively; sibutramine, amantadine, and topiramate have little supportive evidence and a high risk of adverse side-effects.
- *Lifestyle modifications* have been used successfully for weight control in highly motivated subjects and may be complementary to medication (i.e. calorie-controlled diet/regular physical exercise).

Box 23.3 Metabolic syndrome[1] (Syndrome X, insulin resistance syndrome, Reaven's syndrome or CHAOS [Australia])

Essence

Characterized by insulin resistance and abnormal adipose deposition and function. Associated with increased risk of developing atherosclerotic disease (HD and stroke), type 2 diabetes, fatty liver, and cancer. Affects a large number of people (up to 25% in some studies), and prevalence increases with age. Current guidelines allow diagnosis when at least 3 out of the following 5 criteria are present:

- Fasting glucose ≥ 100mg/dL (or receiving drug treatment for hyperglycaemia).
- Blood pressure: ≥130/85mmHg (or receiving drug treatment for hypertension).
- Triglycerides (TG): ≥150mg/dL (or receiving drug treatment for hypertriglyceridaemia).
- High-density lipoprotein cholesterol (HDL-C) <40mg/dL in men or <50mg/dL in women (or receiving drugs for reduced HDL-C).
- Waist circumference ≥102cm in men or ≥ 88cm in women. If **Asian** ethnic group, ≥90cm in men or ≥ 80cm in women.

Aetiology

The cause of the metabolic syndrome is unknown. Debate surrounds whether obesity or insulin resistance is the cause of the metabolic syndrome or if they are consequences of a more far-reaching metabolic derangement. A number of markers of systemic inflammation are often increased, e.g. CRP, fibrinogen, IL-6, TNFα.

Proposed pathophysiology

Development of visceral fat → increased plasma levels of TNFα (as well as adiponectin, resistin, PAI-1) → production of inflammatory cytokines and/or altered cell signalling leading to insulin resistance.

Prevention

Various strategies have been proposed. Usually include increased physical activity (e.g. walking 30min every day) and a healthy, reduced calorie diet.

Treatment

- The first-line treatment is change of lifestyle (i.e. calorie restriction and physical activity).
- If drug treatment is required, the individual disorders that comprise the metabolic syndrome are treated separately: diuretics and ACE inhibitors for hypertension; cholesterol-lowering drugs to lower LDL cholesterol and triglyceride levels and to raise HDL levels; use of drugs that decrease insulin resistance, e.g. metformin and thiazolidinediones, is controversial and local guidelines will apply.

1 The term 'metabolic syndrome' dates back to at least the late 1950s but came into common usage in the late 1970s to describe various associations of risk factors with diabetes that had been noted as early as the 1920s. Confusion arose because the term was used by different authors to describe different, albeit related, syndromes—e.g. Haller (1997) Singer (1977), Phillips (1977, 1978). It was the eponymous Gerald M. Reaven who coined the term 'Syndrome X' in his 1988 Banting lecture. He proposed insulin resistance as the underlying factor and did not include abdominal obesity as part of the condition. Reaven GM (1988) *Diabetes* **37**: 1595–607.

Hyperprolactinaemia with antipsychotics

Essence (see Box 23.4)

Secretion of prolactin (PRL) by the pituitary is under inhibitory control via dopamine from the hypothalamus. Blockade of dopamine D2 receptors on the pituitary lactotroph cells by antipsychotics can raise prolactin levels within minutes to hours of starting treatment. It occurs frequently with FGAs and some SGAs (risperidone, amisulpiride) but is rare with other SGAs (olanzapine > quetiapine, clozapine, ziprasidone, aripiprazole).

Clinical features

Include gynaecomastia, galactorrhoea, erectile dysfunction, loss of libido, and hypogonadism in men and oligo/amenorrhoea, galactorrhoea, infertility, loss of libido, acne, hirsutism, increased risk of osteoporosis, and possibly of breast cancer in women.

Epidemiology

Prevalence of hyperprolactinaemia with 'prolactin-raising' antipsychotics is estimated to be about 34–42% in men and 59–75% in women.

Risk factors

Female sex (women of reproductive age are more at risk than postmenopausal women), postnatal period, children and adolescents.

Differential diagnosis

Diseases of the pituitary (e.g. prolactin-secreting pituitary adenomas) or hypothalamus, severe primary hypothyroidism, liver cirrhosis, end-stage renal disease, acromegaly, stress, pregnancy, post-partum period, chronic cocaine/marijuana use, opiate.

Investigations

- Measure PRL serum level:
  - When PRL-raising antipsychotics are used it is helpful to obtain a pretreatment PRL level.
  - Secretion of PRL is pulsatile and may be raised in response to stress, meals, or post-ictally; hence, blood sample must be taken 1hr after eating or waking.
  - Antipsychotics usually produce PRL elevation of up to six times the upper limit of the reference range.
  - Mild to moderate elevations should be checked with a second sample to exclude physiological surges.
- Look out for signs of chest wall irritation (which can promote galactorrhoea and raise prolactin) and signs of a sellar mass (e.g. headache, visual field defects).
- Check TFTs (exclude hypothyroidism), creatinine/U&Es (exclude renal failure), insulin-like growth factor-1 (exclude acromegaly).
- If history of chronic alcohol misuse, check LFTs and perform abdominal examination to rule out hepatic cirrhosis.

- If clinically suspected, do a pregnancy test unless patient is postmenopausal or has had a hysterectomy.
- If patient is on oral antipsychotics and aetiology remains uncertain, consider diagnostic short-term cessation of medication (72hrs usually suffices for serum PRL to fall to near normal levels).
- Consider CT/MRI and/or a referral to endocrinology.

Management
- Exclude other possible aetiologies.
- Consider a change of medication to a prolactin-sparing antipsychotic (e.g. clozapine, olanzapine, quetiapine, aripiprazole) or reduction in dose if the patient's mental state is stable (monitor closely).
- Another option is augmentation with aripiprazole.
- If problems persist or medication changes are precluded (or not tolerated), refer to endocrinology for consideration of other treatments: combined oral contraceptive (females only), dopamine agonists (amantadine, cabergoline, bromocriptine).
- If patient has been amenorrhoeic for ≥ 1yr, request bone mineral density (BMD) measurement in order to screen for osteoporosis.
- Pre-menopausal women should be advised about resumption of normal menstrual cycle (and return of fertility) when changing antipsychotics, and the use of contraception should be discussed.

Note: asymptomatic hyperprolactinaemia does not warrant (in itself) changes to medication.

Box 23.4 Other drugs reported to cause hyperprolactinaemia

- *Antidepressants:* modest elevation with serotonergic antidepressants, e.g. SSRIs, MAOIs, and some TCAs.
- *Dopamine-depleting agents,* e.g. reserpine, tetrabenazine, methyldopa.
- *Other agents,* e.g. metoclopramide, cimetidine, cyproheptadine, verapamil, oestrogens, antiandrogens.

Sexual dysfunction and psychiatric medication

Degree of sexual dysfunction experienced by patients taking psychiatric medication may be a major source of distress and a significant reason for non-adherence. Clinicians are notoriously poor at enquiring about these problems, despite reports that patients regard sexual side-effects as the most troublesome of all medication-related problems.

Pathophysiology

Not fully understood, but the proposed pharmacological mechanisms of psychotropic-induced sexual dysfunctions are as follows:

Libido Inhibited by dopamine blockade, histamine blockade, prolactin elevation, testosterone decrease.

Arousal (erection or vaginal lubrication) Inhibited by cholinergic blockade, α_1-adrenergic blockade, nitric oxide (NO) decrease, possibly dopamine blockade.

Orgasm Inhibited by dopamine blockade, possibly prolactin elevation.

Ejaculation Inhibited by prolactin elevation, α_1-adrenergic blockade, possibly dopamine blockade.

General points

- Educate patients about possible sexual side-effects and routinely screen for any impairment of sexual performance.
- Be able to distinguish between psychotropic-induced sexual dysfunctions and those related to underlying psychiatric or medical conditions, other concurrent drugs, alcohol/substance misuse, enviromental factors, relationship difficulties.
- Optimal treatment for sexual dysfunctions requires the combination of pharmacological and psychological interventions.
- Complaints of sexual dysfunction may suggest inadequate treatment of underlying mental illness.

Antidepressants

Sexual dysfunction is a possible adverse effect of all antidepressants and all dimensions of sexual functioning can be affected. Clomipramine, SSRIs (paroxetine, sertraline, citalopram, fluoxetine), and venlafaxine appear to be most likely to cause sexual problems (30–60%). Other TCAs show intermediate risk of dysfunction (10–30%). Bupropion, moclobemide, and mirtazapine seem to have the lowest rates of sexual side-effects.

- Spontaneous remission occurs in 10% of patients and partial remission in 11% of cases.
- Dysfunction may be related to increased serotonergic transmission, peripheral α_1-adrenergic blockade, histaminergic antagonism, inhibition of NO, adrenergic/cholinergic imbalance.
- Sexual side-effects are likely to be dose related.
- Paroxetine is more likely to cause disorders of arousal and ejaculatory delay than other SSRIs.

- Serotonergic antidepressants are also employed in the treatment of premature ejaculation and paraphilias.

Management
- Watchful waiting to see if symptoms subside (less likely with SSRIs).
- Reduce antidepressant to minimal effective dose.
- Delay drug intake until after sexual activity.
- 'Drug holidays' or scheduled interruptions in therapy (e.g. weekends).
- Switch to another agent known to have fewer adverse sexual effects (e.g. mirtazapine, bupropion, nefazodone, moclobemide).
- Adjunctive therapy (e.g. mirtazapine, buspirone, bupropion, sildenafil, cyproheptadine, amantadine).

Antipsychotics
The prevalence of sexual dysfunction associated with antipsychotics ranges from 40 to 71%, with reports of problems in all groups of antipsychotic medication (usually reduced libido, impaired sexual arousal, orgasm difficulties, ejaculation problems).
- Dysfunction may be related to dopamine blockade, histaminergic antagonism, anticholinergic effects, hyperprolactinaemia (and 2° decrease in oestrogen and testosterone levels).
- Sexual side effects appear to be dose-dependent.
- $5-HT_{2A}$-blocking property of some of SGAs may facilitate sexual behaviour.
- FGAs (esp. thioridazine) and risperidone can affect all phases of sexual response.
- Clozapine, quetiapine, and aripiprazole seem to have the lowest risk of sexual side-effects.

Management
- Spontaneous remission may occasionally occur.
- Dose reduction where possible.
- Consider switching to a compound with less α_1-blocking properties for ejaculatory/erectile disturbances or to a less anticholinergic drug for disorders of arousal.
- Switching to a prolactin-sparing antipsychotic (e.g. quetiapine, clozapine, aripiprazole) may improve several sexual side-effects.
- Adjunctive treatment with dopamine agonists (e.g. amantadine, bromocriptine) may be tried, but evidence base is poor.
- Consider use of phosphodiesterase inhibitor (e.g. sildenafil) for erectile dysfunction.

Mood stabilizers
Lithium therapy may impair desire and arousal, but does not appear to have a major impact on patient self-satisfaction or subjective sense of pleasure during sexual activity. Although the occurrence of sexual dysfunction is estimated as 10–30%, it is usually mild, not a source of distress, and does not lead to non-compliance.

Carbamazepine and *phenytoin* both increase prolactin and decrease dehydroepiandrosterone and other adrenal androgen levels, making sexual dysfunction likely.

Valproate and *lamotrigine* do not cause these changes, and are associated with a low likelihood of sexual dysfunction.

Priapism

Priapism[1] is defined as a sustained, painful, involuntary erection that cannot be relieved by sexual intercourse or masturbation, and that is unrelated to sexual desire. Without intervention, it usually subsides within a few days, but 50–80% of affected men become permanently impotent. Stasis of blood for more than several hours leads to increased blood viscosity, deoxygenation, and, ultimately, irreversible fibrosis of corporeal smooth muscle and cavernosal artery thrombosis. Thus, **priapism is a urologic emergency requiring immediate intervention**.[2] (Clitoral priapism has also been reported and may be associated with either pain and discomfort or increased libido and orgasmic response.)[3]

Pathophysiology

Not completely understood. One proposed mechanism is penile vascular dysregulation caused by α_1-adrenergic blockade (this, in fact, blocks sympathetic stimuli responsible for penile detumescence), especially if in unbalance with cholinergic transmission (e.g. anticholinergic activity). Drug-induced priapism is the 'low flow', ischaemic form of priapism, whereby venous blood persists in the corpora cavernosa. It is also believed to be an idiosyncratic reaction.

Epidemiology

Drug-induced priapism accounts for 15–41% of all cases of priapism.

Risk factors

History of prolonged erections, concurrent medications (see Box 23.5), chronic cocaine misuse, medical conditions (e.g. sickle cell disease, leukaemia).

Differential diagnosis

Sickle cell disease, other medications (see Box 23.5), other rare causes: thalassaemia, leukaemia, vasculitis, fat embolism, dialysis, prostate cancer, GU bladder cancer, spinal cord stenosis, cauda equina compression.

Investigations

FBC, coagulation screen, penile blood gas analysis.

Management

- Always enquire about sexual side-effects and history of prolonged erections (50% of patients presenting with priapism have a previous history of painless erections lasting for < 1hr).
- Counsel patients about the possibility of developing priapism and educate them about the risks of leaving episodes of priapism untreated and the importance of seeking earlier treatment (time to treatment is the single most important factor affecting outcome).
- Avoid psychotropics with high α_1-adrenergic antagonism (e.g. trazodone, sertraline, chlorpromazine, risperidone, ziprasidone) and polypharmacy with anticholinergic agents.
- Immediate intervention should involve conservative measures such as pain control, vigorous hydration and cold compresses.

- Oral terbutaline can be tried as an early treatment.
- First-line therapy is intracavernosal injection of phenylephrine (the most selective and potent α_1-adrenergic agonist) that usually results in penile detumescence in most patients if < 6hr after onset.
- Aspiration of blood from the penis followed by saline irrigation and, if necessary, injection of phenylephrine.
- If these interventions are unsuccessful, a diluted solution of phenylephrine may be used for irrigation.
- If medical interventions fail, surgical care is warranted.
- Recurrent priapism can be managed with a trial of antiandrogens (only in patients who are fully sexually mature), oral beta-agonists such as terbutaline, a combination of prednisone and ketoconazole.

Box 23.5 Drugs reported to cause priapism

- *Trazodone:* trazodone-induced priapism is rare, occurring in less than 0.1% of patients taking the drug. It is typically seen within the first month of therapy, occurs in all age groups, and may occur even with low daily doses of 50–100mg.
- *Other psychotropics:* antipsychotics (risperidone, olanzapine, quetiapine, ziprasidone, aripiprazole, chlorpromazine, thioridazine, haloperidol, clozapine, zuclopenthixol), SSRIs (especially fluoxetine and sertraline), bupropion, phenelzine, phenytoin.
- *Other medications:* sildenafil, antihypertensives (hydralazine, calcium channel blockers), anticoagulants (heparin, warfarin), adrenergic α-blockers (prazosin, tamsulosin, terazosin), hormones (testosterone, GnRH, tamoxifen), metoclopramide, omeprazole, intracavernosal injection of vasoactive drugs.

---

1 Priapus, the son of Zeus and Aphrodite, was a god with an enormous penis who symbolized the earth's fertility.

2 Banos JE, Bosch F, and Farre M (1989) Drug-induced priapism. Its aetiology, incidence and treatment. *Med Toxicol Adverse Drug Exp* **4**: 46–58.

3 Patel AG, Mukherji K, and Lee A (1996) Priapism associated with psychotropic drugs. *Br J Hosp Med* **55**: 315–19.

Antipsychotic-induced Parkinsonism

Essence

A frequent adverse effect found in full form in at least 20% of patients treated with antipsychotic medication. Characterized by tremor, rigidity, and bradykinesia; the presentation is similar to that of idiopathic Parkinson's disease (📖 p. 168), although bradykinesia and resting tremor may be less prominent, micrographia, and festinant gait are less frequently observed, and symptoms are always bilateral. Is more common in elderly females and in those with pre-existing brain damage. Generally occurs within 4wks of treatment, is dose-dependent, and is a major cause of non-compliance.

Assessment

Routine inquiry and clinical examination is generally sufficient to detect the onset of symptoms and should be carried out frequently in the first 3mths of treatment. Monitoring may help establish the minimally effective dose of antipsychotic needed by individual patients, reducing discomfort and improving compliance.

Pathophysiology

D_2 receptor blockade in the nigrostriatal pathway.

Differential diagnosis

Many drugs have been associated with Parkinsonism (see Box 23.5) and some may increase the likelihood of problems (e.g. prednisolone). Other differentials include: idiopathic Parkinson's disease, dementia (e.g. DLB), negative symptoms of schizophrenia, psychomotor retardation (e.g. in depression).

Treatment

Several strategies may be used, including:
- Dose reduction.
- Switching to another antipsychotic agent, e.g. clozapine/quetiapine < olanzapine/aripiprazole < risperidone (<8mg/day).
- Use of anticholinergic agents (e.g. procyclidine, orphenadrine, trihexyphenidyl) or amantadine (a dopamine agonist so beware of potential worsening of psychosis). Of note, symptoms are usually absent during sleep so night-time dose may not be required.
- When treatment is by depot, there is some evidence that pipotiazine palmitate, flupentixol, or zuclopenthixol decanoate may be better tolerated. Risperidone/paliperidone depot may be considered as another option.

Note: anticholinergic agents are often used in younger patients. However, older patients may not be able to tolerate the side-effects of blurred vision, dry mouth, constipation, urinary retention, and particularly cognitive impairment. This has led to the use of amantadine, which is better tolerated, or more frequent use of the newer antipsychotics, especially when patients already have early signs of Parkinson's disease.

Follow-up

If anticholinergics are prescribed, the need for their continued use ought to be kept under review. Their slow withdrawal should be attempted after the acute phase of treatment, or following any lowering of antipsychotic dose, as drug-induced Parkinsonism tends to resolve over time and additional medication may no longer be needed.

Box 23.5 Drugs reported to cause Parkinsonism

- Antidepressants (e.g. SSRIs, MAOIs, TCAs).
- Lithium.
- Anticonvulsants (e.g. carbamazepine, valproate).
- Analgesics (e.g. NSAIDs, opiates).
- Drugs of abuse (e.g. cocaine, PCP).
- Cardiovascular drugs (e.g. amiodarone, diazoxide, diltiazem, methyldopa, metirosine, nifedipine, tocainide).
- GI drugs (e.g. cimetidine, domperidone, metoclopramide, prochlorperazine).
- Anti-infection drugs (e.g. aciclovir, chloroquine).
- Respiratory drugs (e.g. antihistamines, salbutamol, terbutaline).
- Hormones (e.g. medroxyprogesterone).
- Cytotoxics (e.g. ciclosporin, interferons).
- Others (e.g. cyclizine, ondansetron, levodopa, tetrabenazine).

Akathisia

Essence

Akathisia derives from the Greek meaning 'not to sit still' and describes an unpleasant, distressing side-effect of antipsychotic treatment. Characteristically manifests with a subjective component—a feeling of inner restlessness (with the drive to engage in motor activity, esp. involving lower limbs and trunk), and an objective component—movements: such as pacing constantly; inability to stand, sit, or lie still; rocking; crossing/uncrossing legs. Subjective distress may dominate in the absence of any prominent motor phenomena.

Clinical presentations

- *Acute akathisia* occurs within hours to weeks of commencing an antipsychotic or increasing its dose.
- *Acute persistent akathisia* is the chronic form of primary akathisia.
- *Tardive akathisia* usually develops after ≥ 3mths of treatment and can persist or even get worse when antipsychotic medication is discontinued or reduced. Can be associated with less intense subjective restlessness and dyskinetic movements. Is poorly responsive to anticholinergics.
- *Pseudoakathisia* may occur in older, male, schizophrenic patients with prominent negative symptoms and presents with overt motor restlessness without subjective distress.

Pathophysiology

Not yet fully understood. Theories include: dopaminergic/noradrenergic interactions (DA under-activity in the nucleus accumbens increases NE input from the locus coeruleus), imbalance of dopaminergic/serotonergic transmission ($5-HT_{2A}$ agonism inhibits DA release in the striatum), reduced GABAergic transmission in the globus pallidus due to dopamine antagonism.

Risk factors (see Box 23.6)

Use of high-dose and/or high-potency antipsychotics, chronic use of antipsychotics, rapid increase/sudden withdrawal of antipsychotics, use of intramuscular depot preparations, history of organic brain disease (e.g. dementia, alcoholism, HIV), history of previous akathisia, concomitant use of predisposing drugs (e.g. lithium, SSRIs).

Differential diagnosis

Anxiety/agitation (primary or secondary to other psychiatric disorders), drug withdrawal/discontinuation syndromes, acute confusional states, encephalitis/meningitis, Parkinsonism/dystonia/tardive dyskinesia, serotonergic syndrome (early symptoms), toxicity due to other drugs (e.g. recreational drugs—amfetamine, MDMA, cocaine; antidepressants; antihistamines; sympathomimetics; salicylate), restless legs syndrome, iron deficiency anaemia, endocrine disorders (e.g. thyrotoxicosis, hypo/hyperglycaemia, phaeochromocytoma).

Investigations

FBC, LFTs, U&Es, glucose, TFTs, and urine drug screen.

Management

- Review history/medication to identify possible causative agent(s) and rule out any organic aetiology.
- Beware of akathisia possibly leading to increase/worsening of suicidality, non-adherence to treatment, violent behaviour, substance misuse, long-term risk of tardive dyskinesia.

If antipsychotic-related, treatment strategies are as follows:

Change antipsychotic drug regimen

- Reduce dose of antipsychotic medication.
- Try a low-potency FGA (e.g. chlorpromazine).
- Switch to SGA with low akathisia liability (e.g. quetiapine).
- Consider use of clozapine in cases of intractable akathisia.

Add an anti-akathisia agent

- Try beta-blocker (propranolol 40–80mg/day) or low-dose mirtazapine (5-HT$_{2A}$ receptor antagonist) 15mg/day as first-line.
- Alternative option is mianserin (15mg/day) or cyproheptadine (8–16mg/day) (both 5-HT$_{2A}$ receptor antagonists).
- If patient has concurrent Parkinsonism consider use of anticholinergic agents (e.g. benzatropine, orphenadrine, procyclidine, trihexyphenidyl).
- Consider benzodiazepines (e.g. clonazepam, diazepam, lorazepam) alone or with propranolol esp. in chronic akathisia.
- Amantadine (100mg/day) or clonidine (up to 0.15mg/day) may be tried if these treatments are ineffective.

Course/prognosis

Most cases will respond to treatment and usually the response will be seen after a few days. Chronic or tardive cases may be more difficult to treat, and it should be borne in mind that therapeutic benefit (e.g. of propranolol) can take up to 3mths.

Follow-up

- Once the akathisia has settled, any specific treatment ought to be kept under review.
- Slow withdrawal of any additional agent should be attempted after a few weeks (in the case of benzodiazepines) or after several months (for other agents).
- If akathisia recurs, long-term therapy may be necessary. Little data exists for agents other than propranolol (original optimism for long-term benefit has not been borne out) or anticholinergics.
- The need for continued use of high-dose, high-potency antipsychotics should also be reviewed in the light of any change in the clinical presentation of the primary psychiatric disorder.

Box 23.6 Drugs reported to cause akathisia

- *Antipsychotics (usually high-potency)* Chlorpromazine (less likely), haloperidol, pipothiazine, prochlorperazine, promazine, thioridazine (less likely), trifluoperazine, zuclopenthixol, SGAs (risperidone/ziprasidone/aripiprazole > olanzapine > quetiapine/clozapine).
- *Antidepressants* Citalopram, duloxetine, fluoxetine, fluvoxamine, imipramine (and other TCAs), mianserin, paroxetine, sertraline, venlafaxine (withdrawal).
- *Anxiolytics* Alprazolam, buspirone, lorazepam.
- *Others* Diltiazem, interferon alfa, levodopa, lithium, melatonin (withdrawal), metoclopramide, ondansetron, verapamil.

Tardive dyskinesia

Essence
Late onset (mean 7yrs), involuntary, repetitive, purposeless movements, occurring with long-term antipsychotic treatment (although also has been reported in *untreated* schizophrenic patients). Importantly, patients are often unaware of the movements, which are first detected by friends and family members. Operational diagnostic criteria are ≥1 movement of moderate intensity or ≥2 movements of mild intensity after at least 3mths (1mth if > 60yrs) of antipsychotic treatment or within 4wks (8wks for depot) of its discontinuation.

Symptoms/signs
Peri-oral movements are the most common (e.g. tongue, lips, jaw), hence the alternative terms: oral–lingual, orofacial, oro–bucco–facial, or buccal–lingual–masticatory dyskinesia. Other movements may include: axial—trunk twisting, torticollis, retrocollis, shoulder shrugging, pelvic thrusting; limbs—rapid movements of the fingers or legs, hand clenching (and sometimes choreoathetoid movements). Symptoms can be consciously suppressed, worsen with distraction, are exacerbated by stress and anti-Parkinsonian agents, and disappear during sleep. Peripheral TD is more frequently associated with comorbid acute movement disorders (akathisia, tremor, Parkinsonism) than orofacial TD.

Pathophysiology
Not yet fully understood. Theories include: striatal dopaminergic/cholinergic imbalance, up-regulation/supersensitivity of postsynaptic dopamine D_2 receptors in the basal ganglia following chronic blockade, imbalance of D_1 and D_2 receptors leading to striatal disinhibition of the thalamocortical pathway, striatal GABA hypofunction leading to enhanced DA transmission.

Epidemiology
Prevalence is 15–30% of chronically treated patients but may be as high as 70% in the 'high-risk' population. Approximately 50% of cases are reversible.

Risk factors (see Box 23.7)
Chronic use of antipsychotics (particularly in high dose), change/cessation of chronic treatment (especially intermittent treatment), concomitant anticholinergic treatment, elderly (over 60), female (♀:♂ = 1.7:1), history of organic brain disease (e.g. dementia, learning disability, epilepsy), previous head injury, alcoholism, comorbid mood disorder, negative symptoms of schizophrenia, diabetes mellitus, history of previous drug-induced akathisia/Parkinsonism/dystonias, concomitant use of predisposing drugs (e.g. lithium, antidepressants, stimulants).

Differential diagnosis
Stereotypies, tic disorders, other causes of dyskinesia (e.g. Parkinson's disease or use of anti-Parkinsonian agents), hyperthyroidism (choreiform

movements of the limbs), other causes of chorea/athetoid movements (e.g. Sydenham's/Huntington's chorea, Wilson's disease), epilepsy.

Investigations FBC, LFTs, U&Es, TFTs, Ca^{2+}, serum copper, serum coeruloplasmin, ANA, ANCA.

Management

- Review history/medication to identify possible causative agent(s).
- Reduce dose of potential causative agent, to achieve minimum effective dose that adequately controls psychotic symptoms.
- Anticholinergic agents will exacerbate the problem and should also be slowly reduced and stopped if possible.
- If residual symptoms are tolerable, it is best to 'wait and see' before considering additional treatment, as TD tends to improve with time.
- If residual symptoms are severe, interfere significantly with functional abilities, or may be life-threatening, consider an alternative antipsychotic—clozapine (reportedly effective in up to 43% of refractory cases), then quetiapine > olanzapine > risperidone.
- Otherwise temporarily raising the dose of antipsychotic may give immediate relief, whilst addition of a specific treatment may be commenced (dose of antipsychotic should then be reduced again).

Adjuvant agents

- First line—tetrabenazine (a monoamine-depleting agent) 25–200mg/day, but beware of its depressogenic effect.
- Dopamine agonists (e.g. low-dose bromocriptine 0.75–7.5mg/day, levodopa [L-dopa], amantadine).
- Benzodiazepines (e.g. clonazepam if dystonia also present), but evidence base is poor.
- Calcium-channel blockers.
- Anticonvulsants (e.g. gabapentin, levetiracetam).
- Antioxidants (e.g. vitamin E, though efficacy disputed).
- Other (e.g. botulinum toxin, donepezil, amino acids, ondansetron, melatonin, pyridoxine).
- There is case report evidence for use of TMS (see 📖 p. 298).

Course/prognosis

- Symptoms typically wax and wane, remission rates ~30%/yr with 50% clinically improved after 5yrs, even without treatment.
- Response to treatment often requires the striking of a balance between reduction in dyskinesia vs. control of psychotic symptoms.

Follow-up

- Closely monitor residual symptoms.
- Regularly review the need for continued antipsychotic treatment.
- Clearly record TD symptoms and management plan in case notes.

Box 23.7 Drugs reported to cause tardive dyskinesia

- *Antipsychotics:* phenothiazines, haloperidol, loxapine, pimozide, rarely SGAs (quetiapine, olanzapine, amisulpiride, risperidone).
- *Non-antipsychotic medications:* anticholinergics, antidepressants (phenelzine, sertraline, fluoxetine, trazodone, amitriptyline, amoxapine, imipramine), anti-emetics (metoclopramide, prochlorperazine), anti-epileptics (carbamazepine, phenytoin), antihistamines, lithium, amfetamines, methylphenidate, anti-Parkinson agents (bromocriptine, L-dopa).

Dystonic reactions

Essence
Syndrome of sustained, often painful muscular spasms, producing repetitive, twisting movements, or abnormal postures, that develop following exposure to antipsychotic medication.

Aetiology
Remains unclear. Various mechanisms have been proposed such as alteration in dopaminergic–cholinergic balance in basal ganglia or, paradoxically, increased nigrostriatal dopaminergic activity as a compensatory response to dopamine receptor blockade.

Risk factors
Previous/family history of dystonia, younger age group[1] (rare in patients >45yrs), ♂ > ♀ (most likely due to use of higher doses of antipsychotics in men), liver failure, clinically severe schizophrenia (esp. with marked negative symptoms), use of high-potency antipsychotics, hypocalcaemia, recent cocaine misuse.

Acute dystonia
Usually occurs within 1wk of commencing or rapidly increasing the dose of the antipsychotic medication, or of reducing the anticholinergic medication prescribed to treat it. 50% of cases occur within 48hrs, rising to 90% within 5 days of exposure.

Incidence 3–10% of patients exposed to all antipsychotics (up to 30% with high-potency drugs).

Symptoms/signs Muscles of head and neck are most commonly affected with torticollis, trismus, jaw opening, forceful protrusion of the tongue, blepharospasm, grimacing, oculogyric spasm, opisthotonus. Trunk and limbs are less commonly affected, and involvement of pharyngeal and laryngeal muscles can cause serious symptoms such as dysphagia and laryngospasm. Usually more generalized in younger patients (may be confused with fits, esp. in children) and more localized (head and neck) in older patients.

Course May fluctuate over hours, but most last minutes to hours without treatment.

Tardive dystonia
Develops days to months following exposure to dopamine receptor blocking agents and does not improve rapidly with anticholinergic treatment.

Incidence 1.5–4%.

Symptoms/signs are similar to those seen in acute dystonia. It may present with a unique syndrome of retrocollis, opisthotonus, internal arm rotation, elbow extension with wrist flexion.

Course tends to be chronic and symptoms can persist even when offending medication is removed.

Differential diagnosis

May resemble catatonia, tetany, temporal lobe epilepsy, malingering, conversion disorder.

Management

- If severe, discontinue suspected agent.
- Emergency treatment with IM anticholinergic agents (e.g. procyclidine 5mg, benzatropine 2mg). Intravenous administration is necessary only if dystonic reaction is life threatening.
- Continue use of anticholinergic prophylactically for 5 to 7 days in addition to antipsychotic medication and taper it off over 2–3wks (long-term treatment may predispose to TD).
- Consider switching to antipsychotic with low propensity to cause EPSEs (see Box 23.8).
- Alternative treatment includes use of amantadine (fewer side-effects than other agents).
- Oculogyric crisis that is unresponsive to anticholinergic drugs may benefit from treatment with clonazepam.
- If treatment is unsuccessful check serum calcium concentrations in order to exclude hypocalcaemia.
- Routine prophylaxis should be considered for patients with a history of previous drug-induced dystonic reaction.
- Tardive dystonia may respond to botulinum toxin, ECT, and deep brain stimulation (see 🕮 p. 299).

Box 23.8 Agents reported to cause dystonias

- *Antipsychotics:* aripiprazole, clozapine (rare/abrupt withdrawal), flupentixol decanoate, haloperidol, olanzapine (rare), prochlorperazine, quetiapine, sulpiride, risperidone (rare), alimemazine, zuclopethixol.
- *Other psychotropics:* benzatropine (rare), bupropion, buspirone, gabapentin, carbamazepine, cocaine (+ withdrawal), disulfiram (rare), mirtazapine, fluoxetine, midazolam, paroxetine, phenelzine, sertraline, TCAs.
- *Other (mostly rare/isolated cases):* amiodarone, azapropazone, diphenhydramine, domperidone, ergotamine, indometacin, metoclopramide, nifedipine, penicillamine, prochlorperazine, promethazine, propranolol, sumatriptan.

---

1 *Note:* in contrast with most medication side-effects, acute dystonias are more common in the young than the elderly. This may be related to asymptomatic loss of dopaminergic neurons in later life.

Neuroleptic malignant syndrome

Essence
A rare, life-threatening, idiosyncratic reaction to antipsychotic (and other) medication (see Box 23.9), characterized by: fever, muscular rigidity, altered mental status, and autonomic dysfunction.

Note: if diagnosed in a psychiatric setting, transfer patient to acute medical services where intensive monitoring and treatment are available.

Pathophysiology
Theories: 2° to DA activity in the CNS—i.e. striatum (rigidity), hypothalamus (thermoregulation)—by blockade of D_2-receptors or ↓ DA availability; impaired Ca^{2+} mobilization in muscle cells leads to rigidity (like malignant hyperthermia[1]); sympathetic nervous system activation or dysfunction.

Epidemiology
Incidence 0.07–0.2% (pooled data); ♀:♂ = 2:1.

Mortality
5–20%—death usually due to respiratory failure, cardiovascular collapse, myoglobinuric renal failure, arrhythmias, or disseminated intravascular coagulation (DIC).

Morbidity
Rhabdomyolysis, aspiration pneumonia, renal failure, seizures, arrhythmias, DIC, respiratory failure, worsening of primary psychiatric disorder (due to withdrawal of antipsychotics).

Symptoms/signs
Hyperthermia (>38°C), muscular rigidity, confusion/agitation/altered level of consciousness, tachycardia, tachypnoea, hyper/hypotension, diaphoresis/sialorrhoea, tremor, incontinence/retention/obstruction, creatinine kinase (CK)/urinary myoglobin, leukocytosis, metabolic acidosis.

Risk factors
↑ Ambient temperature; dehydration; patient agitation or catatonia; rapid antipsychotic initiation/dose escalation; withdrawal of anti-Parkinsonian medication; use of high-potency agents/depot IM preparations; history of organic brain disease (e.g. dementia, alcoholism), affective disorder, previous NMS; predisposing drugs (e.g. lithium, anticholinergic agents).

Differential diagnosis
Catatonia (see Table 23.3); malignant hyperthermia[1]; encephalitis/meningitis; heat exhaustion; Parkinsonism/acute dystonia; serotonergic syndrome; toxicity due to other drugs (e.g. amfetamine, MDMA, cocaine, antidepressants, antihistamines, sympathomimetics, salicylates); delirium tremens (DTs); rhabdomyolysis; septic shock; haemorrhagic stroke; tetanus; phaeochromocytoma; strychnine poisoning.

Investigations
FBC, blood cultures, LFTs, U&Es, calcium and phosphate levels, serum CK, urine myoglobin, ABGs, coagulation studies, serum/urine toxicology, CXR (if aspiration suspected), ECG; consider head CT (intracranial cause), LP (to exclude meningitis).

Management
- BDZs for acute behavioural disturbance (📖 p. 988) (*Note:* use of restraint and IM injection may complicate the interpretation of serum CK.)
- Stop any agents thought to be causative (esp. antipsychotics), or restart anti-Parkinsonian agents.
- Supportive measures: oxygen, correct volume depletion/hypotension with IV fluids, reduce the temperature (e.g. cooling blankets, antipyretics, cooled IV fluids, ice packs, evaporative cooling, ice-water enema).
- Rhabdomyolysis—vigorous hydration and alkalinization of the urine using IV sodium bicarbonate to prevent renal failure.
- Pharmacotherapy to reduce rigidity—dantrolene (IV 0.8–2.5mg/kg qds; PO 50–100mg bd), lorazepam (up to 5mg); *2nd line:* bromocriptine (PO 2.5–10mg tds, increase to max 60mg/day), amantadine (PO 100–200mg bd); *3rd line:* nifedipine; consider ECT (*Note:* ↑ risk of fatal arrhythmias).

Course
May last 7–10 days after stopping oral antipsychotics and up to 21 days after depot antipsychotics (e.g. fluphenazine).

Prognosis
In the absence of rhabdomyolysis, renal failure, or aspiration pneumonia, and with good supportive care, prognosis is good.

Follow-up
Monitor closely for residual symptoms. Once symptoms have settled allow 2+wks (if possible) before restarting medication (use low-dose, low-potency, or atypical agents). Consider prophylaxis (bromocriptine). Inform patient about risk of recurrence if given antipsychotic medication. Ensure this is recorded prominently in their medical notes.

Box 23.9 Drugs reported to cause symptoms characteristic of NMS

- **Antipsychotics:** aripiprazole, chlorpromazine, clozapine (rarely), flupentixol, fluphenazine, haloperidol, olanzapine, promazine, quetiapine (rarely), risperidone, thioridazine.
- **Anti-Parkinsonian agents:** amantadine (+ withdrawal), anticholinergics (withdrawal), levodopa (+ withdrawal).
- **Antidepressants:** amoxapine, clomipramine, desipramine, phenelzine, trimipramine, venlafaxine.
- **Other:** carbamazepine (+ withdrawal), ganciclovir, ferrous sulphate, lithium, methylphenidate, metoclopramide, oral contraceptives.

Table 23.3 Differentiating NMS from catatonia

Feature	NMS	Catatonia
Patient taking antipsychotics	Usually	Not usually
Echo phenomena*	Rare	Yes
Ambitendency*	Rare	Yes
Posturing*	Rare	Yes
Hyperthermia	Usually before stupor	Usually before/during severe agitation
Muscle rigidity	Yes	Yes
Raised WCC	Yes	No
Raised CK	Yes	Yes

*Catatonia symptoms.

1 A rare disorder associated with exposure to inhaled aesthetics and succinylcholine. Genetic linkage found to chromosome 19. Possibly due to a muscle membrane defect, leading to ↓ intracellular Ca^{2+} and intense muscle contractions. Temperature rises rapidly (up to 1°C/5min).

Serotonin syndrome (SS)

Essence

A rare, but potentially fatal syndrome occurring in the context of initiation or dose increase of a serotonergic agent, characterized by altered mental state, agitation, tremor, shivering, diarrhoea, hyperreflexia, myoclonus, ataxia, and hyperthermia. Although SSRIs are commonly linked to SS, many other drugs (e.g. amfetamines, MAOIs, TCAs, lithium) have the potential of causing hyperserotonergic symptoms. SS can occur as a result of overdose, drug combinations (including over the counter medications), and rarely with therapeutic doses.

Pathophysiology

A variety of mechanisms can potentially increase the quantity or activity of serotonin: ↑ production of serotonin due to ↑ availability of precursors (L-tryptophan-containing substances); ↓ metabolism of serotonin (MAOIs, selegiline); ↑ release of stored serotonin (amfetamine, cocaine, fenfluramine, MDMA, pethidine); reuptake inhibition (SSRIs, TCAs, SNRIs, NaSSAs, MDMA, dextromethorphan, pethidine, St John's wort); direct stimulation of serotonin receptors (buspirone, LSD); unknown mechanisms (lithium).

Epidemiology

Incidence 71% for SSRIs (moderate/major symptoms; mild symptoms may be common, but tend to go unreported); mortality <1 in 1000 cases.

Symptoms/signs (see Box 23.10)

- *Psychiatric/neurological:* confusion, agitation, coma.
- *Neuromuscular:* myoclonus, rigidity, tremors (including shivering), hyperreflexia (usually lower rather than upper limbs), ataxia.
- *Autonomic:* hyperthermia (may be 2° to prolonged seizure activity, rigidity, or muscular hyperactivity), GI upset (nausea, diarrhoea), mydriasis, tachycardia, hyper/hypotension.

Differential diagnosis

NMS (see Table 23.4), malignant hyperthermia, infections (encephalitis/meningitis, sepsis), metabolic disturbances, substance abuse (cocaine)/withdrawal/overdose (LSD, PCP).

Investigations

FBC, U&Es, LFTs, glucose, pH, biochemistry (including calcium, magnesium, phosphate, anion gap), CK, drug toxicology screen, CXR (if evidence of respiratory distress/possible aspiration), ECG monitoring (arrhythmia/conduction problems—prolonged QRS or QTc interval).

Treatment

- If severe, requires immediate transfer to emergency department for supportive treatment and active management.
- If overdose, consider gastric lavage and/or activated charcoal.
- IV access—to allow volume correction (dehydration: insensible fluid loss due to hyperthermia) and reduce risk of rhabdomyolysis.

- *Rhabdomyolysis:* Should be dealt with quickly, with emphasis on maintaining a high urine output combined with alkalinization using sodium bicarbonate (target urine pH of 6). If necessary, reduce the temperature (e.g. cooling blankets, antipyretics, cooled IV fluids, ice packs, evaporative cooling, ice-water enema).
- *Pharmacotherapy:* Agitation, seizures, and muscular rigidity/myoclonus best managed using a *BDZ* (e.g. lorazepam IV [slow] 1–2mg every 30min; clonazepam). *Serotonin receptor antagonists* may be considered in selected cases (e.g. cyproheptadine PO 4–8mg every 2–4hr [max 0.5mg/kg/day], chlorpromazine [risk of reduced seizure threshold], mirtazapine, methysergide, propranolol [mild 5-HT antagonist]). *Antihypertensives* are usually unnecessary unless the hypertension is persistent and clinically significant (e.g. glyceryl trinitrate IV 2mg/kg/min).

Course and prognosis

Onset is usually acute; however, recurrent mild symptoms may occur for weeks before the appearance of severe symptoms. Most cases resolve without sequelae within 24–36hrs with adequate supportive measures. Following an SSRI overdose, a patient who remains asymptomatic for several hours is unlikely to need further medical management.

Box 23.10 Sternbach's diagnostic criteria[1]

- Other potential causes excluded (e.g. infection, metabolic, substance abuse, withdrawal).
- No concurrent antipsychotic dose changes prior to symptom onset.
- At least three of the following:
  - Agitation/restlessness.
  - Sweating.
  - Diarrhoea.
  - Fever.
  - Hyperreflexia.
  - Ataxia.
  - Mental state changes (confusion, hypomania).
  - Myoclonus.
  - Shivering.
  - Tremor.

1 Sternbach H (1991) The serotonin syndrome. *Am J Psychiat* **148**: 705–13.

Table 23.4 Distinguishing SS from NMS

Although the clinical presentation of these two syndromes is very similar (i.e. autonomic dysfunction, alteration of mental status, rigidity, and hyperthermia), differentiation is very important as specific management may differ (e.g. use of chlorpromazine in SS, which may worsen NMS)

	NMS	SS
Associated Rx	Antipsychotics (idiosyncratic/normal dose)	Serotonergic agents (OD/drug combination)
Onset	Slow (days to weeks)	Rapid
Progression	Slow (24–72hrs)	Rapid
Muscle rigidity	Severe ('lead pipe')	Less severe
Activity	Bradykinesia	Hyperkinesia

Antidepressant discontinuation[1] syndrome

Discontinuation symptoms can occur with *all* antidepressants and differ between antidepressant classes. However, they usually share three common features: abrupt onset within days of stopping the antidepressant, a short duration when untreated, and quick resolution when the original antidepressant is reintroduced. It is estimated at least a third of patients experience discontinuation symptoms. They are usually mild and self-limiting but in a minority of cases they can be severe and prolonged.

Clinical features[2]

SSRIs and related discontinuation syndrome

- *Sensory symptoms:* paraesthesia, visual disturbance, shock-like sensations and numbness.
- *Disequilibrium symptoms:* most common: dizziness, vertigo, and lightheadedness.
- *General somatic complaints:* flu-like symptoms (myalgias and chills), fatigue, headache, sweating, and tremor.
- *GI symptoms:* diarrhoea, vomiting, and nausea/emesis.
- *Affective symptoms:* irritability, anxiety/agitation, low mood, and tearfulness.
- *Sleep disturbance:* nightmares, vivid dreams, and insomnia.

TCAs discontinuation syndrome Similar to SSRIs, but sensory and disequilibrium symptoms are less common with TCAs.

MAOIs discontinuation syndrome More severe than with other antidepressants and includes worsening of depressive symptoms, acute confusion, hallucinations, paranoid delusions, and anxiety symptoms with depersonalization.

Uncommon clinical presentations Rare syndromes such as mania/hypomania (see 📖 p. 308) and Parkinsonian symptoms (see 📖 p. 945) may occur with all antidepressants.

Course and duration

Usually develops after 1mth of treatment, within 2–5 days after antidepressant discontinuation or dose reduction. Onset of symptoms is unusual after more than 1wk. If untreated, duration is variable (1 day to 3wks). Resolution of symptoms usually occurs within 24hrs if antidepressant is reinstated.

Aetiology

Not completely understood. Various underlying mechanisms have been postulated, such as acute decrease in synaptic serotonin in the face of down-regulated or desensitized serotonin receptors, loss of inhibitory 5-HT tone on NE neurons, and cholinergic rebound.

Risk factors

Short half-life drugs (e.g. venlafaxine, paroxetine), duration of treatment ≥8wks (plateau in incidence afterwards), high dose stopped, anxiety symptoms at the start of treatment, previous history of discontinuation symptoms, young age.

Differential diagnosis

Discontinuation symptoms can be misdiagnosed for:
- Recurrence of depressive/anxiety symptoms.
- Treatment ineffectiveness due to covert non-adherence.
- Adverse reaction to new drug when switching across antidepressant classes.

Other possibilities to be excluded are:
- Underlying physical disorder.
- Withdrawal from drugs of abuse/alcohol.
- Mania/hypomania (timing of onset and symptoms such as dizziness and paraesthesia strongly suggest 'discontinuation mania').

Management

- Tapering antidepressant is recommended to reduce the risk of developing discontinuation syndrome (use of liquid preparations may be helpful in allowing greater flexibility). However, guidelines on the optimum rates of dose reduction are at best *empirical* (see 📖 p. 268) and a cautious approach is advised (over a 4-wk period if duration of treatment ≥8wks).
- If mild–moderate and short-lived, symptoms can generally be tolerated by the patient, allowing for successful discontinuation of antidepressant.
- If severe, reintroduction of the original antidepressant rapidly resolves the symptoms. However, the syndrome may recur in up to 75% of patients when the same antidepressant is later discontinued.
- Awareness of risk factors and symptoms of discontinuation syndrome, and education of patients prior to stopping or tapering an antidepressant, should prevent unnecessary and expensive medical investigations.
- Some symptoms of moderate severity can be treated symptomatically (e.g. hypnotic for insomnia, anti-muscarinic agents for cholinergic rebound following TCA discontinuation).
- For SSRI and SNRI discontinuation symptoms another option is to switch to fluoxetine (due to its long elimination half-life).
- If previous history of severe discontinuation symptoms and poor adherence to treatment, choice of antidepressant with low propensity to cause discontinuation symptoms (e.g. fluoxetine) should be considered.

1 The term 'discontinuation' is usually preferred to 'withdrawal' since the latter implies dependence and there is no evidence antidepressants have a significant dependence liability according to internationally accepted criteria.
2 Haddad PM and Anderson IM (2007) Recognizing and managing antidepressant discontinuation symptoms. *Adv Psychiat Treat* **13**: 447–57.

Hyponatraemia and antidepressants

Essence

Low serum sodium (Na^+<135mmol/L) is a rare, idiosyncratic side-effect of all antidepressants which may have serious consequences if undiagnosed. It is probably not dose-related and its onset usually occurs within the first month of treatment.

Aetiology

Incompletely understood, but probably due to the syndrome of inappropriate secretion of anti-diuretic hormone (SIADH) with resultant euvolaemic hypotonic hyponatraemia. It has been postulated serotonin may be involved in the regulation of ADH release.

Risk factors

Previous SIADH, history of hyponatraemia; low BMI, female gender, age >80yrs; physical co-morbidity: diabetes mellitus, hypertension, head injury, hypothyroidism, impaired renal function, COAD; other medications (e.g. thiazides > loop diuretics, chemotherapy, NSAIDs, carbamazepine).

Antidepressants

- *Highest risk (>1% incidence):* citalopram, escitalopram, fluoxetine, sertraline.
- *Medium risk (0.5–1% incidence):* amitriptyline, clomipramine, dosulepine, doxepin, imipramine, lofepramine, moclobemide, paroxetine, venlafaxine.
- *Lowest risk (<0.5% incidence):* nortriptyline, trazodone, phenelzine, tranylcypromine, mirtazapine, reboxetine.

Clinical features

Depend upon the severity, duration, and rate of change in serum sodium. May be asymptomatic, or display symptoms and signs ranging from nausea, muscle cramps/weakness, malaise to hypertension, lethargy, confusion, and, if severe, seizures and coma.

Investigations

Check renal, hepatic, cardiac, thyroid, adrenal function; volume status; serum lipids and protein (to exclude pseudohyponatraemia); serum glucose (raised in hypertonic hyponatraemia); urine osmolality (>100mOsm/L indicates impaired free water excretion); serum osmolality; urinary sodium concentration (usually >20–40mmol/L with SIADH).

Differential diagnosis

- *Psychogenic polydipsia.*
- *Severe malnutrition.*
- *Antipsychotic-induced* (water intoxication, SIADH, severe hyperlipidaemia/hyperglycaemia).
- *Cirrhosis*; *alcoholism.*
- *Nephrotic syndrome, heart failure.*
- *Malignancy,* e.g. lung small-cell, pancreas, prostate, lymphoma.

- *CNS disorders*, e.g. meningoencephalitis, abscess, stroke, subarachnoid/ subdural haemorrhage, head injury, Guillain–Barré, vasculitis.
- *Respiratory disorders*, e.g. TB, pneumonia, abscess, aspergillosis.
- *Endocrine/metabolic disease*, e.g. severe hypothyroidism, hypoadrenalism, pituitary insufficiency, porphyria.
- *Drugs*, e.g. opiates, chlorpropramide, cytotoxic agents, diuretics, carbamazepine, NSAIDs, MDMA.

Management

Prevention Baseline U&Es prior to commencing antidepressant, with monitoring for those at high risk (at 2 and 4wks, then every 3mths).

Treatment

- If serum Na$^+$ is <125mmol/L: refer to specialist medical care and withdraw offending agent immediately.
- If serum Na$^+$ is >125mmol/L: continue to monitor U&Es daily until >135mmol/L.
- Consider a lower risk antidepressant (mirtazapine appears to have the lowest risk) or, if treatment urgent, ECT may be an option.
- Consider fluid restriction and/or careful use of demeclocycline under specialist advice.
- If necessary, rechallenge may be possible without recurrence (low dose, gradual increase, close monitoring).

Prescribing in pregnancy

Data is limited (and often conflicting) regarding the safety of psychotropic drugs in pregnancy. There have been reports that psychotropics may be associated with an increased risk of birth defects or neonatal adverse events. However, also untreated mental illness during pregnancy is an independent risk factor for major congenital malformations (MCMs) and obstetric complications (see Box 23.11 for guidance).

Antipsychotics
- Based on the available evidence no definitive association has been found between *in utero* antipsychotic exposure and an increased rate of MCMs and abnormal postnatal development.
- FGAs are usually considered to have minimal teratogenic potential.
- For SGAs, most evidence is with olanzapine and clozapine (increased rate of gestational diabetes, but no increased risk of MCMs).
- Depot formulations and anticholinergic drugs should be avoided.

Antidepressants
- Untreated affective illness in pregnant women may be associated with an increased risk of pre-term delivery, low birth weight, and poorer long-term developmental outcomes.
- TCAs and SSRIs do not seem to be major teratogens but can cause neonatal withdrawals (agitation, irritability) if used in 3rd trimester.
- Among TCAs, nortriptyline is recommended since it is less anticholinergic and hypotensive than amitriptyline and imipramine.
- SSRIs (most experience is with fluoxetine; less safe is paroxetine) may be associated with low birth weight, spontaneous abortion and, if used in 3rd trimester, neonatal pulmonary hypertension.
- MAOIs and other antidepressants should be avoided.

Anxiolytics
- Neonatal respiratory depression, hypothermia, hypotonia ('floppy baby syndrome') and withdrawal syndromes may occur when benzodiazepines (BDZs) are used close to delivery.
- High doses and use in the 1st trimester increase the teratogenic risk.
- There may be an association between 1st trimester exposure to BDZs (esp. diazepam) and an increased risk of facial clefts.
- Short-term use and minimum effective dose are recommended if BDZs are necessary. Promethazine is often preferred.
- NICE advises the use of low-dose chlorpromazine and amitriptyline.

Mood stabilizers
- All commonly used mood stabilizers are teratogenic and, where possible, should be avoided, at least in the first trimester.
- *Lithium* has been associated with an increased risk (1:1000) of Epstein's anomaly (downward displacement of the tricuspid valve into the right ventricle) and detailed ultrasound/foetal echocardiography is indicated at 16–18wks.

- Relapse rates on discontinuation (50% within 2–10wks) generally regarded to preclude stopping lithium therapy in pregnancy.
- Serum monitoring, dosage adjustment, and ensuring adequate hydration are essential (particularly after delivery).
- Neonatal problems include 'floppy baby syndrome', non-toxic goitre, hypothyroidism, nephrogenic diabetes insipidus, and cardiac arrhythmias.
- *Valproate*, and to a lesser extent *carbamazepine*, are associated with neural tube defects (hence, folic acid supplementation is recommended for women of child-bearing age, although evidence for benefit is inconclusive). Valproate has also been associated with increased risk of long-term cognitive deficits and craniofacial, cardiac, or limb defects.
  - Detailed ultrasonography should be carried out at 16–18wks, and maternal serum α-fetoprotein (AFT) levels measured.
  - There is also an increased risk of neonatal haemorrhage, and vitamin K should be given to mothers in the last month of gestation (and to neonates at birth).
- *Lamotrigine* may be associated with increased rate of cleft palate.

Box 23.11 Guiding principles

For all women of child-bearing age
- Always consider (and ask about) the possibility of pregnancy.
- Pregnancy test recommended before starting any teratogenic drug.
- Counsel the patient about the necessity of adequate contraception.
- Advise further consultation if pregnancy is planned.

For a planned conception
- Discuss risks/benefits of discontinuation/continuation of medication (e.g. relapse vs. teratogenicity, possible time it may take to conceive, no decision is risk-free).
- Avoidance of all drugs during the first trimester (max teratogenic potential is between wks 2–9) is ideal, but often not achievable.

In pregnancy
- Consider switching to a lower risk drug if possible, use the lowest viable dose, avoid polypharmacy, and monitor closely.
- Pregnancy may alter the pharmacokinetics of drugs, hence dosages may need to be adjusted (e.g. lithium).
- Gradual withdrawal of some compounds (e.g. BDZs, TCAs, SSRIs) in the weeks prior to delivery may help avoid 'withdrawal' effects in the newborn baby.

Unexpected pregnancy
- If after week nine, no urgent decision needs to be made as major risk has passed.
- Consider reducing dose if possible and prescribe nutritional supplements (e.g. folic acid).
- Do not stop lithium abruptly and use caution with some SSRIs and anticonvulsants.

Prescribing in lactation

⚠ **Absolute contraindications**

Psychotropic drugs should be avoided if the infant is premature or suffers from renal, hepatic, cardiac, or neurological disorders.

General points

- All psychotropic medication should be regarded as passing into breast milk (to a greater or lesser degree).
- The benefits of breastfeeding to the mother and the infant must be carefully weighed against the risks of neonatal exposure to drugs.
- Of the limited studies examining this problem, the general findings are that levels of most psychotropic drugs in breast milk are relatively low, and infant serum levels (ILs) may be *undetectable*.
- Although infant exposure may be relatively low from breast milk (much lower than *in utero* exposure if mother was taking medication during pregnancy), there is a risk of both withdrawal symptoms and adverse effects on development.
- Evidence may be lacking for *specific* risks, nonetheless, caution should be exercised.
- Monitoring of the infant should include biochemical (renal and liver function tests) and behavioural measures, with the involvement of a paediatrician to ensure development is within normal parameters.

Choice of medication in nursing mothers

- Where possible, consider non-pharmacological treatments.
- If medication is necessary, the lowest effective therapeutic dose should be used and polypharmacy should be avoided.
- Unless otherwise contraindicated, consider continuing with the psychotropic used during pregnancy in order to minimize any withdrawal effects in the newborn.
- Avoid the use of drugs which are sedating and with long half-lives.

Antipsychotics

- Limited data preclude any conclusive prediction on the long-term safety of the available antipsychotics in lactation.
- Among FGAs, most evidence is with haloperidol and chlorpromazine and has not shown any clear adverse infant effects.
- A few case reports indicate low breast milk levels with risperidone, quetiapine, and olanzapine.
- There is one case report of cardiomegaly, jaundice, and sedation with olanzapine but this finding may be spurious.
- Clozapine should not be used as there is a risk of agranulocytosis and seizures in the infant.

Antidepressants

- Available evidence is reassuring with regard to the safety of SSRI use in lactating women, with few reports of adverse effects on exposed infants.

- Low ILs have been found with all SSRIs but higher concentrations have been reported with fluoxetine and citalopram, which should therefore be used with caution.
- Sertraline and paroxetine should be considered first-line since they are usually associated with undetectable ILs.
- Low ILs and no adverse effects in the nursing infant are also reported with TCAs, with imipramine and nortriptyline being recommended as drugs of choice.
- Limited data is available on other antidepressants.

Anxiolytics
- Benzodiazepines (BDZs) are excreted in breast milk and have lower infant milk/plasma ratios than other psychotropic medications.
- Adverse effects such as sedation, lethargy, and weight loss have been reported with the use of BDZs.
- BDZs with a short half-life such as lorazepam and oxazepam are preferable to longer acting ones (e.g. diazepam).

Mood stabilizers
- Valproate and carbamazepine are regarded as compatible with breastfeeding. However, some adverse effects have been noted, hence close monitoring of the infant is advised.
- Previous case reports found high ILs and adverse infant effects (such as cyanosis, hypotonia, heart murmur, lethargy) being associated with lithium.
- However, recent data have shown no serious adverse event and relatively low ILs.
- Infants may be more susceptible to dehydration and lithium toxicity owing to immature renal function.
- In the light of the recent findings, there is no absolute contraindication to the use of lithium in lactating women but caution and careful monitoring are recommended.
- Lamotrigine is not recommended due to theoretical risk of life-threatening Stevens–Johnson syndrome.

Strategies to minimize infant exposure
- Breastfeeding should be avoided at the time when serum levels in the mother are likely to be at their peak (check drug information for these values).
- If possible, medication should be given as a single dose before the infant's longest sleep period.
- Breastfeeding should occur immediately *before* taking the next due dose.
- Alternatively, breast milk may be expressed when serum levels are at their lowest.

Prescribing for patients with cardiovascular disease

General points

In considering a suitable psychotropic drug the main issues revolve around the propensity of that drug to interact with other medications the patient may be taking, to affect blood pressure, or lead to cardiac conduction problems (see Box 23.12). Due to the unpredictability of drug interactions, polypharmacy is best avoided.

Specific contraindications

BDZs and clomethiazole in pulmonary insufficiency; disulfiram and lithium in heart failure or sick sinus syndrome; lofexidine in post-MI patients. Pimozide is best avoided in most conditions.

Myocardial infarction

- *Antidepressants:* best avoided in the first 2mths; if clinically indicated— SSRIs (sertraline is drug of choice), rather than TCAs (but avoiding fluvoxamine and citalopram/escitalopram). If sedation required consider use of a small dose of trazodone at night.
- *Antipsychotics:* high doses should be avoided; phenothiazines are generally more hypotensive than butyrophenones; clozapine should be used with caution in the 1st year post-MI; of the newer antipsychotics, olanzapine may offer best risk–benefit balance.

Heart failure

Where possible, hypotensive agents (β-blockers, clozapine, risperidone, TCAs) and drugs causing fluid retention (carbamazepine, lithium) should be avoided.

Angina/IHD
Avoid hypotensive agents and those known to cause tachycardia (phenothiazines, clozapine, risperidone).

Hypertension
Avoid agents that may raise blood pressure (MAOIs, low-dose TCAs, phenothiazines, clozapine, high-dose venlafaxine).

Arrhythmias (see Box 23.12)

- *Antidepressants:* SSRIs should be first choice (but not fluvoxamine or citalopram/escitalopram).
- *Antipsychotics:* high doses should be avoided; if essential, use of sulpiride and olanzapine is recommended.

Box 23.12 The QT^c question

Awareness of QT prolongation, as measured by the corrected QT interval (QT^c), has been heightened because of the potential (but relatively rare) risk of fatal arrhythmias (e.g. torsade de pointes), highlighted recently by the withdrawal of thioridazine as a first-line antipsychotic (and now contraindicated in patients with a history of, or at risk of, arrhythmias) and specific new cautions regarding high-dose citalopram/escitalopram.

QT^c is derived by dividing the QT interval by the square root of the cycle length i.e.:

$$QT^c = \frac{QT}{\sqrt{R-R}}$$

Normal QT^c is 380–420ms; if prolonged to 450ms—some concern; if >500–520ms—'at risk'.

Causes of prolonged QT interval

Acute myocardial ischaemia, myocarditis, bradycardia (e.g. AV block), head injury, hypothermia, electrolyte imbalance (K$^+$ ↑, Ca^{2+} ↓, Mg^{2+} ↓), congenital, sotalol, antihistamines, macrolides (e.g. erythromycin), amiodarone, antipsychotics (esp. phenothiazines), antidepressants (esp. TCAs).

General advice

Good practice dictates use of routine ECG prior to commencement of antipsychotic medication (esp. pimozide, zotepine, thioridazine, and other phenothiazines) or other psychotropics with known cardiac side-effects (e.g. fluvoxamine, citalopram/escitalopram), and regular monitoring, particularly when high doses are prescribed.

Prescribing for patients with liver disease

General points

- Almost all psychotropic drugs are metabolized by the liver.
- Exceptions to this rule include lithium, gabapentin, sulpiride, and amisulpiride, which have minimal (or no) liver metabolism.
- Most drugs are highly protein-bound (with the exception of citalopram, escitalopram, sulpiride, and amisulpiride) and plasma levels may be *increased* in liver disease.
- In liver disease, when using drugs with high first-pass clearance (e.g. imipramine, amitriptyline, desipramine, doxepin, haloperidol), initial doses should be low.
- Where possible, phenothiazines (e.g. chlorpromazine), hydrazine, and MAOIs (may be hepatotoxic) should be avoided.
- Avoid drugs that are very sedative and constipating (anticholinergic) due to increased risk of precipitating hepatic encephalopathy.
- LFTs can be a poor marker of hepatic metabolic impairment; hence always consider the clinical presentation too.

Risk factors for drug-induced hepatotoxicity are: older age, alcohol intake, female sex, obesity, genetic vulnerability, concomitant prescription of enzyme-inducing drugs.

Antidepressants

- Always start with lowest possible dose and titrate slowly.
- *TCAs:* best evidence for use of imipramine; avoid amitriptyline, dosulepin, and lofepramine (most hepatotoxic).
- *SSRIs:* some evidence for paroxetine and citalopram; avoid sertraline. Also increased risk of bleeding with all SSRIs.
- *MAOIs:* when clinically necessary, use 30–50% usual dose.
- *Others:* venlafaxine (use 50% of usual dose), mirtazapine (cautious use), reboxetine (extensively metabolized, very low starting dose), trazodone (highly protein bound so low starting dose).

Antipsychotics

- Best evidence for low-dose haloperidol (considered 'drug of choice'), with sulpiride a close second (only 5% liver metabolism).
- Few problems reported for flupenthixol/zuclopenthixol.
- Clozapine dose should be kept low (some evidence of hepatotoxicity).
- Amisulpiride is predominantly excreted by the kidneys, but there is little literature on its use in liver disease.
- For the newer agents recommendations suggest:
  - Aripiprazole should be used cautiously esp. in severe disease.
  - Olanzapine (up to 7.5mg) may be safe (but does induce transaminases).
  - Risperidone doses should be kept low (start 0.5mg bd, max 4mg/day).

- Quetiapine is extensively metabolized (hence, start low—25mg).
- Zotepine should only be used with caution (start 2.5mg bd, max 75mg/day, monitor LFTs weekly for at least 3mths).

Mood stabilizers

- Lithium is the 'drug of choice', with gabapentin as second choice.
- Valproate is *contraindicated* in severe liver disease, but may be used with caution in mild–moderate impairment.
- Caution should also be exercised with carbamazepine and lamotrigine, which are *contraindicated* in severe and acute liver disease.

Anxiolytics

- Where necessary, use low doses of short-acting BDZs (e.g. lorazepam, oxazepam, temazepam).
- A low dose of zopiclone 3.75mg can be used with care in moderate hepatic impairment.
- If clomethiazole is to be used, the dose should be reduced to ~30%.

Prescribing for patients with renal impairment

General points

- Renal impairment generally leads to accumulation of drugs (or active metabolites) that are predominantly cleared by the kidney. This will lead to higher serum levels, and increased risk of dose-related side-effects (e.g. postural hypotension, sedation, EPSEs).
- Hence, all psychotropics should be started at a low (or divided) dose, increased slowly, and carefully monitored (for efficacy and tolerability).
- When patients are receiving dialysis, seek specific advice from manufacturer—dosages should usually be reduced by at least 50% and dosing separated in time from dialysis itself.

Classification of chronic renal failure (CRF)

See Box 23.13 for estimation of GFR. CRF may be classified as *mild* (glomerular filtration rate [GFR] 60–89mL/min), *moderate* (GFR 30–59mL/min), *severe* (GFR 15–29mL/min), or *end-stage* (GFR <15mL/min).

Antidepressants

- In severe renal failure avoid duloxetine, fluoxetine, venlafaxine, and lofepramine (unless the patient is on dialysis).
- Otherwise cautious use, beginning low and gradually increasing the dose is advised.
- No specific therapeutic dose adjustments are necessary for MAOIs (except for isocarboxazid), RIMAs, mianserin, tryptophan, trazodone, or TCAs.

Antipsychotics

- Lower doses are recommended to avoid dose-related side-effects (particularly with the phenothiazines, which may be best avoided).
- Highly anticholinergic agents should be avoided due to risk of urinary retention.
- Clozapine is contraindicated in severe renal impairment.
- Avoid amisulpiride/sulpiride (primarily renally excreted) and use caution with risperidone and zotepine.
- Some authorities recommend haloperidol, but accumulation is possible, so careful monitoring is still necessary.

Mood stabilizers

- Lithium is relatively contraindicated in renal failure, but its use may often be necessary, and dose reduction (e.g. to 50–75% for mild–moderate and 25–50% for severe renal failure) with close monitoring of plasma levels is recommended. In dialysis, 600mg ×3/wk (after dialysis) has been shown to maintain therapeutic plasma levels.
- No specific problems are reported for valproate or carbamazepine, although in severe renal failure, serum levels should be monitored.

Box 23.13 Estimating glomerular filtration rate (GFR)

GFR

Normal value approx. 125mL/min, is the volume of fluid filtered by the glomeruli per minute (mL/min) and can be directly measured by collection of urine over 24hr or estimated in adults in two ways:

- *Creatinine clearance (CrCl)*: Using the Cockcroft and Gault equation:

  CrCl (mL/min) = F(140 − age [in yrs] × ideal body weight [kg])/serum creatinine (μmol/L)

  F = 1.23 (men) and 1.04 (women).

CrCl is not accurate in conditions where plasma creatinine is unstable (pregnancy, children, diseases raising creatinine plasma level) and in severe renal failure.

- *Estimated GFR (eGFR)*: Using the Modification of Diet in Renal Disease (MDMR) formula. It gives an eGFR for a 1.73 m^2 body surface area (if the body surface area is more or less than 1.73 m^2 then eGFR is less accurate).

  eGFR (mL/min/1.73m^2) = 175 × ([serum creatinine (μmol/L)/84.4]$^{-1.154}$) × age(yrs)$^{-0.203}$

  × 0.742 if female

  × 1.21 if African American or African Caribbean

Online calculator is available at ✆ www.renal.org/eGFRcalc/GFR

Note: most current drug dose recommendations are based on the CrCl estimations from Cockcroft and Gault. However, the most widely used method for estimating GFR is the MDMR equation, as this has proved the most robust and accurate.

- Gabapentin requires specific dose adjustments and manufacturer's recommendations should be sought.
- Lamotrigine should be used cautiously, particularly in severe renal impairment.

Anxiolytics/hypnotics

- BDZs (with the exception of chlordiazepoxide) tend to accumulate, with increasing CNS side-effects (particularly sedation)—hence use low doses.
- Buspirone is contraindicated in moderate–severe renal failure.
- β-blockers should be started at low dose as they may complicate renal failure by reducing renal blood flow.
- Zopiclone and zaleplon require no dosage adjustment. However, the half-life of zolpidem may be doubled in renal failure.

Others

- *Anticholinergics, disulfiram*: use cautiously.
- *Acamprosate*: contraindicated if serum creatinine >120μmol/L.
- *Anticholinesterases*: no reported problems.

Prescribing for patients with epilepsy

General points

In considering a suitable psychotropic there are two related considerations:

- The propensity of that drug to interact with other medications the patient may be taking (justifying serum monitoring where possible).
- Risk of lowering seizure threshold and exacerbating the condition.
- As these effects appear dose-related, daily dose of any drug should be kept as low as possible. Greater caution is necessary when:
  - Other psychotropics are also being given (e.g. regular *plus* 'as required' antipsychotics).
  - Patients may be withdrawing from CNS depressants (e.g. BDZs, barbiturates, or alcohol).

Risk factors for psychotropic-induced seizures include: history of epilepsy, old age, polypharmacy, reduced drug clearance, pre-existing EEG abnormalities, cerebral arteriosclerosis, neurological impairment.

Antidepressants

- All TCAs appear to lower seizure threshold, although there appears to be greater risk with amitriptyline, clomipramine, and dothiepin.
- Tetracyclics (maprotiline and amoxapine) also appear pro-convulsant, as does bupropion.
- The other antidepressants appear less likely to cause problems, and a usual first choice is often an SSRI (may be anticonvulsant at therapeutic doses).

Antipsychotics

- Greatest risk of seizures is associated with the use of phenothiazines (esp. chlorpromazine), zotepine, olanzapine, and particularly clozapine.
- The risk of seizures with clozapine rises from 1% (at doses <300mg/day), to 2.7% (300–600mg/day), to 4.4% (>600mg/day). EEG changes are seen in up to 75% of people taking clozapine, with ~40% showing paroxysmal discharges.[1] Because of this risk it is quite common to cover high doses of clozapine with concomitant use of valproate. Hence, greater caution is needed when clozapine is used in individuals with epilepsy.
- Lowest risk is associated with haloperidol (best choice), sulpiride, zuclopenthixol, amisulpiride, pimozide, quetiapine, and risperidone.

Mood stabilizers

- Lithium does cause seizures in overdose. However, a therapeutic dose has a low pro-convulsive effect.
- If in doubt, anticonvulsants provide useful alternatives. However, clinical efficacy must be weighed against any potential risks of using lithium.

Anxiolytics/hypnotics

- Generally these drugs are *anticonvulsant*.
- Exceptions include buspirone, zolpidem, and β-blockers, although there is no evidence that they are epileptogenic.

Others

- *Anticholinergics, acamprosate:* no problems reported.
- *Disulfiram:* caution is recommended.
- *Anticholinesterases:* care is needed with donepezil and rivastigmine. However, galantamine appears safe.

1 Pacia SV and Devinsky O (1994) Clozapine-related seizures: experience with 5,629 patients. *Neurology* **44**: 2247–9.

Difficult and urgent situations

Dealing with psychiatric emergencies

It is a common misconception that there are no *real* emergencies in psychiatry. The billowing white coat may be gone, but then so is the back-up of the arrest team. Dealing with acute situations can feel like a lonely business, and doubts about the best management of given situations may prevent you getting that much-needed rest period.

As a psychiatrist, you are primarily a doctor, and you should ensure that you are up to date with basic resuscitation procedures. Familiarize yourself with the procedures in place for the management of medical emergencies in your hospital, as the level of on-site facilities will vary.

There is no substitute for experience, but hopefully some of the guidance in the following section (and the other pages they refer to) will allow a rational approach to a number of common (and not so common) difficult and urgent situations in a psychiatric setting.

Keep the following principles in mind:

'Primum non nocere': above all, do no harm

- Always ensure your own and other staff's safety.
- If necessary facilities or expertise are not available, make appropriate arrangements to get the patient to them as soon as possible.
- Always suspect (and as far as possible exclude) potential organic causes for psychiatric presentations.
- Remember—patient confidentiality does not override issues of threatened harm to themselves or other individuals.

Assess

- Always make the fullest assessment possible—do not fail to ask about important issues just because you feel a person may not wish to talk about them.
- Ensure that you have the best quality information available. If other sources of information are available (e.g. previous notes, third-party information), use them!
- Don't dawdle—if a situation requires immediate action, act.

Consult

- Do not *assume* anything. If in doubt, consult a senior colleague. Remember you are part of a team, and if there is a difficult decision to make, do not make it alone.

Keep contemporaneous records

- Clearly record your assessment, decisions made (*and* reasons), and the names of any other colleagues involved or consulted. Legally, if it's not been recorded, it's not been done.

What to do if summoned to a crisis situation/negotiation principles

First principles
- Speak to the staff who originated the call.
- Obtain as much information as possible about the situation prior to seeing the patient.
- Establish what your expected role is.
- Keep your own safety uppermost in your mind (no heroics).

General aims
- Attempt to put the patient at their ease; explain who you are and why you have been asked to speak to them.
- Be clear in any questions you need to ask.
- Elicit useful information.
- Achieve a safe, dignified resolution of the situation.

Important communication principles
- Be conscious of both verbal and non-verbal language.
  - Listen actively—assimilate and understand what is actually being said and interpret the various underlying meanings and messages.
  - Feedback—go back over what the patient has said with them to assure them that you understand what they are saying.
  - Empathy—show you appreciate them sharing their thoughts, feelings, and motives.
  - Content and feeling—note any difference between what is said verbally and what message is really being given.
- Use checkpoint summaries—brief reviews of the main points discussed, about issues, and any demands.

Important suggestions
- Use open questions to give the patient an opportunity to ventilate what is on their mind (this may help relieve tension, keep the patient talking, and allow you to assess the mental state).
- Listen carefully to what the patient is saying. This may provide further clues as to their actions. It also demonstrates concern for the patient's problem.
- Be honest, up front, and sincere—develop a trusting relationship.
- Be neutral—avoid approval or disapproval unless necessary.
- Orientate the patient to looking for alternative solutions together, without telling them how to act (unless asked).
- Try to divert any negative train of thought.
- Check with other team members before making any commitments.
- If the police have been called, present the reason for their presence realistically, but neutrally.
- Do not involve family members in negotiations.

Some suggestions for dealing with particular patients

The patient responding to paranoid ideas/delusions

- Avoid prolonged eye contact and do not get too close.
- The patient's need to explain may allow you to establish a degree of rapport. Allow them to talk, but try to stay with concrete topics.
- Do not try to argue them out of their delusions—ally yourself with their perspective without sounding insincere (e.g. 'What you are saying is that you believe…x…y…z').
- Avoid using family members who may be part of the delusional system.
- Try to distance yourself from what may have happened in the past (e.g. 'I'm sorry that was your experience before…maybe this time we could manage things better…').
- Be aware that your offer of help may well be rejected.

The patient with antisocial traits

- A degree of flattery may facilitate discussion of alternative solutions (show you understand their need to communicate, how important their opinions are, your desire to work together to resolve things).
- Encourage them to talk about what has led up to this situation.
- Try to convince them that other ways of achieving their aims will be to their advantage—keep any negotiation reality-oriented.
- Focus their attention on you as the means to achieve their aims.

The patient with borderline traits

- Provide 'understanding' and 'uncritical acceptance'.
- Help them find a way to sort things out without having 'failed again'.
- Try to build self-esteem (e.g. 'You have done well coping with everything up to now…')
- Once trust is gained, it may be possible to be more directive.
- Use the patient's desire to be accepted (e.g. 'I really think it would be best if we…').
- Bear in mind that often the behaviour will be attention-seeking, and it may be worth asking: 'What is it you feel you need just now?'
- Do not be surprised if the patient acts impulsively.

The depressed patient

- Psychomotor retardation may slow response time—be patient.
- The presence of friends or relatives may worsen their feelings of worthlessness and guilt.
- Focus on the 'here and now'—avoid talking abstractly.
- Acknowledge that they probably cannot imagine a positive future.
- Be honest and straightforward—once rapport has been established, it may be appropriate to be explicitly directive.
- Try to postpone the patient's plans, rather than dismiss them (e.g. 'Let's try this…and see how you feel in the morning…').
- Be prepared to repeat reassurances.

The patient experiencing acute stress

- Allow ventilation of feelings.
- Try to get them to describe events as objectively as possible.
- Have them go back over the options they have ruled out.
- Review the description of events, and present a more objective, rational perspective.

Managing suicide attempts in hospital

Attempted overdose

In psychiatric wards, the most likely means of attempted self-poisoning involves building up a stock of prescribed medication or bringing into the ward tablets to be taken at a later date (e.g. while out on pass). Often patients will volunteer to trusted nursing staff that they have taken an overdose, or staff will notice the patient appears overtly drowsy and when challenged the patient admits to overdose.

- Try to ascertain the type and quantity of tablets taken (look for empty bottles, medication strips, etc.).
- Establish the likely timeframe.
- If patient is unconscious or significantly drowsy, arrange immediate transfer to emergency medical services. Inform medical team of patient's diagnosis, current mental state, current status (informal/ formal), any other regular medications.
- If patient asymptomatic, but significant overdose suspected, arrange immediate transfer to emergency services:
  - Do not try to induce vomiting.
  - If available, consider giving activated charcoal (single dose of 50g with water) to reduce absorption (esp. if NSAIDs or paracetamol).
- If patient asymptomatic, and significant overdose unlikely:
  - Monitor closely (general observations, level of consciousness, evidence of nausea/vomiting, other possible signs of poisoning).
  - If paracetamol or salicylate (aspirin) suspected: perform routine bloods (FBC, U&Es, LFTs, HCO_3, INR) and request specific blood levels (4hr post-ingestion level for paracetamol).
  - If other psychiatric medications may have been taken, consider urgent blood levels (e.g. lithium, anticonvulsants—see 🕮 p. 928).
  - Be aware that LFTs may be abnormal in patient on antipsychotic or antidepressant medication.
  - If in doubt, get advice, or arrange for medical assessment.

Deliberate self-harm

Most episodes of deliberate self-harm involve superficial self-inflicted injury (e.g. scratching, cutting, burning, scalding) to the body or limbs. These may be easily treated on the ward with little fuss (to avoid secondary reinforcement of behaviour).

- Any more significant injuries (e.g. stabbing, deep lacerations) should be referred to emergency medical services, with the patient returning to the psychiatric ward as soon as medically fit.
- Medical advice should also be sought if:
  - You do not feel sufficiently competent to suture minor lacerations.
  - Lacerations are to the face/other vulnerable areas (e.g. genitals) or where you cannot confirm absence of damage to deeper structures (e.g. nerves, blood vessels, tendons).
  - The patient has swallowed/inserted sharp objects into their body (e.g. vagina, anus).
  - The patient has ingested potentially harmful chemicals.

Attempted hanging

Most victims of attempted hangings in hospitals do not use a strong enough noose or sufficient drop height to cause death through spinal cord injury ('judicial hanging'). Cerebral hypoxia through asphyxiation is the probable cause of death and should be the primary concern in treatment of this patient population.

On being summoned to the scene

- Support the patient's weight (if possible enlist help).
- Loosen/cut off ligature.
- Lower patient to flat surface, ensuring external stabilization of the neck and begin usual basic resuscitation (ABCs, IV access, etc.).
- Emergency airway management is a priority:
  - Where available, administer 100% O_2.
  - If competent and indicated: use nasal or oral endotracheal intubation.
- Assess conscious level, full neurological examination, and degree of injury to soft tissues of the neck.
- Arrange transfer to emergency medical services as soon as possible.

Points to note

- Aggressive resuscitation and treatment of post-anoxic brain injury is indicated even in patients without evident neurological signs.
- Cervical spine fractures should be considered if there is a possibility of a several foot drop or evidence of focal neurological deficit.
- Injury to the anterior soft tissues of the neck may cause respiratory obstruction. Close attention to the development of pulmonary complications is required.

Attempted asphyxiation

- Remove source (ligature, polythene bag, etc.).
- Give 100% O_2.
- If prolonged period of anoxia, or impaired conscious level, arrange immediate transfer to emergency medical services.

After the event

Patient

- Once the patient is fit for interview, formally assess mental state and conduct assessment of further suicide risk (p. 784).
- Establish level of observation necessary to ensure patient's safety, clearly communicate your decision to staff, and make a record in the patient's notes. (*Note*: Hospital policy may vary, but levels of observation will range from timed checks (e.g. every 15mins to having a member of staff within arm's length of the patient 24hrs/day).

Staff

For particularly traumatic events, it may be necessary to arrange a 'critical incident review' (at a later date) where all staff involved participate in a confidential debriefing session. This is not to apportion blame, but rather to review policy and to consider what measures (if any) might be taken to prevent similar events occurring in the future.

Severe behavioural disturbance

This covers a vast range of presentations, but will usually represent a qualitative acute change in a person's normal behaviour, that manifests primarily as antisocial behaviour—e.g. shouting, screaming, increased (often disruptive/intrusive) activity, aggressive outbursts, threatening violence (to others or self).

In extreme circumstances (e.g. person threatening to commit suicide by jumping from a height [out of a window, off a roof], where the person has an offensive weapon, or a hostage situation), this is a *police* matter and your responsibility does not extend to risking your own or other people's lives in trying to deal with the situation.

Common causes
- Acute confusional states (see delirium 🕮 p. 790).
- Drug/alcohol intoxication.
- Acute symptoms of psychiatric disorder (anxiety/panic, 🕮 p. 358, mania, 🕮 p. 310, schizophrenia/other psychotic disorders, 🕮 p. 186).
- 'Challenging behaviour' in brain-injured or LD patients (🕮 p. 766).
- Behaviour unrelated to primary psychiatric disorder—this may reflect personality disorder, abnormal personality traits, or situational stressors (e.g. frustration).

General approach
- Sources of information will vary depending on the setting (e.g. on the ward, in outpatients, emergency assessment of new patient). Try to establish the context in which the behaviour has arisen.
- Follow the general principles outlined on 🕮 p. 990.
- Look for evidence of possible psychiatric disorder.
- Look for evidence of possible physical disorder.
- Try to establish any possible triggers for the behaviour— environmental/interpersonal stressors, use of drugs/alcohol, etc.

Management
This will depend upon assessment made:
- If physical cause suspected:
  - Follow management of delirium (🕮 p. 790).
  - Consider use of sedative medication (see 🕮 p. 990) to allow proper examination, facilitate transfer to medical care (if indicated), or to allow active (urgent) medical management.
- If psychiatric cause suspected:
  - Consider pharmacological management of acute behavioural disturbance (see 🕮 p. 990).
  - Consider need for compulsory detention.
  - Review current management plan, including observation level.
- If no physical or psychiatric cause suspected, and behaviour is dangerous or seriously irresponsible, inform security or the police to have person removed from the premises (and possibly charged if a criminal offence has been committed, e.g. assault, damage to property).

Pharmacological approach to severe behavioural disturbance

There are often local protocols for rapid tranquillization and for control and restraint and these should be followed where available. In situations requiring rapid tranquillization or control and restraint, discuss management with a senior colleague as soon as possible.

In the guide (Box 24.1) the doses quoted are appropriate for young, physically fit patients who have previously received antipsychotic medication. In patients who are elderly, have physical health problems, or are 'antipsychotic naïve', dosage should at least be halved (refer to BNF for further guidance).

Potential risks

• Over-sedation causing loss of consciousness or alertness.
• Compromise of airway.
• Cardiovascular or respiratory collapse (raised risk where there is stress or extreme emotion or extreme physical exertion).
• Interaction with prescribed or illicit medication.
• Damage to therapeutic relationship.
• Other (related or coincidental) physical disorders (e.g. congenital prolonged QTc syndromes, patient on medication lengthening QTc).

Dos and don'ts

• Follow local protocols where these are available.
• Document all decisions/actions.
• Have a low threshold for obtaining senior advice.
• Always prescribe oral and IM doses separately to avoid confusion.
• Do not use two different drugs of the same class for rapid tranquillization.
• Document maximum total daily dose and maximum dosage frequency on the prescription kardex.
• Do not mix medications in the same syringe.

Aftercare

• Respiration, pulse, and blood pressure should be monitored within an hour of drug administration and regularly thereafter.
• Look for extra-pyramidal side-effects, particularly acute dystonia (see 📖 p. 954); possible NMS (see 📖 p. 956).
• Remember: fatalities have occurred during emergency restraint.

Issues of consent

Giving emergency medication for acute behavioural disturbance is essentially treatment under common law (📖 p. 874). The justification rests on the judgement that no other management options are likely to be effective, and that tranquillization will prevent the patient harming themselves or others. Harm may include behaviour that is likely to endanger the physical health of the patient (e.g. not consenting to urgent treatment or investigations that are likely to be life-saving) when capacity to give consent is judged to be impaired (📖 p. 872).

Box 24.1 A guide to rapid tranquillization

First-line treatments (allow sufficient time between doses for assessing clinical response)

Non-psychotic context: Consider oral lorazepam 1–2mg.

Psychotic context: Consider oral lorazepam 1–2mg and oral anti-psychotic, e.g. haloperidol 10–20mg, chlorpromazine 50–100mg.

Second-line treatments—oral medication failed/refused/not indicated (allow sufficient time between doses for assessing clinical response)

Non-psychotic context: Consider IM lorazepam 1–2mg.

Psychotic context
- Consider IM lorazepam 1–2mg + IM haloperidol 10–20mg.
- Consider IM olanzapine 5–10mg for moderate disturbance (do not give IM lorazepam within 1hr of IM olanzapine).
- Consider IM chlorpromazine 25–100mg (*Note*: danger of postural hypotension and fatality if given inadvertently by IV injection.
- Consider IM depot zuclopenthixol acetate (Clopixol acuphase®) 50–150mg—repeat every 2–3 days if necessary up to max total dose 400mg. (This is a rapidly acting, sedating, depot antipsychotic which is best avoided in antipsychotic-naïve or inexperienced patients because of long half-life.)

Exceptional circumstances—immediate tranquillization necessary
- Consider IV benzodiazepines, e.g. diazepam 10mg by slow IV bolus (*Note*: ensure flumazenil available in case of respiratory depression).
- Consider IV haloperidol 2–10mg (high risk of dystonia—max daily dose 18mg may sometimes be given as single dose).

Third-line treatments
- Other treatments (e.g. paraldehyde) or combinations of the above may be suggested in some centres.
- Always consult senior medical advice before administering these interventions.

The catatonic patient

Catatonia is certainly less common in current clinical practice, thanks to the advent of effective treatments for many psychiatric disorders and earlier interventions. Nonetheless, the clinical presentation may be a cause for concern, particularly when a previously alert and oriented patient becomes mute and immobile. The bizarre motor presentations (e.g. posturing) may also raise concerns about a serious acute neurological problem (hence these patients may be encountered in a medical/liaison setting), and it is important that signs of catatonia are recognized. Equally, the 'excited' forms may be associated with sudden death ('lethal' or 'malignant' catatonia), which may be preventable with timely interventions.

Clinical presentation

Characteristic signs
- Mutism
- Posturing
- Negativism
- Staring
- Rigidity
- Echopraxia/echolalia

Typical forms
- Stuporous/retarded
- Excited/delirious

Common causes

- **Mood disorder** More commonly associated with mania (accounts for up to 50% of cases) than depression. Often referred to as manic (or depressive) stupor (or excitement).
- **General medical disorder** Often associated with delirium:
  - Metabolic disturbances
  - Endocrine disorders
  - Viral infections (including HIV)
  - Typhoid fever
  - Heat stroke
  - Autoimmune disorders
  - Drug-related (antipsychotics, dopaminergic drugs, recreational drugs, BDZ withdrawal, opiate intoxication)
- **Neurological disorders**
  - Postencephalitic states
  - Parkinsonism
  - Seizure disorder (e.g. non-convulsive status epilepticus)
  - Bilateral globus pallidus disease
  - Lesions of the thalamus or parietal lobes
  - Frontal lobe disease
  - General paresis
- **Schizophrenia** (10–15% of cases) Classically catalepsy, mannerisms, posturing, and mutism (see **catatonic schizophrenia**, 📖 p. 179).

Differential diagnosis

- **Elective mutism** Usually associated with pre-existing personality disorder, clear stressor, no other catatonic features, unresponsive to lorazepam.
- **Stroke Mutism** associated with focal neurological signs and other stroke risk factors. 'Locked-in' syndrome (lesions of ventral pons and cerebellum) is characterized by mutism and total immobility (apart from vertical eye movements and blinking). The patient will often try to communicate.
- **Stiff-person syndrome** Painful spasms brought on by touch, noise, or emotional stimuli (may respond to baclofen, which can induce catatonia).
- **Malignant hyperthermia** Occurs following exposure to anaesthetics and muscle relaxants in predisposed individuals (📖 p. 956).
- **Akinetic Parkinsonism** Usually in patients with a history of Parkinsonian symptoms and dementia—may display mutism, immobility, and posturing. May respond to anticholinergics, not BDZs.

Other recognized catatonia (and catatonia-like) subtypes

- **Malignant catatonia** Acute onset of excitement, delirium, fever, autonomic instability, and catalepsy—may be fatal.
- **Neuroleptic malignant syndrome (NMS)**— 📖 p. 956.
- **Serotonin syndrome (SS)**— 📖 p. 960.

Management

Assessment

- Full history (often from third-party sources), including recent drug exposure, recent stressors, known medical/psychiatric conditions.
- Physical examination (including full neurological).
- Investigations—temperature, BP, pulse, FBC, U&Es, LFTs, glucose, TFTs, cortisol, prolactin, consider CT/MRI and EEG.

Treatment

- Symptomatic treatment of catatonia will allow you to assess any underlying disorder more fully (i.e. you will actually be able to talk to the patient).
- Best evidence for use of BDZs (e.g. lorazepam 500 mcg–1mg oral/ IM—if effective, given regularly thereafter), barbiturates (e.g. amobarbital [amytal] 50–100 mg), and ECT.
- Alone or in combination these effectively relieve catatonic symptoms regardless of severity or aetiology in 70–80% of cases.[1,2]
- Address any underlying medical or psychiatric disorder.

1 Bush G, Fink M, Petrides G, et al. (1996) Catatonia II: treatment with lorazepam and electroconvulsive therapy. Acta Psychiat Scand 93: 137–43.
2 Ungvari GS, Kau LS, Wai-Kwong T, et al. (2001) The pharmacological treatment of catatonia: an overview. Eur Arch Psychiat Clin Neurosci 251(Suppl. 1): 31–4.

The manipulative patient 1

Manipulation is a term that is generally used pejoratively, although some ethologists regard manipulative behaviour as 'selfish but adaptive' (i.e. the means by which we use others to further our own aims—which may be entirely laudable). In the context of psychiatric (and other medical) settings, manipulative behaviours are usually maladaptive and include:

- Inappropriate or unreasonable demands:
  - More of your time than any other patient receives.
  - Wanting to deal with a *specific* doctor.
  - Only willing to accept one particular course of action (e.g. admission to hospital, a *specific* medication or other form of treatment).
- Behavioural sequelae of failing to have these demands met:
  - Claims of additional symptoms they failed to mention previously.
  - Veiled or explicit threats of self-harm, lodging formal complaints, litigation, or violence.
  - Passive resistance (refusing to leave until satisfied with outcome of consultation).
  - Verbal or physical abuse of staff/damage to property.
  - Actual formal complaints relating to treatment (received or refused), or false accusations of misconduct against medical staff.

Key points

- Patients DO have the right to expect appropriate assessment, care, and relief of distress.
- Doctors DO have the right to refuse a course of action they judge to be inappropriate.
- Action should always be a response to clinical need (based on a thorough assessment, diagnosis, and best evidence for management), NOT threats or other manipulative behaviours.
- It is entirely possible that a patient who demonstrates manipulative behaviour DOES have a genuine problem (it is only their way of seeking help that is inappropriate).
- Some of the most difficult patients tend to present at 'awkward' times (e.g. the end of the working day, early hours of the morning, weekends, public holidays, intake of new staff)—this is no accident!
- Admitting a patient to hospital overnight (when you are left with no other option) is not a failure—some patients are very good at engineering this outcome. At worst it reinforces inappropriate coping behaviours in the patient. (Critical colleagues would probably have done the same themselves in similar circumstances.)
- If you have any doubts about what course of action to take, consult a senior colleague and discuss the case with them.

Management principles

1. New case

- Make a full assessment to establish:
  - Psychiatric diagnosis and level of risk (to self and others).
  - Whether other agencies are required (e.g. specific services: drug/alcohol problems; social work: housing/benefits/social supports;

counselling: for specific issue—debt/employment/bereavement/
alleged abuse).
- Ask the patient what they think is the main problem.
- Ask the patient what they were hoping you could do for them, e.g.
  - Advice about what course of action to take.
  - Wanting their problem to be 'taken seriously'.
  - Wanting to be admitted to hospital.
  - Wanting a specific treatment.
- Discuss with them your opinion of the best course of action, and
establish whether they are willing to accept any alternatives offered
(e.g. other agencies, outpatient treatment).

2. The 'frequent attender'/chronic case
- Do not take short cuts—always fully assess current mental state and
make a risk assessment.
- When available—always check previous notes, any written care plan,
or 'crisis card'.
- Establish the reason for presenting *now* (i.e. what has changed in their
current situation).
- Ask yourself 'Is the clinical presentation significantly different so as to
warrant a change to the previously agreed treatment plan?'
- If not, go with what has been laid out in the treatment plan.

See Box 24.2 for pitfalls and how to avoid them.

Box 24.2 Pitfalls (and how to avoid them)
- Try not to take your own frustrations (e.g. being busy, feeling
'dumped on' by other colleagues, lack of sleep, lack of information,
vague histories) into an interview with a patient—your job is to
make an objective assessment of the person's mental state and to
treat each case you see on its own merits.
- Try not to allow any preconceptions or the opinions of other
colleagues colour your assessment of the current problems the
patient presents with (people and situations have a tendency to
change with time, and what may have been true in the past may no
longer be the case).
- Watch out for the patient who appeals to your vanity by saying
things like: 'You're much better than that other psychiatrist I saw…I
can really talk to you…I feel you really understand'. They probably
initially said the same things to 'that other psychiatrist' too!
- Do not be drawn into being openly critical of other colleagues;
remember you are only hearing one side of the story. Maintain a
healthy regard for the professionalism of those you work beside—
respect their opinions (even if you really don't agree with them).
- If you encounter a particularly difficult patient, enlist the support of a
colleague and conduct the assessment jointly.
- NEVER acquiesce to a 'private' consultation with a patient of the
opposite sex; do not make 'special' arrangements; and NEVER give
out personal information or allow patients to contact you directly.

The manipulative patient 2

Specific situations

Patient demanding medication
- There are really only two scenarios where there is an urgent need for medication:
  - The patient who is acutely unwell and requires admission to hospital anyway (e.g. with acute confusion, acute psychotic symptoms, severe depression, high risk of suicide).
  - The patient who is known and has *genuinely* run out of their usual medication (for whom a small supply may be dispensed to tide them over until they can obtain a repeat prescription).

Patient demanding immediate admission
- Clarify what the patient hopes to achieve by admission, and decide whether this could be reasonably achieved, or if other agencies are better placed to meet these requests (see 🕮 p. 6).
- If the patient is demanding admission due to drug/alcohol dependence, emphasize the need for clear motivation to stop, and offer to arrange outpatient follow-up (the next day) (see 🕮 p. 556).
- Always ask about any recent trouble with the police; it is not uncommon for hospital to be sought as a 'sanctuary' from an impending court appearance (but remember this can be a significant stressor for patients with current psychiatric problems).

Additional complications

Demanding relatives/other advocates
- Assess the patient on their own initially, but allow those attending with the patient to have their say (this may clarify the 'why now' question, particularly if it involves the breakdown of usual social supports).
- Ask the patient for their consent to discuss the outcome of your consultation with those accompanying them (to avoid misunderstandings and improve compliance with the proposed treatment plan).

Patient 'raising the stakes'
- If a patient is dissatisfied with the outcome of your consultation, they may try a number of ways to change your mind (see 🕮 p. 994); they may even explicitly say: 'What do I have to do to convince you?' before resorting to other manipulative behaviours.
- This type of response only serves to confirm any suspicions of attempted manipulation and should be recorded as such in the notes (verbatim if possible).
- Stick to your original management plan, and if the behaviour becomes passively, verbally, or physically aggressive, clearly inform them that unless they desist, you will have no other option than to have them removed (by the police, if necessary).
- Equally, any threats of violence towards individuals present during the interview or elsewhere should be dealt with seriously and the police (and the individual concerned) should be informed—patient

confidentiality does not take precedence over ensuring the safety of others.

Suspected factitious illness

- Try to obtain corroboration of the patient's story (or confirmation of your suspicions) from third-party sources (e.g. GP, relative, previous notes, including other hospitals they claim to have been seen at).
- If your suspicions are confirmed, directly feed this information back to the patient, and clearly inform them of what course of action you plan to take (e.g. recording this in their notes, informing other agencies, etc.).
- Do not feel 'defeated' if you decide to admit them to hospital. Record your suspicions in the notes and inform the psychiatric team that the reason for admission is to assess how clinically significant the reported symptoms are (it will soon become clear in a ward environment and it may take time to obtain third-party sources).

Patient threatening suicide by telephone

- Keep the person talking (see 📖 p. 984).
- Try to elicit useful information (name, where they are calling from, what they plan to do, risk to anyone else).
- If you judge the patient to be at high risk of suicide, encourage them to come to hospital—if they refuse or are unable to do so, organize for emergency services to go to their location and bring them to hospital.
- If the patient refuses to give you any information, inform the police who may have other means to determine the source of the call and respond.
- Always document phone calls in the same way as you would any other patient contact (see **Closure**).

Closure

- Clearly document your assessment, any discussion with senior colleagues, the outcome, and any treatment plan.
- Record the agreement/disagreement of the patient and any other persons attending with them.
- If appropriate, provide the patient with written information (e.g. appointment details, other contact numbers) to ensure clear communication.
- Ensure that you have informed any other necessary parties (e.g. keyworkers/psychiatric team already involved with the patient, source of referral—which may be the GP, other carers, social workers, etc.).
- If the assessment occurs out of hours, make arrangements for information to be passed on to the relevant parties in the morning (ideally try to do this yourself).
- If you have suggested outpatient follow-up for a new patient, make sure you have a means of contacting the patient, to allow the relevant service to make arrangements to see them as planned.
- If you think it is likely the patient will re-present to other services, inform them of your contact with the patient and the outcome of your assessment.

Issues of child protection

The treating doctor has a responsibility to consider the welfare not only of their patient, but also of the patient's dependants (in most cases, their children). Where there are concerns relating to the welfare of children, this responsibility may be discharged both through actions you take yourself (e.g. admitting the patient to hospital), and through involvement of appropriate statutory agencies (e.g. child and family social services). Each case should be individually assessed; however, a number of scenarios can be recognized:

• **Necessary absence** When a patient is brought into hospital (e.g. for emergency assessment) the admitting doctor should clarify whether they have dependent children, and if so, what arrangements have been made for their care. If these are unsatisfactory, or are disconcertingly vague (e.g. 'with a friend'), child and family social services should be consulted.

• **Neglect of childcare responsibilities** In some circumstances, as a result of mental disorder, patients' ability to provide the appropriate level of physical or emotional care may be impaired. This may relate to functional impairments (e.g. poor memory), continuing symptomatology (and medication side-effects), or dependence on drugs or alcohol. Having a mental disorder does not preclude being a parent—what is important is that individual patients receive appropriate assessment to ascertain the type of additional support they may need and the level of monitoring required.

• **Risk of positive harm to child** Certain disorders carry the risk of harm to the child by acts of *commission*, rather than *omission*. These include:
  • Psychotic disorders in which the patient holds abnormal beliefs about their child.
  • Severe depressive disorder with suicidal ideas, which involve killing the child (usually for altruistic reasons).
  • Drug misuse where there are drugs or drug paraphernalia left carelessly in the child's environment.

In these cases, a joint approach should be adopted involving mental health (optimizing the patient's management) and social services (addressing issues of child protection and welfare).

Patients acting against medical advice 1: guiding principles

In certain situations, doctors are faced with deciding whether or not to act against a patient's stated wishes. This most commonly occurs when:
- A patient does not consent to a particular treatment plan.
- A patient wishes to leave hospital, despite medical advice that this is not in their best interests.
- Some common clinical scenarios are discussed in Box 24.3 (see 📖 p. 1002).

Fundamental principles
- An adult has the right to refuse treatment or to leave hospital should they wish.
- Doctors have a responsibility to discuss what they are proposing with the patient fully, to ensure that the patient is informed of the options, risks, and the preferred management (but not to enforce or coerce).

Special circumstances

In some circumstances, doctors have the power to act without the patient's consent or override a patient's expressed wishes when:
- Consent cannot be obtained in an *emergency* situation and treatment may be given under *common law* (📖 p. 974).
- A patient's *capacity* is either temporarily or permanently impaired (📖 p. 970) and they are unable to give *informed* consent. The responsible doctor should act in the patient's *best interest* (📖 p. 874)—consider treatment using incapacity legislation (📖 pp. 876–9).
- They are suffering from a mental disorder and their capacity to take decisions is impaired. Use of the MHA may be necessary to ensure their own (or other persons') safety.

Points to note
- When a *capable* patient disagrees with a proposed course of action, this should be recorded clearly in the notes (with the reasons given by the patient). If this involves discharge from hospital, a 'discharge against medical advice' form may be useful (as a written record of the patient's decision), even though such forms have no special legal status.
- In emergency situations, the definition of 'mental disorder' is that of a layperson, not whether ICD-10 or DSM-IV criteria are satisfied.
- Incapacity legislation does not allow for detention in hospital; equally detention under the MHA does not allow for compulsory treatment of physical disorders.
- Always consider the balance of risks: ask yourself 'what am I more likely to be criticized (or sued) for?'
- Although the final decision in non-mentally ill, capable adults rests with them, in 'close-call' situations it is better to err on the side of safety, and review again later. (Such situations should always be discussed with a senior colleague.)

Patient wanting to leave a psychiatric ward

The duty psychiatrist is often called to psychiatric wards when patients wish to take their own discharge. Although *not* wanting to be in a psychiatric ward may often seem the most rational response—particularly when there are other more behaviourally disturbed patients in the same ward—a pragmatic approach should be adopted (i.e. balancing the need for assessment/inpatient treatment against the additional stress caused by admission). Follow the general principles detailed here, focusing on managing risk and acting in the patient's 'best interests'. Note especially:

- Deciding whether a patient is permitted to leave the ward will be informed by both an assessment of their current mental state and knowledge of any established management plans.
- Often decisions regarding the course of action to take will have already been discussed by the responsible consultant with nursing staff. When there are concerns, the default position is often reassessment at the time the patient is asking to leave.
- When a patient does elect to leave against medical advice, record this clearly in the notes with, at the very minimum, an agreement for a planned review (e.g. as an outpatient, by the GP) and the recommendation that, should the patient (or their relatives) feel the situation has become unsustainable at home, they should return to the hospital.

Patients acting against medical advice 2: clinical scenarios

Box 24.3 Some examples of clinical scenarios

52-yr-old ♂ admitted with chest pain, who ought to remain in the hospital for overnight telemetry, cardiac enzymes, and repeat ECG (in the morning), but does not wish to do so. He is not incapable and not suffering from a mental disorder.

The decision rests with him (he has a right to refuse—even if you think he is acting foolishly).

22-yr-old ♀ who admits to ingesting 56 aspirin, brought to GP by a concerned friend, now refusing to get in an ambulance to go to hospital.

Most people would agree that she is possibly suffering from a mental disorder (suggested by her recent OD), hence there are grounds for use of MHA, with emergency treatment under common law.

18-yr-old ♀ admitted after a paracetamol overdose who needs further treatment, but wishes to leave. She has some depressive features and may possibly be under the influence of alcohol.

There is sufficient suspicion of mental disorder to detain under the MHA (perhaps more than in the previous scenario); treatment would be under common law.

34-yr-old ♀ with long history of anorexia nervosa, current weight under 6st, with clear physical complications of starvation (and biochemical abnormalities), refusing admission for medical management.

Clear mental disorder, as well as 'risk to themselves'—detain under the MHA; emergency treatment under common law.

53-yr-old ♂ previously seen in A&E following a fall whilst intoxicated, brought back up to A&E 6 days later by spouse with fluctuating level of consciousness (also has been drinking heavily)—suspected extradural, but angrily refusing CT head.

Capacity impaired both by alcohol and potentially serious underlying treatable physical disorder. Necessary urgent investigation warranted as in patient's best interests—with use of sedation (if necessary) under common law.

67-yr-old ♂ with post-operative URTI who presents as confused, wishing to leave the ward because he is 'late for his brother's wedding'.

There is a clear mental disorder and he ought to be detained under the MHA; treat under common law (sedate if necessary).

23-yr-old ♂ admitted with psychotic illness, who wants to go home to confront the neighbours whom he believes have conspired with the police to get him 'banged up in a nut hut'.

Clear mental disorder. Detain under MHA; emergency treatment if required under common law.

The mental health of doctors

'Quis custodiet ipsos custodes?' Who will watch the watchmen?

In general, doctors are in a pretty good state of health, with a lower prevalence of smoking, cardiovascular disease, cancer, and a longer life expectancy than the general population. With respect to mental health, however, the situation is reversed—with the incidence of most psychiatric disorders *higher* in doctors:

- Surveys have found ~25% of doctors to have significant depressive symptoms, with increased risk in: junior house officers/interns; junior doctors in O&G and psychiatry; radiologists, anaesthetists, surgeons, and paediatricians.
- Suicide rates are high, with depression, alcohol, and drug misuse significant contributory factors. Specialties over-represented include anaesthetics, GP, psychiatry, and emergency medicine.
- Problems of drug and alcohol dependence may affect as many as 1 in 15 doctors in the UK.

Why are doctors more likely to have mental health problems?

Individual factors

- Personality—many of the qualities that make a 'good doctor' may also increase the risk of psychiatric problems (e.g. obsessionality, perfectionism, being ambitious, self-sacrifice, high expectations of self, low tolerance of uncertainty, difficulty expressing emotions).
- Ways of thinking/coping styles, e.g. being overly self-critical, denial, minimization, rationalization, drinking culture, need to appear competent ('no problems').

Occupational factors

- Long and disruptive work hours.
- Exposure to traumatic events—dealing with death, ethical dilemmas.
- Lack of support (particularly from senior colleagues).
- Competing needs of patients and family.
- Increasing expectations with diminishing resources.
- Professional and geographic isolation.

Barriers to seeking help

Doctors are notoriously bad at seeking help for their own medical problems—particularly psychiatric problems—often only presenting when a crisis arises. Reasons for this include:

- Symptom concealment due to fears of hospitalization, loss of medical registration, exposure to stigmatization.
- Negative attitudes to psychiatry, psychiatrists, and people with psychiatric problems.
- Lack of insight being a feature of many psychiatric disorders.

This may lead to delayed referral, misdiagnosis, and not receiving the benefits of early interventions.

What to do if you suspect a colleague has a problem

You have a duty to take action (see Box 24.4), both in the interests of patient care and of your colleague's health (such actions are both ethically responsible and caring). Not to do so could both put patients at risk and potentially deny your colleague treatment which might prevent further deterioration in health and performance. Usually a staged approach works best:

- Confirm your suspicions through informal discussion with other colleagues.
- If a clear pattern of behaviour is present, first consider discussing this observation with the colleague in question.
- It is better if face-to-face discussion is conducted by someone of the same grade.
- If face-to-face discussion yields no results, speak to an impartial senior colleague and/or seek further advice about local procedures (see Box 24.4).
- If the colleague is YOU, remember: *responsible* physicians put their patients first and take pride in looking after their own health (see 📖 p. 1006).

Box 24.4 Duty to take action[1,*]

You must protect patients from risk of harm posed by another colleague's conduct, performance or health. The safety of patients must come first at all times. If you have concerns that a colleague may not be fit to practise, you must take appropriate steps without delay, so that the concerns are investigated and patients protected where necessary. This means you must give an honest explanation of your concerns to an appropriate person from your employing or contracting body, and follow their procedures.

If there are no appropriate local systems, or local systems do not resolve the problem, and you are still concerned about the safety of patients, you should inform the relevant regulatory body. If you are not sure what to do, discuss your concerns with an impartial colleague or contact your defence body, a professional organization, or the GMC for advice.

If you know that you have, or think that you might have, a serious condition that you could pass on to patients, or if your judgement or performance could be affected by a condition or its treatment, you must consult a suitably qualified colleague. You must ask for and follow their advice about investigations, treatment and changes to your practice that they consider necessary. You must not rely on your own assessment of the risk you pose to patients.

[1] **General Medical Council** (2006) *Good medical practice*, paragraphs 43,44 and 79.

* It is worth noting that doctors referred to the GMC because of mental health problems can continue to practise, provided their problems are not judged to affect their professional abilities, and they are suitably supervised in an agreed treatment regime.

Looking after your own mental health

You have a duty to yourself and your patients to act promptly if you feel there are early warning signs that your health may be affecting your performance.

Signs to watch out for
- Difficulties sleeping.
- Becoming more impatient or irritable.
- Difficulties concentrating.
- Being unable to make decisions.
- Drinking or smoking more.
- Not enjoying food as much.
- Being unable to relax or 'switch off'.
- Feeling tense (may manifest as somatic symptoms, e.g. recurrent headache, aches and pains, GI upset, feeling sweaty, dry mouth, tachycardia).

Developing good habits
- **Learn to relax** This can involve learning methods of progressive relaxation, or simply setting aside time when you are not working to relax with a long bath, a quiet stroll, listening to music. It also means living life less frantically—going to bed at a regular time and getting up 15–20min earlier to prevent the feeling of 'always being in a rush'.
- **Take regular breaks at work** This includes regular meal breaks (away from work). Even when work is busy, try to give yourself a 5–10min break every few hours.
- **Escape the pager** In the day and age of being always obtainable, it is a good idea to be 'unobtainable' once or twice a week, to give yourself time to be alone and reflect.
- **Exercise** There is no doubt that regular exercise helps reduce levels of stress. It will also keep you fit, helps prevent heart disease, and improve quality of sleep.
- **Drugs** Tobacco and other recreational drugs are best avoided. Caffeine and alcohol should be used only in moderation.
- **Distraction** Finding a pursuit that has no deadlines, no pressures, and which can be picked up or left easily can allow you to forget about your usual stresses. This might be a sport, a hobby, music, the movies, the theatre, or books. The important point is that it is not work-related.

Organizing your own medical care
- Register with a GP! Two-thirds of junior doctors have not done this.
- Allow yourself to benefit from the same standards of care (including expert assessment, if this is felt to be necessary) you would expect for your patients.
- If you are having difficulties related to stress, anxiety, depression, or use of substances, consult your GP sooner rather than later.
- Be willing to take advice. In particular, do not rely on your own judgement of your ability to continue working.

- If your GP suggests speaking to a psychiatrist, and you feel uncomfortable with being seen locally, ask for an out-of-area consultation.
- Utilize other sources of help and advice—both informal (friends, family, self-help books) and formal (see **Sources of support and advice**.) Remember you are certainly not the first doctor to have encountered these sorts of difficulties.

Sources of support and advice

- The **National Counselling Service for Sick Doctors** is a confidential independent service supported by the Royal Colleges, the Joint Consultants Committee, the BMA, and other medical professional bodies. (Tel: 0870 21 0535).
- The **Doctors' Support Network**. (Tel: 07071 223 372).
- The **BMA** offers free expert advice for members who may be affected by illness through '**Doctors for doctors**' (Tel: 020 7383 6739) and a free telephone counselling service (Tel: 0645 200 169).
- The **Sick Doctors' Trust** runs a 24-hr helpline for doctors with addiction problems. Callers are put in touch with the nearest member of the **Addicted Physicians Programme (APP)**, an independent and free service. The **British Doctors and Dentists Group** is an affiliated organization, running support groups in local areas throughout the UK and Eire. For further information contact: Isis, 126 Weybourne Road, Farnham, Surrey, GU9 9HD (Tel: 020 7487 4445; Helpline: 01252 345163).

Useful resources

Resources for patients

Education of the patient and their relatives and carers is an important part of the management of mental disorders. Equally, contact with fellow sufferers can be an invaluable source of help and support to patients. This applies particularly if the disorder is chronic or is only partially treatment-responsive. The following list of patient organizations, websites, helpline numbers, and books is one which we have found useful in our clinical practice. You should familiarize yourself with the service provided by each resource before recommending it to patients. You should also find out about local services available in your area.

General mental health problems

The Samaritans
℠ http://www.samaritans.org.uk
jo@samaritans.org
08457 90 90 90

Confidential emotional support for those experiencing feelings of distress, despair, or thoughts of suicide.

MIND
℠ http://www.mind.org.uk
15–19 Broadway, London, E15 4BQ
0300 123 3393 (helpline)
020 8519 2122 (professional contact)

Mental health charity which runs support networks, campaigns on behalf of sufferers from mental health problems, and provides information services.

Royal College of Psychiatrists—leaflets and self-help advice
℠ http://www.rcpsych.ac.uk/info
Leaflets Department, The Royal College of Psychiatrists, 17 Belgrave Square, London, SW1X 8PG

Wide range of information and self-help advice.

SANE
℠ http://www.sane.org.uk
1st Floor, Cityside House, 40 Adler Street, London, E1 1EE
0845 767 8000 (helpline)
020 7375 1002 (professional contact)

Mental health charity which campaigns on behalf of patients with mental illness, funds and carries out research, and provides information services.

Affective disorders: patient organizations

Association for Post Natal Illness
℠ http://www.apni.org
145 Dawes Road, Fulham, London, SW6 7EB
020 7386 0868

Information and advice about postnatal depression.

Beyond Blue
🖰 http://www.beyondblue.org.au

Self-help and information about depression from the Australian National Depression Initiative.

Manic Depression Fellowship (MDF)
🖰 http://www.mdf.org.uk
21 St George's Road, London, SE1 6ES
020 7931 6480

Charity which provides information and support to those with bipolar disorder online and via local self-help groups.

Books

Copeland M and McKay M (1993) *The depression workbook: a guide for living with depression and manic depression.* Oakland: New Harbinger.
Burns D (1981): *The feeling good handbook.* London: Penguin.
Butler G and Hope T (2007) *Manage your mind: the mental fitness guide.* Oxford: Oxford University Press.
Westbrook D *Managing depression.* Oxford: Oxford University Press. From the Oxford Cognitive Therapy Centre. Available at: 🖰 http://www.octc.co.uk
Greenberger D and Padesky CA (1995) *Mind over mood.* London: Guilford Press.
Gilbert P (2009) *Overcoming depression: a self-help guide using cognitive behavioural techniques.* London: Robinson.

Bereavement: patient organizations

Compassionate Friends
🖰 http://www.tcf.org.uk
08451 23 23 04 (Great Britain)
0288 77 88 016 (Northern Ireland)

Befriending and support by and for bereaved parents.

CRUSE Bereavement Care
🖰 http://www.cruselochaber.freeuk.com/canhelp.html
Cruse House, 126 Sheen Road, Richmond, Surrey, TW9 1UR
0870 167 1677 (helpline)
020 8939 9530 (professional contact)

Counselling and support for those who have experienced bereavement.

CRUSE Bereavement Care Scotland
🖰 http://www.crusescotland.org.uk
3 Rutland Square, Edinburgh, EH1 2AS
0845 600 2227 (helpline)
01738 444 178 (professional contact)

Counselling and support for those who have experienced bereavement.

Children and parents: patient organizations

Attention Deficit Disorder Information and Support Service (ADDISS)
℡ http://www.addiss.co.uk
020 8952 2800

Information, training, and support for parents, sufferers, and professionals in the fields of ADHD, and related learning and behavioural difficulties.

Childline
℡ http://www.childline.org.uk
0800 1111

National helpline for young people in trouble or danger.

Children 1st
℡ http://www.children1st.org.uk
0131 446 2300

Helps families with children at risk of abuse.

Education and Resources for Improving Childhood Continence (ERIC)
℡ http://www.eric.org.uk
0845 370 8008 (helpline)

Education and resources for improving childhood continence.

Family Lives (formerly Parentline)
℡ http://familylives.org.uk/
0808 800 2222 (helpline)

Charity offering help and support to parents.

National Autistic Society
℡ http://www.autism.org.uk/
0845 070 4004 (helpline)

Information, advice, and support for individuals with autism and their families.

One Parent Families Scotland
℡ http://www.opfs.org.uk
0800 018 5026 (helpline)

Counselling, information, and self-help groups.

Tourette Syndrome (UK) Association
℡ http://www.tourettes-action.org.uk/
0300 777 8427 (helpline)

A charity which offers advice and support to Tourette's sufferers and funds research into the condition.

YoungMinds
℡ http://www.youngminds.org.uk
102–108 Clerkenwell Road, London, EC1M 5SA
020 7336 8445

Charity providing advice and training and campaigning to improve the mental health of children and young people.

Self-harm/borderline personality disorder: patient organizations

BPD Resource Center

🖰 http://bpdresourcecenter.org/

Extensive range of information and links to other resources for borderline personality disorder.

BPD World

🖰 http://www.bpdworld.org
4 King Street, Wakefield WF1 2SQ

Online information, support, and advice on borderline personality disorder, self-harm, and related issues.

FirstSigns

🖰 http://www.firstsigns.org.uk

Information and support network for those who self-harm.

National Self Harm Network

🖰 http://www.nshn.co.uk
PO Box 7264, Nottingham NG1 6WJ

Online support and self-help for people who self-harm.

Books
Schmidt U and Davidson K (2004) *Life after self-harm: a guide to the future.* New York: Brunner-Routledge.
Kennerley H (2000) *Overcoming childhood trauma.* London: Robinson.

Domestic abuse and violence: patient organizations

Domestic Abuse Helpline

🖰 http://www.domesticabuse.co.uk
0800 027 1234

Advice and information for people who have experienced or are experiencing domestic abuse.

Books
McKay M and Rogers P (2009) *The anger control workbook.* Oakland: New Harbinger.
Davies W (2009) *Overcoming anger and irritability.* London: Robinson.

Drug and alcohol problems: patient organizations

Al-Anon

🖰 http://www.al-anonuk.org.uk
61 Great Dover Street, London, SE1 4YF
020 7403 0888 (England and Wales)
0141 339 8884 (Scotland)
028 9068 2368 (Northern Ireland)
00353 1 873 2699 (Republic of Ireland)

Helpline and meetings for families and friends of those with a drink problem.

Alcoholics Anonymous (AA)
🖰 http://www.alcoholics-anonymous.org.uk
PO Box 1, Stonebow House, Stonebow, York YO1 7NJ
0845 769 7555 (national helpline)

Alcohol Concern
🖰 http://www.alcoholconcern.org.uk
020 7928 7377

Range of information about alcohol problems.

Drinkline
0800 917 8282

National, confidential helpline for alcohol problems.

Narcotics Anonymous
🖰 http://www.ukna.org
UK Service Office, 202 City Road, London, EC1V 2PH
0300 999 1212 (helpline)
020 7251 4007 (professional contact)

Group based self-help recovery programmes based on the '12 step' model.

National Drugs Helpline
🖰 http://www.talktofrank.com
Tel: 0800 77 66 00

Department of Health website with information and advice about drug problems.

Books
Fanning P and O'Neil J (1996) *The addiction workbook: step-by-step guide to quitting alcohol and drugs.* Oakland: New Harbinger.

Dementia: patient organizations

Alzheimer's Society (England, Wales, and Northern Ireland)
🖰 http://www.alzheimers.org.uk
Gordon House, 10 Greencoat Place, London, SW1P 1PH
0845 300 0336 (helpline)
020 7306 0606 (professional contact)

Local and telephone support services for those affected by dementia.

Alzheimer Scotland—Action on Dementia
🖰 http://www.alzscot.org
22 Drumsheugh Gardens, Edinburgh, EH3 7RN
0808 808 3000 (helpline)
0131 243 1453 (professional contact)

Local and telephone support services for those affected by dementia.

Eating disorders: patient organizations

Beating Eating Disorders
℘ http://www.b-eat.co.uk
Wensum House, 103 Prince of Wales Road, Norwich NR1 1DW
0845 634 1414 (helpline)
0845 634 7650 (under-18 helpline)

Information and self-help for people with eating disorders.

Overeaters Anonymous
℘ http://www.oa.org
PO Box 19, Stretford, Manchester M32 9EB
07000 784985 (helpline)
01236 825507 (local meeting information)

Supportive fellowship for people with compulsive overeating, following the 12-step programme.

Books

Cooper P (1993) *Bulimia nervosa and binge-eating.* London: Robinson.
Schmidt U and Treasure J (1993) *Getting better bit(e) by bit(e).* London: Brunner-Routledge.
Freeman C (2009) *Overcoming anorexia nervosa.* London: Robinson.
McCabe R (2004) *The overcoming bulimia workbook.* Oakland: New Harbinger.
Gauntlett-Gilbert J and Grace C (2005) *Overcoming weight problems.* London: Robinson.

Learning disability: patient organizations

Down's Syndrome Association
℘ http://www.downs-syndrome.org.uk
Langdon Down Centre, 2a Langdon Park, Teddington, TW11 9PS
0845 230 0372 (helpline)
Information, education, and training about Down's syndrome.

Down's Syndrome Scotland
℘ http://www.dsscotland.org.uk
158/160 Balgreen Road, Edinburgh, EH11 3AU
0131 313 4225

Advice, information, advocacy, and local group support for individuals with Down's syndrome and their families.

Fragile X Society
℘ http://www.fragilex.org.uk
Rood End House, 6 Stortford Road, Great Dunmow, Essex, CM6 1DA
01371 875 100

Charity offering information and supporting research.

Mencap
℘ http://www.mencap.org.uk
123 Golden Lane, London, EC1Y 0RT
020 7454 0454

National charity offering housing support, education, and employment and local groups for individuals with learning disability.

Prader Willi Syndrome Association UK
🖰 http://pwsa.co.uk
125a London Road, Derby, DE1 2QQ
01332 365 676

Charity supporting sufferers and carers.

Rett Syndrome Association UK
🖰 http://www.rettuk.org/
113 Friern Barnet Road, London, N11 3EU
01582 798 911

Charity offering information, advice, and practical help to people with Rett syndrome, their families, and carers.

Neurotic disorders: patient organizations

Anxiety UK
🖰 http://www.anxietyuk.org.uk/
08444 775 774

Information and self-help guides on a range of anxiety disorders.

OCD Action
🖰 http://www.ocdaction.org.uk
0845 390 6232

Information and advice for people suffering from OCD and related disorders.

OCD-UK
🖰 http://www.ocduk.org
0870 126 9506

Information and self-help advice for people suffering from OCD.

Panic Center
🖰 http://www.paniccenter.net

Information and web-based self-help programme for overcoming panic attacks.

Books

Pollard A and Zuercher-White E (2003) *Agoraphobia workbook*. Oakland: New Harbinger.

Bourne E (2011) *Anxiety and phobia workbook*. Oakland: New Harbinger.

Kennerley H *Managing anxiety: a user's manual*. Oxford: Oxford University Press. From the Oxford Cognitive Therapy Centre, 01865 223986. Available at: 🖰 http://www.octc.co.uk

Westbrook D and Morrison N *Managing obsessive-compulsive disorder*. Oxford: Oxford University Press. From the Oxford Cognitive Therapy Centre, 01865 223986. Available at: 🖰 http://www.octc.co.uk

Beckfield D (2004) *Master your panic and take back your life*. USA: Impact.

Davis M and Eshelman ER (2008) *Relaxation and stress reduction workbook*. Oakland: New Harbinger.

Hyman B and Pedrick C (2010) *OCD workbook*. Oakland: New Harbinger.

Kennerley H (2009) *Overcoming anxiety*. London: Robinson.

Veale D and Willson R (2009) *Overcoming obsessive compulsive disorder.* London: Robinson.

Silove D (1997) *Overcoming panic.* London: Robinson.

Sanders D *Overcoming phobias.* Oxford: Oxford University Press. From the Oxford Cognitive Therapy Centre, 01865 223986. Available at: ℘ http://www.octc.co.uk

Butler G (2009) *Overcoming social anxiety and shyness.* London: Robinson.

Herbert C and Wetmore A (2008) *Overcoming traumatic stress.* London: Robinson.

Williams M-B and Poijula S (2002) *PTSD workbook.* Oakland: New Harbinger.

Antony M and Swinson R (2008) *Shyness and social anxiety workbook.* Oakland: New Harbinger.

Foa E and Wilson R (2001) *Stop obsessing!* USA: Bantam.

Kuchemann C, Sanders D *Understanding health anxiety.* Oxford: Oxford University Press. From the Oxford Cognitive Therapy Centre, 01865 223986. Available at: ℘ http://www.octc.co.uk

Westbrook D and Rouf K *Understanding panic.* Oxford: Oxford University Press. From the Oxford Cognitive Therapy Centre, 01865 223986. Available at: ℘ http://www.octc.co.uk

Herbert C *Understanding your reactions to trauma.* Blue Stallion. From the Oxford Cognitive Therapy Centre, 01865 223986. Available at: ℘ http://www.octc.co.uk

Schizophrenia: patient organizations

Rethink (previously National Schizophrenia Fellowship)
℘ http://www.rethink.org
Head Office, 5th floor, Royal London House, 22–25 Finsbury Square, London, EC2A 1DX
0300 5000 927 (national advice line)
0845 456 0455 (professional contact)

Charity running support groups, carer support, advocacy services, residential and rehabilitation services and supported housing.

Books

Torrey F (2001) *Surviving schizophrenia: a family manual.* New York HarperCollins.

Somatization

Books

Campling F and Sharpe M (2008) *Chronic fatigue syndrome: the facts.* Oxford: Oxford University Press.

Fennell P (2011) *The chronic illness workbook.* Albany Health Management Publishing.

Shepherd C (1999) *Living with M.E.: the chronic, post-viral fatigue syndrome.* Vermilion.

Frances C and MacIntyre A (1998) *M.E./chronic fatigue syndrome—a practical guide.* Thorsons Health.

Burgess M and Chalder T *Overcoming chronic fatigue.* London: Robinson.

Cole F, MacDonald H, Carus C (2005) *et al. Overcoming chronic pain.* London: Robinson.

Online clinical resources

Over the last decade a huge amount of clinically useful information has become available online. Most major journals, professional bodies, governmental organizations and clinical authorities now publish new material online and more historical material is digitized and added each month.

Database portals

HON (Health on the Net Foundation)
Portal to quality assessed medical information, based in Geneva.
🖰 http://www.hon.ch

NHS Evidence in Health and Social Care
National NHS e-library
🖰 https://www.evidence.nhs.uk/

Intute: Health and Life Sciences
Catalogue of hand-selected and evaluated Internet resources in health and medicine (formerly known as OMNI).
🖰 http://www.intute.ac.uk/healthandlifesciences/medicine

The Knowledge Network
NHS Education for Scotland e-Library.
🖰 http://www.knowledge.scot.nhs.uk

PubMed
Medline searches via the US National Library of Medicine.
🖰 http://www.pubmed.gov

TRIP (Turning Research Into Practice)
Allows simultaneous searches of multiple databases.
🖰 http://www.tripdatabase.com

Evidence-based medicine resources

Centre for Evidence-Based Medicine
Oxford-based centre promoting the practice of evidence-based health care.
🖰 http://www.cebm.net

Clinical Evidence
This 'evidence formulary' from the *BMJ* aims to supply the best available current evidence of therapeutic effectiveness.
🖰 http://www.clinicalevidence.com

Cochrane Library
Evidence from systematic reviews of the results of medical research studies.
🖰 http://www.cochrane.org

NHS Centre for Reviews and Dissemination
Database of Abstracts of Reviews of Effects, NHS Economic Evaluation Database, and the Health Technology Assessment Database.
🖰 http://www.york.ac.uk/inst/crd/

Online journals

Directory of Open Access Journals
Free, full text, scientific and scholarly journals across all topics.
🔗 http://www.doaj.org

Free Medical Journals
Online, full text journals.
🔗 http://www.freemedicaljournals.com

PubMed Central Journal Archive
US National Institutes of Health's free digital archive of biomedical and life sciences journal literature.
🔗 http://www.pubmedcentral.nih.gov

Science Direct
Large electronic collection of science, technology and medicine full text and bibliographic information.
🔗 http://www.sciencedirect.com

Wiley Interscience
International resource with scientific, technical, medical, and professional content.
🔗 http://www3.interscience.wiley.com

American Journal of Psychiatry
The journal of the American Psychiatric Association.
🔗 http://ajp.psychiatryonline.org

British Journal of Psychiatry
The 'yellow journal', published monthly by the Royal College of Psychiatrists.
🔗 http://bjp.rcpsych.org

British Medical Journal
General Medical Journal published by the British Medical Association.
🔗 http://bmj.bmjjournals.com

Journal of the American Medical Association (JAMA)
Published weekly by the American Medical Association.
🔗 http://jama.ama-assn.org

New England Journal of Medicine
High impact factor general medical journal.
🔗 http://www.nejm.org/

Clinical guidelines

NICE (National Institute for Health and Clinical Excellence)
Organization responsible for providing national guidance on promoting good health and preventing and treating ill health.
🔗 http://www.nice.org.uk

Healthcare Improvement Scotland
Organization providing advice and guidance to NHS Scotland on effective clinical practice.
🖰 www.healthcareimprovementscotland.org/

SIGN (Scottish Intercollegiate Guidelines Network)
Organization for the development of national clinical guidelines containing recommendations for effective practice.
🖰 http://www.sign.ac.uk

US National Guideline Clearinghouse
American resource for evidence-based clinical practice guidelines.
🖰 http://www.guideline.gov

Search engines

Google Scholar
Searches of peer-reviewed papers, theses, books, preprints, abstracts and technical reports.
🖰 http://scholar.google.com

Scirus
A science-specific web search engine owned by Elsevier.
🖰 http://www.scirus.com/srsapp

Online professional resources

British Association for Behavioural and Cognitive Psychotherapists
Directory of accredited cognitive behavioural psychotherapists.
⅏ http://www.babcp.org.uk

British Association for Counselling
Directories and other information.
⅏ http://www.bac.co.uk

British Association for Psychopharmacology
Journal, membership, and training events.
⅏ http://www.bap.org.uk

British Confederation of Psychotherapists
⅏ http://www.bcp.org.uk

British Medical Association
The professional association for doctors in the UK.
⅏ http://www.bma.org.uk

British Psychological Society
The professional body for psychologists in the UK.
⅏ http://www.bps.org.uk

General *Medical Council*
The governing authority for medicine in the UK which maintains the medical register and sets standards for good practice.
⅏ http://www.gmc-uk.org

Royal College of Psychiatrists
The professional and educational body for psychiatrists in the UK and Republic of Ireland.
⅏ http://www.rcpsych.ac.uk

ICD-10/DSM-IV index

ICD-10 Classification of Mental and Behavioural Disorders (1992)

The following index lists the mental and behavioural disorders in their ICD-10 order and provides ICD-10 coding information, the 'equivalent' DSM-IV coding, and a page reference within this volume (where available).

Because 'mental and behavioural disorders due to psychoactive substance abuse' is so dissimilar in organization to DSM-IV (i.e. separate coding for substance use and substance-induced disorders), equivalent codings have not been included.

F00–F09 Organic, including symptomatic, mental disorders

ICD-10	DSM-IV	Disorder	Page
F00	**290**	**Dementia in Alzheimer's disease**	*134*
F00.0	290.10	Early onset	
F00.1	290.0	Late onset	
F00.2	294.1	Atypical or mixed type	
F00.9	294.1	Unspecified	
F01	**290.40**	**Vascular dementia**	*144*
F01.0	290.40	Acute onset	
F01.1	290.40	Multi-infarct	
F01.2	290.40	Subcortical	
F01.3	290.40	Mixed cortical and subcortical	
F02.0	290.10	Dementia in Pick's disease	*142*
F02.1	290.0	Dementia in Creutzfeldt–Jakob disease	*146*
F02.2	294.1	Dementia in Huntington's disease	*170*
F02.3	294.1	Dementia in Parkinson's disease	*168*
F02.4	294.9	Dementia in HIV disease	*160*
F02.8	294.1	Dementia in other specified diseases	
F03	**294.8**	**Unspecified dementia**	
F04	**294.0**	**Organic amnesic syndrome, not induced by alcohol and other psychoactive substances**	*148*
F05	**293.0**	**Delirium**	*790*
F05.0	293.0	Delirium not superimposed on dementia	
F05.1	293.0	Delirium superimposed on dementia	
F06	**293.8**	**Mental disorders due to brain damage, dysfunction, and physical disease**	
F06.0	293.82	Hallucinosis	
F06.1	293.89	Catatonic disorder	*992*
F06.2	293.81	Delusional (schizophrenia-like) disorder	*132*
F06.3	293.83	Mood (affective) disorders	*130*
F06.4	293.84	Anxiety disorder	*131*
F06.5	293.9	Dissociative disorder	*806*
F06.6	293.9	Emotionally labile (asthenic) disorder	
F06.7	294.9	Mild cognitive disorder	

F07	310.1	**Personality and behavioural disorders due to brain disease, damage, or dysfunction**	
F07.0	310.1	Organic personality disorder	154
F07.1	310.1	Post-encephalitic syndrome	164
F07.2	310.1	Post-concussional syndrome	154
F09	**293.9**	**Unspecified organic or symptomatic mental disorder**	

F10–F19 Mental and behavioural disorders due to psychoactive substance abuse

ICD-10	Drug	Page
F10	**Alcohol**	566
F11	**Opioids**	582
F12	**Cannabinoids**	588
F13	**Sedatives and hypnotics**	582
F14	**Cocaine**	584
F15	**Stimulants including caffeine**	585
F16	**Hallucinogens**	586
F17	**Tobacco**	
F18	**Solvents**	589
F19	**Multiple or other**	589

Notes: A 4th character denotes the clinical condition and a 5th modifies it:

F1x.0—Acute intoxication
F1x.0—.00 uncomplicated
F1x.0—.01 with trauma or other bodily injury
F1x.0—.02 with other medical complications
F1x.0—.03 with delirium
F1x.0—.04 with perceptual distortions
F1x.0—.05 with coma
F1x.0—.06 with convulsions
F1x.0—.07 pathological intoxication
F1x.1—Harmful use
F1x.2—Dependence syndrome
F1x.2—.20 currently abstinent
F1x.2—.21 currently abstinent but in a protected environment
F1x.2—.22 on a clinically supervised maintenance or replacement regime
F1x.2—.23 currently abstinent, but receiving treatment with aversive or blocking drugs
F1x.2—.24 currently using
F1x.2—.25 continuous use
F1x.2—.26 episodic use
F1x.3—Withdrawal state
F1x.3—.30 uncomplicated
F1x.3—.31 convulsions
F1x.4—Withdrawal state with delirium
F1x.4—.40 with convulsions
F1x.4—.41 without convulsions
F1x.5—Psychotic disorder
F1x.5—.50 schizophrenia-like
F1x.5—.51 predominantly delusional
F1x.5—.52 predominantly hallucinatory
F1x.5—.53 predominantly polymorphic
F1x.5—.54 predominantly depressive
F1x.5—.55 predominantly manic
F1x.5—.56 mixed

F1x.6—Amnestic disorder
F1x.7—Residual and late-onset psychotic disorder
F1x.7—.70 flashbacks
F1x.7—.71 personality or behavioural disorder
F1x.7—.72 residual affective disorder
F1x.7—.73 dementia
F1x.7—.74 other persisting cognitive impairment
F1x.7—.75 late-onset psychotic disorder

F20–F29 Schizophrenia, schizotypal, and delusional disorders

ICD-10	DSM-IV	Disorder	Page
F20	**295**	**Schizophrenia**	*178*
F20.0	295.30	Paranoid	
F20.1	295.10	Hebephrenic	
F20.2	295.2	Catatonic	
F20.3	295.90	Undifferentiated	
F20.4	311	Post-schizophrenic depression	
F20.5	295.60	Residual	
F20.6	295.90	Simple	
F21	**301.22**	**Schizotypal disorder**	*218*
F22	**297**	**Persistent delusional disorder**	*220*
F22.0	297.1	Delusional disorder	
F22.8	297.1	Other persistent delusional disorders	
F23		**Acute and transient psychotic disorders**	*226*
F23.0	298.9	Acute polymorphic psychotic disorder without symptoms of schizophrenia	
F23.1	295.40	Acute polymorphic psychotic disorder with symptoms of schizophrenia	
F23.2	295.40	Acute schizophrenia-like psychotic disorder	
F23.3	297.1	Other acute predominantly delusional psychotic disorders	
F24	**297.3**	**Induced delusional disorder**	*228*
F25	**295.7**	**Schizoaffective disorder**	*218*
F25.0	295.70	Manic type	
F25.1	295.70	Depressive type	
F25.2	295.70	Mixed type	
F28	**298.9**	**Other non-organic psychotic disorders**	*230*
F29	**298.9**	**Unspecified non-organic psychosis**	

Notes: Schizophrenia: a 5th character denotes course: continuous (1), episodic with progressive deficit (2), episodic but stable deficit (3), episodic remittent (4), incomplete remission (5), complete remission (6), other (8), and period of observation less than **1**yr (9).

Acute and transient psychotic *disorders:* a 5th character may be used to identify the presence (1) or absence (0) of acute stress.

F30–F39 Mood (affective) disorders

ICD-10	DSM-IV	Disorder	Page
F30		**Manic episode**	306
F30.0	296.00	Hypomania	
F30.1	296.03	Mania without psychotic symptoms	
F30.2	296.04	Mania with psychotic symptoms	
F31		**Bipolar affective disorder**	314
F31.0	296.40	Current episode hypomanic	
F31.1	296.43	Current episode manic without psychotic symptoms	
F31.2	296.44	Current episode manic with psychotic symptoms	
F31.3	296.52	Current episode mild or moderate depression	
F31.4	296.53	Current episode severe depression without psychotic symptoms	
F31.5	296.54	Current episode severe depression with psychotic symptoms	
F31.6	296.60	Current episode mixed	
F31.7	296.66	Currently in remission	
F32		**Depressive episode**	236
F32.00	296.21	Mild without somatic symptoms	
F32.01	296.21	Mild with somatic symptoms	
F32.10	296.22	Moderate without somatic symptoms	
F32.11	296.22	Moderate with somatic symptoms	
F32.2	296.23	Severe without psychotic symptoms	
F32.3	296.24	Severe with psychotic symptoms	
F32.8	311	Other	*240*
F33		**Recurrent depressive disorder**	*237*
F33.00	296.31	Current episode mild without somatic symptoms	
F33.01	296.31	Current episode mild with somatic symptoms	
F33.10	296.32	Current episode moderate without somatic symptoms	
F33.11	296.32	Current episode moderate with somatic symptoms	
F33.2	296.33	Current episode severe without psychotic symptoms	
F33.3	296.34	Current episode severe with psychotic symptoms	
F33.4	296.36	Currently in remission	

F40–F49 Neurotic, stress-related, and somatoform disorders

ICD-10	DSM-IV	Disorder	Page
F40		**Phobic anxiety disorders**	
F40.00	300.22	Agoraphobia without panic disorder	364
F40.01	300.21	Agoraphobia with panic disorder	358
F40.1	300.23	Social phobias	370
F40.2	300.29	Specific (isolated) phobias	366
F41		**Other anxiety disorders**	
F41.0	300.01	Panic disorder (episodic paroxysmal anxiety)	358
F41.1	300.02	Generalized anxiety disorder	372
F41.2	300.00	Mixed anxiety and depressive disorder	
F41.3	300.00	Other mixed anxiety disorders	
F42		**Obsessive–compulsive disorder**	376
F42.0	300.3	Predominantly obsessional thoughts or ruminations	
F42.1	300.3	Predominantly compulsive acts (obsessional rituals)	
F42.2	300.3	Mixed obsessional thoughts and acts	
F43		**Reaction to severe stress and adjustment disorders**	
F43.0	308.3	Acute stress reaction	382
F43.1	309.81	Post-traumatic stress disorder	390
F43.2	309.9	Adjustment disorders	386
F44		**Dissociative (conversion) disorders**	806
F44.0	300.12	Dissociative amnesia	
F44.1	300.13	Dissociative fugue	
F44.2	300.15	Dissociative stupor	
F44.3	300.15	Trance and possession disorders	
F44.4	300.15	Dissociative motor disorders	
F44.5	300.15	Dissociative convulsions	
F44.6	300.15	Dissociative anaesthesia and sensory loss	
F44.7	300.15	Mixed dissociative (conversion) disorders	
F44.80	300.11	Ganser syndrome	97
F44.81	300.14	Multiple personality disorder	100
F44.82	300.11	Transient dissociate (conversion) disorders occurring in childhood and adolescence	

F45		**Somatoform disorders**	
F45.0	300.81	Somatization disorder	*802*
F45.1	300.82	Undifferentiated somatoform disorder	
F45.2	300.7	Hypochondriacal disorder	*808*
F45.3	300.82	Somatoform autonomic dysfunction	
F45.4	307.80	Persistent somatoform pain disorder	*804*
F48		**Other neurotic disorders**	
F48.0	300.82	Neurasthenia	*812*
F48.1	300.6	Depersonalization-derealization syndrome	*394*

Notes:

Somatoform autonomic dysfunction: 5th character denotes organ or system: unspecified (0), heart and cardiovascular system (1), upper gastrointestinal tract (2), lower gastrointestinal tract (3), respiratory system (4), genitourinary system (5), other (8), multiple (9).

F50–F59 Behavioural syndromes associated with physiological disturbance and physical factors

ICD-10	DSM-IV	Disorder	Page
F50		**Eating disorders**	
F50.0	307.1	Anorexia nervosa	*398*
F50.1	307.1	Atypical anorexia nervosa	*398*
F50.2	307.51	Bulimia nervosa	*406*
F50.3	307.51	Atypical bulimia nervosa	*406*
F50.4	307.50	Overeating associated with other psychological disturbances	
F50.5	307.50	Vomiting associated with other psychological disturbances	
F51		**Non-organic sleep disorders**	
F51.0	307.42	Insomnia	*424*
F51.1	307.44	Hypersomnia	*430*
F51.2	307.45	Disorder of the sleep–wake schedule	*436*
F51.3	307.46	Sleepwalking (somnambulism)	*444*
F51.4	307.46	Sleep terrors (night terrors)	*442*
F51.5	307.47	Nightmares	*446*
F52		**Sexual dysfunction, not caused by organic disorder or disease**	
F52.0	302.71	Lack or loss of sexual desire	*474*
F52.1	302.79	Sexual aversion and lack of sexual enjoyment	*474*
F52.2	302.72	Failure of genital response	*476; 478*
F52.3	302.73/4	Orgasmic dysfunction	*476; 478*
F52.4	302.75	Premature ejaculation	*478*
F52.5	306.51	Non-organic vaginismus	*476*
F52.6	302.76	Non-organic dyspareunia	*477; 479*
F52.7	302.9	Excessive sexual drive	*475*
F53		**Mental and behavioural disorders associated with the puerperium, not elsewhere classified**	*468*
F53.0	293.9	Mild	
F53.1	293.9	Severe	

F54	316	**Psychological and behavioural factors associated with disorders or diseases classified elsewhere**
F55	**305**	**Abuse of non-dependence-producing substances**
F55.0	305.90	Harmful use of antidepressants
F55.1	305.90	Harmful use of laxatives
F55.2	305.90	Harmful use of analgesics
F55.3	305.90	Harmful use of antacids
F55.4	305.90	Harmful use of vitamins
F55.5	305.90	Harmful use of steroids or hormones
F55.6	305.90	Harmful use of specific herbal or folk remedies
F55.8	305.90	Harmful use of other substances that do not produce dependence
F59	**300.9**	**Unspecified behavioural syndromes associated with physiological disturbances and physical factors**

F60–F69 Disorders of adult personality and behaviour

ICD-10	DSM-IV	Disorder	Page
F60		**Specific personality disorders**	*494*
F60.0	301.0	Paranoid	
F60.1	301.20	Schizoid	
F60.2	301.7	Dissocial	
F60.30	301.9	Emotionally unstable—impulsive type	
F60.31	301.83	Emotionally unstable—borderline type	
F60.4	301.50	Histrionic	
F60.5	301.4	Anankastic	
F60.6	301.82	Anxious (avoidant)	
F60.7	301.6	Dependent	
F61	**301.9**	**Mixed and other personality disorders**	
F62		**Enduring personality changes, not attributable to brain damage and disease**	
F62.0	301.9	After catastrophic experience	
F62.1	301.9	After psychiatric illness	
F63	**312**	**Habit and impulse disorders**	
F63.0	312.31	Pathological gambling	*410*
F63.1	312.33	Pathological fire-setting (pyromania)	*409*
F63.2	312.32	Pathological stealing (kleptomania)	*408*
F63.3	312.39	Trichotillomania	*410*
F64		**Gender identity disorders**	
F64.0	302.85	Transsexualism	*484*
F64.1	302.85	Dual-role transvestism	*484*
F64.2	302.6	Gender identity disorder of childhood	
F65		**Disorders of sexual preference**	*480*
F65.0	302.81	Fetishism	
F65.1	302.3	Fetishistic transvestism	
F65.2	302.4	Exhibitionism	
F65.3	302.82	Voyeurism	
F65.4	302.2	Paedophilia	
F65.5	302.83/4	Sadomasochism	

F66		**Psychological and behavioural disorders associated with sexual development and orientation**
F66.0	302.6	Sexual maturation disorder
F66.1	302.6	Egodystonic sexual orientation
F66.2	302.6	Sexual relationship disorder
F68		**Other**
F68.0	300.9	Elaboration of physical symptoms for psychological reasons
F68.1	300.19	Intentional production or feigning of symptoms or disabilities, either physical or psychological

Notes:

For F66: psychological and behavioural disorders associated with sexual development and orientation—a 5th character denotes orientation (.x0 heterosexuality, .x1 homosexuality, .x2 bisexuality, .x8 other, including prepubertal).

F70–F79 Mental retardation

ICD-10	DSM-IV	Disorder	Page
F70	317	**Mild mental retardation**	*730*
F71	318.0	**Moderate mental retardation**	*730*
F72	318.1	**Severe mental retardation**	*730*
F73	318.2	**Profound mental retardation**	*730*
F78	319	**Other mental retardation**	
F79	319	**Unspecified mental retardation**	

Notes:

A 4th character may be employed to specify the extent of associated behavioural impairment:

F7x.0 none or minimal.

F7x.1 significant, requiring attention or treatment.

F7x.8 other impairments of behaviour.

F7x.9 unspecified (without mention of impairment of behaviour).

F80–F89 Disorders of psychological development

ICD-10	DSM-IV	Disorder	Page
F80		**Specific developmental disorders of speech and language**	*634*
F80.0	315.39	Specific speech articulation disorder	
F80.1	315.31	Expressive language disorder	
F80.2	315.32	Receptive language disorder	
F80.3	307.9	Acquired aphasia with epilepsy (Landau–Kleffner)	
F80.8	307.9	Other developmental disorders of speech and language	
F81		**Specific developmental disorders of scholastic skills**	*634*
F81.0	315.00	Specific reading disorder	
F81.1	315.2	Specific spelling disorder	
F81.2	315.1	Specific disorder of arithmetical skills	
F81.3	315.9	Mixed disorder of scholastic skills	
F81.8	315.9	Other developmental disorders of scholastic skills	
F81.9	315.9	Developmental disorder of scholastic skills, unspecified	
F82	**315.4**	**Specific developmental disorder of motor function**	
F83	**315.4**	**Mixed specific developmental disorders**	
F84		**Pervasive developmental disorders**	*578*
F84.0	299.00	Childhood autism	*630; 760*
F84.1	299.80	Atypical autism	*630; 760*
F84.2	299.80	Rett's syndrome	*758*
F84.3	299.10	Other childhood disintegrative disorder	*759*
F84.4	299.80	Overactive disorder associated with mental retardation and stereotyped movements	
F84.5	299.80	Asperger's syndrome	*758*
F84.8	299.80	Other pervasive developmental disorders	
F88	**299.80**	**Other disorders of psychological development**	
F89	**299.80**	**Unspecified disorder of psychological development**	

F90–F98 Behavioural and emotional disorders with onset usually occurring in childhood and adolescence

ICD-10	DSM-IV	Disorder	Page
F90		**Hyperkinetic disorders**	626
F90.0	314.9	Disturbance of activity and attention	
F90.1	312.81	Hyperkinetic conduct disorder	
F90.8	314.9	Other hyperkinetic disorders	
F91	**312.8**	**Conduct disorders**	624
F91.0	312.89	Confined to the family context	
F91.1	312.89	Under socialized conduct disorder	
F91.2	312.89	Socialized conduct disorder	
F91.3	313.81	Oppositional defiant disorder	625
F91.8	312.89	Other conduct disorders	
F92		**Mixed disorders of conduct and emotions**	
F92.0	312.89	Depressive conduct disorder	
F92.8	312.89	Other mixed disorders of conduct and emotions	
F93		**Emotional disorders with onset specific to childhood**	
F93.0	309.21	Separation anxiety disorder of childhood	640
F93.1	300.29	Phobic anxiety disorder of childhood	644
F93.2	300.23	Social anxiety disorder of childhood	644
F93.3	V61.8	Sibling rivalry disorder	
F93.8	313.9	Other childhood emotional disorders	
F94		**Disorders of social functioning with onset specific to childhood and adolescence**	
F94.0	313.23	Elective mutism	645
F94.1	313.89	Reactive attachment disorder of childhood	621
F94.2	313.89	Disinhibited attachment disorder of childhood	620
F94.8	313.9	Other childhood disorders of social functioning	
F95		**Tic disorders**	632
F95.0	307.21	Transient tic disorder	
F95.1	307.22	Chronic motor or vocal tic disorder	
F95.2	307.23	Combined vocal and multiple motor tic disorder (de la Tourette)	
F95.8	307.20	Other tic disorders	

The ICD-10 multi-axial system

In multi-axial diagnosis, a patient's problems are viewed within a broader context, which includes: clinical diagnosis, assessment of disability, and psychosocial factors. In ICD-10, multi-axial diagnoses are made along three axes, as follows:

Axis I: clinical diagnoses

This includes all disorders, both psychiatric and physical, including learning disability and personality disorders.

Axis II: disabilities

Conceptualized in line with WHO definitions of impairments, disabilities, and handicaps, this covers a number of specific areas of functioning that are rated on a scale of 0–5 ('no disability' to 'gross disability'):

- *Personal care:* personal hygiene, dressing, feeding, etc.
- *Occupation:* expected functioning in paid activities, studying, home-making, etc.
- *Family and household:* participation in family life.
- *Functioning in a broader social context:* participation in the wider community, including contact with friends, leisure, and other social activities.

Axis III: contextual factors

The factors considered to contribute to the occurrence, presentation, course, outcome, or treatment of the present Axis I disorder(s). They include problems related to:

- Negative events in childhood.
- Education and literacy.
- Primary support group, including family circumstances.
- Social environment.
- Housing or economic circumstances.
- (Un)employment.
- Physical environment.
- Certain psychosocial circumstances.
- Legal circumstances.
- Family history of disease or disabilities.
- Lifestyle or life-management difficulties.

Index

Urgent detention under mental health legislation

Which section?

Jurisdiction	Legislation	Outpatient[1]	Inpatient[2]
England and Wales (p880)	Mental Health Act 1983	s.2 or 3 should be used rather than s.4* unless the situation is such an emergency that to do so would be unsafe.	s.5(2)* can be used immediately. In some cases s. 2 or 3 would be used directly instead.
Scotland (p886)	Mental Health (Care and Treatment) (Scotland) Act 2003	Emergency Detention Certificate* (part 5, section 36) if arranging Short Term Detention (part 6, section 44) would involve undesirable delay. Same procedure for in- and out-patients.	
Northern Ireland (NI) (p890)	Mental Health (Northern Ireland) Order 1986	a.4**	a.7(2)* In some cases patient may be detained directly under a.4**
Republic of Ireland (RoI) (p894)	Mental Health Act 2001	s.9 and 10**	s.23*

1 Patients not currently admitted to hospital—includes day hospital, outpatient department, accident and emergency, and patients attending wards who have not been admitted to a bed yet.

2 Patient in psychiatric or non-psychiatric units, except for RoI where patient must be in an approved centre (i.e. a psychiatric unit).

* Indicates procedures where medical recommendation does not need to be by an approved doctor (England and Wales, Scotland)/appointed doctor (NI) or consultant psychiatrist (RoI).

** Indicates procedures which may be initiated by recommendations from doctors who are not appointed (NI) or consultant psychiatrists (RoI), although soon after admission an assessment from such a doctor is required for the order to stand.

N.B. for the procedures marked * and ** the doctor should be a registered medical practitioner, but need not be a psychiatrist or psychiatric trainee.

Other issues to consider when detaining patients

- Patients should only be detained if it is necessary and there is no alternative less restrictive option
- Before seeing a patient (especially an outpatient), if it seems likely from the available information that detention will be necessary, make appropriate arrangements (e.g. booking a bed, arranging for the necessary medical and social work personnel to arrive at the same time, having staff available to convey the patient, liaising with the police if indicated)
- In some cases getting the person to hospital will be straightforward. However in more difficult cases nursing staff and an ambulance, and where there is potential for violence, the police will be required.